Principles of Goat Disease
and Prevention

Principles of Goat Disease and Prevention

Edited by

Tanmoy Rana
Department of Veterinary Clinical Complex,
West Bengal University of Animal & Fishery Sciences,
Kolkata, India

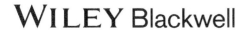

Library of Congress Cataloging-in-Publication Data applied for:

LCCN: 2023006574
Hardback ISBN: 9781119896111
ePDF: 9781119896135
ePUB: 9781119896128
oBook: 9781119896142

Cover Design: Wiley
Cover Images: Courtesy of Tanmoy Rana

Set in 9.5/12.5pt STIXTwoText by Straive, Pondicherry, India

SKY10052557_080723

Contents

Contributors

Rajesh Agrawal
Faculty of Veterinary Sciences & Animal Husbandry
Sher-e-Kashmir University of Agricultural Sciences and
Technology-Jammu
Ranbir Singh Pura, UT Jammu & Kashmir, India

Shailesh K. Bhavsar
Department of Veterinary Pharmacology and Toxicology
College of Veterinary Science and Animal Husbandry
Kamdhenu University
Anand, Gujarat, India

Suman Biswas
Department of Avian Sciences
Faculty of Veterinary & Animal Sciences
West Bengal University of Animal & Fishery Sciences
Mohanpur, West Bengal, India

Antônio C.L. Câmara
Large Animal Veterinary Teaching Hospital
Universidade de Brasília
Brasília, Brazil

Gauri A. Chandratre
Department of Veterinary Public Health and
Epidemiology
College of Veterinary Sciences
Lala Lajpat Rai University of Veterinary
and Animal Sciences
Hisar, Haryana, India

Gaurav Charaya
Department of Veterinary Medicine
College of Veterinary Sciences
Lala Lajpat Rai University of Veterinary and Animal
Sciences
Hisar, Haryana, India

G.K. Chetan Kumar
Department of Veterinary Medicine
Veterinary College Hassan
Karnataka Veterinary, Animal and Fisheries Sciences
University
Hassan, Karnataka, India

Sunita Choudhary
Department of Clinical Veterinary Medicine
College of Veterinary & Animal Sciences
Rajasthan University of Veterinary & Animal Sciences
Bikaner, Rajasthan, India

Bhupamani Das
Department of Clinics
College of Veterinary Sciences & Animal Husbandry
Sardarkrushinagar
Kamdhenu University
Gandhinagar, Gujarat, India

Jasleen Kaur
Department of Veterinary Microbiology
College of Veterinary Sciences
Lala Lajpat Rai University of Veterinary
and Animal Sciences
Hisar, Haryana, India

K. Justin Davis
Department of Veterinary Epidemiology
& Preventive Medicine
College of Veterinary & Animal Sciences
Mannuthy, Kerala, India

Rabjot Kour
Department of Veterinary Parasitology, College of
Veterinary Science
Guru Angad Dev Veterinary and Animal Sciences
University
Rampura Phul, Punjab, India

Savleen Kour
Faculty of Veterinary Sciences & Animal Husbandry
Sher-e-Kashmir University of Agricultural Sciences and Technology-Jammu
Ranbir Singh Pura, UT Jammu & Kashmir, India

Padmanath Krishnan
Tamil Nadu Veterinary and Animal Sciences University
Chennai, Tamil Nadu, India
Veterinary Clinical Complex
Veterinary College and Research Institute
Theni, Tamil Nadu, India

Rohit Kumar
Department of Livestock Production Management
Dr GC Negi College of Veterinary and Animal Sciences
CSKHPKV
Palampur, Himachal Pradesh, India

Chinmoy Maji
North 24 Parganas Krishi Vigyan Kendra
West Bengal University of Animal & Fishery Sciences
Ashokenagar, West Bengal, India

Kruti Debnath Mandal
Teaching Veterinary Clinical Complex
Faculty of Veterinary and Animal Sciences
Institute of Agricultural Science
Benaras Hindu University
Mirzapur, Uttar Pradesh, India

Vipin Maurya
Department of Livestock Production Management
Faculty of Veterinary & Animal Sciences
Institute of Agricultural Sciences
Banaras Hindu University
Mirzapur, Uttar Pradesh, India

Falguni Mridha
Department of Veterinary Clinical Complex
West Bengal University of Animal & Fishery Sciences
Kolkata, West Bengal, India

Pierre-Yves Mulon
Department of Large Animal Clinical Sciences
University of Tennessee
Knoxville, TN, USA

Mohsina Mushtaq
Division of Veterinary Clinical Complex
Faculty of Veterinary Sciences and Animal Husbandry Shuhama
Sher E Kashmir University of Agricultural Sciences and Technology of Kashmir Srinagar, Jammu and Kashmir, India

Simant Kumar Nanda
Fisheries and ARD Department
Government of Odisha
Koraput, Odisha, India

Panikkaparambil Shilpa
Veterinary Surgeon
Veterinary Dispensary, Vilayur
Palakkad, Kerala, India

Oveas R. Parray
Division of Veterinary Medicine
Faculty of Veterinary Sciences and Animal Husbandry Shuhama
Sher E Kashmir University of Agricultural Sciences and Technology of Kashmir Srinagar, Jammu and Kashmir, India

Ranjani Rajasekaran
Department of Veterinary Microbiology
Veterinary College and Research Institute
Theni, Tamil Nadu, India
Tamil Nadu Veterinary and Animal Sciences University
Chennai, Tamil Nadu, India

Tanmoy Rana
Department of Veterinary Clinical Complex
West Bengal University of Animal & Fishery Sciences
Kolkata, West Bengal, India

Kamlesh A. Sadariya
Department of Veterinary Pharmacology and Toxicology
College of Veterinary Science and Animal Husbandry
Kamdhenu University
Anand, Gujarat, India

Pardeep Sharma
Department of Veterinary Medicine
DGCN College of Veterinary and Animal Sciences
CSK Himachal Pradesh Krishi Vishvavidyalaya
Palampur, Himachal Pradesh, India

Pratishtha Sharma
Department of Veterinary Pharmacology and
Toxicology
College of Veterinary & Animal Sciences
Rajasthan University of Veterinary & Animal Sciences
Bikaner, Rajasthan, India

Subir Singh
Department of Veterinary Medicine and
Public Health
Faculty of Animal Science, Veterinary Science and
Fisheries
Agriculture and Forestry University
Rampur Chitwan, Nepal

Joe S. Smith
Department of Large Animal Clinical Sciences
University of Tennessee
Knoxville, TN, USA

Tamanna H. Solanki
Department of Veterinary Pharmacology and
Toxicology
College of Veterinary Science and Animal Husbandry
Kamdhenu University
Anand, Gujarat, India

Benito Soto-Blanco
Department of Veterinary Clinics and Surgery
Veterinary School
Universidade Federal de Minas Gerais
Belo Horizonte, Brazil

Vikrant Sudan
Department of Veterinary Parasitology, College of
Veterinary Science
Guru Angad Dev Veterinary and Animal Sciences
University
Rampura Phul, Punjab, India

Deepak Sumbria
Department of Veterinary Parasitology, College of
Veterinary Science
Guru Angad Dev Veterinary and Animal Sciences
University
Rampura Phul, Punjab, India

Abhinav Suthar
Department of Medicine
College of Veterinary Sciences & Animal Husbandry
Sardarkrushinagar
Kamdhenu University
Gandhinagar, Gujarat, India

Abha Tikoo
Faculty of Veterinary Sciences & Animal Husbandry
Sher-e-Kashmir University of Agricultural Sciences and
Technology-Jammu
Ranbir Singh Pura, UT Jammu & Kashmir, India

Amita Tiwari
Department of Veterinary Medicine
College of Veterinary Science & Animal Husbandry
Nanaji Deshmukh Veterinary Science University
Jabalpur, Madhya Pradesh, India

Shivangi Udainiya
Department of Veterinary Medicine
College of Veterinary Science & Animal Husbandry
Nanaji Deshmukh Veterinary Science University
Jabalpur, Madhya Pradesh, India

Rather I. Ul Haq
Division of Veterinary Medicine
Faculty of Veterinary Sciences and Animal
Husbandry Shuhama
Sher E Kashmir University of Agricultural Sciences
and Technology of Kashmir Srinagar, Jammu and
Kashmir, India

Hridya Susan Varughese
Department of Veterinary Microbiology
Veterinary College, Hebbal
Bangalore, Karnataka, India
Karnataka Veterinary Animal and Fisheries Sciences
University
Bidar, Karnataka, India

Mohammad I. Yatoo
Division of Veterinary Clinical Complex
Faculty of Veterinary Sciences and Animal
Husbandry Shuhama
Sher E Kashmir University of Agricultural Sciences
and Technology of Kashmir Srinagar, Jammu and
Kashmir, India

Preface

Ruminants are mammals that have peculiar and specialized organs that can permit the fermentation of microbes from ingested materials before the process of digestion. The most common examples of ruminants are cattle, goats, and sheep. Goats were one of the first animals to be domesticated globally for the production of milk, meat, and skin. As they are voracious grazers, they are generally more susceptible to various diseases and disorders. This book emphasizes the various diseases that can affect goats, as well as how goats' health may impact human health simultaneously. The book encompasses nutritional management, the etiopathogenesis of goat diseases, diagnostic tools, prevention, and control. The types of diseases described include bacterial, viral, fungal, parasitic, production, and genetic diseases, as well as exotic disease. After completion of this book, readers will have acquired knowledge about the latest new thinking and understanding of a plethora of diseases affecting goats.

The main concept is to give ample information to veterinary surgeons who are actively involved in small farm animal, mixed, or small animal practices. This book will also act as a reference book for undergraduates, postgraduates, academics, and scientists. The book provides a wealth of information about diseases to provide a veterinarian with the support they need when treating caprine patients. It also describes how to improve the health as well as the productivity of goat herds and flocks. I expect the book to be helpful and interesting to clinicians, researchers, veterinary students, extension personnel, animal scientists, herd managers, and hobbyists alike.

Tanmoy Rana
Kolkata, India

Acknowledgments

I am extremely grateful to all contributors involved for contributing chapters to the book in the pandemic situation. I would like to convey my gratitude to Dr. Rituparna Bose, Health Sciences Editor, Jennifer Seward, Managing Editor, and other members of the Wiley staff who actively or indirectly gave me the opportunity to edit this text. Finally, I would like to acknowledge my wife for encouraging the writing and editing of this book as well as tolerating the time and attention that were required of me.

1

Introduction

K. Justin Davis[1], *Sunita Choudhary*[2], *and Tanmoy Rana*[3]

[1] *Department of Veterinary Epidemiology & Preventive Medicine, College of Veterinary & Animal Sciences, Mannuthy, Kerala, India*
[2] *Department of Clinical Veterinary Medicine, College of Veterinary & Animal Sciences, Rajasthan University of Veterinary & Animal Sciences, Bikaner, Rajasthan, India*
[3] *Department of Veterinary Clinical Complex, West Bengal University of Animal & Fishery Sciences, Kolkata, West Bengal, India*

1.1 Introduction

Goats are important domesticated animals in various parts of the globe that have served humankind for centuries. Along with sheep, cattle, and pigs, goats are considered as the first domesticated ungulates and originated from their wild ancestor, the bezoar or *Capra aegagrus* (Naderi et al. 2008). They were domesticated as early as 10 000 years ago in the area around the Zagros Mountains, western Iran. Ancient farmers used wild goats for milk and meat, dung, bones, and hair. Domestication of goats played an important role in the development of agriculture and civilization (Zeder and Hesser 2000). Currently, goats are spread globally, with more than 300 breeds living on every continent except Antarctica (Kumar et al. 2010). Their extraordinary adaptability to desert, mountainous, and tropical areas along with their hardiness led to their rapid spread. The domestication of goats was favored by their body size, which made them more suitable for management, with their earlier puberty and maturity, greater reproduction rate, social nature, and obedient behavior. These animals re raised for meat, milk, and dairy products, and for fiber and skin products. They are tagged the "poor man's cow" or the "bank on the hoof" because of their role in rural economies. There are a large number of goat breeds that are grouped into meat breeds, dairy breeds, dual-purpose breeds, fiber breeds, and pet breeds based on the utility and purpose of rearing them.

1.2 Global Distribution

The world goat population is 1128.10 million, which places them third in the total livestock population after cattle and sheep. The world population of goats has an increasing trend (Figure 1.1), which indicates huge demand for goat products like chevon (goat flesh), fiber, and milk. Asia is the continent with the highest population, representing 51.35% of the world's total goat population. The majority of the total population (94.5%) is distributed in Asia and Africa (FAOSTAT 2020) and the lowest proportion is in Oceana (0.38%). The population density of goats in particular regions may be due to historical and religious reasons. Chevon is more used in Muslim countries where pork is forbidden. In Asia, the highest population is noticed in India (Figure 1.2) where beef is not among traditional foods.

1.3 Advantages of Goat Rearing

Goats can adapt well in areas where other livestock or crops are not suitable (Figure 1.3). They are opportunistic and selective feeders, which makes them thrive well on depleted pastureland and enables them to convert poor-quality forage (Figure 1.4). They can consume, digest, and extract nutrients from tannin-rich browse. Goats are more able to withstand adverse climate conditions like heat stress compared with cattle and sheep. Their bipedal stance helps them access tree leaves that are considered unavailable to other livestock species. Their better feed efficiency than other ruminant species distinguishes them as a good candidate for farming. Goat rearing does not require specialized shelter structures, which along with reduced labor increases its popularity among farmers (Figure 1.5). To meet the growing demands of the human population, scientists have proposed goats, which are climate-adapted animals and are expected to perform better than other species.

Principles of Goat Disease and Prevention, First Edition. Edited by Tanmoy Rana.

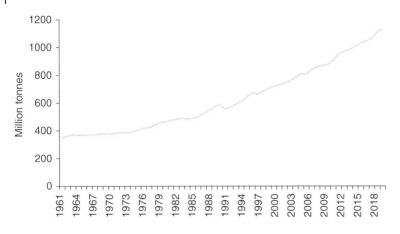

Figure 1.1 Global goat population, 1961–2020.

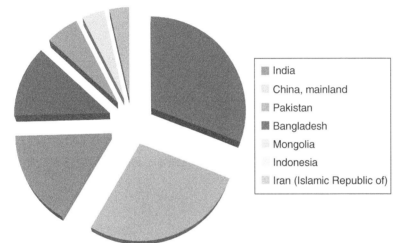

Figure 1.2 Country-wise distribution of largest goat producers in 2020.

India
China, mainland
Pakistan
Bangladesh
Mongolia
Indonesia
Iran (Islamic Republic of)

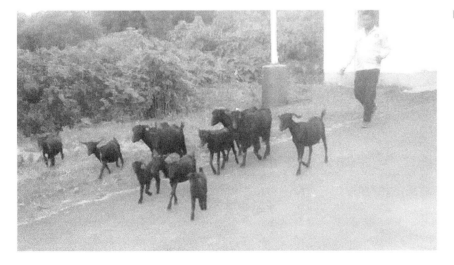

Figure 1.3 A flock of goats.

1.4 Goat Milk and Products

Goat rearing is a major source of income for poor farmers and women in rural areas, especially in developing countries. Goats are considered as the "poor man's cow" and are kept for milk, meat, fiber, or fertilizer. They can thrive well on difficult terrains with a small amount of feed, which, along with their small size, makes them suitable for farming with reduced maintenance costs. Dairy goats are fewer in number than dairy cows, but they contribute 1.3% of world total milk production, while milk produced by cattle is 83.1% (Mazinani and

Figure 1.4 Goats grazing in a field.

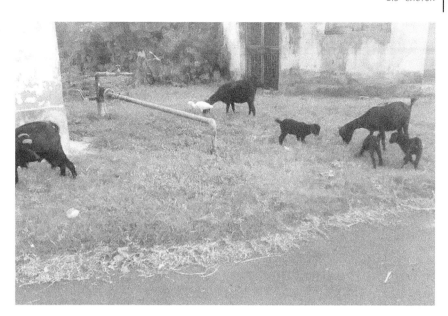

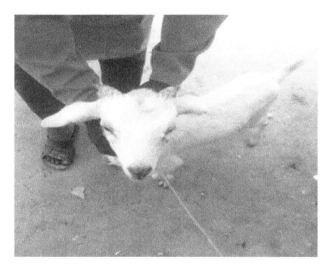

Figure 1.5 An owner with his goat.

Rude 2020). Dairy goats can produce 2.8–3.8 l of milk daily during their peak lactation time.

Goat's milk production is showing an increasing trend due to increased demand for goat's milk and related products. There is a well-organized market for goat's milk in Europe, especially in France, where the goat sector is dedicated to milk production and cheese making. Goat's milk can be a replacement for those who suffer from an allergy or intolerance to cow's milk or other animal milk protein. It is a source of fat, lactose, protein, minerals, and vitamins. Goat's milk is easily digested and more similar to human milk than cow's milk. Fat globules in goat's milk are smaller and have different casein types that are easier to digest. Goat's milk can be used for the preparation of different products like dried milk, cheese, fermented milk, desserts, sweets, whey products, and so on. Cosmetic products are

also produced from goat's milk, including soaps, creams, body lotions, shampoos, hair conditioners, and aftershave lotions, which are marketed in many countries such as the United States and Switzerland (Ribeiro and Ribeiro 2010).

1.5 Chevon

Goats are reared mainly for chevon, goat meat, which serves as a source of fat, amino acids, and several micronutrients such as vitamins and minerals including zinc and iron (Webb 2014). China and India are large chevon producers at 2.3 and 0.55 million tonnes, respectively. Goat meat is rich in essential amino acids, low in cholesterol, high in protein, and a good source of iron. The world consumption of beef is higher than that of chevon, especially in western countries, but goat meat can serve as a great source of protein to humans, especially in developing countries, hence the goat populations are higher in those countries. Per capita meat consumption approximately doubled from 20 to 43 kg globally from 1961 to 2014, with marked variations in direction and rate among countries (Ritchie et al. 2017). Countries that underwent a strong economic transition had the highest variations. China saw a 15-fold increase since 1961 and the rate in Brazil nearly quadrupled, whereas the rate stayed same in India with per capita consumption less than 4 kg per person. Chevon can act as a staple food in countries where there are restrictions on other red meats such as beef and pork. These include Muslim countries where pork is forbidden and in India where beef is not considered a traditional food. China ranks first in production of chevon, followed by India and Pakistan. Most of the goat meat produced is consumed locally in the communities of developing countries, as the market structure has not = developed to trade within the country and internationally.

1.6 Fiber and Other Products

Fiber from goats includes both cashmere and mohair produced by cashmere goats (selectively bred) and angora goats. Cashmere goats produce a double fleece known as guard hair and down hair. Down hair or cashmere gives protection from cold and guard hair covers the animal's body. China and Mongolia are two of the leading producers of cashmere. Cashmere fibers from the beautiful, soft, durable, bright, and elastic downy undercoat of the goat are desirable to the textile industry (Shakyawar et al. 2013). Each animal can contribute from 500 g to 1 kg/head cashmere annually, which can be used for making clothes and fabrics. Mohair is quite different from cashmere, as there is only one type of fleece which does not require dehairing as in cashmere production. One goat can produce around 5–8 kg of mohair a year. It is lustrous, long, and coarse, and is suitable for knitwear, apparel, curtaining, upholstery material, shawls, socks, and accessories.

Tanned leather from goat skin is used for products that require soft hide like gloves, bags, and boots. It has been used for leather book binding and untanned goat skins were traditionally used as containers for water, kefir, wine, and so on (Skapetas and Bampidis 2016). The Black Bengal breed is considered as a high-quality goat skin producer.

Goat manure contains macronutrients as well as micro elements that can be used as an organic soil fertilizer (Sunaryo et al. 2021). Goat manure is considered an excellent source of nitrogen, phosphorus, and potassium, which are essential for plants.

Goats, especially dwarf and pygmy breeds, are commonly used as pets because of their particularly pleasing and fun-loving behavior.

1.7 Goat Production System

Based on fodder and grazing land availability, farmers in different countries have adopted different systems of management for goats (Hegde 2020). In Asia and Africa, where there is the major share of the goat population, they practice the extensive system, semi-intensive system, and intensive system of goat farming. The extensive production system is characterized by a large area with a reduced or low density of animals. This land is not suitable for agriculture and has low rainfall or sometimes extreme temperatures. The economic return will be reduced in this system as there will be

a lower kid crop and the goats will be raised in an adverse climate. There can be a mobile grazing system or a sedentary grazing system. The first system is characterized by movement of the shepherd along with their flock from one place to another in search of feed, whereas the other system involves a farm for keeping animals in during the night. The intensive production system involves confinement of animals with limited access to land. These animals are fed concentrated feeds and have minimal grazing. This requires a high capital income and more labor. The animal density and kid crop are higher in this system than in the extensive system of production. High-producing and fertile animals will be used in the intensive system and it gains more income. The semi-intensive system of goat farming is a combination of the other two systems with limited free-range grazing on fenced pastureland and feeding in stalls. The cost of feed will be higher than in the extensive system.

In Europe intensive management with good use of pastureland is practiced to reduce feed costs, control the weed problem, and maintain natural behavior (Hegde 2020). The extensive system of goat farming is not very common in Europe and North America.

1.8 Constraints in Goat Farming

Even though goat husbandry has so many advantages, it also has some problems, like low body weight gain, disease outbreaks, and mortality, which in turn reduce the production potential of the animal and hence the economics of the farmer. Major constraints in goat farming are in breeding, feeding, healthcare, and marketing, among which marketing is the major constraint, followed by healthcare, feeding, and breeding in India (Patbandha et al. 2018). A structured marketing channel is required to help farmers trade their product with maximum profit. Feed and availability of grazing land are other important limitations in goat farming. Scientific knowledge of farming and inadequate veterinary aids could also act as limitations in goat rearing, especially in developing countries. Planned extension work is mandatory to create awareness among farmers regarding scientific farming. Outbreaks of diseases and mortality can have a severe impact on the economy of the goat farmer. Early detection of disease and prompt control of disease outbreaks are essential to profitable goat farming.

1.9 Economics of Disease in Goats

Even though goats are resistant to many diseases, they are affected by many animal diseases (Figure 1.6). Some of these are zoonotic, like brucellosis, which can be a real

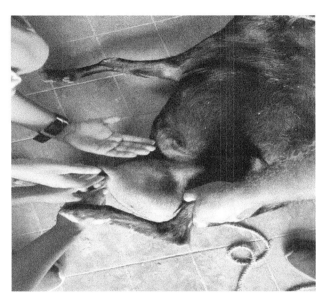

Figure 1.6   Udder inflammation of denoting a disease.

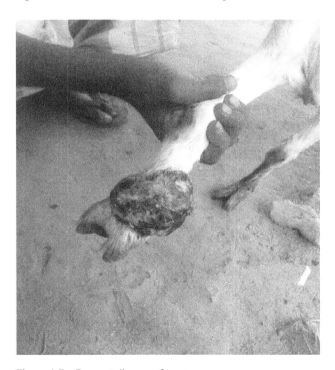

Figure 1.7   Foot rot disease of goats.

threat to humans. The occurrence of diseases will break the back of a goat farmer be due to direct or indirect losses (Sejian et al. 2021). These losses can be due to mortality, loss of wool, reproductive failure, increased inter-kidding period, higher number of abortions, body-weight loss, treatment costs, and opportunity costs. The economic losses are more pronounced in infectious diseases like bacterial, viral, parasitic, and protozoan diseases (Figure 1.7). Morbidity and mortality are high in viral diseases – peste des petits ruminants (PPR), foot and mouth disease (FMD),

sheep and goat pox – as well as bacterial diseases – enterotoxemia, contagious caprine pleuropneumonia (CCP), and anthrax – followed by parasitic diseases like fascioliasis/distomatosis (Singh and Prasad 2008). Limon et al. (2020) reported that overall economic losses due to goat pox at a farm level ranged from US$9.6 to US$6340 depending on the species affected and the production system in northeast Nigeria. The total losses due to PPR have been found to range from US$11.2 in sheep to US$11.55 in goats in Maharashtra, India. The annual financial loss due to diseases in goats was calculated as US$8.17 million in selected areas of Bangladesh. Singh et al. (2014) reported high annual economic losses due to PPR in goats and sheep. Kihu et al. (2015) estimated losses due to PPR in Kenya as US$19.1 million. Vashist et al. (2021) also reported annual economic losses due to PPR.

1.10   Goat Diseases and Public Health

Goats can act as an important source of infection, which can be transmitted directly or indirectly to humans. Most transmission occurs as an occupational hazard affecting breeders, farmers, veterinarians, and slaughterhouse workers. Transmission of these diseases can be prevented by strict biosecurity, scientific management, and mandatory vaccination programs in animals.

1.11   Prevention of Disease

Proper nutrition and management of goats are needed for the prevention of any disease. Nutrition can exert an immense influence on flock reproduction, milk production, and kid growth. Certain diseases like enterotoxemia, polioencephalomalacia, urinary calculi, pregnancy toxemia, and white muscle disease are considered to be associated with nutrition and management. So it is imperative to know about the nutrition and management of goats.

Parasitic diseases might result in significant weight loss in goats as well as moderately high mortality. These diseases are distributed worldwide and are responsible for poor health and low yields. Endoparasites of goat reside in the gastrointestinal tract and include nematodes, cestodes, trematodes, and *Protozoa*. Ectoparasites, like ticks, lice, mites, fleas, and flies, can cause losses through reduced productivity, loss of blood by sucking, and so on.

Bacterial diseases in goats have increased due to intensive and unscientific farming. Diseases like brucellosis, tuberculosis, and anthrax are zoonotic diseases that can be transmitted to humans by handling or close contact with infected animals. Goat farming is practiced commonly in rural areas, where poor scientific knowledge is another factor in the transmission of zoonotic disease. Anthrax, enterotoxemia, gas gangrene, tetanus, listeriosis, caseous lymphadenitis, tuberculosis, Johne's disease, pasteurellosis/mannheimiosis, dermatophilosis, brucellosis, CCP, foot rot, colibacillosis, and salmonellosis are the major bacterial diseases of goats. Goat skin harbors varieties of fungal organisms including dermatophytes and saprophytes like *Aspergillus*, *Penicillium*, *Emericella*, *Alternaria*, and *Cochliobolus* (El-Said et al. 2009). The opportunistic fungus can cause disease in immune-compromised animals. Mycotic abortion, fungal mastitis, and mycotic pneumonia are not rare in goats and are difficult to diagnose in the early stages. Goats are susceptible to many mycotoxins and these can cause serious production losses in the animal. Dermatophytes and yeast (*Malassezia* and *Candida*) are responsible for skin diseases like ringworm and seborrheic dermatosis (Seyed et al. 2018).

Goats are susceptible to many viral infections that can cause a severe economic burden to farmers. PPR, blue-tongue, goat pox, and orf are the common viral diseases in goats.

Transboundary diseases are highly contagious and transmissible epidemic diseases of animals that can disrupt or inhibit trade in animals or animal products within a country or internationally. The majority of these are emerging viral diseases like PPR, FMD, goat pox, and Rift Valley fever. Transboundary, emerging, and exotic diseases are major zoonotic diseases of goats.

Toxicity in the goat is mainly caused by the consumption of toxic plants and the clinical signs vary with the toxic content.

Selection pressure and domestication lead to the occurrence of undesirable traits commonly recognized as due to inherited diseases or disorders. These disorders or diseases occur sporadically and rarely cause a serious economic impact.

Common nutritional or metabolic diseases of goats arise due to insufficient intake of nutrients and their repercussions on the metabolism. Pregnancy toxemia, polioencephalomalacia, urolithiasis, subacute ruminal acidosis, lactational ketosis, hepatic lipidosis, hypocalcemia, low milk-fat syndrome, and vitamin E or selenium deficiency are major diseases.

Different methods are available for accurate diagnosis of diseases in goats, which is an integral part of disease identification and management.

The temporal and spatial distribution of infectious disease can vary in different countries. Awareness of the diseases and the availability of veterinary services are the main factors in prevention of infectious diseases. Reduced vaccination coverage is also attributed to economic loss due to disease. Knowledge about a disease and its transmission helps the farmer to effectively control the disease. Even though goats are resistant to many infections, intensive farming, reduced pasture facilities, and climatic changes make them more vulnerable.

Vaccination can increase immunity against most bacterial and viral infections among goats. The effectiveness of a vaccination program depends on several factors, including general health, nutrition, stresses, and so on. A vaccine should be administered to a systemically healthy animal. Deworming prior to vaccination is recommended. Vaccines against bacteria (clostridial diseases types C, D, and T; foot rot; *Brucella* for caseous lymphadenitis; *Campylobacter fetus* and *Campylobacter jejuni* bacterin; bacterial pneumonia from *Mannheimia haemolytica* and *Pasteurella multocida*; chlamydia; and anthrax) and viruses (sore mouth, bluetongue, PPR, goat pox, FMD, and rabies) are commonly used in goats as a control measure.

Effective biosecurity measures should be employed to control the transmission of disease from outside and the spread of disease inside a flock. These are a set of protocols intended to control the spread of disease. The transmission of disease can be multifactorial. It depends on the epidemiological triad: host factors (health status, immune status), environmental factors (temperature, pasture condition, etc.), and the disease agent (virulence, pathogenicity). The fundamental goal of biosecurity is either to break the transmission of disease or to minimize its effect. Biosecurity controls disease transmission not only among animals, but also from animals to human and vice versa.

Multiple-Choice Questions

1 Which among the following are ancestors of goats?
   A Bezoars
   B Aurochs
   C Hyracotherium
   D Wild boar

2 Currently, goats are spread globally, with more than 300 breeds living on every continent except which one?
   A Antarctica
   B Asia
   C Africa
   D Americas

3 Which among these species are highest in number worldwide?
- **A** Sheep
- **B** Goat
- **C** Cow
- **D** Pig

4 What is goat meat known as?
- **A** Mutton
- **B** Chevon
- **C** Venison
- **D** Beef

5 Where is the highest population of goat seen?
- **A** China
- **B** India
- **C** Pakistan
- **D** Bhutan

6 What is known as the poor man's cow?
- **A** Goat
- **B** Cow
- **C** Buffalo
- **D** Sheep

7 Which country contributes the highest production of goat milk?
- **A** India
- **B** China
- **C** Afghanistan
- **D** Estonia

8 Which country is the largest producer of chevon?
- **A** India
- **B** China
- **C** Nepal
- **D** Pakistan

9 What breed of goat produces mohair?
- **A** Angora
- **B** Cashmere
- **C** Gadi
- **D** Malabari

10 How much cashmere can each goat contribute annually?
- **A** 100–250 g
- **B** 500 g–1 kg
- **C** 1–2 kg
- **D** 2.5–5 kg

References

El-Said, A.H., Sohair, T.H., and El-Hadi, A.G. (2009). Fungi associated with the hairs of goat and sheep in Libya. *Mycobiology* 37 (2): 82–88. https://doi.org/10.4489/MYCO.2009.37.2.082.

FAOSTAT (2020). Food and agriculture data. https://www.fao.org/faostat/en/#home

Hegde, N.G. (2020). Goat development: an opportunity to strengthen rural economy in Asia and Africa. *Asian Journal of Research in Animal and Veterinary Sciences* 5 (4): 30–47.

Kihu, S.M., Gitao, G.C., Bebora, L.C. et al. (2015). Economic losses associated with Peste des petits ruminants in Turkana County Kenya. *Pastoralism* 5: 9. https://doi.org/10.1186/s13570-015-0029-6.

Kumar, S., Rama Rao, C.A., Kareemulla, K., and Venkateswarlu, B. (2010). Role of goats in livelihood security of rural poor in the less favoured environments. *Indian Journal of Agricultural Economics* 65 (4): 761–781.

Limon, G., Gamawa, A.A., Ahmed, A.I. et al. (2020). Epidemiological characteristics and economic impact of lumpy skin disease, sheep pox and goat pox among subsistence farmers in northeast Nigeria. *Frontiers in Veterinary Science* 7: 8. https://doi.org/10.3389/fvets.2020.00008.

Mazinani, M. and Rude, B. (2020). Population, world production and quality of sheep and goat products. *American Journal of Animal and Veterinary Sciences* 15 (4): 291–299.

Naderi, S., Rezaei, H.R., Pompanon, F. et al. (2008). The goat domestication process inferred from large-scale mitochondrial DNA analysis of wild and domestic individuals. *Proceedings of the National Academy of Sciences of the United States of America* 105 (46): 17659–17664. https://doi.org/10.1073/pnas.0804782105.

Patbandha, T.K., Gamit, V.V., Odedra, M.D. et al. (2018). Constraints in goat farming under extensive production system in western Gujarat. *Indian Journal of Animal Production Management* 34 (3–4): 1–6.

Ribeiro, A.C. and Ribeiro, S.D.A. (2010). Specialty products made from goat milk. *Small Ruminant Research* 89 (2–3, 233): 225.

Ritchie, H., Rosado, P., and Roser, M. (2017). Meat and Dairy Production. *Our WorldInData*. https://ourworldindata.org/meat-production.

Sejian, V., Silpa, M.V., Reshma Nair, M.R. et al. (2021). Heat stress and goat welfare: adaptation and production considerations. *Animals* 11: 1021. https://doi.org/10.3390/ani11041021.

Seyedmousavi, S., Bosco, S.M.G., de Hoog, S. et al. (2018). Corrigendum: Fungal infections in animals: a patchwork of different situations. *Medical Mycology* 56 (8): e4. https://doi.org/10.1093/mmy/myy028.

Shakyawar, D.B., Raja, A.S.M., Kumar, A. et al. (2013). Pashmina fibre-production, characteristics and utilization. *Indian Journal of Fibre & Textile Research* 38: 207–221.

Singh, B. and Prasad, S. (2008). Modelling of economic losses due to some important diseases in goats in India. *Agricultural Economics Research Review* 21: 297–302.

Singh, B., Bardhan, D., Verma, M.R. et al. (2014). Estimation of economic losses due to PPR in small ruminants in India. *Veterinary*. *World* 7: 194–199. https://doi.org/10.14202/vetworld.2014.194-199.

Skapetas, B. and Bampidis, V. (2016). Goat production in the world: present situation and trends. *Livestock Research for Rural Development* 28: 200. http://www.lrrd.org/lrrd28/11/skap28200.html.

Sunaryo, Y., Darini, M.T., Cahyani, V.R., and Purnomo, D. (2021). Potential liquid fertilizer made from goat feces to improve vegetable product. In: *Goat Science: Environment, Health and Economy* (ed. S. Kukovics). London: IntechOpen, ch. 12. https://doi.org/10.5772/intechopen.99047.

Vashist, V.S., Yadav, A.K., Rajak, K.K. et al. (2021). Flock level economic loss due to Peste Des Petits ruminants outbreak in transhumance sheep and goat population in Himachal Pradesh (India). *Indian Journal of Animals Research* B-4386: https://doi.org/10.18805/IJAR.B-4386.

Webb, E.C. (2014). Goat meat production, composition, and quality. *Animal Frontiers* 4 (4): 33–37. https://doi.org/10.2527/af.2014-0031.

Zeder, M.A. and Hesse, B. (2000). The initial domestication of goats (*Capra hircus*) in the Zagros mountains 10,000 years ago. *Science* 287 (5461): 2254–2257. https://doi.org/10.1126/science.287.5461.2254.

2

Nutrition and Management of Goats

Rohit Kumar

Department of Livestock Production Management, Dr GC Negi College of Veterinary and Animal Sciences, CSKHPKV, Palampur, Himachal Pradesh, India

Goat rearing started around 11 000 years ago and has played an important role to support humankind in terms of the production of milk, meat, cashmere/pashmina, mohair, skin, and manure. Further, goats' low costs of maintenance, high fecundity, easy marketing, and the social acceptance of their meat resulted in their being an ideal livelihood option for underprivileged rural households. There are around one billion goats and about 300 breeds worldwide. In India, there are 148.88 million goats (20th livestock census, 2019) and 37 registered breeds, which indicates the country's good indigenous stock in comparison to the rest of the world. The meat obtained from the goat is termed chevon, which makes up around 5% of the world's total meat consumption. The goat has long been a very popular animal in India and is known as the "poor man's cow," representing 13.72% of total meat and 2.95% of total milk production in the country. These animals are highly fertile with superior reproductive potential in comparison to other livestock species. However, poor management can lead to failure of conception, loss of estrous cycles, and a decrease in the number of offspring in their lifetime. Scientific feeding, breeding, and management can play a key role in successful goat farming. This further depends upon an understanding of the fundamental scientific knowledge applicable in goat husbandry about their nutrition and management during different stages of their life.

2.1 Essential Nutrients for Goats

The six classes of nutrients that are essential in goat nutrition are protein, carbohydrates, fat, vitamins, minerals, and water. These are necessary to sustain life and play an essential role in their growth, productivity, and reproductive performance.

2.1.1 Protein

The basic structure of a protein involves amino acids, which are utilized by the animal body to produce all the proteins required for growth, production, and maintenance. Generally, protein supplements are fed to ruminants to make up for dietary shortfalls. Much of the protein consumed is degraded by the rumen bacteria into amino acids, which are used to form bacterial protein. Bacterial protein can also be formed from non-protein nitrogen (NPN) sources. Urea is the main NPN source used in ruminant feeding. However, goats are not fed with urea as frequently as cattle, as goats may be more prone to urea toxicity. Goats appear to be more efficient at nitrogen recycling from the body to the rumen in comparison to other species provided that sufficient energy is available. This helps to reduce the amount of protein required in the goat diet. Therefore, when goats are on low-quality forage, a grain supplement may also help in the improvement of protein status by providing additional energy to ruminal microbes for microbial protein synthesis. Protein is required in higher amounts during growth (kids), milk synthesis (lactation), and mohair growth.

2.1.2 Carbohydrates

Carbohydrates are the major source of energy in goats. They can be simple (e.g. sugars) or complex (e.g. starch found in grains, or cellulose, i.e. fiber). Generally, goats consume high levels of cellulose in the form of grasses, leaves, forbs, and other plant species that must be digested in the rumen to provide energy. Feedstuffs with a lower level of fiber have a higher level of digestible energy. However, a certain minimum level of fiber is necessary for healthy rumen function. Fresh pastures and young plants may have highly digestible fiber and provide high energy compared to older plants. Energy requirements vary during different physiological stages in animals. It is essential to provide high-energy rations at the time of breeding, late gestation, and lactation. Lactating does have the highest energy demand.

In addition, goats are not easily adapted to high-concentrate diets, in comparison to cattle and sheep. They are predisposed to conditions like acidosis, founder, urinary calculi, and enterotoxemia if kept on high-concentrate diets. To prevent such problems when placing goats on a high-concentrate diet, there should be a gradual increase of concentrate and a minimum of 12% crude fiber should be maintained in the diet, or around half of the diet should be grass, browse, or hay.

2.1.3 Fats

Fats are high energy sources. They provide more than twice the energy on a weight basis in comparison to carbohydrates. Goat diets are generally low in fat content as the animals mainly thrive on plants. They consume fats in the form of plant waxes while grazing or browsing, but these are also not digested in their rumen. Fat can increase the energy content of their diet if it is treated to be inactive in the rumen, as it can depress fiber digestion. These treated fat sources are called "bypass fat" and may be used in the diets of dairy goats but generally not those of meat goats. Fat supplementation may not be a cost-effective idea for goat production.

2.1.4 Vitamins and Minerals

Vitamins and minerals are required for maintenance as well as for the proper functioning of the physiological systems in goats. Vitamin B is synthesized in sufficient quantity by the rumen flora. Therefore, it is not required to add sources of this vitamin to the goats' diet. Fat-soluble vitamins (A, D, E, K) are required to be included in goat feeding due to the animal's inability to make these vitamins. In addition, vitamin C is essential for the immune system to work efficiently.

Minerals can be classified as macrominerals and microminerals. Minerals play an important role in various functions, for instance feeding calcium (Ca) and phosphorous (P) (2 : 1) provides better structural and bone strength, while other minerals play important roles in the nervous and reproductive systems. Free-choice loose minerals and salt supplementation always work well. However, adding minerals into the feed should be based on the quality of the forage, as some forage can be high in some minerals and low in others. If there is enough salt present in the supplied minerals then one should be careful when providing separate free-choice salt. Goats tend to be copper (Cu) deficient, therefore there must be enough Cu (10–80 ppm) in their diets. Selenium (0.1–3 ppm) is another mineral required for goats that are reared in areas where the soil is deficient in it.

2.1.5 Water

Water is the cheapest feed ingredient available. Insufficient intake of water may affect the production, growth, and general performance of goats more severely than any other dietary insufficiency. Goats are among the most efficient domesticated livestock in terms of their use of water; however, a water loss of only ~10% from their body may prove fatal.

Various factors influencing the water consumption in goats include the water content of the forage consumed, the environmental temperature, the amount of exercise, the stage of production (growth, maintenance, lactation, etc.), and the salt and mineral content of the diet. When kept on a high-protein ration they consume more water. Goats kept on lush green pasture or forage soaked with rain or heavy dew may consume less water in comparison to those feeding on dry hay. Still, it is necessary to provide ad lib water for all goats, as some animals in the flock such as lactating does may need it more and it is difficult to work out the individual water requirement of goats in a flock.

Not just the quantity but the quality of the water must also be good. Clear fresh water flowing in streams is preferred over stagnant water with a potentially high blue algae content, which may be toxic for goats. Nitrate content is another matter of concern in the case of livestock. Safe levels for drinking water are less than 100 ppm for nitrate nitrogen, less than 443 ppm for nitrate ion, and less than 607 ppm for sodium nitrate.

2.2 Nutrition and Management of Kids

Today's kids are tomorrow's well-grown goats and their management starts with excellent care and adequate nutrition immediately after birth. Kids should nurse from their mothers in the first eight hours of their life to consume colostrum at a minimum rate of 10–20% of their body weight, preferably within two to three hours after birth. It is recommended that kids should be fed colostrum within half an hour after birth. Colostrum is the first secretion of mammary glands obtained from the dam after her kidding and it has an essential role in the development of a kid's immunity. Losses are low in colostrum-fed kids worldwide. The colostrum is enriched with immune components including immunoglobins (IgG, IgM, IgE), lactoferrin, lysozyme, cytokines, growth factors, and hormones. The concentrations of these components are found to be elevated during the first 72 hours when the changes in the milk composition of transition milk are proceeding toward normal milk. IgG is the most dominant immunoglobin found in colostrum and helps in providing passive immunity to newborns. The other components like lactoferrin, lysozyme, growth factors, and other metabolites help to enhance the immune system and overall body composition. This saves the kids from many diseases including enterotoxemia and tetanus.

There is a phenomenon that occurs at a gradual pace in the epithelium of the intestine termed "gut closure," due to which a kid may lose its ability to absorb immunoglobins 20–28 hours after birth. Some evidence states that this ability may persist longer in starved kids, but the maximum potential for absorption is during the early hours after birth, and "gut closure" may even be started if we feed a small amount of colostrum, which can affect the kid's ability to absorb immunoglobin. Therefore, it must be ensured during the initial feedings that the kid gets the proper amount of colostrum. This will maximize immunoglobin absorption, which may be less in case of low colostrum consumption or any delay in colostrum feeding. This makes it obvious that the effective transfer of immunoglobins from colostrum to the kid's plasma is a function of the concentration of immunoglobins available for absorption, the level of colostrum intake by the kid, and the time of colostrum consumption in relation to its birth. Further, it is also recommended that the newborn be allowed to suckle its mother up to three to four days after birth, because the availability of the different nutritive bioactive components for absorption is much higher during the initial days after kidding (colostrum followed by transition milk) and decreases as the transition occurs toward the normal milk (Figure 2.1). Kids born as twins and triplets may need colostrum from other high-producing does. Colostrum can be stored in the freezer if a newborn dies and can be used for feeding twins and triplets of the flock or orphan kids. Thawing of frozen colostrum at room temperature is sufficient and it should not be thawed using high heat or a microwave, as this can denature the nutrients. Replacement kids should be allowed to stay with their milking mothers as long as possible because their early weaning can leave them undernourished, which can affect their production potential.

The following points must be kept in mind for the care and management of kids:

- Immediately after birth, the nasal passage of the kid should be cleared and there should not be any entangling membrane or mucous present in the passage, as it can lead to suffocation.
- If there is a breathing problem, artificial means of breathing should be adopted.
- If extra mucous membrane has adhered to the body after birth it should be removed and the kid should be cleaned and dried.
- The navel should be dipped in tincture iodine or swabbed with an antiseptic solution to prevent navel ill. If the umbilical cord is intact, it should be severed with a sterile knife/blade about 4–7 cm from the umbilicus. The severed end should be swabbed with tincture iodine.
- The kid's birth weight should be recorded.
- It is recommended to feed colostrum within 30 minutes after kidding as it has a role in immunity development and the expulsion of the meconium (first fecal material) during early life.

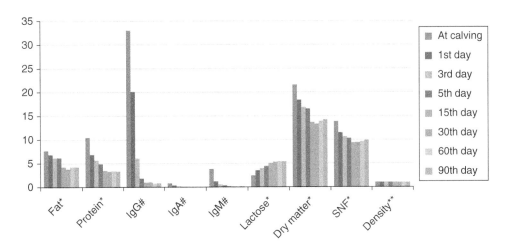

Figure 2.1 Comparison in the composition of colostrum with mature milk from the first day of calving up to the 90th day after calving. *, values in %; **, values in g/ml; #, values in mg/ml. *Source:* The average values in the graph are adapted from Sánchez-Macías et al. (2014).

Table 2.1 Feeding of goat kids (0–90 days).

Age of kids (d)	Body weight (kg)	Milk (ml)	No. of feedings	Creep feed (g)	Forage, green/day (g)
0–7	1–3	Free choice	With mother	–	–
8–30	3–5	200–350	2–3	Free choice	Free choice
31–60	5–7	300–400	2	Free choice	Free choice
61–90	6–10	200	2	100–150	Free choice

- Later milk should be fed daily, depending upon the kid's body weight.
- An identification number must be given to each kid at an early age.
- Feeding of kid starters should be begun at the age of 3 weeks to 1 month old. It should be introduced gradually in the diet and the amount should be increased at a rate at which the kids can consume it without upsetting their digestion.
- Chaffed greens and hay should be offered to the kids.
- Milk feeding can be discontinued by the age of 3–4 months or possibly sooner if the kids start consuming grass or hay and concentrate.
- Overfeeding and underfeeding must be avoided and taken care of, as this may cause digestive problems and may affect the kid's growth performance.
- At the age of 4 weeks, the kid should get its first dewormer, and after that it should be dewormed periodically.
- Male kids, not required for breeding purposes, should be castrated before weaning.
- Kids should be weaned at the age of 90 days (Table 2.1).

2.2.1 Feeding of Kids from 3 Months to 1 Year of Age

- Grazing under pasture should be allowed for around eight hours a day.
- Provide concentrate mixture (protein 16–18%) @ 100–200 g/kid/day.
- Dry fodder should be provided during the night (in summer and rainy months).

2.3 Nutrition and Management of Goats

Goats are generally reared under an extensive system and this is the most widely followed system practiced all over the world. It includes migratory, transhumance, free-range, pasture, and range grazing. One can combine pasturage with a stall feeding system (semi-intensive system) or rear the goats by the method of "soiling," which is keeping the goats constantly in houses and providing all of the required rations in the houses themselves (intensive system). Adoption of this depends on whether the farmer owns pasturage or not. Unless a farmer has good pastureland that is of the right sort, the goats will flourish better and live for longer time under a stall feeding system. The only demerit of goat rearing where there is no grass or pasturage is the extra cost of feeding.

The most up-to-date feeding standards are published by the National Research Council (NRC) of the National Academy of Sciences, USA. Rations for different classes and categories of goats can be formulated by using these standards and proper use of available feedstuffs. Nutrient requirements for ration formulation may be calculated using the following formulae (Ranjhan 1998):

$$DM\,(g/d) = 76\,g\,/\,Wkg^{0.75}$$
$$DCP\,(g/d) = 3\,g\,/\,Wkg^{0.75}$$
$$TDN\,(g/d) = 30\,g\,/\,Wkg^{0.75}$$

where DM is dry matter, DCP is digestible crude protein, and TDN is total digestible nutrients. $Wkg^{0.75}$ means per kg metabolic body weight.

The DM intake is higher in goats in comparison to large farm animals and it varies from 3% (meat goat) to 4–6% (dairy goat) in different breeds in India. The following are the points that should be kept in mind while feeding goats:

- The ration should include approximately 60–70% green fodder, 20–30% dry fodder, and 5–10% concentrate feed. This combination should provide 16–20% DCP and 65% TDN to goats.
- Additional concentrate feed should be provided for pregnant and lactating does and also for breeding bucks.
- Green fodder provided to goats should include legumes like guar, cowpea, lucerne, berseem, and stylosanthes; non-legumes or cereals (oats, maize, sorghum, pearl millet, etc.); grasses (Napier hybrid, Anjan grass, guinea grass, etc.), and fodder trees (Sesbania, Subabul, Gliricidia, etc.).
- Concentrate feed may be prepared using a combination of grains, maize, soybean, green grams, or cereals

(30–40%), oilcake (20–30%), bran or husk (30–40%), mineral mixture, and salt (1–2%).

- Goats can also be fed low-grade roughage/residues that are treated by the following methods: physical and mechanical (soaking, chopping, grinding, pelleting, steaming, and irradiation); chemical (sodium hydroxide, urea/ammonia, etc.); and biological (fungi).
- A minimum quantity of 250 g of concentrate along with 5 g of mineral mixture and 5 g of common salt should also be included daily in the goat diet.

2.3.1 Feeding of Adult Goats

- Feeding of adult goats depends on the availability of pasture: if it is good then concentrate supplementation is not required.
- Under poor grazing conditions, the goats may be provided with 150–350 g of concentrate/goat/day, depending on their age, pregnancy, and lactation status.
- The DCP level of the concentrate mixture for feeding adults is 12%.

2.3.2 Care and Management of Pregnant Does

- The doe comes into heat every 18–24 days (average 21 days). The duration of the heat period is 2–3 days. Generally, the breeding season is spread throughout the year and under good breeding and management conditions two pregnancies in a year are possible. A doe is ready to conceive at 10–20 months of age. Body weight at this age depends on the breed: smaller breeds like Barbari have a range of 15–25 kg and larger breeds like Beetal, Jamunapari, Jakhrana, and Kalawari have a range of 30–40 kg.
- A pregnant doe should be separated from the flock and kept in a kidding pen as she approaches kidding.

- Adequate nutrition including fresh clean water, green fodder, and feed is necessary and should be given the utmost importance after the 90th day of gestation for the developing fetus.
- Hooves should be trimmed.
- As the doe completes her gestation period (145 ± 5 days), she should be kept under observation at least one week before the expected date of kidding and the visible signs of parturition should be looked for.
- The signs usually noticed are enlargement of the udder, loosening of the vulva (three days before kidding), a distinct depression on either side of the tail, a hollow appearance in the flank area, visible behavior of pawing on the floor, lying down and getting up at frequent intervals, restlessness and nervousness, frequent low bleating sounds, and a slight opaque yellowish discharge from the vagina. Any of these indicates that kidding has started (Table 2.2).

2.3.3 Care and Management at Kidding

- The kidding pen should be prepared by cleaning, disinfecting, and using fine bedding to prevent the kids from getting any infections.
- The day before kidding, substitute part of the grain with a warm wet wheat bran mash, which has a laxative action and will clean out the digestive tract, and also help in kidding.
- The doe should be left alone and should be checked every half an hour. Does should be given a chance to kid without assistance.
- The placenta will usually be passed out 30 minutes to 4 hours after the kids are born. If this does not happen within 6 hours of parturition the assistance of the veterinarian should be sought.

Table 2.2 Scientific feeding schedule for pregnant goats under intensive and semi-intensive systems.

Feed components (g)	0–2 mo		2–3.5 mo		3.5–5 mo	
	Smaller doe	Larger doe	Smaller doe	Larger doe	Smaller doe	Larger doe
Under intensive system						
Concentrate ration	200	300	300	400	400	500
Hay	400	600	400	600	500	800
Green (fodder/leaves)	1000	1200	1000	1200	1200	1500
Under semi-intensive system						
Concentrate ration	200	250	250	350	300	400
Hay	300	500	400	600	500	700
Browse/grazing	5–6 h/d					

2.3.4 Care and Management of Bucks

- Bucks become fertile at the age of 7 months and are capable of breeding then.
- Male goats that are not worth retaining should be castrated.
- The buck should be in good condition and well suited for breeding. He should be kept on the range and made to cover 3–5 km each day for sufficient exercise.
- Hooves should be trimmed regularly to avoid lameness or foot rot.
- Bucks should always be kept separate from does.

2.4 Goat Management during the Breeding Season

To achieve maximum reproductive potential, goats must be maintained in a healthy and disease-free condition with a proper body condition score (BCS) at the start of the breeding season. Besides this, breeding should be delayed until they attain 60–70% of their adult body weight at a BCS of 3–3.5. A doe that does not kid by the time they are 2 years of age should be culled. A successful breeding period depends on mating appropriate numbers of sound bucks to the reproductively active doe and keeping them under surveillance to identify any problems. There are various factors like the numbers, ages, and nutritional status of the animals involved, mating management, and so on. The literature frequently mentions a mating ratio of 1 buck per 30–50 does. It should be kept in mind that the buck used should be experienced, good for breeding, and should be between 2.5 and 3.5 years old. The buck serving the does must have a good nutritional status, because keeping a buck in a poor or underfed condition can result in a reduction in testicular size and fewer sperm per gram of testicular tissue, which can affect fertility.

2.4.1 Management of Does

There are various management practices during the breeding season that can result in successful kidding. Practices such as age-wise distribution of does, health and soundness examinations, and flushing during the breeding season can be beneficial in supporting a higher ovulation rate, a better conception rate, and reducing early embryonic mortality.

2.4.1.1 Age-Wise Distribution

All livestock species reach a stage in their lifespan when they are most productive. Does are most productive when they are 3–4 years of age. All the animals in a herd or flock do not usually fall within the category 3–4 years of age at the same time. Ages in a flock or herd may vary from 1 to 5 years or even older, as animals aged 6 years or more can be present in the same flock. Younger animals in a flock or herd that have not yet reached their mature size at the time of breeding often need extra care in terms of feeding. Similarly, older animals in a flock or herd that have been kept sometimes for an extra year may require some extra care as their teeth start to spread, and also it is more economic if the farmer sells them and saves the feed resources for the younger and most productive animals in the flock or herd, thus gaining more economic benefits. For these reasons, the animals may be grouped according to their age during the breeding season. Therefore, animals between the ages of 2, 3, and 4 years may be kept together in a group and this will make their management more efficient.

2.4.1.2 Health and Soundness

For successful breeding females, ensuring sound health is an important management practice. Unfit does with teeth malformations, excessive wear on their teeth like a broken mouth or gums, does with unsound udders and non-functional teats, and animals that are not sound on their feet and legs should be removed before the beginning of the breeding season. Besides this, the animals should be taken care of to ensure they are free from all diseases including parasites. They must be provided with the appropriate dose of a dewormer prescribed by the veterinarian.

2.4.1.3 Flushing

Flushing is an important management tool that influences the profitability of the farm because it is directly related to the flock's kidding rate. It can increase the kidding rate by 10–20% and also increases the chances of twins and triplets during the kidding season. An extra amount of ration such as good-quality hay, with fresh pasture and concentrate, is provided to the breeding doe around 15–30 days before the onset of the breeding season. This temporary increase in the level of nutrition has the purpose of boost the ovulation, conception, and embryo implantation rates and also decreasing early embryonic mortality by strengthening fetal membrane integrity. It may also lead to an increase in the incidence of estrus occurrence in the flock. Doe with a normal BCS do not need to be flushed. Similarly, no benefits were seen in does with an excessive BCS before and during the breeding season, nor do overly thin does respond to flushing. A doe should have a BCS between 3.0 and 3.5 at the time of breeding. Further, it is best to flush a doe with a BCS of 2–2.5 to raise its BCS to 3–3.5. Such does shed more ova than does on a steady nutritional plane. One can identify the animals most suitable for flushing by looking at their BCS. It takes around three weeks to increase a BCS by a half-score for a doe kept on a rising nutritional plane. Therefore, the required length of time essential for bringing does in below-average condition up to the ideal BCS for breeding will be about 9, 6, 3, and 2 weeks for BCS 1.5, 2.0, 2.5, and 3, respectively.

Besides these management practices, the farmer can opt for breeding manipulation practices like estrus stimulation and synchronization. Estrus in does can be stimulated by utilizing the "buck effect" where vasectomized males are kept in direct contact or through fence-line contact with breeding females around 10 days to 2 weeks before breeding. Estrus stimulation leads to a large number of females ovulating in the early part of the breeding season. The phenomenon of synchronization can also be applied either naturally or hormonally. Natural synchronization is the traditionally practiced method in which complete weaning of lambs/kids is done at the same time for all batches, which results in synchronization to some extent. In hormonal synchronization, progesterone or its analog is administered through feed, implants, or sponges, and prostaglandin is given through the intramuscular route. After the administration of progesterone for 14 days, the hormone is withdrawn and following that the doe comes into heat within 3 days. In the case of prostaglandin F2 alpha or its synthetic analogs, two intramuscular injections at 10 mg dose each at an interval of 10 days can bring all the administered animals into heat within 72–96 hours. Hormonal synchronization is generally practiced in institutions for research purposes, but at a commercial level it is not used to a large extent. Hormonal synchronization can also be utilized for breeding of animals during the off-season (out-of-season breeding). However, poor availability of feeding resources and unfavorable environmental conditions during the off-season can have a negative impact on newborn kids (poor health, mortality, etc.) as well as on the mother's health.

2.4.2 Management of Bucks

The selection of breeding bucks is primarily based on their phenotype or genotype. Despite that, it must be ensured that they are genitally sound, free from physical abnormalities, and also free from certain specific diseases. If there is a need to purchase breeding bucks from other farms, then purchase and transport to the farm must be done at least eight weeks before the start of the breeding season, because factors influencing scrotal temperature, like transportation, stress, or crowding, can affect spermatogenesis and semen quality. These animals are kept in the quarantine area of the farm and should undergo

Table 2.3 Essential interventions for management of breeding bucks.

Intervention	Details
Nutrition	Provide 250–500 g of concentrate/day as per body weight. This practice should be started 6 weeks before the breeding season and continued during the breeding season also
Housing	Cool housing facilities during the summer season and warm housing facilities during the winter season should be provided
General management	Deworming with proper dose
	Hoof trimming and inspection for foot rot or other diseases
	Hair trimming around the prepuce
	Shearing 2 weeks before onset of the breeding season
Breeding soundness evaluation	Physical examination
	Inspection of the reproductive organs
	Semen collection and its evaluation

administration of a suitable anthelmintic and an appropriate vaccination program and be examined for diseases such as foot rot. Despite their economic value, breeding rams and bucks are often ignored outside their breeding period, but it is essential to give attention to their health, particularly to their nutrition, parasite control, and foot health issues all through the year. The provision of shade during the summer season and warm houses during winter could reduce the stress level in these animals. Similarly, shearing of breeding males two weeks before the onset of the breeding season could have a beneficial effect in terms of improving semen quality by reducing the stress caused to animals due to the prevailing higher environmental temperature, which affects semen quality. Annual breeding soundness examinations (BSEs) are also recommended to ensure they are healthy and sound for breeding (Table 2.3).

2.5 Housing Management of Goats

A goat prefers a clean, dry, and well-ventilated house. The housing facilities should be located on higher-level ground for efficient drainage, should be well-lit and free from parasites, and their long axis should be in an east–west direction. There must be some provision to protect the animals against inclement weather conditions like rain, cold, direct sunshine, and wind. Comfortable housing for a goat is one where the inside temperature remains between 15 and 25 °C. In rural conditions, a house of 2.1 m in length and 1.5 m in width may be sufficient to sustain three to five goats.

In hot and humid areas, slatted floor-type housing is preferred for goats. In this type of housing an elevated bamboo or wooden floor is constructed approximately 1 m (3–3.5 ft) above the ground. Bamboo or wooden slats 3 in. thick and 1 in. wide (7.5 cm and 2.5 cm, respectively) are used as flooring material and are laid one after the other, leaving about a 1 cm gap in between. In this system, a space of 2 ft 6 in. × 4 ft 6 in. (0.75 m × 1.35 m) is required for each goat. The advantage of the slatted floor type of housing is that it facilitates easy cleaning operations as the urine and feces fall away from the main flooring that is in direct contact with the animals, therefore the goats do not come into direct contact with urine and feces, preventing various parasitic and respiratory diseases. The ideal width of such a kind of sheds is 3–3.5 m with a 90 cm wide manger running through the center. Goats can be tied on either side with a floor space of 1.5 m^2/adult goat. Feeding racks and water troughs can also be arranged in the houses. Bamboo or timber may be used as raw material for making walls with a provision for adequate ventilation. A thatched type of roofing or roofing with asbestos sheets can be chosen, which can maintain a more or less equitable temperature in all seasons. These sheds should be attached to an open fenced area for loafing purposes.

When constructing a commercial goat farm, the following sheds can be constructed for different groups of animals:

- **General flock shed**: This shed is for adult breeding. Each shed should accommodate around 50–60 does and should be partitioned to make pens to accommodate 10–12 does/pen.
- **Buck shed**: Bucks must be kept in separate sheds and should not be kept with milking does.
- **Kidding shed**: Pregnant animals are housed individually in these sheds. In the winter season, some warming devices like room heaters should be provided here. These pens should be protected from the entry of birds like crows, etc.
- **Kid shed**: Kids are kept in these houses from weaning up to the attainment of maturity, preferably in groups.
- **Segregation shed**: Provision for a small segregation shed (sick animals shed) of about 3.6 m^2 is desirable when the herd is large (Figures 2.2–2.5 and Table 2.4).

2.6 General Goat Husbandry Practices

These practices should be carried out periodically as they are necessary for a successful goat business.

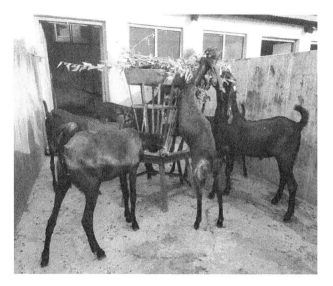

Figure 2.2   Feeding of Beetal goats (hexagonal feeder).

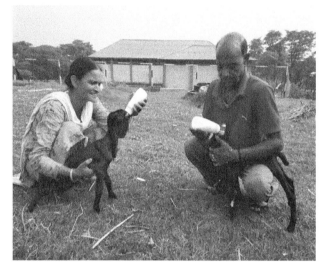

Figure 2.3   Bottle feeding to Beetal twin kids.

2.6.1 Identification of Animals and Data Recording

Identification of goats at an early age using a suitable method (e.g. tattooing, ear tag) is an important husbandry practice that should be carried out along with proper maintenance of performance records of individual goats. This record ultimately helps in the selection of superior animals. For this purpose various records are required to be maintained:

- Herd strength register
- Birth register
- Growth register
- Service and kidding
- Disease and treatment
- Death record

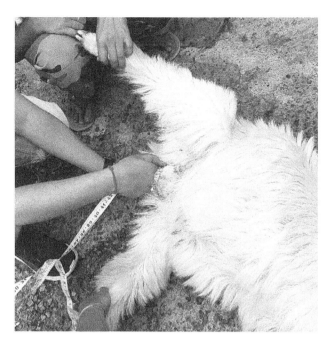

Figure 2.4 Testicular biometry recording of a Gaddi buck during breeding soundness examination.

2.6.2 Disbudding

The presence of horns can create a nuisance under extensive and semi-intensive systems of goat rearing. Disbudding helps to make the handling of bucks safe, prevents injuries to other animals, and helps in the prevention of a goaty smell by removing the scent or musk glands at the base of the horns.

The age for disbudding in the male kid is 4–5 days and in the female kid is 10–12 days. It can be done by using a caustic potash (KOH) stick or an electric dehorner (at a temperature of 198 °C for 8 seconds).

2.6.3 Castration

Castration is an important practice from the point of view of meat production as well as breeding practices. It is best carried out at the age of 3 months by the Burdizzo technique or by the open method in male kids.

Castration is associated with higher body weight gain as well as good-quality meat. It also plays an important role in selection procedures, as inferior male kids cannot produce the next generation if they are castrated.

2.6.4 Hoof Trimming

It is important to remove the overgrown hooves of goats periodically. Overgrown hooves may predispose the animals to various foot-related disorders, which may lead to lameness. Materials like sharp knives, curved hand pruning shears, hoof knives, a hoof rasp, and electric hoof trimmers are available on the market to carry out hoof trimming. It should be practiced three to four times a year in flocks reared in confinement. Only a trained and experienced person should be allowed to trim the hooves, as serious injuries can occur and may become a reason for the unnecessary culling of the animals.

Periodic hoof trimming gives the following advantages:

- Keep the overgrowth of hooves in check.
- Keeps animal fit to walk.

Figure 2.5 Dipping of Gaddi goats for prophylaxis against ectoparasites.

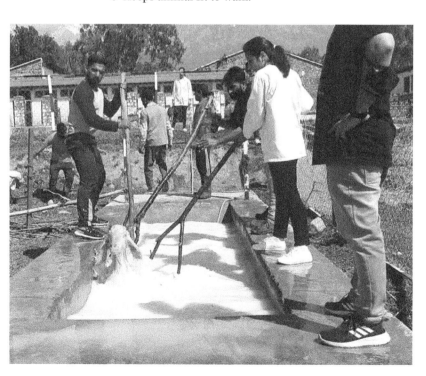

Table 2.4   Floor space, feeding, and watering space for goats.

Category	Floor space (m²)	Maximum animals/pen	Shed height (cm)	Feeding space/ animal (cm)	Watering space/ animal (cm)
Kids	0.5–1	20–25	300[a] 220[b]	30–35	3–5
Adult female	1–1.5	60	300[a] 220[b]	40–50	4–5
Pregnant/ lactating doe	2	8–10	300[a] 220[b]	40–50	4–5
Adult male	2	1	300[a] 220[b]	40–50	4–5

[a] In dry areas.
[b] In heavy rainfall areas.

- Prevents leg weakness.
- Prevents foot rot and other foot-related problems that may damage the hoof structure and lower milk production.
- Promotes the well-being of the animal.

2.6.5 Grooming

It is good practice to groom goats that are constantly kept under a stall feeding system with little or no exercise. Brushing them down with a stiff dandy brush every morning or combing goats with long hair (e.g. Gaddi) has many advantages. Grooming for animals can be compared to what is a bath for the human being:

- Grooming helps in the removal of dirt that collects on the skin's surface every day.
- It helps in the prevention of ectoparasites to a great extent. It is more of a preventive approach than a cure. If there are high numbers of ectoparasites, other means to exterminate them should be adopted (e.g. dipping).
- It promotes health by leading to better blood circulation.
- It gives the goat a sleek and glossy appearance.

2.6.6 Culling

Culling animals is an important procedure from an economic point of view. Goats may need to be culled for the following reasons:

- Slow growth rate
- Congenital defects
- Old age (8–9 years)
- Chronic debilitating diseases

2.7 Conclusion

Scientific knowledge regarding adequate nutrition, proper care, and management of goats can play a key role in successful goat farming. In addition to this, an emphasis given to proper housing, management of bucks and does during the breeding season, and implementing general goat husbandry-related practices can further help in obtaining better productive, reproductive, and overall health performance from goats.

Multiple-Choice Questions

1 What is dry matter intake in dairy goats?
   A 3% of their body weight
   B 4–6% of their body weight
   C 2–2.5% of their body weight
   D None of the above

2 What may flushing in goats result in?
   A Increased kidding rate
   B Increase chances of twins and triplets
   C Decreased early embryonic mortality
   D All of the above

3 What is the length of time required to bring a doe with BCS 2.0 up to the ideal body condition for breeding?
   A Nine weeks
   B Three weeks
   C Two weeks
   D Six weeks

4 Breeding should be delayed in female goats until they attain which body weight?
   A 50% of their adult body weight
   B 60–70% of their adult body weight
   C 40% of their adult body weight
   D None of the above

5 What is the digestible crude protein (DCP) level of the concentrate mixture for feeding adult goats?
   A 12%
   B 20%
   C 10%
   D 16%

6 At what age should kids be weaned?
   A 60 days
   B 90 days
   C 30 days
   D 180 days

7 Which vitamin is not required to be supplemented in a goat's ration?
   A Vitamin C
   B Fat-soluble vitamins (A, D, E, K)

C Vitamin B
D Both a and b are correct

8 What might be a reason for castrating a kid?
   A Higher body weight gain
   B Selection of breeding males
   C Both a and b are correct
   D None of the above

9 What may regular grooming of goats be associated with?
   A Better circulation
   B Removal of ectoparasites
   C Sleek and glossy hair coat
   D All of the above

10 When should colostrum be fed to kids?
   A 30 minutes after birth
   B 10 hours after birth
   C 24 hours after birth
   D 28 hours after birth

References

Ministry of Fisheries, Animal Husbandry & Dairying (2019). *20th Livestock Census: All India Report*. New Delhi: Animal Husbandry Statistics Division https://dahd.nic.in/sites/default/filess/20th-Livestock-census-2019-All-India-Report.pdf.

Ranjhan, S.K. (1998). *Nutrient Requirements of Livestock and Poultry*, 2e. New Delhi: ICAR.

Sánchez-Macías, D., Moreno-Indias, I., Castro, N. et al. (2014). From goat colostrum to milk: physical, chemical, and immune evolution from partum to 90 days postpartum. *Journal of Dairy Science* 97 (1): 10–16.

Further Reading

Ensminger, M.E. (2002). *Sheep & Goat Science*. Danville, IL: Interstate Publishers.

ICAR-NIANP (2013). *Nutrient Requirements of Sheep, Goat and Rabbit*. New Delhi: Indian Council of Agricultural Research.

NRC (2007). *Nutrient Requirements of Small Ruminants*. Washington, DC: National Academy of Sciences.

Pegler, H.S.H. (2005). *Goats and Their Profitable Management*. New Delhi: Biotech Books.

Prasad, J. (2014). *Goat, Sheep and Pig: Production and Management*. Ludhiana: Kalyani Publishers.

Reddy, D.V. (2019). *Applied Nutrition: Livestock, Poultry, Rabbits and Laboratory Animals*. New Delhi: CBS Publishers & Distributors.

Ridler, A.L., Smith, S.L., and West, D.M. (2012). Ram and buck management. *Animal Reproduction Science*. 130: 180–183.

Sagar, R. (2009). *Commercial Goat Farming*. Makhdoom: Central Institute for Research on Goats.

Sastry, N.S.R., Pearson, R.A., and Thomas, C.K. (2021). *Livestock Production Management*, rev. ed. Ludhiana: Kalyani Publishers.

3

Handling and Restraining of Goats

Falguni Mridha

Department of Veterinary Clinical Complex, West Bengal University of Animal & Fishery Sciences, Kolkata, West Bengal, India

Handling and restraining are an indispensable part of goatery. For the health aspect, being able to restrain and care during handling, treatment, and weighing are the key aspects (King et al. 2006). As goats are curious in nature with a good memory, it is easy to train them in handling (Figure 3.1).

3.1 Purposes of Handling and Restraining

- **Physical examination**: There are four components of physical examination: inspection, palpation, percussion, and auscultation. In small ruminants like goats, accuracy of physical examination depends on handling and proper restraining of the animal using patience, perseverance, expressiveness, and practice by the clinician. Many times a sick goat may become very restless and may react while being approached during an examination. Constant practice and prolonged experience of handling can resolve the situation.
- **Administration of medicine and vaccine**: Different drugs and vaccines are applied by three routes: surface application, administration through natural orifices, and parenteral administration. Before applying a surface application, the animal should be restrained in such a way that it cannot lick the medicine. In myiasis (maggot infestation) when a spray is applied the animal should be handled carefully to avoid accidental entry of the spray through eyes, anus, genitalia, or nostrils.
- **Surgical intervention**: Generally small ruminants like goats are not good subjects for general anesthesia. Local anesthesia (anesthesia of the target site) and regional anesthesia (anesthesia around a nerve trunk) are popular for goats and require skillful restraining of the animal, particularly for paravertebral and epidural anesthesia. Castration, dehorning, and other surgical procedures need proper restraining.
- **Identification of the animal**: Common methods of identification like branding, tattooing, ear tagging, and ear notching in goats need proper restraining. Improper handling or restraining may lead to faulty identification, undesired damage of subcutaneous tissue, unnecessary bleeding, and so on.
- **Feeding of ailing animals and orphan kids** (Hoppe et al. 2010).
- **Shearing**: Shearing is removing wool from goats like from sheep, and requires proper handling for quick, complete, and easy removal of the wool with minimal discomfort for the animal and operator.
- **Transportation of livestock**: Repeated improper handling during transportation and disturbances associated with it causes serious weight loss in goats.

3.2 Basics of Animal Behavior Associated with Handling

Animal behavior is the response of an animal to the environment and stimuli. Goats are generally considered as stubborn and misbehaved, but they can be managed more easily after their behavior is understood (Bourguet et al. 2011; King et al. 2006).

There are many circumstances where farm animals have to be handled, restrained, or transported due to different needs and conditions. When some animals are restrained they react with more disturbed behavior, and elevated cortisol, glucose, or lactate levels (Zavy et al. 1992).

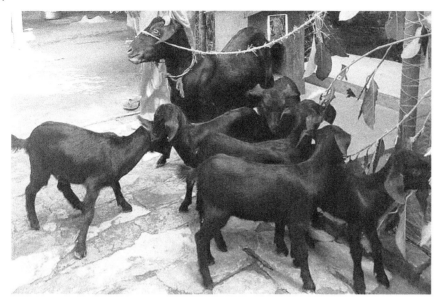

Figure 3.1 Goats are herd animals by nature.

3.2.1 Experience of Handler

A major factor that is connected to the intensity of either a physiological or behavioral response during handling is the previous experience of the handler. Handling for veterinary procedures may be very stressful for one animal and for another animal it may involve relatively low stress, depending on the experience and approach of the handler concerned. Simply handling a goat by holding a stick may cause stress to the animal. For a cautiously acclimated animal, a restraint mechanism (Grandin et al. 1986) or procedure may be associated with food treats and either physiological or behavioral indicators of stress will be lower (Dantzer and Mormede 1983).

3.2.2 Food Treats

The animal's reaction during handling may be influenced by its prior experience with handling and restraint. A watchfully acclimated animal will probably have a positive affective state. The animal can be motivated to enter a restrainer to get a food treat. Another animal that is handled in a cruel way such as shocking or dragging will be frightened and have a negative affective state. Aversive handling causes fear and reduces milk production and the productivity of the herd.

3.2.3 Separation Distress and Fear

The stress reaction (Bourguet et al. 2015) is influenced by the animal's previous experiences, its temperament (Café et al. 2010), and other inherited behavioral characteristics (Apple et al. 1993). Procedures for gentling young kids by

separating them from the mother goat are problematic rather than letting them become accustomed to the mother (Rivaland et al. 2007). More reactive breeds may have higher cortisol levels and show more restless behavior during handling. The stria terminalis in the brain is concerned with separation distress (Rault et al. 2011) and can be mediated by brain opioids (LeDoux 2000). This system is activated when the mother and young are separated or a single animal is isolated from the herd or flock. Generally behavior changes during handling (Boissey et al. 2005) are due to fear and separation distress. The two emotional systems in the brain that would be most likely to have a bearing on an animal's physiological or behavioral reaction to restraint and handling are the fear system and the panic system. The amygdala is the brain's fear center (Davis 1992). When the amygdala is stimulated, stress hormones such as corticosterone are secreted, causing a fear response like when an animal learns to avoid a place where it has received a shock. When goats are handled or restrained, they are frequently separated from other animals. Segregation from herd mates is often highly stressful (Grandin et al. 1994; Panksepp 1998, 2011). An isolated single goat may respond with either agitated behavior, increased physiological indicators of stress, or vocalization (Grandin 1980, 1989, 1997, 1998, 2001, 2014).

3.3 Methods to Assess Reaction to Handling or Restraining

There are several different types of behavioral tests to evaluate animal behavior during routine handling (Baszczak et al. 2006) and restraint. Calmer goats are often selected for breeding or other day-to-day purposes because they gain weight more easily and are safer to handle.

- **Chute scoring**: The animal's behavior is noted while it is restrained in a single animal scale, squeeze chute, or headgate. Independent observers score each animal on a point scale with scores ranging from stands still, to highly agitated, and struggling. The scale ranges from 1 to 3, such that 1 = calm, when the animal moves its head and body gently; 2 = agitated, when the animal moves a lot; and 3 = struggling to escape. It is likely that this test will determine fearfulness. Extremely agitated animals will lose weight (Hall et al. 2011) and have poorer meat quality (Akinmoladun et al. 2020; Grignard et al. 2001; Warriss et al. 1994).
- **Exit speed scoring**: The animal's behavior is noted while the speed at which it exits from a squeeze chute is electronically measured. Those with fast exit speeds show lower weight gain and higher physiological indicators of stress (Vetters et al. 2013). Exit speed can also be counted by scoring the exit gait as walk, trot, or canter. Exit scores (1–3) were determined as follows: 1 = walk, a four-beat gait; 2 = trot, a two-beat diagonal gait; and 3 = run, a three-beat gait where the front hooves strike the ground.
- **Pen scoring**: Animals are held in a tiny enclosure and a handler deliberately invades their flight zone. The test can be done in two ways: it can be used to judge the flight distance or used to decide if the animal will charge and attempt to hit the handler.
- **Vocalization scoring**: The animal's behavior is measured as its vocal response to handling or restraint (Lawrence et al. 1991). Vocalization during handling of goats is associated with higher physiological stress measurements. Goat will vocalize loudly when they become separated from other goats.
- **Aversion test**: This test is generally done to determine the comfort level of the animal to a particular handling procedure. It evaluate the animal's sensitivity to handling and restraint to measure its willingness to reenter a place where it was previously handled or restrained (Abbott et al. 1997). Goats have long memories for bad experiences. A year later they may be reluctant to enter somewhere they were restrained harshly like by shouting or hitting, which are highly aversive to goats. For instance, when a race led to a shouting person, animals moved more slowly through it the next time they entered.

3.4 Advantages and Procedures of Adapting Goats to Handling and Restraint

Different studies have proved benefit use of adapting farm animals to handling. Animal movement through a race was enhanced by providing barley feed rewards when the animals exited the system. Handling young animals with adult animals made the adult animals calmer (Faure and Mills 1998).

When an animal is going through a painful procedure while held in a restrainer, their escape behavior may increase and they will be more difficult to move through the race. Adaptation of the handling procedure makes the situation easier for the handler as well as the animal. When restraint or any kind of veterinary procedure or examination does not hurt or is only slightly painful, the animal may acclimate and become increasingly willing to come into the squeeze chute or restrainer.

Adaptation to handling before artificial insemination enhanced conception rates, decreased temperament, lowered cortisol levels, and decreased timing to puberty, which ultimately makes a huge difference to the productivity of a farm (Petherick et al. 2009).

A regular practice of handling with an understanding of animals' natural behavior can give clues to their affective state during various procedures (Cooke et al. 2009; Reale et al. 2007). Adapting non-painful measures of animal stress not only develops the quality of production (Boissey and Lee 2014; Cooke et al. 2012; Cooke and Kunkle 2014), it can also improve animal welfare (Andreson et al. 2013; Kauppinen et al. 2012).

Walking fattening animals in a trip or having people walk with them when being moved produced goats that were easier to move and handle. Repeated improper handling during transportation and related disturbances causes serious weight loss in goats. During movement by walking, the handler must accompany the trip from beginning to end. In the case of a large trip, several handlers must be there to direct the goats from beginning to middle and end to make feel them safe.

A goat's first experience of handling and restraint should be positive, as their memory of a negative handling situation can last a long time (Waiblinger et al. 2002). As goats have very strong memories, kicking, dragging, yelling, and so on may cause annoying experiences for them during handling, which may lead to difficulties in further handling (Waiblinger et al. 2004). A passive human presence was sufficient to familiarize goats with humans, though moderate handling was better at habituating them to active human procedures.

So after understanding animal behavior associated with handling and restraining, it is necessary to judge the ability of the animal to adjust to the handling procedure. Goats need special care during handling and restraining due to their special characteristics.

Above all, learning about animals is actually very specific. Learning about goats in a specific subject area helps when applying that particular subject. So training goats in a particular situation may help in the same kind of situation, but it may not help in other situations.

3.5 Points to Be Kept in Mind while Handling Goats

- **Herd animals**: Goats generally like the company of other animals or humans as they are herd animals. So it is easier to handle or manage a herd of four goats rather than a single goat.
- **Female-dominant herd**: A goat herd is generally led by a dominant female and a dominant male goat, where the female generally leads the herd regarding grazing, sleeping, rest, and so on. She takes food first, before the others. She protects the herd from predators.
- **Male leader**: In a herd of goats the dominant male goat retains his position according to his strength and dominance. Horn and body size play an important role in determining his dominance in the herd. He mates with the females in season and protects the herd alongside the female leader.
- **Inquisitive and aggressive**: Goats are curious by nature and generally show aggressiveness to dominate others by lowering their head and pointing their horns at other goat.
- **Fundamental behavior**: Like with other animals, hunger, thirst, maternal instinct, and sickness play an important role in handling of goats. A good handler must consider these factors when handling the goats.
- **Environment**: Goats generally develop a comfortable attachment to their environment such as pastures and farm buildings. Forcible changing of the surrounding environment or an approach by an unfamiliar person may cause an unexpected outcome in terms of production.
- **Moving objects**: Moving objects like a swinging cloth or harsh-sounding fan make the handling procedure difficult.
- **Frustrating situation**: As goats have very strong memories, kicking, dragging, or yelling may cause a frustrating experience for them during handling, which may create difficulties for the next handling.

So it is necessary for the clinician, handler, or farmer to approach the goat properly considering the purposes for which it is to be handled and its likely behavior.

3.6 Approach

It is often necessary on goat farms to apprehend individual goats or groups of goats temporarily for different purposes. Sometimes a goat may become restless, reacting with violence and vocalization during the approach. The goat may show inappropriate responses when approached in an altered environment or by an unfamiliar person (Reale et al. 2007; Rushen and DePassille 1999). Constant practice and experience can help in such conditions (Wickham et al. 2015). The handler must not catch, lift, or pull the goat's hair, leg, head, ear, or tail (Figures 3.2 and 3.3).

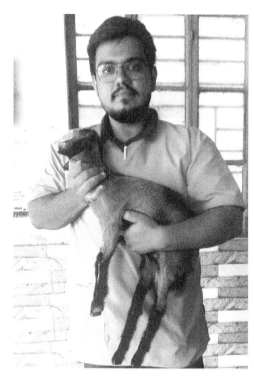

Figure 3.2 Holding a kid.

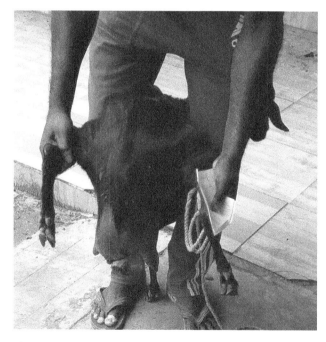

Figure 3.3 Holding a goat between the handler's knees to show the posterior.

The handler must be very friendly to the goat while approaching it. As goats' eyes are situated on the side of the head, approaching a goat must be from the side of the animal rather than the front. During the approach, calling the animal and speaking before touching are common practice. It is not necessary to put the hands over the goat's head or horn, which may cause panic.

When a goat is approached it can be rewarded by giving it some food or grass.

After approaching, the goat has to be handled or restrained as required in such a way that no harm comes to either the goat(s) being handled or the handler to fulfill the purpose of handling or restraining.

3.7 Different Methods for Handling and Restraining Goats

- **Halter**: Halters for goats are generally made from rope. A small halter and a 5 × 1 m length of soft 1 cm diameter rope are generally used for restraining goats. A lasso can be used as an improvised halter. There are different types of halters, like rope halter, alternate rope halter, lasso halter, and so on.
- **Collar**: Collars are commonly used to handle small animals like goats and sheep. While holding a goat one can hold the collar from the animal's side to stop the animal running away (Figure 3.4).
- **Flank hold**: The goat should be held by the handler holding a skin fold of the lower flank gently, standing at the back or side of the animal.
- **Restraining by holding the jaw**: The goat should be held by the handler standing on its left or right side, placing one hand under its jaw and keeping the other hand free to place behind its buttock to prevent the animal running backward.
- **Rumping**: This method enables the animal to sit on its rump without its feet being in contact with the ground. It prevents the animal struggling and it becomes submissive to the handler (Figure 3.5).
- **Horn restraint**: Horned animals can be restrained by head restraining. The horn should be restrained near its base.
- **Restraining a kid on the lap**: Sternal recumbency holding the kid on the handler's lap by folding the kid's front legs beneath it is preferred. The handler's forearms are placed on the kid's back and pressed down.
- **Horizontal hold**: Holding the side of the goat with knees of any fore limb, shoulders, and with a hand hold on the top legs.

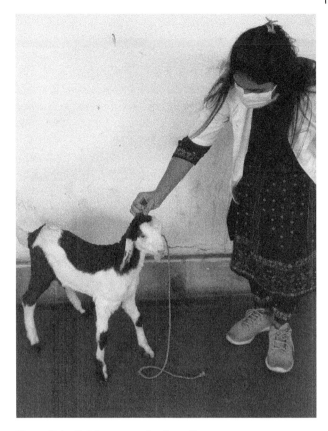

Figure 3.4   Holding a goat by the collar.

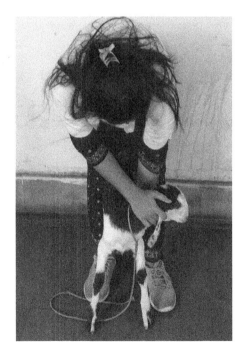

Figure 3.5   Rumping.

- **Leg holding**: Holding the neck region of the goat between the handler's legs while holding the goat's two hind legs at the hock joint.

3.8 Handling Kids

A few hours after birth is the best time to handle kids (Ellingsen et al. 2014). It makes the relation with the handler less fearful and less stressful, particularly when different procedures need to be done (Figure 3.2). Hold tight so that the kid can feel secure. Holding the chest closely with one hand and wrapping the kid with the other arm is the normal procedure. Gently cleaning away mucus after birth with clean sterilized cloths is necessary, particularly from the nostrils, eyes, and mouth. Cleaning the nostrils by holding the hind legs, putting the head lower to the side, and shaking gently is necessary for normalization of respiration. The navel cord should be tied 2.5 cm from the body with sterilized thread and regular application of tincture iodine to the area is a healthy practice. The kid should be fed with colostrum for at least five days after birth according to its body weight.

3.9 Handling Goats during Transportation

The animals should not be restrained unless there is a risk of their jumping out; tying of legs should not be permitted (Miranda dela-Lama 2018). During loading, excessive temperatures of day or night should be avoided. Proper ramps should be arranged for loading and unloading the animals (Stockman et al. 2011). The ramp should be at least 0.75 m in width with a raised side at least 0.75 m high. The floor of the ramp should be at about 15 cm height so the animals do not slide as they climb or descend it. In case of a railway carriage, when the loading is done on the platform, the dropped door of the wagon can be used as a ramp. In such cases bales or bags of hay or feed may be positioned on each side of the dropped door to avoid the animals getting their legs between the sides of the wagon and the platform. Space requirements during transport are outlined in Table 3.1.

Table 3.1 Space requirements during transport.

Approximate weight of animals (kg)	Space required (m^2)
<20	0.18
21–25	0.20
26–30	0.23
>30	0.28

3.10 Handing Goats for Administration of Medication

3.10.1 Surface Application of Medication

Drugs can be applied to the body surface as topical medication against certain pathogens of different origins. During application care should be taken so that the medication does not enter through the goat's mouth, eyes, or genitalia. Other problems are irritation from topical medicines, the sound produced by a spray machine, and the smell of topical medicines. Restraint may be a positive experience associated with food rewards in this type of case. Different holding procedures like rumping or holding by the jaw are helpful in this situation.

3.10.2 Oral Administration of Medication

During oral administration of medicines by drenching, using a balling gun, stomach tubing, or as an electuary, it is necessary to avoid drenching pneumonia and choking (Figures 3.6 and 3.7). During drenching, hold the head of the animal by the horn or jaw and slightly raised. The medicine must be poured onto the middle of the tongue or into the cheek beside the teeth. While using a balling gun or

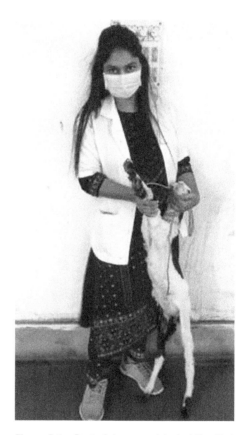

Figure 3.6 Restraining a goat by holding its jaw.

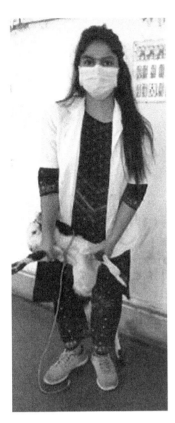

Figure 3.7   Restraining a goat by holding its jaw and forelegs.

manual feeding of a bolus, it is necessary to hold the head to push the bolus over the back of the tongue. Inserting a stomach tube is also possible if the head is held properly by passing the tube along the base of the tongue on the left side of the animal. Goats are very prone to choking on powder medication, especially kids. Holding newly born kids on the lap and spoon feeding or bottle feeding the medication is preferred.

3.10.3   Administration of Medication by the Rectal or Vulval Route

An enema to counteract constipation is introduced to the rectum by a douche can and the vulval route is used for a uterine wash in metritis, cervicitis, repeat breeding, and so on. The animal is controlled in both cases by holding the neck between the handler's legs and elevating the animal by holding both stifles.

3.10.4   Parenteral Administration of Medication

During intramuscular administration, restraint is applied by holding the jaw, holding the animal from its side, or rumping. Loose skin is used for subcutaneous injection (Muller et al. 2008). For irritant or oily drugs, holding the

goat by rumping or holding the jaw is preferred. The jugular vein is the intravenous route for goats. Jaw restraint and rumping are the normal procedures for holding during intravenous administration. In a case of an extremely emaciated animal, holding the four legs in the handler's hands with the neck extended is the normal procedure.

3.10.5   Local and Regional Anesthesia

The major hazards of general anesthesia in goats are ruminal tympany, regurgitation, and aspiration, so regional anesthesia is preferred. For cornual nerve block to desensitize the horns, the goat is restrained by holding the horns at their base. In case of epidural anesthesia, the goat is restrained in lateral recumbency with the sacral spine in full flexion. Other forms of local and regional anesthesia are given by holding the goat accordingly in lateral recumbency, holding the jaw, holding the animal from its side, rumping, or in a standing position pressing the goat against a wall.

3.11   Handling and Restraining Goats during Shearing

Goats should not be held by catching their wool or pulling the wool during shearing. The animal should be held firmly to prevent struggling and kicking. As goats have bony rumps, they are not usually placed sitting upright like sheep during shearing. Goats are generally held during shearing either standing up with a head cradle to keep animal still or lying the goat on its side and leaning the animal well back.

3.12   Restraining Animals Using Drugs

Narcosis (the stage of deep sleep with analgesia) or subnarcosis can be attained by administering certain drugs to goats with special precautions for restraint. Before administration of the drug, the goat should be starved for 18–24 hours. Induction of such a drug in an animal with a full stomach may lead to the hazard of aspiration. Distension of the rumen in small ruminants affects ventilation and leads to other respiratory problems like hypoxemia and hypercapnia. Water should be withheld from the goat for 12 hours before administration of the drug for restraint. Very vicious and nervous large goats are restrained for different procedures by administering a tranquilizer like chlorpromazine hydrochloride or an alpha-2 adrenoreceptor agonist like xylazine.

- **Chlorpromazine hydrochloride**: An antiemetic, central depressant drug. It causes sedation with a calming effect in goats to minimize struggling. Sometimes it produces delayed recovery. It can be used with local analgesics. Dose: 1–1.5 mg/kg by the intramuscular route.
- **Xylazine hydrochloride**: A very potent non-narcotic sedative (causes a calming effect in a nervous, vicious, or excited animal), analgesic, and muscle relaxant. After administration sometimes it causes decreased respiration and heart rate. The advantage of xylazine is its wide margin of safety. Dose: 0.005–0.01 mg/kg by the intramuscular route.

3.13 Good Stockmanship

Stockmanship is the art and science of the proper handling of farm animals. The benefits of good stockmanship lead to increased productivity for the farm (Hemsworth and Coleman 2010; Bates et al. 2014; Caroprese et al. 2012). Animals that are scared and move away from handlers are less productive. Young kids that were subjected to mild handling and stroking and those that experienced aversive treatment slaps and shocks showed considerable differences in productivity. Aversively treated goats had a lower growth rate (Hemsworth and Barnett 1991). Shouting, slapping, and dragging also resulted in lower milk yields compared to soft talking and stroking. Animals can learn to recognize individual people. However, when people treat it roughly, an animal may become afraid of all people. People with a positive approach using good stockmanship toward the animals they are handling or raising are calmer, leading to more productive animals.

The stress and trauma of handling and restraint may be partially determined by how the goats observe it. For one goat restraint may be a positive incident associated with food rewards, and for another animal with different prior experiences being restrained may be frustrating. Temperament, environment, and overall reactivity have an impact on relations between animals and humans. Positive human interactions have significant advantageous effects on animals and can potentially compensate for bad experiences. Gentle physical contact, such as rubbing kids, simulates play behavior between animals (Becker and Lobato 1997); maternal behavior such as licking can make the situation easier (Rutherford et al. 2012; Stephens and Toner 1975). Above all, good stockmanship increases not only the animal's comfort and the safety of the handler, but also the margin of productivity of the farm and the welfare of the animals by attaining proper handling and restraining.

Multiple-Choice Questions

1 What are the advantages of adaptation to handling before artificial insemination?
   - **A** Enhanced conception rates
   - **B** Decreased temperament
   - **C** Lowered cortisol levels
   - **D** All of the above

2 Shouting, slapping, and dragging result in lower milk yield compared to which of the following?
   - **A** Soft talking
   - **B** Stroking in goats
   - **C** Both of the above
   - **D** None of the above

3 During oral administration of medicines by drenching, using a balling gun, stomach tubing, or via an electuary, which of the following is it necessary to avoid?
   - **A** Drenching pneumonia and choking
   - **B** Stomatitis
   - **C** Facial paralysis
   - **D** Swallowing

4 What is the preferred intravenous route for a goat?
   - **A** Cephalic vein
   - **B** Saphenous vein
   - **C** Ear vein
   - **D** Jugular vein

5 Where can horned animals be restrained?
   - **A** Anywhere on the horn
   - **B** Near the base of the horn
   - **C** Tip of the horn
   - **D** Middle of the horn

6 What is the drug of choice for restraining goats?
   - **A** Magnesium sulfate
   - **B** Chloral hydrate
   - **C** Ketamine
   - **D** Chlorpromazine hydrochloride

7 What is rumping generally used for?
   - **A** Controlling the animal by holding the flank
   - **B** Controlling the animal by sitting it on its rump
   - **C** Controlling the animal by holding its legs
   - **D** Controlling the animal by holding its jaw

8 What material is generally used for halters for goats?
 A Metal
 B Leather
 C Rope
 D Chain

9 What is stockmanship?
 A The stocking of products
 B The art and science of proper handling of farm animals
 C Using field knowledge in selling
 D A profit policy

10 Where is the muzzle?
 A Head
 B Tail
 C Neck
 D Flank

11 What does a goat prefer during handling?
 A Feed
 B Scratching
 C Both a and b
 D Being held by its legs

12 What is holding the goat's chest closely with one hand and wrapping the animal with the other arm normal procedure for?
 A Buck
 B Doe
 C Pregnant goat
 D Kid

13 Which of the following is very easy to handle or manage?
 A A herd of four goats
 B A single goat
 C Both of the above
 D Goats with sheep

14 What are the purposes of handling and restraining?
 A Physical examination
 B Medication
 C Increasing production
 D All of the above

15 When approaching, a goat handler must not catch, lift, or pull which part of the goat?
 A Leg
 B Hair
 C Head, ear, or tail
 D All of the above

16 Why may kicking, dragging, yelling, etc. cause a frustrating experience for the goat during handling?
 A They have strong reactions
 B They have a good memory
 C They have a vicious nature
 D They have a tendency to run

17 What is the space requirement during transport for a 35 kg goat?
 A $0.24\,m^2$
 B $0.40\,m^2$
 C $0.28\,m^2$
 D $1\,m^2$

18 How does the goat experience segregation from its herd mates?
 A As stressful
 B As normal
 C As encouraging
 D As likely to increase playfulness

19 What does the adoption of good handling procedures do?
 A Makes the situation easy for the handler
 B Makes the situation easy for the animal
 C Both a and b
 D Makes no difference in handling

20 Which of the following behavioral tests evaluate animal behavior during routine handling and restraint?
 A Chute scoring
 B Pen scoring
 C Aversion test
 D All of the above

21 Before administration of a restraining drug, how long should a goat be starved for?
 A 18–24 hours
 B 48 hours
 C 32 hours
 D 4–8 hours

22 What is common practice when approaching an animal?
 A Calling the animal
 B Speaking before touching
 C Both a and b
 D Shouting

23 Who is a goat herd generally led by?
 A A dominant female
 B A dominant male goat
 C Both a and b
 D A kid

24 What does repeated improper handling of goats during transportation and related disturbances cause?
A Increased production
B Serious weight loss
C Higher conception rate
D Increased production of milk

25 Why should a goat's first experience of handling and restraint be positive?
A Their nature is to be calm
B Their nature is to be annoying
C Their memories of a negative handling situation can last a long time
D None of the above

References

Abbott, T.A., Hunger, E.J., Guise, J.H., and Penny, R.H.C. (1997). The effect of experience of handling on a pig's willingness to move. *Applied Animal Behaviour Science* 54: 371–375. https://doi.org/10.1016/S0168-1591(97)00045-2.

Akinmoladun, O.F., Fon, F.N., and Mpendulo, C.T. (2020). Stress indicators, carcass characteristics and meat quality of Xhosa goats subjected to different watering regimen and vitamin C supplementation. *Livestock Science* 238: 104083.

Andreson, S.N., Wernelsfelder, F., Sandoc, P., and Forkman, B. (2013). The correlation between qualitative behavioral assessments with welfare quality protocol outcomes in on-farm assessments of dairy cattle. *Applied Animal Behaviour Science* 143: 9–17.

Apple, J.K., Minton, J.E., Parsons, K.M., and Unruh, J.A. (1993). Influence of repeated restraint and isolation stress and electrolyte administration on pituitary adrenal secretions, electrolytes and other blood constituents of sheep. *Journal of Animal Science* 71: 71–77.

Baszczak, J., Grandin, T., Bruber, S.L. et al. (2006). Effects of ractopomine supplementation on behavior of British continental and Brahman crossbred steers during routine handling. *Journal of Animal Science* 84: 3410–3414.

Bates, L.S.W., Ford, E.A., Brown, S.N. et al. (2014). A comparison of handling methods relevant to the religious slaughter of sheep. *Animal Welfare* 23: 251–258.

Becker, B.G. and Lobato, J.E.P. (1997). Effect of gentle handling on the reactivity of zebu crossbred calves to humans. *Applied Animal Behaviour Science* 53: 219–224.

Boissey, A. and Lee, C. (2014). How assessing relationships between emotions and cognition can improve farm animal welfare. *Revue Scientifique et Technique* 33: 103–110.

Boissey, A., Bouix, J., Orgeur, P. et al. (2005). Genetic analysis of emotional reactivity of sheep: effects of genotype of the lambs and their dams. *Genetics, Selection, Evolution* 37: 381–401.

Bourguet, C., Deiss, V., Tannugi, E.C., and Terlouw, E.M.C. (2011). Behavioral and physiological reactions of cattle in a commercial abattoir and relationships with organizational aspects of the abattoir and animal characteristics. *Meat Science* 88: 158–168.

Bourguet, C., Deiss, V., Boissy, A., and Terlouw, E.C. (2015). Young blond d'Aquitaine, Angus and Limousin bulls differ in emotional reactivity: relationships with animal traits, stress reactions at slaughter and post-mortem muscle metabolism. *Applied Animal Behaviour Science* 164: 41–55.

Café, L.M., Robinson, D.L., Ferguson, D.M. et al. (2010). Cattle temperament, persistence of assessments, and associations with productivity, efficiency carcass, and meat quality traits. *Journal of Animal Science* 89: 1452–1465.

Caroprese, M., Napolitano, R., Boivin, X. et al. (2012). Development of affinity to the stockperson in lambs of two breeds. *Physiology & Behavior* 105: 251–256.

Cooke, R.F. and Kunkle, B.E. (2014). Interdisciplinary beef symposium: temperament and acclimation to human handling influenced growth, health, and reproductive responses in cattle. *Journal of Animal Science* 92: 5325–5333.

Cooke, R.F., Arthington, J.D., Austin, B.R., and Yellich, J.V. (2009). Effects of acclimation to handling on performance, reproductive and physiological responses of Brahman crossbred heifers. *Journal of Animal Science* 87: 3403–3412.

Cooke, R.F., Ohmart, D.W., Cappellozza, B.J. et al. (2012). Effects of temperament and acclimation to handling on reproductive performance of *Bos taurus* beef females. *Journal of Animal Science* 90: 3547–3555.

Dantzer, R. and Mormede, P. (1983). Stress in farm animals: a need for re-evaluation. *Journal of Animal Science* 57: 6–18.

Davis, M. (1992). The role of amygdala in fear and memory. *Annual Review of Neuroscience* 15: 353–375.

Ellingsen, K., Coleman, G.J., Lund, V., and Mejdell, C.M. (2014). Using qualitative behaviour assessment to explore the link between stock person behavior and dairy calf behavior. *Applied Animal Behaviour Science* 153: 10–17.

Faure, J.M. and Mills, A.D. (1998). Improving the adaptability of animals by selection. In: *Genetics and the Behavior of Domestic Animals* (ed. T. Grandin), 235–264. San Diego, CA: Elsevier.

Grandin, T. (1980). Livestock behavior as related to handling facilities design. *International Journal for the Study of Animal Problems* 1: 39–52.

Grandin, T. (1989). How to improve livestock handling and reduce stress. In: *Improving Animal Welfare: A Practical Approach*, 2e (ed. T. Grandin), 69–95. Cambridge: CABI Publishing.

Grandin, T. (1997). Assessment of stress during handling and transport. *Journal of Animal Science* 75: 240–257.

Grandin, T. (1998). The feasibility of vocalization scoring as an indicator of poor welfare during slaughter. *Applied Animal Behaviour Science* 56: 121–128.

Grandin, T. (2001). Cattle vocalizations are associated with handling and equipment problems in slaughter plants. *Applied Animal Behaviour Science* 71: 191–201.

Grandin, T. (2014). Handling facilities and restraint in extensively raised range cattle. In: *Livestock Handling and Transport*, 4e (ed. T. Grandin), 94–115. Cambridge: CABI Publishing.

Grandin, T., Curtis, S.E., Widowski, T.M., and Thurmon, J.C. (1986). Electro-immobilization *versus* mechanical restraint in an avoid–avoid choice test for ewes. *Journal of Animal Science* 62: 1469–1480.

Grandin, T., Odde, K.G., Schutz, D.N., and Behrens, L.M. (1994). The reluctance of cattle to change a learned choice may confound preference tests. *Applied Animal Behaviour Science* 39: 21–28.

Grignard, L., Bovin, X., Boissy, A., and LeNeindre, P. (2001). Do beef cattle react consistently to different handling situations? *Applied Animal Behaviour Science* 71: 263–276.

Hall, N.L., Buchanan, D.S., Anderson, V.L. et al. (2011). Working chute behavior of feedlot cattle can be an indicator of cattle temperament and beef carcass composition and quality. *Meat Science* 89: 52–57.

Hemsworth, P.H. and Barnett, J.L. (1991). The effects of aversively handling pigs either individually or in groups on their behavior, growth and corticosteroids. *Applied Animal Behaviour Science* 30: 61–72.

Hemsworth, P.H. and Coleman, G.J. (2010). *The Stockperson and the Productivity and Welfare of Intensively Farmed Animals*, 2e. Cambridge: CABI Publishing.

Hoppe, S., Brandt, H.R., Konig, S. et al. (2010). Temperament traits in beef calf measured under field conditions and relationships on performance. *Journal of Animal Science* 88: 1982–1989.

Kauppinen, T.K., Vesala, K.M., and Valros, A. (2012). Farmer attitude towards improvement of animal welfare is correlated with piglet production paameters. *Livestock Production Science* 143: 142–150.

King, D.A., Schuehle-Pfeiffer, C.E., Rnadel, R. et al. (2006). Influence of animal temperament and stress responsiveness on the carcass quality and beef tenderness of feedlot cattle. *Meat Science* 74: 546–556.

Lawrence, A.B., Terlouw, E.M.C., and Illius, A.D. (1991). Individual differences in behavioral responses of pigs exposed to non-social and social challenge. *Applied Animal Behaviour Science* 30: 73–78.

LeDoux, J.E. (2000). Emotion circuits in the brain. *Annual Review of Neuroscience* 23: 155–184.

Miranda-dela Lama, G.C. (2018). Goat handling and transport. In: *Livestock Handling and Transport*, 5e (ed. T. Grandin), 271–289. Cambridge: CABI Publishing.

Muller, R., von Keyserlinkg, M.A.G., Shah, M.A., and Schwartzkopf-Genswein, K.S.B. (2008). Effect of neck injection and handler visibility on behavioral reactivity of beef steers. *Journal of Animal Science* 86: 1215–1222.

Panksepp, J. (1998). *Affective Neuroscience: The Foundations of Human and Animal Emotions*. Oxford: Oxford University Press.

Panksepp, J. (2011). The basic emotional circuits of mammalian brains: do animals have emotional lives? *Neuroscience and Biobehavioral Reviews* 35: 1791–1804.

Petherick, J.C., Doogan, V.J., Venus, B.K. et al. (2009). Quality of handling and holding yard environment and beef cattle temperament, consequences for stress and productivity. *Australian Journal of Experimental Agriculture* 42: 389–398.

Rault, J.L., Boissey, A., and Bouivin, X. (2011). Separation distress in artificially reared lambs depends on human presence and number of conspecifics. *Applied Animal Behaviour Science* 132: 42–50.

Reale, D., Reader, S.M., Sol, D. et al. (2007). Integrating animal temperament into ecology and evolution. *Biological Reviews* 82: 291–318.

Rivaland, E.T.A., Charles, I.J., Turner, A.J. et al. (2007). Isolation and restraint stress results in differential activation of cortitrophin releasing hormone and arginine vasopressin neurons in sheep. *Neuroscience* 145: 1048–1058.

Rushen, J. and DePassille, A.M.B. (1999). Fear of people by cows and effects on milk yield, behavior and heart rate at milking. *Applied Animal Behaviour Science* 82: 720–727.

Rutherford, K.M.D., Donald, R.D., Lawrence, A.B., and Wemelsfelder, L.F. (2012). Qualitative behavioral assessment of emotionality in pigs. *Applied Animal Behaviour Science* 139: 218–224.

Stephens, D.M. and Toner, J.N. (1975). Husbandry influence on some physiological parameters of emotional responses in calves. *Applied Animal Behaviour Science* 1: 233–243.

Stockman, C.A., Collins, T., Barnes, A.L. et al. (2011). Qualitative behavioral assessment and quantitative physiological measurement of cattle naive and habituated to road transport. *Animal Production Science* 51: 240–249.

Vetters, M.D.D., Engle, T.E., Ahola, J.K., and Grandin, T. (2013). Comparison of flight speed and exit score as measurements of temperament in beef cattle. *Journal of Animal Science* 91: 374–381.

Waiblinger, S., Menke, C., and Coleman, G. (2002). The relationship between attitudes, personal characteristics and behavior of stock people and subsequent behavior and production of dairy cows. *Applied Animal Behaviour Science* 79: 195–219.

Waiblinger, S., Menke, C., Korf, J., and Bueher, A. (2004). Previous handling and gentle interactions affect behaviour and heartrate of dairy cows during veterinary procedures. *Applied Animal Behaviour Science* 85: 31–42.

Warriss, P.D., Brown, S., Adams, S.J.M., and Conett, T.R. (1994). Relationship between subjective and objective assessment of stress at slaughter and meat quality in pigs. *Meat Science* 38: 329–340.

Wickham, S.L., Collins, T., Barnes, A.L. et al. (2015). Qualitative behavioral assessment of transport naive and transport habituated sheep. *Journal of Animal Science* 90: 4523–4535.

Zavy, M.T., Juniewicz, P.E., Phillips, W.A., and von Tungeln, D.L. (1992). Effect of initial restraint, weaning and transport stress on baseline and ACTH stimulated cortisol responses in beef calves of different genotypes. *Australian Journal of Veterinary Research* 53: 551–557.

4

Clinical Findings of Diseases of Goats

Sunita Choudhary[1], K. Justin Davis[2], G.K. Chetan Kumar[3], and Pratishtha Sharma[4]

[1] *Department of Clinical Veterinary Medicine, College of Veterinary & Animal Sciences, Rajasthan University of Veterinary & Animal Sciences, Bikaner, Rajasthan, India*
[2] *Department of Veterinary Epidemiology and Preventive Medicine, College of Veterinary & Animal Sciences, Mannuty, Kerala, India*
[3] *Department of Veterinary Medicine, Veterinary College Hassan, Karnataka Veterinary, Animal and Fisheries Sciences University, Hassan, Karnataka, India*
[4] *Department of Veterinary Pharmacology and Toxicology, College of Veterinary & Animal Sciences, Rajasthan University of Veterinary & Animal Sciences, Bikaner, Rajasthan, India*

4.1 Diagnosis of Skin Diseases by Clinical Findings

The character of the skin and hair coat is a good indicator of general health in the goat. Many skin diseases of the goat have identical lesions, so a scientific approach is required to reach a preliminary diagnosis. A history of the occurrence of skin lesions followed by thorough clinical examination of animals and the skin is very helpful to reach a cause. The collection of appropriate samples is necessary for a definite diagnosis to be made. The prognosis depends on the correct diagnosis followed by appropriate treatment. A rough, unglossy, or dry coat; excessive dander or flakiness; and failure to shed in the spring are all suggestive of parasitism, poor nutritional status, or other chronic diseases. The skin should be examined for lice, ticks, fleas, nodules, swellings, crusts, eczema, necrosis, neoplasia, photosensitization, sunburn, and focal or regional alopecia. Various conditions that lead to these lesions are discussed here.

The location and intensity of skin lesions are characteristic of the particular disease and close attention should be paid to primary skin lesions that directly indicate the underlying cause. The primary skin lesions are papules, vesicles, pustules, and nodules.

- **Papules** with folliculitis suggest fungal, bacterial, or parasitic diseases. Papules without a hair follicle at the center are typical of allergy and an ectoparasitic infestation. Papules as initial lesions may occur in chorioptic, sarcoptic, and psoroptic mange, pox and orf virus infection, and malignant catarrhal fever.

- **Vesicles and pustules** are seen in autoimmune, irritant, or viral etiologies. Pemphigus is an autoimmune condition in which the primary lesion is a pustule that ruptures soon after formation, resulting in erosions and epidermal collarettes (rings of the exfoliating superficial epidermis), scale, and crust. The lesions may or may not be associated with pruritus or pain. Demodicosis is a common pustular disease in goats. In bacterial infection, the primary lesion is a non-follicular or follicular papule that develops into a pustule. Viral diseases in which vesicles are present include capripox, foot and mouth disease, vesicular stomatitis, and contagious ecthyma (Figure 4.1). In capripox, cutaneous lesions are found on the external nares and lips.

4.1.1 Pruritus

Pruritus leads to excoriation and secondary lesions. Sarcoptic or chorioptic mange leads to severe pruritus. Dermatophilosis, also known as "lumpy wool disease" in sheep or Streptothricosis, is a contagious skin condition caused by the bacterium *Dermatophilus congolensis* and, in severe cases, pruritis causes animals to scratch constantly. Other causes can be ectoparasites such as lice and fleas, hypersensitivity to other insects such as Culicoides, zinc deficiency, pemphigus, and photosensitization. Apart from this, fungal and bacterial dermatitis can be pruritic.

Migration of *Parelaphostrongylus tenuis* through the spinal cord or dorsal nerve root causes linear vertical excoriation. Acute pruritus is suggestive of pseudorabies (Shope 1931; Baker et al. 1982), whereas chronic pruritus has been reported in one goat affected with rabies (Tarlatzis 1954). Scrapie in goats is pruritic, as

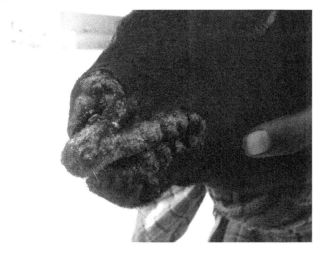

Figure 4.1 Dry crusty lesions of contagious ecthyma on the lips of a goat.

demonstrated by biting and rubbing at the legs, flanks, lumbar region, and neck, and by alopecia in these areas (usually without scab formation).

4.1.2 Hyperkeratosis

Hyperkeratosis is seen in many chronic skin diseases like ectoparasitisms, seborrhea, zinc-responsive disease, dermatophytosis, and dermatophilosis. Goats that survive the acute phase of peste des petits ruminants (PPR) may develop labial scabs that persist for up to 14 days; histologically, acanthosis and hyperkeratosis are evident.

4.1.3 Abscesses, Nodules, Scales, and Crust

Scales and crust indicate that exudation has occurred and have many causes like dermatophyte hyphae, dermatophilosis, and pemphigus complex. *D. congolensis* infects the skin causing matted tufts of hair or wool, with progress to scab formation. Later it forms a wart-like accumulation on the skin. Lesions mainly appear on dense scabs along the topline, below the rectum or vulva, or adjacent to the udder; moist lesions with thickened, folded skin may occur and tend to ooze. Other affected areas of the body include the muzzle, nose, feet, scrotum, and underside of the tail (Mémery 1960; Yeruham and Hadani 2003; Loria et al. 2005; Scott 2007). This happens because these skin areas are frequently exposed to moisture or mild abrasion from vegetation. Caseous lymphadenitis is a very common bacterial disease in goats caused by *Corynebacterium pseudotuberculosis* and is characterized by one or more abscesses involving lymph nodes, typically associated with nodes in the head and neck. In cases of alopecia, scaling, and crusty lesions, budding yeasts are sometimes found in goats (Scott 1988). Mostly these are secondary opportunists (Reuter et al. 1987).

Infection with *Malassezia* has also been reported in goats from teat and udder lesions and also from greasy, seborrheic lesions over the trunk. In bluetongue viral infection, chronic lesions include necrosis, ulceration, and crusting on the lips, tongue, coronary band, and teats. Nodules on the face or eyelids occur in caprine herpesvirus infection.

4.1.4 Alopecia

Alopecia in goats may be due to several reasons, including external parasites and bacterial, fungal, and nutritional causes. Alopecia due to external parasites generally appears as patches of missing hair accompanied by scabs, redness, and roughness of skin. Following the parasitic activity, a secondary bacterial infection also causes hair loss. *D. congolensis* causes hair loss and can form extensive colonies of filament-like branches, resulting in crust and exudate formation at the base of the hair. *Staphylococcus aureus* causes staphylococcal dermatitis that appears as lesions, scaling, and hair loss. Sometimes viral infections also combine with bacteria, causing ulcerative dermatitis and alopecia. Ringworm lesions in goats consist of scaling, erythema, alopecia, and crusts. They typically involve the neck, external ears, face, or limbs, and may be annular in shape (Scott 2007). Pruritus is not common but has been reported according to Chineme et al. (1981).

Nutritional deficiencies or imbalances such as high calcium with low zinc have been noted in alopecia (van der Westhuysen et al. 1988). Zinc deficiency usually appears with the goat losing hair in the nose area (Figure 4.2). Iodine

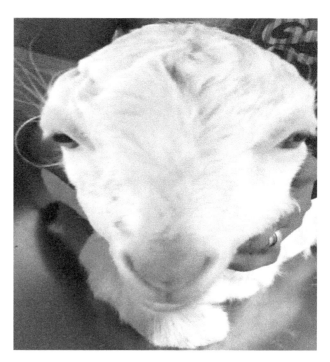

Figure 4.2 Alopecia on the nose of a goat.

deficiency also causes hair loss, particularly in young goats. In vitamin E and selenium deficiency, alopecic exfoliative dermatitis can be seen as periorbital alopecia. It can also be seen due to self-excoriation when pruritus is present or can be the result of grooming by pen mates. Thickening of skin and hair loss on the head, neck, flanks, lower limbs, and the perineal area may be associated with vitamin A deficiency. Stress or hormonal imbalance may be one of the causes of alopecia. In these conditions, hair loss generally occurs on the back and shoulders (Smith and Sherman 2009).

4.1.5 Pigmentary Changes

Copper deficiency can lead to decoloration of hair, since a copper-containing enzyme is necessary for melanin production.

4.1.6 Body Localization of Skin Lesions as an Aid to Diagnosis

The entire body surface should be examined. Lesions on various body areas can be helpful to diagnose the particular disease (Table 4.1). For instance, contact dermatitis or parasite invasion causes lesions only on the ventral part of the body. Photosensitization or sunburn causes lesions only on non-pigmented skin.

4.2 Diagnosis of Diseases by Clinical Findings of the Gastrointestinal System

The gastrointestinal (GI) system is the system in the goat most prone to disorders because of unscientific feeding, infectious diseases, and parasitism. The clinical signs specific to the GI system are elaborated here.

4.2.1 Frothing at the Mouth

Excessive chewing and salivation cause frothing at the mouth. This commonly occurs during convulsions in goat. Drugs like levamisole at higher doses can induce frothing. *Cadabaro tundifolia* and *Cestrum aurantiacum* are toxic plants that can cause hemorrhagic gastroenteritis in goats, and are also responsible for frothing at the mouth (El Dirdiri et al. 1987). This particular non-specific clinical sign is also seen in infectious diseases like PPR, orf, or enterotoxemia, and non-infectious diseases like severe tympany, uneven teeth, or vitamin B1 deficiency.

4.2.2 Excessive Salivation or Drooling

Excessive salivation or drooling, known as ptyalism, may be caused by hypersialosis or pseudoptyalism. Hypersialosis is increased secretion of saliva, whereas pseudoptyalism is secondary to disorders in goats producing a normal quantity of saliva. This can be from a conformational abnormality or a swallowing disorder. Salivation in goats can occur due to stomatitis, neurological disease, systemic poisonings, or obstructions of the digestive tract distal to the oral cavity. Stomatitis can be infectious or non-infectious. Infectious causes include contagious ecthyma, goat pox, unclassified viral dermatitis, foot and mouth disease, bluetongue, vesicular stomatitis, rinderpest, PPR, caprine herpesvirus, necrotic or ulcerative stomatitis caused by *Fusobacterium necrophorum* infection, and alveolar periostitis. Non-infectious causes of stomatitis include chemical irritants, traumatic injuries, plant and chemical poisonings, and possibly neoplasia. Salivation or drooling is an evident clinical sign in neurological diseases such as rabies and polioencephalomalacia, caprine arthritis encephalitis virus infection, listeriosis, botulism, migrations of the

Table 4.1 Diagnosis of skin diseases based on lesions seen on various body areas.

Lesions on lips, face, and neck	Lesions on ears	Lesions on feet	Lesions on udder
Contagious ecthyma	Dermatophilosis	Contagious ecthyma	Contagious ecthyma
Capripox	Dermatophytosis	Foot and mouth disease	*Staphylococcal* folliculitis
Peste des petits ruminants	Sarcoptic mange	*Staphylococcal* folliculitis	Zinc deficiency
Bluetongue	Ear mites	*Dichelobacter* infection (foot rot)	Hyperpigmentation from exposure to the sun
Staphylococcal folliculitis	Photodermatitis	Dermatophilosis	Neoplasia
Dermatophilosis	Squamous cell carcinoma	Sarcoptic mange	
Dermatophytosis	Frostbite	Chorioptic mange	
Sarcoptic mange	*Pemphigus foliaceus*	*Pelodera* dermatitis	
Zinc deficiency		*Besnoitia* dermatitis	
Pemphigus foliaceus		Zinc deficiency	
Prototheosis		Contact dermatitis	
		P. foliaceus	

nematode parasite *Parelaphostrongylus tenuis*, and trauma to the facial nerve. Poisoning condition such as organophosphate, carbamate, acute chlorinated hydrocarbon, and cyanide poisoning are also responsible for drooling in goats. Similarly, nutritional muscular dystrophy, or white muscle disease, also can cause drooling due to necrosis of muscles of the tongue and pharynx. Physical obstruction of the esophagus or pharynx will affect the swallowing of saliva and hinder the normal flow of saliva, which may lead to excess salivation in animals.

4.2.3 Dysphagia

Dysphagia is difficulty in swallowing, clinically manifested by prolonged chewing, retaining food in the mouth, and dropping food from the mouth. This condition is manifested in focal neurological diseases such as listeriosis, brain abscess, parasitic larval migration, caprine arthritis, and encephalitis. These conditions may damage cranial nerve roots VII, IX, X, or XII, which in turn cause dysphagia. Rabies, tetanus, botulism, and polioencephalomalacia are other diseases where dysphagia is evident. Excessive tooth wear due to chronic exposure to fluoride and associated pain can produce signs of dysphagia. Additional dental problems that may lead to dysphagia include overeruption of teeth, broken teeth, vestigial teeth, and displaced, rotated, or migrated teeth (Rudge 1970). Some plant toxins like honey mesquite (*Prosopis glandulosa*) are also attributed as causing dysphagia in goats (Washburn et al. 2002).

4.2.4 Regurgitation, Retching, or Projectile Vomiting

Vomiting is not a common symptom in goats, but it may be noticed in obstruction of the upper GI tract or toxicity. Partial or complete obstructions of the pharynx or esophagus can lead to regurgitation of food in goats (Fleming et al. 1989). Acute copper toxicity results in vomiting with other clinical signs like abdominal pain, muscle fasciculations, labored breathing, tachycardia, and frothing at the mouth before death (Shlosberg et al. 1978). Ingestion of toxin plants containing grayanotoxin (also referred to as andromedotoxin), which acts primarily on the autonomic nervous system, stimulates the vomiting center via the vagus nerve and produces hypotension (Smith 1978; Gibb 1987; Knight 1987).

4.2.5 Rumen Atony

Rumen atony or ruminal hypomotility is mainly associated with digestive system pathologies like simple indigestion, bloat, rumen acidosis caused by acute carbohydrate engorgement, and rumen alkalosis associated with urea poisoning. Apart from this, plant and chemical poisonings frequently lead to rumen atony. Rations low in coarse roughage and high in finely ground concentrate may lead to rumen atony or hypomotility.

Pain from any source, severe dehydration, electrolyte or acid–base imbalances, hypocalcemia, high fever, and toxemias are extra-digestive system factors that can trigger rumen atony. Rumen motility is also changed according to the excitement or fearfulness of the animal. Use of drugs like atropine, anesthetics and depressants such as barbiturates reduces rumen contractions.

4.2.6 Abdominal Distension

Abdominal distension in the goat may be due to a fetus, abnormal accumulations of food, foreign bodies, gas or fluid in the abdominal cavity, or herniation of the abdominal wall. Ruminal tympany (both frothy and free gas bloat), left displacement of the abomasum, and acute carbohydrate engorgement are the major causes of abdominal distension in the goat (Figure 4.3). Rumen impaction causes lower left abdominal distension, whereas lower right abdominal distension is seen in late pregnancy or abomasal disorders like abomasal impaction or abomasal bloat due to an abrupt change in feeding. Bilateral ventral distension can be observed in acute duodenal obstruction caused by a phytobezoar or due to accumulation of ascites fluid secondary to hypoproteinemia or cardiac insufficiency. Pseudopregnancy, hydrometra, hydroallantois, or hydramnios in female breeding goats are common causes of bilateral ventral abdominal distension. A ruptured bladder in male goats due to obstructive urolithiasis may lead to accumulation of urine in the abdominal cavity, thereby causing abdominal distension.

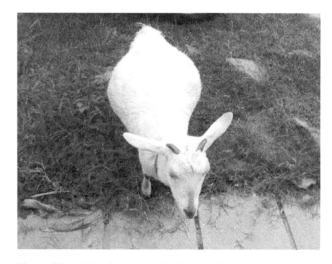

Figure 4.3 Abdominal distension in a goat.

Intestinal and ovarian adenocarcinomas in aged female goats are responsible for progressive abdominal distension. Severe peritonitis and sporadic intestinal accidents can lead to generalized ileus and may lead to secondary abdominal distension. Umbilical hernia and spontaneous or traumatic ruptures of the abdominal wall are other causes of focal distortion of the abdomen.

4.2.7 Abdominal Pain or Colic

Abdominal pain in goats is clinically manifested by restlessness, depression, bleating, reluctance to move, teeth grinding, increased shallow respiration, increased heart rate, tenesmus, or an abnormal posture with an arched back and tucked-up abdomen. Kicking at the belly or rolling is a less common sign in a goat with colic. Abdominal pain may be due to mechanical reasons, infection, toxicity, or obstruction.

Mechanical causes are common in young kids due to feeding cold milk or a greater amount of milk, cecal torsion, intussusception (Mitchell 1983), and torsion of the root of the mesentery (Thompson 1985).

The foremost infectious causes that lead to abdominal pain are from acute *Clostridium perfringens* type D enterotoxemia along with other clinical signs like diarrhea, screaming, and convulsions. This may also be observed in young goats with acute coccidiosis, before the onset of diarrhea.

Peritonitis can produce abdominal pain in addition to ileus, abdominal distension, and fever. Peritonitis in goats may be due to rumen trocharization, uterine tears associated with dystocia, and extension of metritis from the uterus to the abdominal cavity. It can also occur as a sequela to rumenitis after acute carbohydrate engorgement. Streptococci, staphylococci, *Escherichia coli, F. necrophorum,* and *Clostridium* spp. are responsible for infectious peritonitis in goats. Systemic mycoplasmosis causes serositis-arthritis disease complex along with peritonitis in goats (DaMassa et al. 1983). Non-infectious peritonitis may be caused by intraperitoneal injections of sulfa drugs or calcium solutions, or talc from surgical gloves used on goats (Hall 1983).

Toxicities due to ingestion of plants and chemical toxins can produce abdominal pain. Obstructive urolithiasis is the most common cause of abdominal pain in male goats.

4.2.8 Absence of Feces or Constipation

These conditions are seen in case of any hindrance in normal motility in the GI tract of animals. Volvulus, intussusception, incarceration, or luminal obstructions by a foreign body are the major cause of absence of feces or constipation in goats. Atresia ani and atresia coli must be considered when there are no feces in neonates.

Constipation can be a side effect in normal pregnancy or in pregnancy toxemia during late gestation (Pinsent and Cottom 1987). Limited access to water or a fibrous diet, a poor-quality diet, extraluminal compression of the intestine by intra-abdominal abscesses due to *C. pseudotuberculosis,* or subclinical coccidiosis can lead to constipation.

4.2.9 Diarrhea

Diarrhea is the frequent voiding of loose, watery, and unformed feces in goats, which may be due to infectious and non-infectious agents, as illustrated in Figure 4.4.

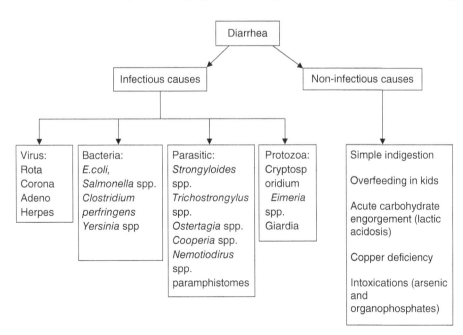

Figure 4.4   Causes of diarrhea.

4.3 Diagnosis of Diseases by Clinical Findings of the Respiratory System

Rate of respiration, dyspnea, respiratory sounds, cough, and nasal discharge are the common clinical signs associated with respiratory diseases.

4.3.1 Respiratory Rate

An increased respiratory rate in a goat is noticed in fever, metabolic disturbances, or pain. Metabolic disturbances include pregnancy toxemia, lactational ketosis, rumen acidosis, and diarrhea. An altered respiratory rate is observed in listeriosis or other brainstem disease due to acidosis from loss of saliva or lesions in the respiratory centers of the brain.

4.3.2 Dyspnea

Dyspnea, difficult or labored breathing, can be inspiratory, expiratory, or mixed type. Dyspnea or tachypnea is seen in conditions like anemia, rumen acidosis, bloat, pregnancy toxemia, ketosis, nasal obstruction (tumor or foreign body), progressive interstitial retroviral pneumonia (caprine arthritis encephalitis virus, CAEV), heatstroke, urolithiasis, PPR, pasteurellosis, septicemia, internal caseous lymphadenitis, contagious caprine pleuropneumonia, inhalation pneumonia, congenital heart malformation, tuberculosis, lungworms (*Dictyocaulus*), nutritional muscular dystrophy, nitrate poisoning, cyanide poisoning, and other assorted toxicities.

4.3.3 Externally Audible Sounds

Sneezing is observed when the nasal mucosa is irritated by accumulations of exudates, secretions, or foreign matter. Constriction in the upper respiratory tract leads to stenotic sounds. Nasal-origin snuffling sounds are loudest during inspiration, whereas pharyngeal-origin sounds are loudest on expiration, and laryngeal stenosis sounds are more pronounced on inspiration.

4.3.4 Coughing

Goats exhibit dry and powerful coughing if irritation lies in the upper respiratory tract; if there is a deep-seated bronchopneumonia, the cough may be moist and feeble. Causes of coughing include dusty or moldy hay, a tight collar, tracheal stenosis, dysphagia (nutritional muscular dystrophy, neurological disease), contagious caprine pleuropneumonia, CAEV, parainfluenza virus (PI3), pasteurellosis, heart failure, ammonia and other fumes, an abscessed retropharyngeal lymph node, cryptococcosis, and lungworm (*Dictyocaulus*) infestation.

4.3.5 Nasal Discharge

Nasal discharge could be seen due to nose bots (*Oestrus ovis*), which cause a chronic catarrhal to purulent discharge; cleft palate; powdery feed causing foreign body rhinitis; irritant fumes (ammonia, smoke); atrophic rhinitis (toxigenic strains of *Pasteurella multocida*); regurgitation due to nutritional muscular dystrophy; or nasal adenoma (affected animals show profuse seromucous nasal exudate, coughing, dyspnea, and stertor). PPR, rinderpest, PI3, respiratory syncytial virus, and caprine herpesvirus cause clear nasal discharge that may turn into purulent nasal discharge because of secondary bacterial infection. Pulmonary adenomatosis (jaagsiekte) and mycoplasma infections like infectious keratoconjunctivitis, possibly due to *Mycoplasma conjunctivae*, cause mucopurulent nasal discharge. Atrophic rhinitis associated with toxigenic strains of *Pa. multocida* shows purulent nose bleeding and nasal discharge.

4.3.6 Pneumonia

Pneumonia in goats can be caused by a virus (respiratory syncytial virus, progressive interstitial retroviral pneumonia, ovine pulmonary adenocarcinoma, sheep pulmonary adenomatosis, jaagsiekte, PPR, or goat pox), bacterial (*Pasteurella* and *Mannheimia* pneumonia, caseous lymphadenitis abscesses in the lungs, tuberculosis, melioidosis and rhodococcal pneumonia), fungal (cryptococcosis), parasitic (*Dictyocaulus* pneumonia, protostrongylids, *Eimeria*, echinococcosis, hydatidosis, liver flukes, schistosomosis), mycoplasma (contagious caprine pleuropneumonia, pleuropneumonia, non-specific mycoplasma pneumonia), chlamydia, or rickettsial pneumonia (Q fever).

4.4 Diagnosis of Diseases by Clinical Findings of the Urinary System

Clinical signs associated with urinary tract diseases are abnormal appearance of urine, anuria, oliguria, polyuria, dysuria, pollakiuria, stranguria, uremia, and abdominal distension. These symptoms are explained here.

4.4.1 Abnormal Appearance of Urine or Abnormal Urinalysis

Normal urine of the goat is clear and pale to dark yellow. Cloudy urine is usually associated with inflammation caused by pyelonephritis, cystitis, or possibly vulvovaginitis.

Hematuria or hemoglobinuria leads to pink, red, or coffee-color urine. Hematuria can occur due to obstructive urolithiasis, pyelonephritis, cystitis, or an infiltrative carcinoma at the neck of the urinary bladder. Hemoglobinuria is seen in case of excessive intravascular hemolysis or in excessive water consumption, which may lead to hypotonicity and hemolysis (Middleton et al. 1997). A goat that has died due to anthrax may have oozing of unclotted blood from all natural orifices. Brown urine results from myoglobinuria, which can be seen in nutritional muscular dystrophy and in certain plant poisonings resulting in muscle necrosis. Brownish yellow urine in bilirubinuria is poorly documented in goats. Proteinuria accompanies inflammatory conditions of the urogenital tract and bacterial endotoxemia.

Proteinuria, in conjunction with prolonged weight loss, is a hallmark of renal amyloidosis characterized by deposition of fibrillar amyloid protein in the glomeruli. Ketonuria is diagnostic for pregnancy toxemia in the non-lactating, pregnant doe, but it can occur in lactational ketosis also.

Glucosuria is recorded in enterotoxemia caused by *Cl. perfringens* type D and also in cases where goats are stressed by other serious disease problems, including convulsions from any cause. It can be iatrogenic from administration of venous dextrose or xylazine.

Crystalluria can be observed in cases of obstructive urolithiasis, or after consumption of ethylene glycol or plants high in oxalates. Casts in the urine indicate tubular damage in the kidney, usually because of poor renal perfusion, toxins, or drugs. Urine sediments containing increased numbers of red cells, white cells, and epithelial cells indicate inflammation. Sperm may be observed in the urine of sexually active bucks.

4.4.2 Anuria, Oliguria, or Polyuria

Anuria or oliguria is more common in bucks because of the anatomic peculiarity of their urinary tract. Male goats with obstructive urolithiasis may produce no urine, but dysuria is more common. Instances of anuric renal failure are poorly documented in goats. In most documented cases of toxic nephropathy, affected goats were oliguric initially and later polyuric.

4.4.3 Dysuria, Pollakiuria, and Stranguria

Dysuria is difficult painful urination, pollakiuria is frequent urination, and stranguria is slow and painful urination or straining to pass urine. Dysuria in males can be seen in ulcerative posthitis cases and due to scabbing over of the preputial orifice or "hair rings," accumulations of loosely matted hairs encircling the penis behind the glans. In females, cystitis and vulvovaginitis lead to abnormal urination. Stranguria was seen due to obstructive uropathy from trauma and adhesions of the urinary tract due to dystocia (Morin and Badertscher 1990). Pollakiuria has been seen in cases of hydrometra and in uterine enlargement due to neoplasia (Pfister et al. 2007).

4.4.4 Uremia

Uremia is failure to remove byproducts of protein metabolism through the kidney. Uremia can be prerenal, renal, or postrenal. Prerenal uremia is due to dehydration or poor renal perfusion, which may result from a variety of causes not related to the urinary system. Uremia of renal origin is mainly decreased renal function or kidney failure. Postrenal uremia is most commonly reported in goats and is associated with obstructive urolithiasis.

4.4.5 Abdominal Distension

Abdominal distension related to the urinary system is most commonly due to rupture of the urinary bladder secondary to obstructive urolithiasis with bilateral and ventral distension of the abdomen. It is more common in males than in females.

A similar "pot-bellied" appearance may be seen due to obstructions of the forestomachs, infectious peritonitis, GI parasitism, and reproductive conditions leading to distension of the uterus.

4.4.6 Subcutaneous Swelling

Obstructive urolithiasis can cause rupture of the urethra, which in turn leads to subcutaneous pooling of urine in either the perineal or preputial area, or it can be seen due to trauma to the urethra during forceful bladder catheterization or congenital urethral diverticulum.

Preputial swelling may be seen in cases of ulcerative posthitis, balanoposthitis due to venereal caprine herpesvirus infection and also due to hypoproteinemia causing subcutaneous ventral edema involving the prepuce.

4.5 Diagnosis of Diseases by Clinical Findings of the Musculoskeletal System

The musculoskeletal system includes bones, cartilage, ligaments, tendons, and connective tissues. The skeleton provides a framework for muscles and other soft tissues. Together, they support the body's weight, maintain the posture, and help the animal to move. Various conditions that affect feet, joints, limbs, and gait of the goat are described here.

4.5.1 Abnormalities of Feet or Sore Feet

In goats, infectious diseases causing sore feet include foot scald, foot rot, foot abscess, foot and mouth disease, bluetongue, and dermatophilosis. Dermatophilosis, or mycotic dermatitis and mange mite infestations, particularly chorioptic mange, affects the feet and distal limbs as well as other areas of skin. Metabolic and nutritional causes of sore feet include zinc deficiency and laminitis. Laminitis can be in an acute or chronic form. In acute laminitis feet are predominantly sore and hot, while in chronic laminitis they are malformed and overgrown. In toxic causes only chronic selenosis leads to abnormal appearance of feet.

A sore foot can occur due to traumatic causes like overgrown hooves secondary to inadequate trimming, puncture wounds of the foot, foreign bodies such as stones or wood chips lodged between the claws, and bruising of the sole.

4.5.2 Stiff, Painful, or Abnormal Gait

Abnormalities of gait can be caused by neurological dysfunction or musculoskeletal diseases. Primary musculoskeletal diseases can be seen in any of the causes of painful feet or swollen joints, which can contribute to development of a stiff, abnormal, or painful gait. Additional causes of muscular origin include nutritional muscular dystrophy in its early or mild stages, parasitic myositis involving tapeworm cysts of the muscle, and myotonia congenita. Painful gait will also be observed in enzootic calcinosis caused by ingestion of *Trisetum flavescens* or yellow oat grass, which causes calcification of tendons and ligaments.

Skeletal-origin causes leading to pain and abnormal gait include fibrous osteodystrophy associated with excessive phosphorus in the diet, and chronic fluorosis resulting in abnormal bone growth and bone pain. Goats affected with chronic fluorosis were physically weak, showed mild to severe intermittent lameness in hind limbs, were indolent, and were reluctant to move. In these goats stiffness of the leg tendons and wasting of the main mass of the hind quarters were also observed. During walking, these animals showed a lowering of the neck indicating pain (Choubisa 2015). In kids, bone pain is associated with abnormal osteogenesis and subsequent bone fragility.

4.5.3 Arthritis

Arthritis is an inflammatory condition of one or more joints. Infectious causes of arthritis include various *Mycoplasma* spp., CAE virus, and a variety of bacterial agents among which *Erysipelothrix* and *Chlamydophila* are the most common. Nutritional and metabolic causes include rickets and osteopetrosis. Traumatic injury causing swelling of joints occurs secondary to avulsions of tendons and ligaments, hemarthrosis, and dislocations.

Swelling may develop around and above the coronary bands of hind limbs during late pregnancy. Very old goats can develop degenerative osteoarthritis, which can also be seen in goats with excessive straight-leggedness in the hind limb.

4.5.4 Weakness and Recumbency

Only primary muscle and skeletal problems that cause weakness and recumbency are listed here. Muscular diseases include nutritional muscular dystrophy, clostridial myositis, milk fever or hypocalcemia, and ingestion of myodegenerative plants such as *Cassia roemeriana* or *Karwinskia humboldtiana*. Deficiency of selenium and vitamin E causes white muscle disease, which is a nutritional myopathy leading to degeneration of skeletal and heart muscle in which kids become recumbent and are depressed, reluctant to move, and appear stiff, with a "sawhorse" stance. Acute mycoplasma arthritis is especially associated with recumbency in goats. Severe hoof diseases, mainly laminitis, foot rot, and chronic selenosis, can keep the goat recumbent.

Bone abnormalities can produce recumbency due either to bone pain or secondary fracture. Metabolic bone diseases leading to recumbency include rickets and fibrous osteodystrophy. Traumatic fractures, especially those of the vertebral canal, can cause the goat not to rise. Osteomyelitis if involving the vertebrae can also predispose to fracture and recumbency.

4.5.5 Failure to Extend Limb

In newborn goats, arthrogryposis, congenital fixation of multiple joints, has been reported to result from infectious (Akabane virus, Cache Valley virus, border disease virus), toxic, and genetic causes that affect the developing fetus. Severely flexed fore limbs and overextended hind limbs are seen in affected animals. Other conditions are contracted tendons associated with positional constraints in utero during fetal growth or possible congenital lupinosis. In Australian Angora goats, an inherited tendon shortening also occurs. In older kids, flexor contracture of the fore limbs may occur in enzootic ataxia.

In mature animals, CAE virus arthritis commonly causes ankylosis of joints. Apart from this any traumatic or infectious cause of arthritis may result in a reduced range of motion when chronic in nature. Dislocations or luxations may also cause pain on extension of joints.

4.5.6 Non-weight Bearing on a Limb

In this case animals are able to extend the affected limb but unwilling to bear weight on that limb. Differential diagnoses include fractures, dislocations, severe arthritis involving a single joint, puncture wounds of the foot, severe foot rot, foot scald, or foot abscesses. Fractures may be primarily traumatic in origin or may be predisposed to by increased bone fragility such as in rickets, fibrous osteodystrophy, copper deficiency, and chronic fluorosis. Osteomyelitis may also predispose to fracture or cause sufficient pain to result in non-weight bearing.

4.5.7 Bowed Limbs

Bowing of the fore limbs is seen primarily in metabolic bone diseases. Main causes include rickets, epiphysitis, and phosphorus deficiency causing bowie or bent leg. Zinc deficiency may cause bowing of hind limbs in goats. Weak attachments of the shoulder assembly may lead to winged-out elbows and the appearance of bowed limbs.

4.5.8 Conditions of the Fore Limb

In goats luxation of the scapulohumeral joint may be common. Shoulder instability can result in either luxation or subluxation of the scapulohumeral joint. These are traumatic injuries that likely result from severe abduction of one of the front limbs by fighting with other males or attempting to breed a non-receptive female. They are usually presented with non-specific, non-localizing signs of lameness. Goats maintained on rough, hard flooring may commonly develop carpal hygromas.

4.5.9 Conditions of the Hind Limb

Conditions that affect the hind limbs include white muscle disease, which leads the hind limb muscles to become firm and painful to the touch. Patellar luxation (PL) is a musculoskeletal affection characterized by deviation of the patella from its normal sliding movement on the trochlear groove. In PL, one or both of the trochlear ridges flattens, allowing the patella to slide from its normal pathway (Di Dona et al. 2018). The patella deviates in either a medial, lateral, dorsal, or rarely ventral direction (Burnei et al. 2020). Abhushhiwa et al. (2021) has reported the first observation of lateral PL in Hejazi goats bred in Libya.

4.6 Diagnosis of Nervous System Diseases by Clinical Findings

Nervous system disorders are defined as disorders that affect the brain, nerves, and spinal cord. Structural, electrical, or biochemical abnormalities in the brain, spinal cord, or nerves can result in a range of symptoms. Examples of symptoms include behavior changes, exhibiting involuntary activity, and change in gait or posture.

4.6.1 Behavior Changes

4.6.1.1 Excitation

Goats with behavior changes have signs of excitation or mania, which are clinically exhibited as excessive bleating, aimless running, resistance or overreaction to touch or handling, head pressing, hyperesthesia, obvious fear or aggression, fluttering of the eyelids, constant chewing, teeth grinding, frenzy, or compulsive walking.

There are multiple causes that can lead to change in behavior. Infectious causes include pseudorabies, rabies, scrapie, Borna disease, cowdriosis (heartwater), and bacterial meningoencephalitis. Possible parasitic causes include trypanosomosis, coenurosis (gid), aberrant *O. ovis* larval migration into the brain (false gid), and *Strongyloides papillosus*. Metabolic causes include pregnancy toxemia, hypomagnesemic tetany, and polioencephalomalacia. Hepatoencephalopathy can produce hyperesthesia or head pressing. Toxic agents that can cause excitation in goats include urea, chlorinated hydrocarbons, cyanide, organophosphates, nitrates, nitrofurans, and the coyotillo plant (*Karwinskia humboldtiana*).

4.6.1.2 Coma

Coma is a state of prolonged unconsciousness that can be caused by various diseases. Infectious causes that can lead to coma are enterotoxemia, pseudorabies, and meningoencephalitis. Metabolic causes for coma include polioencephalomalacia, milk fever, and pregnancy toxemia. Systemic disease like hepatoencephalopathy and uremia can also cause coma. Salt poisoning, organophosphate, carbamate, or chlorinated hydrocarbon insecticide toxicities, milkweed (*Asclepias*) poisoning, and oxalate poisoning are toxic causes for coma.

4.6.2 Involuntary Activity

4.6.2.1 Muscle Tremors

Tremor is an involuntary and rhythmic contraction of muscle leading to shaking movements in one or more parts of the body. Infectious causes of tremors include bacterial meningoencephalitis, rabies, scrapie, border disease, Borna disease, and CAE. Tremors can also be seen as an early sign of tetanus. Metabolic and nutritional causes include enzootic ataxia or swayback. Hypoglycemia, hypomagnesemic tetany, hepatoencephalopathy, and polioencephalomalacia. Toxicological causes include plant poisoning, cyanide poisoning, organophosphate, carbamate or chlorinated hydrocarbon insecticide poisoning, oxalate poisoning, nitrate poisoning, salt poisoning, boron ingestion, urea poisoning, levamisole overdose, and diesel fuel consumption.

4.6.2.2 Convulsions (Seizures)

A seizure is defined as a transient occurrence of physical signs with a finite duration and a tendency to begin and end abruptly, caused by abnormal excessive or synchronous neuronal activity in the brain (Trinka et al. 2015). According to the International League Against Epilepsy (ILAE), seizures are classified as genetic, structural or metabolic, and unknown, based on etiology (Berg and Scheffer 2011).

Causes of seizures can be infectious, which include pseudorabies, enterotoxemia, cowdriosis, tetanus, bacterial meningoencephalitis, and Borna disease. *Mycoplasma mycoides* subspecies *capri* was found to be an unusual cause of meningitis leading to convulsions and other neurological signs like nystagmus and circling (Schumacher et al. 2011; Johnson et al. 2019). Parasitic causes such as coccidiosis, coenurosis, and *O. ovis* migration into the brain (false gid) lead to convulsion. Metabolic causes include hypomagnesemic tetany, pregnancy toxemia, hypoglycemia, polioencephalomalacia, and hepatoencephalopathy.

Toxic causes include poisonous plants, copper intoxication, organophosphate, carbamate, and chlorinated hydrocarbon insecticides, levamisole overdose, dinitro herbicides, and pentachlorophenol wood preservatives.

Lidocaine in sheep produces convulsive signs at an approximate dose of 6 mg/kg intravenously and circulatory collapse at a dose of 37 mg/kg intravenously (Morishima et al. 1981). Olcott et al. (1987) reported partial epilepsy of unknown origin as a cause of convulsions in an adult Nubian doe.

Other causes include hypernatremia, bronchopneumonia, trauma, cortical thermal necrosis secondary to disbudding, brain abscess, leukoencephalomalacia of the cerebral cortex associated with vasculitis secondary to sepsis caused by *Escherichia coli* metritis, meningoepithelial hyperplasia, systemic sarcosporidiosis, and suspected hereditary central nervous system spongiform myelinopathy (Chigerwe and Aleman 2016).

4.6.2.3 Nystagmus

Nystagmus is an involuntary rhythmic side-to-side, up-and-down, or circular motion of the eyes that occurs with a variety of conditions. Infectious causes of nystagmus include otitis, CAE, rabies, brain abscess, and listeriosis. Parasitic causes for it are cerebrospinal nematodiasis with *Setaria digitata*, *Parelaphostrongylus tenuis*, or *Elaphostrongylus* spp. and coenurosis. One metabolic cause of nystagmus is polioencephalomalacia. Toxic causes include salt poisoning and consumption of locoweeds (*Astragalus* spp.). In newborn kids hereditary beta-mannosidosis causes nystagmus. It can also be caused by certain poisonous plants such as bracken, rock fern, or mulga fern in goat kids.

4.6.2.4 Pruritus

All the neurogenic causes of pruritus in goats are of infectious or parasitic origin and include scrapie, rabies, pseudorabies, *Parelaphostrongylus tenuis*, and *Elaphostrongylus* spp.

4.6.3 Change in Gait

4.6.3.1 Ataxia (Incoordination)

Ataxia is a neurological sign in which a lack of voluntary coordination of muscle movement leads to gait abnormalities. Ataxia can be seen in cases of spinal cord lesions, vestibular, cerebellar, and occasionally cerebral lesions. Infectious causes for ataxia include scrapie, rabies, bacterial (or thermal) meningoencephalitis, brain abscess, cowdriosis, CAE, and listeriosis. Parasitic causes include cerebrospinal nematodiasis with either *Parelaphostrongylus tenuis*, *Elaphostrongylus* spp., or *Setaria digitata*; coenurosis; aberrant *O. ovis* migration into the brain; tick paralysis; trypanosomosis; and possibly *Strongyloides papillosus*. Metabolic and nutritional causes include milk fever, enzootic ataxia, hypomagnesemic tetany, and polioencephalomalacia. Toxic causes include plant poisonings, bromide, lead, salt, oxalate, urea, cyanide, or nitrate poisonings; organophosphate, carbamate, or chlorinated hydrocarbon insecticide intoxications; diesel fuel consumption; and nitrofuran or levamisole overdosage. Neoplastic causes of ataxia have been reported sporadically. Lymphosarcoma associated with the brain or meninges has resulted in incoordination (Craig et al. 1986).

Congenital or hereditary causes include congenital vertebral or spinal abnormalities such as hemivertebra in which only one half of the vertebral body develops (Rowe 1979). Progressive paresis in Angora goats is also a heritable disorder showing spastic paresis and ataxia, which progress to recumbency within a few weeks. Multisystem neuronal degeneration is seen at necropsy. There is a report of atlanto-axial malarticulation in two young Angora goats that led to spinal cord degeneration at the level of the atlantoaxial joint resulting in ataxia (Robinson et al. 1982). Polyradiculoneuritis and caprine encephalomyelomalacia also produce ataxia, but the etiology is unknown.

4.6.3.2 Circling

Circling in goats is cerebral or vestibular in origin. Animals with circling caused by cerebral disease usually have other abnormalities of behavior or mental status. Signs associated with circling caused by vestibular lesions are usually more localized and may be limited to hemiparesis, head tilt, nystagmus, and other specific cranial nerve deficits such as facial nerve paralysis.

4.6.3.3 Hypermetria

Hypermetria is characterized by a high stepping gait with overflexion of joints. It has been reported in scrapie, coenurosis, coyotillo poisoning, and enzootic ataxia. It is also seen in alpha-mannosidosis in goats caused by the swainsonine-containing plant *Ipamoea verbascoidea* (Mendonça et al. 2012).

4.6.4 Change in Posture

4.6.4.1 Opisthotonus

Opisthotonus is a backward arching of the head and neck caused by spasm of extensor muscles. This condition can be observed in infectious diseases like tetanus, rabies, CAE, enterotoxemia, bacterial meningoencephalitis, and brain abscess. Disseminated toxoplasmosis and trypanosomosis are protozoan infections causing opisthotonos in goats. Metabolic and nutritional diseases in which it is observed are hypomagnesemic tetany and polioencephalomalacia (Figure 4.5). It can also be observed in toxic causes like plant poisonings, salt poisoning, and chlorinated hydrocarbon toxicity.

4.6.4.2 Paresis

Paresis refers to a condition in which voluntary muscle movement becomes weakened or impaired. Paresis through neurological impairment of motor function can be due to lesions of the brainstem, spinal cord, peripheral nerves, or neuromuscular junctions. There could be tetraparesis, paraparesis, hemiparesis, or monoparesis.

Infectious causes of paresis include listeriosis, rabies, CAE or visna, and botulism. Parasitic causes include cerebrospinal nematodiasis with either *Parelaphostrongylus*

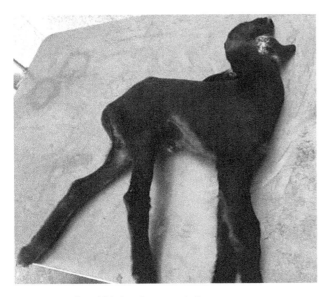

Figure 4.5 Goat kid showing an opisthotonus posture.

tenuis, *Setaria digitata*, or *Elaphostrongylus* spp.; coenurosis; and tick paralysis. Metabolic and nutritional causes include pregnancy toxemia, milk fever, and enzootic ataxia or swayback. Toxic causes include plant poisonings, salt poisoning, organophosphate and carbamate, bromide intoxication, insecticide poisoning, boron toxicity, and pentachlorophenol toxicity. Neoplastic causes of paresis include lymphosarcoma sporadically associated with the brain or meninges (Craig et al. 1986) and malignant melanoma metastasized to the vertebral canal (Sockett et al. 1984).

Hydrocephalus and progressive paresis of Angora goats are due to congenital or inherited causes of paresis. Paraparesis or tetraparesis is also observed in caprine encephalomyelomalacia, a disease of unknown etiology.

4.6.4.3 Paralysis

Paralysis is the complete loss of motor function in any part of the body. Conditions that cause paresis can lead to paralysis. Tetraplegia, paraplegia, or hemiplegia may be observed in limbs due to paralysis, which could be flaccid or spastic depending on the location of the lesions. Flaccid paralysis is associated with hyporeflexia and the spastic type leads to hyperreflexia.

Causes are similar to those of paresis. Trauma is the usual cause of peripheral nerve injuries leading to paralysis, most commonly trauma to the sciatic nerve. Sciatic nerve injury causes flaccid carriage of the entire hind limb. A case of hind limb paralysis caused by a metastatic malignant melanoma of the sciatic nerve has also been reported (Sockett et al. 1984).

Radial nerve paralysis related to trauma can occur in goats. Trauma to the vertebral column can lead to paralysis by damage to the spinal cord due to vehicular injuries or fighting between goats. An abscess or osteoporosis associated with rickets predisposes to fractures of the vertebrae, which can lead to paralysis.

4.6.5 Diagnosis of Hemic-lymphatic Diseases by Clinical Findings

4.6.5.1 Bleeding Disorders

Bleeding disorders can result due to platelet disorders, vasculitis, or coagulopathies, which clinically present with petechial or ecchymotic hemorrhages of mucous membranes, prolonged bleeding from venipuncture sites or surgical wounds, passage of blood from body orifices, or development of subcutaneous or periarticular swellings.

In a family of Saanen goats, inherited afibrinogenemia has been reported (Breukink et al. 1972). In a case of anthrax there will be bleeding from all natural orifices. In African trypanosomosis thrombocytopenia is a consistent

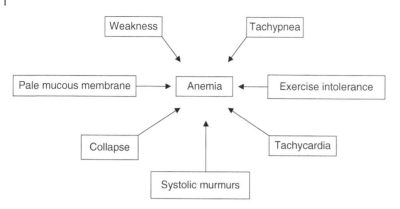

Figure 4.6 Clinical findings in anemia.

finding in all affected species, including goats (Davis 1982). Bracken fern (*Pteridium aquilinum*) ingestion by cattle can lead to a syndrome of anemia, thrombocytopenia, and pancytopenia with leukopenia, but no signs of hemorrhage were observed in naturally occurring bracken fern toxicity in goats (Tomlinson 1983).

4.6.5.2 Anemia

Anemia is a decrease in production of red blood cells that are needed to carry oxygen and nutrients to the cells of the body. Due to anemia a variety of clinical findings can be observed, illustrated in Figure 4.6.

In cases of intravascular anemia other clinical signs can also be observed like jaundice and hemoglobinuria. Signs of anemia are frequently accompanied by signs of hypoproteinemia such as ascites, intermandibular edema, and weight loss.

4.6.5.2.1 *Causes of Hemolytic Anemia* Common causes of hemolytic anemia in goats include the hemoparasitic diseases anaplasmosis, babesiosis, eperythrozoonosis, and theileriosis; nutritional disorders including copper toxicity, kale ingestion, and consumption of other, regional poisonous plants; and an infectious cause, leptospirosis.

Other suspected causes of hemolytic anemia in goats include infections due to *Cl. perfringens* type A and *Clostridium novyi* type D (*C. hemolyticum*), as reported in sheep. Experimentally oak tannin poisoning caused marked hemolytic anemia in goats, but naturally occurring oak poisoning is uncommon in this species (Begovic et al. 1978). Sarcocystosis (sarcosporidiosis) produces hemolytic anemia when induced experimentally (Dubey et al. 1981).

Hypophosphatemia was reported in two female goats suggested as the cause of hemolytic anemia and hemoglobinuria, but in two of the three reported cases serum inorganic phosphorus levels were in the normal range (Setty and Narayana 1975; Samad and Ali 1984).

4.6.5.2.2 *Causes of Blood Loss Anemia* Blood loss anemia is mostly seen in parasitic infestations by *Haemonchus* spp. and liver flukes, especially *Fasciola hepatica*. External parasites like sucking lice, ticks, and fleas also cause anemia (Schillhorn van Veen and Mohammed 1975).

Nutritional causes that lead to anemia include iron, copper (Brain 1983; Black et al. 1988), and cobalt deficiencies (Mgongo et al. 1981). Toxic causes include fluorosis and possibly bracken fern ingestion. Chronic infections like paratuberculosis can also lead to anemia in goats.

Nonregenerative anemia has been documented in chronic fluorosis of goats grazing near a superphosphate factory in Egypt (Karram et al. 1984).

4.6.6 Lymphadenopathy

Swelling of regional lymph nodes can be expected in common, localized infections such as mastitis, or subsequent to vaccinations. Persistent lymphadenopathy, however, is a major clinical finding in many important caprine diseases including caseous lymphadenitis, lymphosarcoma tuberculosis, melioidosis, nocardiosis, trypanosomosis, theileriosis, and trypanosomosis.

4.7 Diagnosis of Disease by Clinical Findings of the Udder

4.7.1 Mastitis

Mastitis is clinically characterized by an inflamed, hot, painful, and swollen udder, which may occur through several different bacteria, mainly *Staphylococcus* spp., but also *Streptococcus* spp., *Pasteurella haemolytica*, and *C. pseudotuberculosis* (caseous lymphadenitis), mycoplasma, and *E. coli*. Most common is *S. aureus*, which produces gangrenous mastitis that is characterized by inflamed, bluish discoloration of the udder and the skin of the teat (Tariq et al. 2014) (Figure 4.7).

Figure 4.7 Inflamed, bluish discoloration of the udder and skin of the teat of a goat affected with gangrenous mastitis.

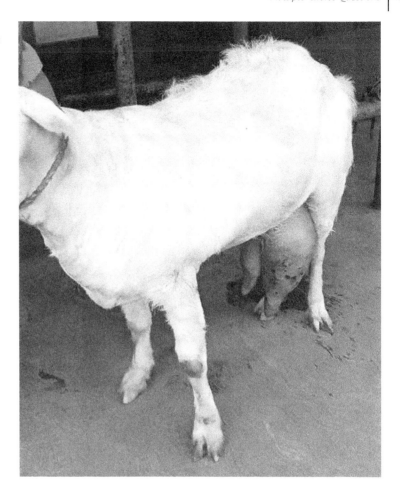

Multiple-Choice Questions

1 What cause of disease is suggested by papules with folliculitis?
   A Fungal
   B Bacterial
   C Parasitic
   D All of the above

2 What is pruritus caused by prion?
   A Lice
   B Sarcoptic
   C Scrapie
   D Photosensitization

3 What is lumpy wool disease caused by?
   A *Dermatophilus congolensis*
   B Photosensitization
   C Parasite
   D Fungus

4 Decoloration of hair is due to deficiency of which mineral?
   A Iron
   B Zinc
   C Cobalt
   D Copper

5 What is bilateral ventral distension in goats due to?
   A Fetus
   B Acute duodenal obstruction
   C Food
   D Gas

6 What is the cause of ascites?
   A Hypoproteinemia
   B Urinary bladder rupture
   C Peritonitis
   D Hydrometra

7 Which is an obstructive cause of abdominal pain?
 A Cecal torsion
 B Urolithiasis
 C *Escherichia coli*
 D Ileus

8 Deficiency of which mineral can lead to diarrhea in goats?
 A Zinc
 B Copper
 C Manganese
 D Calcium

9 When are pharyngeal-origin sounds loudest?
 A Inspiration
 B Expiration
 C Both of the above
 D None of the above

10 Hemoglobinuria is seen in a case of what?
 A Urolithiasis
 B Cystitis
 C Carcinoma
 D Intravascular hemolysis

11 Glucosuria is caused by which bacterial disease?
 A *Clostridium perfringens* type D
 B Anthrax
 C *Escherichia coli*
 D Salmonellosis

12 Of what is ketonuria diagnostic?
 A Amyloidosis
 B Pregnancy toxemia
 C Enterotoxemia
 D Muscular dystrophy

13 What is stranguria?
 A Difficulty in urination
 B Frequent urination
 C Slow painful urination
 D Absence of urination

14 What is uremia of renal origin due to?
 A Poor renal effusion
 B Dehydration
 C Renal failure
 D Urolithiasis

15 White muscle disease is due to deficiency of what?
 A Selenium and vitamin E
 B Calcium

C Phosphorus
 D Iron

16 What does arthrogryposis refer to?
 A Congenital fixation of multiple joints
 B Severely flexed fore limbs
 C Overextended hind limbs
 D Contracted tendon

17 Polioencephalomalacia occurs due to deficiency of what?
 A Glucose
 B Magnesium
 C Thiamine
 D Copper

18 In a case of coenurosis, what clinical sign is seen?
 A Convulsions
 B Diarrhea
 C Dyspnea
 D Pruritus

19 In pregnancy toxemia, clinical signs observed are related to which system?
 A Lymphatic
 B Nervous
 C Musculoskeletal
 D Gastrointestinal

20 When are convulsions seen?
 A Hypoglycemia
 B Hypomagnesemia
 C Hepatoencephalopathy
 D All of the above

21 Nutritional anemia is caused by deficiency of what?
 A Iron
 B Copper
 C Cobalt
 D All of the above

22 What is gangrenous mastitis caused by?
 A *Streptococcus* spp.
 B *Staphylococcus* spp.
 C *Escherichia coli*
 D *Mycoplasma*

23 What is the cause of nonregenerative anemia in goats?
 A External parasites
 B Hypophosphotemia
 C Chronic flurosis
 D Haemoprotozoa

24 What does braken fern poisoning lead to?
  A Anemia
  B Thrombocytpopenia
  C Pancytopenia
  D All of the above

25 When is the condition of hypermetria seen?
  A Scrapie
  B Gid
  C Enzootic ataxia
  D All of the above

References

Abushhiwa, M.H., Alrttib, A.M., Elmeshreghi, T.N. et al. (2021). Patellar luxation in Hejazi goats. *Open Veterinary Journal* 11 (2): 295–300.

Baker, J.C., Esser, M.B., and Larson, V.L. (1982). Pseudorabies in a goat. *Journal of the American Veterinary Medical Association* 181: 607.

Begovic, S., Duaic, E., Sacirbegovic, A., and Tafro, A. (1978). Study of etiology and pathogenesis of function disturbances of haematopoietic system in alimentary intoxications with tannins. *Veterinaria, Yugoslavia.* 27 (4): 459–470.

Berg, A.T. and Scheffer, I.E. (2011, 2011). New concepts in classification of the epilepsies: entering the 21st century. *Epilepsia* 52: 1058–1062.

Black, H., Hutton, J.B., Sutherland, R.J., and James, M.P. (1988). White liver disease in goats. *New Zealand Veterinary Journal* 36: 15–17.

Brain, L.T.A. (1983). Cobalt deficiency in a young goat. *Goat Veterinary Society Journal* 4: 45.

Breukink, H.J., Hart, H.C., von Arkel, C. et al. (1972). Congenital afibrinogenemia in goats. *Zentralblatt für Veterinärmedizin, Reihe A* 19: 661–676.

Burnei, G., Raducan, I., Lala, C. et al. (2020). Patellar dislocation: etiopathogenic diagnosis and treatment methods. *Clinics in Surgery* 5: 1–8.

Chigerwe, M. and Aleman, M. (2016). Seizure disorders in goats and sheep. *Journal of Veterinary Internal Medicine* 30 (5): 1752–1757.

Chineme, C.N., Adekeye, J.O., and Bida, S.A. (1981). Ringworm caused by *Trichophyton verrucosum* in young goats: a case report. *Bulletin of Animal Health and Production in Africa* 29: 75–78.

Choubisa, S.L. (2015). Industrial fluorosis in domestic goats (*Capra Hircus*), Rajasthan, India. *Fluoride* 48 (2): 105–112.

Craig, D.R., Roth, L., and Smith, M.C. (1986). Lymphosarcoma in goats. *Compendium on Continuing Education for the Practicing Veterinarian* 8: S190–S197.

DaMassa, A.J., Brooks, D.L., and Adler, H.E. (1983). Caprine mycoplasmosis: widespread infection in goats with *Mycoplasma mycoides* subsp mycoides (large-colony type). *American Journal of Veterinary Research* 44 (2): 322–325.

Davis, C.E. (1982). Thrombocytopenia a uniform complication of African trypanosomosis. *Acta Tropica* 39: 123–134.

Di Dona, F., Della, V.G., and Fatone, G. (2018). Patellar luxation in dogs. *Veterinary Medicine (Auckl)* 9: 23–32.

Dubey, J.P., Weisbrode, S.E., Speer, C.A., and Sharma, S.P. (1981). Sarcocystosis in goats: clinical signs and pathologic and hematologic findings. *Journal of the American Veterinary Medical Association* 178: 683–699.

El Dirdiri, N.I., Barakat, S.E.M., and Adam, S.E.I. (1987). The combined toxicity of *Aristolochia bracteata* and *Cadaba rotundifolia* to goats. *Veterinary and Human Toxicology* 29: 133–137.

Fleming, S.A., Dallman, M.J., and Sedlacek, D.L. (1989). Esophageal obstruction as a sequela to ruptured esophagus in a goat. *Journal of the American Veterinary Medical Association* 195: 1598–1600.

Gibb, M.C. (1987). Lily of the valley poisoning in an Angora goat. *New Zealand Veterinary Journal* 35: 59.

Hall, A. (1983). Digestive disorders—part 1. Diagnosing bloat, compaction and peritonitis. *Dairy Goat Guide* 6: 17–18.

Johnson, G.C., Fales, W.H., Shoemake, B.M. et al. (2019). An outbreak of *Mycoplasma mycoides* subspecies *capri* arthritis in young goats: a case study. *Journal of Veterinary Diagnostic Investigation* 31 (3): 453–457.

Karram, M.H., Amer, A.A., and Ibrahim, H.A. (1984). Aplastic anaemia in caprine fluorosis. *Assiut Veterinary Medical Journal* 12: 167–171.

Knight, A.P. (1987). Rhododendron and laurel poisoning. *Compendium on Continuing Education for the Practicing Veterinarian* 9: F26–F27.

Loria, G.R., La Barbera, E., Monteverde, V. et al. (2005). Dermatophilosis in goats in Sicily. *Veterinary Record* 156: 120–121.

Mémery, G. (1960). La streptothricose cutanée. II. Sur quelques cas spontanés chez des caprins dans la région de Dakar. *Revue D'élevage et de Médecine Vétérinaire Des Pays Tropicaux* 13: 143–153.

Mendonça, F.S., Albuquerque, R.F., Joaquim, E.N. et al. (2012). Alpha-mannosidosis in goats caused by the swainsonine-containing plant ipomoea verbascoidea. *Journal of Diagnostic Investigation* 24 (1): 90–95.

Mgongo, F.O.K., Gombe, S., and Ogaa, J.S. (1981). Thyroid status in cobalt and vitamin B12 deficiency in goats. *Veterinary Record* 109: 51–53.

Middleton, J.R., Katz, L., Angelos, J.A., and Tyler, J.W. (1997). Hemolysis associated with water administration using a nipple bottle for human infants in juvenile pygmy goats. *Journal of Veterinary Internal Medicine* 11 (6): 382–384.

Mitchell, W.C. (1983). Intussusception in goats. *Veterinary Medicine, Small Animal Clinician* 78: 1918.

Morin, D.E. and Badertscher, R.R. (1990). Ultrasonographic diagnosis of obstructive uropathy in a caprine doe. *Journal of the American Veterinary Medical Association* 197: 378–380.

Morishima, O.H. et al. (1981). Toxicity of lidocaine in adult, newborn and fetal sheep. *Anesthesiology* 55: 57–61.

Olcott, B.M., Strain, G.M., and Kreeger, J.M. (1987). Diagnosis of partial epilepsy in a goat. *Journal of the American Veterinary Medical Association* 191: 837–840.

Pfister, P. et al. (2007). Pollakisuria in a dwarf goat due to pathologic enlargement of the uterus. *Veterinary Quarterly* 29 (3): 112–116.

Pinsent, J. and Cottom, D.S. (1987). Metabolic diseases of goats. *Goat Veterinary Society Journal* 8: 40–42.

Reuter, R., Bowden, M., Besier, B. et al. (1987). Zinc responsive alopecia and hyperkeratosis in Angora goats. *Australian Veterinary Journal* 64: 351–352.

Robinson, W.F., Chapman, H.M., Grandage, J., and Bolton, J.R. (1982). Atlanto-axial malarticulation in angora goats. *Australian Veterinary Journal* 58 (3): 105–107.

Rowe, C.L. (1979). Hemivertebra in a goat. *Veterinary Medicine, Small Animal Clinician* 74: 211–214.

Rudge, M.R. (1970). Dental and periodontal abnormalities in two populations of feral goats (*Capra hircus* L.) in New Zealand. *New Zealand Journal of Science* 13: 260–267.

Samad, A. and Ali, M.S. (1984). Non-febrile haemoglobinuria in goats—a record of two cases. *Livestock Advisor* 9: 53–55.

Schillhorn van Veen, T.W. and Mohammed, A.N. (1975). Louse and flea infestations on small ruminants in the Zaria area. *Nigerian Veterinary Medical Association* 4: 93–96.

Schumacher, V.L., Hinckley, L., Xiaofen, L. et al. (2011). Meningitis caused by *Mycoplasma mycoides* subspecies capri in a goat. *Journal of Veterinary Diagnostic Investigation* 23 (3): 565–569.

Scott, D.W. (1988). *Large Animal Dermatology*. Philadelphia, PA: W.B. Saunders.

Scott, D.W. (2007). *Color Atlas of Farm Animal Dermatology*. Ames, IA: Blackwell.

Setty, D.R.L. and Narayana, K. (1975). A case of non-febrile haemoglobinuria in a she goat. *Indian Veterinary Journal* 52: 149.

Shlosberg, A., Egyed, M.N., and Huri, J. (1978). Acute copper poisoning in a herd of goats. *Refuah Veterinarith* 35: 15.

Shope, R.E. (1931). An experimental study of "mad itch" with especial reference to its relationship to pseudorabies. *Journal of Experimental Medicine* 54: 233–248.

Smith, M.C. (1978). Japanese pieris poisoning in the goat. *Journal of the American Veterinary Medical Association* 173: 78–79.

Smith, M.C. and Sherman, D.M. (2009). *Goat Medicine*, 2e. New York: Wiley Blackwell.

Sockett, D.C., Knight, A.P., and Johnson, L.W. (1984). Malignant melanoma in a goat. *Journal of the American Veterinary Medical Association* 185: 907–908.

Tariq, A., Shahzad, A., Kuasar, R. et al. (2014). Gangrenous mastitis: an important *Staphylococcus aureus* related problem in goat husbandry. *Advances in Animal and Veterinary Sciences* 2 (1): 46–49.

Tarlatzis, C.B. (1954). Un cas de rage prurigineuse chez la chèvre. *Annales Méd. Vét.* 98: 87–89.

Thompson, K.G. (1985). Enteric diseases of goats. In: *Proceedings of a Course in Goat Husbandry and Medicine*, Publication no. 106, Veterinary Continuing Education, 78–85. Palmerston North: Massey University.

Tomlinson, C.J. (1983). Bracken poisoning/PGE. *Goat Veterinary Society Journal* 4: 43–44.

Trinka, E., Cook, H., Hesdorffer, D. et al. (2015). A definition of status epilepticus – report of the ILAE task force on classification of status epilepticus. *Epilepsia* 56: 1515–1523.

Washburn, K.E., Breshears, M.A., Ritchey, J.W. et al. (2002). Honey mesquite toxicosis in a goat. *Journal of the American Veterinary Medical Association* 220 (12): 1837–1839.

van der Westhuysen, J.M., Wentzel, D., and Grobler, M.C. (1988). *Angora Goats and Mohair in South Africa*, 3e. Port Elizabeth: NMB Printers.

Yeruham, I. and Hadani, A. (2003). Self-destructive behaviour in ruminants. *Veterinary Record* 152: 304–305.

5

Collection, Preservation, Processing, and Dispatch of Clinical Material of Goats
Gauri A. Chandratre

Department of Veterinary Public Health and Epidemiology, College of Veterinary Sciences, Lala Lajpat Rai University of Veterinary and Animal Sciences, Hisar, Haryana, India

The goat is called the poor man's cow. Generally goats are resistant to many diseases. Small ruminant farming is being adopted by many farmers nowadays for meat and milk purposes. However, when we rear a higher number of animals in one place with insufficient pasture facilities, an intensive system of rearing leads to the spread of many diseases. Various factors like an increase in herd size, reduced ventilation, and poor husbandry practices can predispose to disease (Pfeiffer 2010). Diseases like peste des petits ruminants (PPR), foot and mouth disease (FMD), enterotoxemia, tetanus, gas gangrene, caseous lymphadenitis, listeriosis, tuberculosis, Johne's disease, dermatophilosis, pasteurellosis/mannheimiosis, and brucellosis affect goats and can cause various ailments. These causes reduce production potential and lead to higher mortality, which in turn results in heavy economic losses to farmers. Hence identification of diseases in goats and their diagnosis, treatment, and prevention are very important.

The collection of clinical material from diseased and dead animals for laboratory diagnostic procedures is an important task since an exact diagnosis can be determined only by the use of laboratory diagnostic procedures. The specimen collected should be appropriately preserved, labeled for proper identification, and dispatched.

The information required along with the specimen intended for submission that will aid in diagnosis include the following:

- Species identification.
- Clinical history.
- Relevant clinical/necropsy findings.
- Nature of the sample collected and the mode employed in collection and preservation.

- Disease suspected or type of examination requested.
- Date and time of death and sample collection if collected from a dead animal in case of a disease outbreak.

It is the responsibility of the examiner to notify relevant government offices where the specimen is collected from a suspected case of a highly contagious, zoonotic, or exotic disease. Adequately labeled specimens taken from such cases warn others about the potential of spreading the infection or of posing a danger to the biological system, or to the courier of the specimen if improper handling occurs. The method of collection of tissues and preservative for different examinations are discussed in the following.

5.1 Why Are Samples Collected?

There are several reasons why samples may need to be collected for detection of diseases, including but not restricted to:

- Outbreak investigation: diagnosis of PPR, enterotoxemia, fasciolosis, hemorrhagic septicemia, etc.
- Serological surveillance programs to estimate the prevalence of disease in an endemic situation.
- Serological surveillance programs to demonstrate freedom from infection or transmission.
- Postvaccination monitoring.
- Research purposes.

The type of sample to be collected depends on purpose of the investigation, the timing of sample collection in relation to any clinical disease, and the vaccination status of the population under investigation.

5.2 Who Should Collect the Samples?

In an outbreak situation, samples should generally be collected by veterinary officers appointed to investigate the outbreak. Whoever is appointed to collect samples should be aware of this responsibility before the outbreak occurs and be adequately trained to carry out this role.

5.3 Sample Collection and Emergency Preparedness

Preparations for successful sample collection and submission should be in place in readiness for possible disease outbreaks rather than starting at the time of the outbreak. When samples are collected in an outbreak situation there will be little warning and it is therefore important to have trained personnel and suitable equipment prepared in advance. It is also important that field veterinarians are able to make contact with laboratories for advice if needed. Therefore, current contact details for local, national, and reference laboratories should be made available to field staff at all times.

5.4 Various Samples and Sample Collection Methods from Diseased Goats

5.4.1 Sampling Lesions

Lesions represent the richest source of infectious agents, so they are the sampling area of choice for detection of the causative agent, virus, bacteria, or fungi. It is important that animals are restrained well for sample collection (and sedated if considered necessary for personnel safety and animal welfare), as the lesions will be painful and the animal will resist handling of the affected areas.

Some principles should be followed for collection and handling of samples from lesions:

- Samples should be as fresh as possible and should be sent to the laboratory urgently and by the most direct route.
- Always contact the laboratory beforehand to inform its staff that the samples are being sent and the estimated time of arrival.
- Ensure samples are suitably labeled as hazardous biological material.
- Samples should be kept cool but not frozen (unless advised by the laboratory) from collection until delivery to the laboratory.
- Use of buffered media/proper preservative (as described later) is recommended.

- Adequate quantities of tissue/fluid should be collected and submitted.
- Use of a separate tube/container for each animal is advised.
- Labeling packaging and transportation keeping the sample at the proper temperature is very important for good results and correct diagnosis.

5.4.2 Epithelium in Cases of Foot and Mouth Disease

Epithelium can be taken from vesicles (either unruptured or recently ruptured) or from around the edges of erosions (Figure 5.1). Fresher vesicles are the preferable sites for sample collection. Up to $2\,cm^2$ or $1\,g$ of epithelium is ideal from foot, mouth, or teat lesions. If this is not available, then as much as possible should be collected for submission. Samples from fresh lesions may rub off or you may need to gently grasp the epithelium with forceps before cutting a section away (Britton 2015). On collection, the epithelial samples should be placed in a suitable transport media that maintains the epithelium within the required pH range. Kitching and Donaldson (1987) recommend that the specimens are suspended in a mixture of equal amounts of glycerine and $0.04\,M$ phosphate buffer pH 7.2–7.6, preferably with added antibiotics. There will be considerable loss of viability if samples are sent in buffer outside of this pH range.

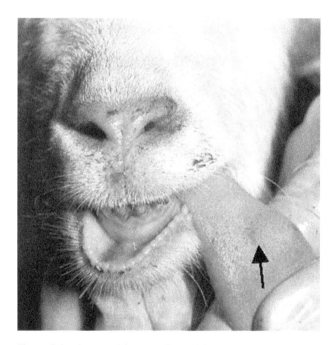

Figure 5.1 A goat with a two-day-old foot and mouth disease lesion (arrow). *Source:* Department for Environment Food & Rural Affairs / CC BY 4.0.

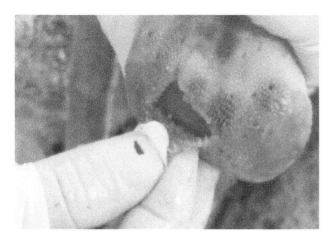

Figure 5.2 Sample collection from a ruptured vesicle. *Source: World Organisation for Animal Health/https://rr-asia.woah.org/wp-content/uploads/2020/02/seacfmd-manual-7.pdf.*

5.4.3 Vesicular Fluid

If an unruptured vesicle is observed on the tongue of an affected goat (Figure 5.2), fluid can be withdrawn from within the vesicle and submitted in a plain tube or sterile sample container. Up to 5 ml fluid can be collected and should be placed in a container that is suitable for the volume of fluid to allow for easier recovery of the fluid from the container at the laboratory (Britton 2015). The fluid should be collected using a sterile needle (narrow gauge) and syringe.

5.4.4 Sampling Whole Blood

Whole blood samples are generally collected for hematology, clinical chemistry, toxicology, direct examination for bacteria or parasites, polymerase chain reaction (PCR) testing, immunological testing, or for culture for bacteria or viruses. Dependent on testing needs, whole blood, blood cells, and/or plasma samples can be obtained from whole blood collected in appropriate anticoagulants. In selecting the anticoagulant to be used, the collector must be aware of the laboratory tests, including PCR-based diagnostics, clinical chemistry, and toxicology, which may be negatively affected by the presence of specific anticoagulants or preservatives. Ethylenediaminetetraacetate (EDTA) is a good anticoagulant for routine diagnostic tests. To be effective, anticoagulants require that the collected blood be thoroughly mixed with the chosen anticoagulant during or immediately following its sampling from the animal.

5.4.5 Sampling Blood (for Serum)

Serum may be used for identification of the agent during an active outbreak, and for detection of antibody following a suspected outbreak. It is also used in serological surveillance studies and postvaccination monitoring for detection of antibodies resulting from exposure to infectious agents or vaccine. Most of the time serum separated from blood gets hemolyzed, so proper process should be followed:

- Blood collection should be done from the jugular vein using a sterile needle and syringe or a plain vacutainer (no anticoagulant should be added) (Figures 5.3 and 5.4).
- At least 2–3 ml of serum should be submitted to the laboratory for investigation. Therefore, it is preferable to collect at least 5–10 ml of whole blood.
- Ensure that the area from which the sample is collected is clean (free from gross contamination).
- Sterile technique should be used during sample collection.
- Blood is usually collected from the jugular vein, based on the restraint methods generally available. After collecting the blood the sample is allowed to stand (in a cool area, out of direct sunlight) for at least 15 minutes to allow clot formation.
- Clear fluid, i.e. serum, should be separated before submission to the laboratory. The sample should be centrifuged or, if this is not available, stood in an upright position overnight.
- During this time, the sample should be kept in a refrigerator or cool box. If a cool box is used, the icepacks should be sealed to prevent wetting of the sample.
- If dispatch to a laboratory is delayed, serum samples should be frozen and stored at −20 °C.

5.4.6 Feces

Feces should be collected freshly voided or preferably directly from the rectum/cloaca for testing for the presence of microorganisms, parasite examination, or fecal occult blood determination. It can also be collected for culture and molecular-based diagnostics from the rectum/cloaca using cotton or gauze-tipped swabs, dependent on the volume of sample required by the specific test methodology. Samples collected on swabs should be kept moist by placing them in the transport medium. The transport medium depends on the type of test to be done on fecal samples, which may range from sterile saline to culture media containing antimicrobials or stabilizers. Fecal specimens should be kept chilled (e.g. refrigerated at 4 °C or on ice) and tested as early as possible after collection to minimize the negative impacts on test results caused by death of the targeted microorganism, bacterial overgrowth, or hatching of parasite eggs. Double packaging of fecal samples in screw-cap or sealable containers that are subsequently contained within sealed plastic bags is mandatory to prevent cross-contamination of samples and associated packaging materials.

Stopper Color	Additive	Sample Obtained	Intended Use/Disadvantages
Red	None	Serum	Routine use for all tests. Prolonged clot exposure results in decreased glucose and Ca and increased phosphorus. Hemolysis problems usually occur.
Gray	Na Fluoride or K Oxalate	Serum	Glycolytic inhibitor for sensitive glucose analysis
Royal Blue	Plastic Stopper Na Heparin	Serum, Plasma, or Whole Blood	Trace mineral analysis, especially Zn
Lavender	EDTA	Whole Blood, Plasma	Routine use for Complete Blood Count/ EDTA chelates Ca, Mg and decrease enzyme activities
Green	Na Heparin	Plasma, Whole Blood	Routine analyses for either plasma or whole blood/No effect on metabolites
Red and Gray	Serum Separator plug	Serum	During centrifugation gel plug moves completely separate the serum from the clot/hemolysis can be a problem

Figure 5.3 Types of blood collection tubes. *Source:* Reproduced by permission of Abu Dhabi Agriculture and Food Safety Authority from www.adafsa.gov.ae/English/PolicyAndLegislations/AdvisoryGuidlines/Documents/Guideline%207%20of%202019%20 Collection%20and%20Shipment%20of%20Animal%20Biological%20Samples.pdf.

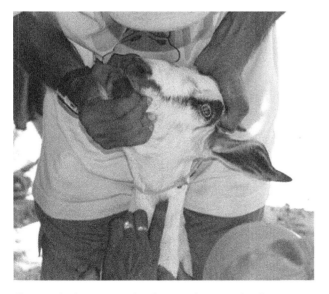

Figure 5.4 Blood collection from the jugular vein of a goat. *Source:* World Organisation for Animal Health / https://rr-asia. woah.org/wp-content/uploads/2020/02/seacfmd-manual-7.pdf.

5.4.7 Ocular Sampling

The surface of the eye can be sampled by swabbing or ocular scraping, ensuring that cells rather than mucopurulent discharge or lachrymal fluids are collected for testing. Specimens from conjunctiva are typically collected by holding the palpebra apart and gently swabbing the area using cotton. Such swabs should be kept moist in saline or transport medium specifically recommended for use with the testing to be performed.

5.4.8 Sampling the Reproductive Tract

Preputial and vaginal washings/fluids and swabs of the cervix and urethra are used as specimens for investigation of reproductive diseases. Semen specimens are typically obtained by use of an artificial vagina or by extrusion of the penis and artificial stimulation. Avoid contamination of the specimen with antiseptic or detergent solutions used to prepare the animal/site for sampling.

5.4.9 Environment and Feed

Environment sampling may be of litter, water from troughs and drinkers, or feed that has been exposed to urine, feces, and/or saliva of the affected animal.

Bacterial and viral diseases like anthrax, enterotoxemia, tetanus, gas gangrene, caseous lymphadenitis, listeriosis, tuberculosis, Johne's disease, pasteurellosis, brucellosis, foot rot, contagious caprine pleuropneumonia, PPR, FMD, and pox affect goats and can cause various ailments. Some diseases can cause heavy mortality, leading to huge economic losses to the farmer. Table 5.1 shows a list of important diseases of goats, their clinical signs, and samples to be collected antemortem and postmortem.

Table 5.1 Important diseases of goat, their clinical signs, and samples collected antemortem and postmortem.

Disease	Symptoms	Antemortem samples collected for diagnosis	Postmortem samples collected for diagnosis
Bacterial disease			
Anthrax	Sudden fever and death Dark colored bloody discharge from natural orifices such as nose, anus, and vagina	Smears from ear vein, discharge from swelling Whole blood with or without anticoagulant	Smear of blood from ear vein or caudal vein Whole blood should be collected from ear vein/caudal vein Exudate or blood-mixed soil should be placed in a sealed pack Pieces of ear or muzzle should be placed in a sterile container for Ascoli's test
Hemorrhagic septicemia	Fever, dysentery, swelling of lower mandible, death More occurrences in rainy season	Smears from ear vein, discharge from swelling Whole blood with or without anticoagulant Nasal swab	Blood smears or exudates obtained from edematous swelling using sterile syringe Heart blood with or without anticoagulant Portion of lungs, spleen, mediastinal lymph nodes on ice Lungs and other affected tissues in 10% formalin
Brucellosis	Abortion during late pregnancy, infertility, scrotal swelling in male, joint swelling	Serum after 2–3 weeks from abortion Vaginal discharge Discharge from testis of males Seminal plasma	Fetal stomach tied off Pieces of stomach, liver, placenta, aborted fetus on ice Affected tissue in 10% formalin
Enterotoxemia	Sudden death in young growing kids Mucous diarrhea may also be seen during death	Fecal sample in sterile container	Smears from bowel mucus membrane and intestinal loop or samples of ingesta from duodenum, jejunum ileum preserved in 3–4 drops of chloroform Transportation should be immediate
Pneumonia	Respiratory distress, discharge from nostrils	Nasal swabs in sterile container	Tracheal swabs, discharge from lung lesions, impression smears from lung Affected tissues in 10% formalin
Foot rot	Wound in foot region	Pus in sterile container	Impression smears and swabs from affected region, small pieces of affected tissue in 10% formalin
Mastitis	Swelling of udder, change in milk quality and quantity	Milk sample in sterile vial	Impression smear and swabs from cut surface of affected region Small pieces of affected tissue in 10% formalin

(Continued)

Table 5.1 (Continued)

Disease	Symptoms	Antemortem samples collected for diagnosis	Postmortem samples collected for diagnosis
Mycoplasmosis/ contagious caprine pleuropneumonia (CCPP)	Chronic coughing	Swabs from sinus/trachea. Nasal and vaginal swabs, preferably in Amies transport medium on ice. Serum samples (paired serum)	Small pieces of affected lung tissues in 10% formalin
Tuberculosis	Chronic coughing	Sputum in a sterile swab, sample of milk from infected udder. Feces in a sterile container	Smear from enlarged lymph nodes showing nodular lesions. Lungs, lymph glands, intestine, mesenteric lymph glands should be collected if lesions are seen, on ice
Johne's disease	Diarrhea, anorexia, weight loss	Rectal pinch, swab/smear	Small pieces of, intestine, lungs, lymph nodes in 10% formalin
Tetanus	Difficulty in walking	Smear from exudates or wounds	Muscles, spinal cord, and brain on ice and in 10% formalin separately
Viral diseases			
Peste des petits ruminants (PPR)	Fever, ocular and nasal mucous discharge, mouth lesions, respiratory distress	Ocular, buccal, rectal, nasal swabs on ice, no preservative should be added. Paired serum samples	Pieces of spleen, lymph nodes, lungs, liver on ice. Lungs, liver, spleen, tonsil in 10% formalin for histopathology
Foot and mouth disease	Vesicular lesions on mouth and feet, excess salivary secretion, difficult in walking, fever	Oral swab, pharyngeal swabs, vesicular fluid, foot lesion scrapings	Lymph nodes, kidney, adrenal gland, heart, thyroid gland on ice and in 10% formalin
Goat pox	Fever, ocular and nasal mucous discharge, respiratory distress, pox lesion in unhairy parts such as lips, thigh, udder	Swabs from pox lesions	Pieces of skin and other organs in 10% formalin
Endoparasitic diseases			
Flukeworm	Emaciation, anemia, edema in lower jaw	Fecal sample	Whole parasites observed in liver and other organs. Small pieces of affected organ in 10% formalin
Tapeworm	Reduced growth, fever, kid mortality	Fecal sample	Worms as such and small pieces of affected tissues in 10% formalin
Roundworm	Fever, anemia, edema in lower jaw, reduced growth	Fecal sample	Worms as such and small pieces of affected tissues in 10% formalin
Coccidiosis	Blood-tinged brownish diarrhea, anemia, kid mortality	Fecal sample	For coccidial oocysts, 2.5% potassium dichromate solution is preferred transport medium
Ectoparasitic infestation			
Ticks, lice, etc.	Reduced growth, loss of skin shine, skin allergy	Skin scrapings from lesions, including some hair roots, unpreserved in tightly sealed container	Affected skin in 10% formalin

5.4.9.1 Collection of Tissue/Other Material for Microbiological Examination

When any bacterial disease is suspected on antemortem or postmortem examination of a goat, the following points should be remembered while collecting samples for microbiological examination:

- Specimens intended for microbiological examination should be collected aseptically. Instruments must be flamed before collecting each specimen or use of separate sterile instruments is advised for the collection of samples.
- Samples from the gut or intestine should be collected last.
- It is recommended to sear the surface of the organ or tissue with a hot spatula, then incise and collect the required material from the deeper portion of solid organs, abscesses, or coagulated masses. From this incision, sterile swabs, tissue fragments, and aspirates may then be taken.
- Place sterile swabs and aspirates in a special transport medium, especially if the suspect organism is a fastidious one. The choice of transport medium depends largely on the microorganism suspected to be present in the specimen.
- Sterile swabs should be taken from body cavities or openings. The swabs should be taken immediately before fully opening this part of the animal cadaver.
- Hollow organs such as segments of the gastrointestinal tract (GIT) are best handled by obtaining via a loop tied at both ends and placed in a sterile petri dish.
- For bacteriological examination, samples should be collected in completely sterile conditions without using any chemical preservative and dispatched on natural ice.
- For viral examination, the preservative is 5–10 volumes of 50% buffered glycerine.
- For mycological studies, skin scrapings are collected in 20% potassium hydroxide solution.

5.4.9.2 Collection of Tissue for Toxicological/Poisoning Examination

Goats are very independent and curious creatures. As part of their curiosity, they explore their world by mouthing and tasting things, which has earned them the unfortunate reputation of eating everything and anything. In fact goats are the most fastidious of eaters. They are mixed feeders and agile and inquisitive animals, so they may gain access to toxic plants. This can occur when the goat escapes from their enclosure into an ornamental garden or if plants grow into the living area. Poisoning may also occur if toxic plants are trimmed and their clippings are fed to goats or left where they can gain access. It is important to identify any plant in the goat's environment and to remove or restrict access to any potential hazards.

There are several plants that can be poisonous to goats. However, the severity of plant poisoning depends on the quantity of the plant that was eaten, the degree of ground moisture, the health of the animal prior to consuming the toxic plant, and the size and age of the animal that consumed the plant. Under normal circumstances, animals will not consume poisonous plants. However, there are some factors that might cause goats to eat poisonous plants. Those factors include starvation, unbalanced rations, overgrazing, and drought; allowing animals to have access to yard waste or newly plowed areas where roots from toxic plants are exposed; allowing the herd to have access to dry or partially dry water hoses; incidental ingestion of toxic plants; and just plain curiosity.Some examples of poisonous plants include azaleas, China berries, sumac, dog fennel, bracken fern, curly dock, eastern baccharis, honeysuckle, nightshade, pokeweed, red root pigweed, black cherry, Virginia creeper, and crotalaria. Milk weed is often eaten during dry seasons when there is not much else to find to eat or if has been cut and baled up in hay. The process of drying out does not reduce its toxicity and as little as 0.25% of the goat's body weight is toxic. Clinical signs such as bloating, dilated pupils, and weakness are observed. Nitrate poisoning is a condition that may affect small ruminants consuming certain forage or water containing an excessive amount of nitrate. Some plants are more likely to accumulate nitrate than others. Crops capable of high levels of nitrate accumulation under adverse conditions include corn, small grains, Sudan grass, and sorghum, which can cause toxicity and produce clinical signs in goats.

Along with plants, pesticides also cause poisoning in goats. Clinical signs exhibited by goats are similar in any poisoning. The earliest signs of poisoning are hypersalivation, abdominal discomfort, diarrhea or constipation, ruminal stasis, and distension. Animals may appear to be disoriented by weakness, depressed, and dull. Initial diuresis is followed by oliguria and collapse, recumbency, and convulsions; death can occur in severe case. Laboratory findings include hyperkalemia, hypophosphatemia, acidosis, raised creatine kinase, and leukocytosis.

To diagnose a case of poisoning sample collection and handling are critical for toxicology analysis. The appropriate sample must be collected and preserved so that accurate analysis can be undertaken. In general for animals that die acutely without clinical signs, collection of urine, stomach contents, and ocular fluid is helpful. In addition to these samples, fresh liver, kidney, fat, and brain should be collected and refrigerated or frozen. Do not formalize any tissues that will be used for toxicology testing.

- Materials taken for toxicological examination should be free from any contaminating chemicals being used during necropsy. Chemicals that may contaminate the specimen include fixatives, detergents, and disinfectants routinely used during necropsy.
- Collect the samples in clean, wide-mouthed, stoppered glass/plastic bottles of 1 l capacity and use separate bottles for each of the materials.
- No chemical preservative should be added to the samples and preferably samples should be sent on dry ice/in refrigerated conditions.

- The materials required for laboratory examination in cases of poisoning are indicated in Table 5.2.

5.4.9.3 Collection of Tissue for Parasitological Examination

There are very high economic losses due to worm infestation, either internal or external, like tapeworms, roundworms, flukes, ticks, and lice. It is a ubiquitous phenomenon affecting all classes of livestock, especially goats, that is hampering the development of the livestock/goat industry. The worm-infested animals become unthrifty, lethargic, and less responsive, and it causes chronic diseases and ultimately the death of both young and older animals.

Table 5.2 Specimens to be collected in suspected cases of poisoning.

S. no.	Suspected material to be collected	Amount and indications
a	Stomach and its contents	About 500–1000 g in large animals and all available contents in small animals
		In suspected cases of poisoning from mycotoxins or certain plants
b	Upper part of small intestine with its contents Any suspicious substance in stomach and intestine	About 500–1000 g in large animals and all available contents in small animals
		In suspected cases of poisoning from mycotoxins or certain plants
c	Liver	About 500–1000 g in large animals or whole liver in small animals
		In suspected cases of poisoning from mycotoxins like aflatoxin present in feed and for confirmation of toxicity conditions affecting the animals, like cyanide, organophosphates, selenium, arsenic, carbamates, and certain plant poisonings
d	Kidney	One complete kidney
		In suspected cases of poisoning from mycotoxins like ochratoxin, other toxicity conditions, and plant poisonings
e	Spleen	Complete or a portion if large
		For confirmation of toxicity conditions affecting the animals like cyanide, organophosphates, selenium, arsenic, carbamates, and certain plant poisonings
f	Urine (all available) and feces in preservative kept separately	Sufficient quantity
		Thymol used for preserving urine if rectified spirit is contraindicated
		For confirmation of toxicity conditions affecting the animal like cyanide, organophosphates, selenium, arsenic, carbamates, and certain plant poisonings such as *Senecio*, *Astragalus*, *Crotolaria*
g	Heart and portion of brain	In suspected cases of poisoning by strychnine
h	Lung tissue and heart blood without adding preservative	In suspected cases of poisoning by carbon monoxide, coal gas, hydrocyanic acid, alcohol, or chloroform
i	Portion of skin and subcutaneous tissue	In suspected cases of poisoning by subcutaneous injection
j	Hair	About 5–10 g in suspected cases of subacute or chronic poisoning by minerals, especially arsenic or lead (most minerals are eliminated through the hair)
k	Portion of long bones	In suspected cases of subacute or chronic poisoning by arsenic and antimony (especially in a case of extreme putrefaction or if the body is exhumed after a long burial)

Irrespective of breed, sex, and age, goats harbor a wide variety of worms: nematodes, cestodes, and trematodes, collectively called helminths; a few species of protozoa; and external infestation with varieties of ticks, lice, mites, fleas, and flies.

The most prevalent nematodes or roundworms identified as species of parasites include *Strongyloides*, *Haemonchus contortus*, *Bunostomum phlebotomum*, *Oesophagostomum* spp., *Cooperia* spp., *Trichostrongylus* spp., *Toxocara vitulorum*, *Ostertagia ostertagi*, and *Nematodirus* spp., rumen worm, and lung worm in the GIT. Among nematodes, *H. contortus* is highly pathogenic and causes mortality too. Among cestodes or tapeworms, *Moniezia* spp. especially *M. expansa* cause disease in small animals (sheep and goats). Among trematodes, flukes like the liver fluke or *Fasciola hepatica* are important in small and large ruminants and cause severe jaundice affecting the liver. Coccidiosis is a protozoan disease that can also infect small ruminants. Among protozoa causing coccidiosis, *Eimeria arloingi*, *E. christenseni*, and *E. ovinoidalis* are highly pathogenic in kids. *E. ninakohlyakimovae* is the commonest one, followed by *E. arloingi*, *E. caprina*, and *E. hirci*. Clinical signs include diarrhea with or without mucus or blood, dehydration, emaciation, weakness, anorexia, and death. It causes enteritis and bloody diarrhea leading to less assimilation of nutrients, anemia, and weight loss. External parasites like ticks, lice, mites, fleas, and flies are important and equally cause losses, low productivity, blood drain/losses, less feed concentration, loss in milk letdown, especially at dusk and dawn, and even loss of life. Hemoprotozoans like *Theileria* are reported in goats and cause severe anemia, leading to the death of the animal.

Only 5–10% of internal parasites actually reside within an individual animal, and the rest are present in the pasture, infecting the animal as it grazes. Therefore it is very important to collect samples from a diseased goat to diagnose parasitic infestation. It will help in proper therapeutic management of the worm load. Ectoparasites and endoparasites are collected during necropsy for identification before opening the carcass from the skin and after opening the carcass from the GIT.

- Ticks, fleas, and lice should be carefully brushed off from the fur and fixed in 10% formalin. To disable these organisms, wet the fur of the animal with a detergent solution.
- In collecting ticks, prevent the mouthparts of the tick from damage by wiping the body part of the tick with ether. This will kill the tick and allow it to drop off.
- Fix the collected specimens in 70% ethyl alcohol or 10% formalin. Information about the degree of ectoparasite infestation should be provided along with the submission.

- Collect mange mites by scraping the affected skin deeply and put the scrapings on a glass slide with a drop of mineral oil. Collect the skin scrapings in 10% potassium hydroxide.
- Roundworms collected from intestinal segments may be fixed in 10% formalin immediately after collection. Allow them to relax by dipping in menthol solution or lukewarm water before fixation to prevent curling of the specimen.
- Tapeworm segments collected should include both mature and immature segments, with the scolex still intact. Never lift the tapeworm from its attachment, as this will break the scolex. The scolex is important in species identification. Excise the part where the scolex is attached and fix it in formalin.
- Press specimens of cestodes between two glass slides held together by a rubber band, a piece of twine, or paper clips before immersion in the fixative.
- For total worm count in ruminants, tie the abomasum at both ends and save all its contents.
- Scraping the deep mucosa of the affected intestinal segment and examining the scrapings as a wet smear make do the diagnosis of coccidial infection. Coccidial oocyst feces are collected in 2.5% dichromate.

5.4.9.4 Collection of Specimens for Cytological Examination

- It is often possible to reach a diagnosis by preparing and examining smears (from cut surfaces of the tumor) and aspirates even before tissue blocks of the tumor tissues are processed by a conventional paraffin embedding technique.
- Allow the smears to dry immediately after collection to preserve the cell architecture.
- Fixation may be done by heat treatment or by dipping in absolute methanol.
- Smears may be prepared from body fluids by putting a few drops onto a glass slide.
- The fluid may be collected and centrifuged and the cell pellet at the bottom of the tube fixed in formalin or methanol and the smears prepared.
- Alternatively, use gelatin or albumin to suspend the cell pellet and then fix the mixture in formalin. This preparation may then be submitted for routine paraffin embedding technique similar to a tissue block.

5.4.9.5 Collection of Body Cavity Fluids

Typically there is little fluid present in the peritoneal, pleural, and pericardial cavities, and thus they are considered potential spaces. These serous body cavities are lined by specialized cells, termed mesothelial cells. Clinical signs of the presence of increased amounts of fluid include abdominal distension, abdominal pain, dyspnea, muffled heart sounds, and cardiac arrhythmia. Collection and evaluation of fluid from these sites may be therapeutic as well as diagnostic for the presence of inflammatory, hemorrhagic, neoplastic, lymphatic, or bilious conditions. Additionally, further diagnostic tests may be indicated by the cytological characteristics. Removal and examination of fluid are highly recommended unless anesthetic risk or bleeding diathesis is present or further injury is likely. The body fluids include blood, urine, cerebrospinal fluid, synovial fluid, serum, and also effusions formed in cavities during the disease process.

5.4.10 Abdominal Fluid

Place the patient in left lateral recumbency and restrained. Clip and surgically prepare an area (e.g. 4–6 in. square) with the umbilicus in the center. The urinary bladder should be emptied before performing paracentesis. Infiltrate a small area with local anesthetic, if desired. Use a 20–22-gauge needle or over-the-needle catheter to penetrate the abdomen. Attempt to obtain fluid in four quadrants, allowing the fluid to flow freely by gravity and capillary action.

5.4.11 Pleural Fluid

For removal of fluid from the thorax, the patient should be standing or in ventral/sternal recumbency. Clip the hair and surgically prepare the thoracic wall from the 5th to the 11th intercostal space. Infiltrate a small area at the 7th–8th intercostal space at the level of the costochondral junction with local anesthetic. Insert the needle or catheter into the chest wall at the surgically prepared site, taking care to avoid the intercostal vessels located just caudal to each rib.

5.4.12 Pericardial Fluid

For removal of fluid from the pericardial sac, sedate the patient if necessary. Surgically prepare an area over the lower to mid-5th–7th intercostal space bilaterally. Place the patient in lateral or sternal recumbency. Infiltrate an area at the costochondral junction, or approximately where the lower and mid-thorax meet, with local anesthetic. Use an over-the-needle catheter or Intrafusor system with a three-way valve to which a 30 ml syringe is attached. Always maintain negative pressure on the syringe as the chest wall is punctured. Carefully advance the needle into the 4th intercostal space through a nick incision in the direction of the heart. Collect the fluid.

- The general rule in collecting body fluids is to obtain samples free from contaminants.
- Body fluids should be collected as the examination progresses if it is anticipated that such an examination is required.

- Urine may be collected directly from the urinary bladder by aspiration.
- Pleural, pericardial, synovial, or cerebrospinal fluid should be collected by aspirating the fluid through a syringe and needle.
- In a case of abortion, particularly in brucellosis, stomach contents from the aborted fetus may be collected with the help of a sterilized syringe or Pasteur pipette.

The fluid should be collected into both a lavender-top tube (EDTA anticoagulant) for cytology and a red-top tube (or any sterile tube without additives) for potential bacterial culture. Also at collection make both direct unconcentrated smears by a squash or blood smear technique and smears from spun samples. Romanowsky-type stains such as Wright stain or an aqueous-based Wright (quick) stain can be used on a few slides for immediate in-house evaluation. The remaining unstained smears, as well as an EDTA and serum tube filled with fluid, should be submitted to the laboratory. This will allow the clinical pathologist evaluating the sample to compare the cellularity of the sample and the appearance of the cells at the time of collection with what was submitted in the tube. Septic causes (e.g. bacterial, fungal, protozoal, viral) and non-septic causes (e.g. bile peritonitis, pancreatitis, steatitis, abscesses, inflammation associated with neoplasia) are responsible for exudate formation as result of infection. Metabolic and deficiency causes can form transudate in the diseased animal. Therefore, collection and evaluation of body cavity fluids is a very important method for diagnosing the disease condition.

5.4.13 Collection of Tissue from Dead Animals

This to be performed by experienced personnel in the discipline of veterinary pathology who are well trained in the correct procedures for examination of the subject species of animal, to select the most favorable organs and lesions for sampling. The purpose of sample collection may include microbiological culture, parasitology, biochemistry, histopathology, immuno-histochemistry, and detection of proteins, prions, or genome nucleic acids.

- For histopathological examinations, the pieces of organs/tissues particularly showing lesions should be collected in 10% neutral buffered formalin immediately during the postmortem examination and these pieces should not be more than 0.5 cm thick.
- Moreover, the tissue should include both the normal and abnormal portion (lesion) of the organ or tissue.
- Collect the tissue using a sharp knife or scissors, taking care not to crush the tissue or allow it to dry, otherwise

this will cause undue distortions on the morphology of cells in the tissues.

- Fix the collected tissue immediately in 20 times the tissue volume of 10% neutral buffered formalin.
- Wash the specimen in physiological saline solution before fixing it in formalin, if it is heavily soiled with debris/blood.
- In the case of brain, the whole brain may be immersed in a large volume of the fixative. Allow it to harden for 24 hours, and then slice the brain and take the desired sections.
- Cut open the segment of the GIT longitudinally before putting it in the fixative to ensure adequate and prompt preservation of the mucosal lining and to increase the surface area for penetration of the fixative.

5.5 Submission/Dispatch of Specimens to the Diagnostic Laboratory

The transport of diagnostic specimens from the place of postmortem to the diagnostic laboratory is required to confirm the diagnosis. These diagnostic specimens must be handled as infectious substances; therefore, proper dispatch of specimens is required so that the material has no possibility of escaping from the package. This is a brief account of labeling, sealing, and packing of specimens:

- **Labeling**: Use a method of labeling that means the specimen cannot be lost or easily destroyed. For example, adhesive tape should go entirely around the vial so that it will not be dislodged by moisture. Writing should be with pencil or waterproof ink. It is advisable to put labeled paper inside the specimen bottle and paste a similar label on the outside of the specimen bottle. The label should carry the following information: (i) case number; (ii) species; and (iii) name of the organ. A piece of absorbent cotton should invariably be placed to keep the tissues moist, particularly for floating tissues, and in case the bottle is broken during transit.
- **Sealing**: Enough care should be taken to seal the mouth of the bottle by paraffin wax so as to make it water tight. Use plastic screw-cap containers instead of glass containers where practical. Electrical tape should be wound around the cap in the same direction as the screw cap is applied.
- **Packing**: Sealed and labeled receptacles containing specimens should be placed in a suitable container along with the history sheet and/or postmortem report bearing the clinical/postmortem diagnosis as the case may be. Enough packing material should be provided to ensure safe delivery of the contents in the laboratory.

5.5.1 Precautions in Forwarding Material

The following methods are erroneous and must be avoided:

- Sending large pieces of tissue such as whole organ. In this case only the surface of the tissues is preserved and the interior undergoes autolysis, rendering the tissue unfit for correct histopathological examinations.
- Forcing large pieces of tissue or a whole organ into a small receptacle. With the hardening effect of fixation like with formalin, it is impossible to remove the material without breaking the bottle; moreover, the tissue is mutilated.
- Sending material from the center of an extensive lesion like suppuration or a tumor, which does not give the maximum amount of information.

5.5.2 Dispatch of Material

The following points must be kept in mind when dispatching material to a laboratory for diagnosis:

- Describe the clinical signs, lesions, tentative diagnosis, and treatment given to the animal in your letter. Also mention the type of test you want with your tentative diagnosis.
- Write the correct address on the letter as well as on the parcel, preferably with the pin/postal code, if the material is sent through the post.
- Mark the parcel "Biological material," "Handle with care," "Glass material," "Fragile," etc. in order to avoid damage to the parcel. Also mark the side to be kept uppermost with arrows.
- Seal the container so that it cannot leak in transit.
- Try to send the material as soon as possible after its collection from the animal.
- Keep one copy of the cover letter inside the parcel and send another copy by hand or post in a separate envelope.
- Keep adequate material such as thermocol (polystyrene) in the parcel to save the material from outside pressure or jerking.
- Use dry ice if available, or ice in sealed containers.

5.5.3 Biosecurity

Strict biosecurity precautions should be taken by personnel involved when visiting outbreak areas for the purposes of sample collection, or even when samples are collected from apparently healthy animals for routine monitoring purposes. It is very important that everyone implements good personal biosecurity measures as well as thorough cleaning and disinfection of any vehicles or equipment used so that they do not transmit the infectious agent.

Multiple-Choice Questions

1 Which of the following is used as a preservative for tissues collected for histopathological examination?
   A 10% neutral buffered formalin
   B Acetone
   C Ether
   D None of the above

2 If PPR virus is to be isolated, which preservative will be used for storage of pneumonic lungs?
   A Chloroform
   B Formalin
   C 50% buffered glycerine
   D All of the above

3 If a goat is suffering from fungal infection of skin, which of the following examinations is needed?
   A Histopathological examination
   B Virological examination
   C Skin scraping examination
   D Toxicological examination

4 If a goat is suspected to have died due to ochratoxicosis, which of the following tissue samples must be collected for isolation of ochratoxin?
   A Brain
   B Skin
   C Kidney
   D Spleen

5 Why are clinical samples collected?
   A To investigate an outbreak
   B To estimate the prevalence of disease in an endemic situation
   C To demonstrate freedom from infection or transmission
   D All of the above

6 Which of the following is the sample of choice to diagnose FMD in goats?
   A Vesicular lesions
   B Liver tissue
   C Urine
   D None of the above

7 What should samples collected for bacteriological examination be transported on/in?
   A Formalin
   B Chloroform
   C Ether
   D Ice

8 In a case of abortion, particularly in brucellosis, which of the following is the sample of choice for diagnosis?
   A Stomach contents of fetus
   B Kidney contents of fetus
   C Skin of fetus
   D None of the above

9 What must ticks collected from the body of a goat with dermatitis be preserved in?
   A 70% ethanol
   B 10% formalin
   C 5% ether
   D Both a and b

10 If a goat is suspected to have died due to arsenic poisoning, which of the following samples should be collected for diagnosis?
   A Eye
   B Hair
   C Brain
   D None of the above

11 For coccidial oocysts, which solution is the preferred transport medium?
   A 2.5% potassium dichromate
   B 2% ether
   C 1% sodium hypochlorite
   D All of the above

12 For mycological studies, which solution are skin scrapings collected in?
   A 20% potassium hydroxide
   B 5% potassium hydroxide
   C 2% potassium hydroxide
   D Saturated potassium hydroxide

13 For toxicological analysis, which preservative should be added to the sample collected?
   A No preservative
   B 10% formalin
   C 5% ether
   D Saturated sodium hydroxide

14 To diagnose Johne's disease antemortem, which of the following samples will be preferred?
    A Rectal pinch
    B Voided feces
    C Urine
    D Nasal swab

15 To diagnose mastitis in goats, which sample should be collected?
    A Milk
    B Tissue
    C Feces
    D Urine

References

Britton, S. (2015). *Foot and mouth disease – laboratory samples for diagnosis or exclusion*. Australia: Department of Primary Industries, New South Wales Government.

Kitching, R.P. and Donaldson, A.I. (1987). Collection and transportation of specimens for vesicular virus investigation. *Revue Scientifique et Technique de L'Office International Des Epizooties* 6 (1): 263–272.

Pfeiffer, D. (2010). *Veterinary Epidemiology: An Introduction*. Chichester: Wiley-Blackwell.

6

Parasitic Diseases of Goats

G.K. Chetan Kumar

Department of Veterinary Medicine, Veterinary College Hassan, Karnataka Veterinary, Animal and Fisheries Sciences University, Bidar, Karnataka, India

Parasitic diseases are quite common in goat populations. Goats are popularly known as "walking banks" for farmers, because farmers can sell them whenever they are in need. Parasitic infestation can lead to huge economic losses in terms of milk, meat, and hair/skin if this area is neglected in farming practice. In this chapter we discuss common parasitic infections of the goat.

6.1 Common Trematode Diseases of Goats

6.1.1 Fasciolosis

- **Etiology and parasite description**: The leaf-shaped *Fasciola hepatica* is the largest liver fluke, measuring about 30 mm in length and 13 mm in width. *F. hepatica* has a small oral sucker and a larger acetabulum at the anterior end. *F. gigantica* is much larger than *F. hepatica* and can measure up to 7.5 cm in length. The outer surface or tegument of these flukes is made up of scleroproteins, which give protection from the digestive juices of the definitive host. The digestive system of these flukes is blind and they do not have any external segmentation (Barger and MacNeill 2015). These flat, oval-shaped flukes are hermaphrodites; that is, they have both female and male reproductive organs.
- **Synonyms**: *F. hepatica* is called the common liver fluke/ sheep liver fluke/beef liver fluke, whereas *F. gigantica* is called the tropical liver fluke. The disease is otherwise called liver rot or distomatosis.
- **Predilection sites**: Bile duct and gallbladder.
- **Host and susceptibility**: In goats, fasciolosis is caused by *F. hepatica* and *F. gigantica*. Compared to cattle, goats and sheep are highly susceptible to fasciolosis because they lack both fluke rejection on first exposure and acquired immunity for subsequent exposures for

F. hepatica, although for *F. gigantica* goats have the ability to develop protective immunity (Figure 6.1). Mostly the condition is chronic in nature in goats, and rarely occurs in an acute form leading to huge mortality and morbidity.

- **Geographic distribution**: Fasciolosis is one of the important zoonotic diseases found on all five continents, and is most prevalent in humid temperate climatic regions of the world.
- **Life cycle**: The life cycle of the liver fluke is complex. It requires an intermediate snail host for immature fluke development before entering the definitive host (Figure 6.2). Eggs laid by adult parasites in the definitive host are passed in the stool. These eggs remain dormant in the environment until temperature and humidity become optimum. Then miracidium will be released from embryonated eggs. Miracidium has a life span of 12 hours in which to find a suitable mollusk intermediate host like a snail. Within the snail, a single miracidium develops into hundreds of cercariae and these are released into the environment. In the environment cercariae encyst to become metacercariae and attach to vegetation. The definitive host gets the infection by ingestion of vegetation. In the duodenum of the definitive host excystation occurs and the immature flukes released will penetrate the liver capsule and migrate into the liver parenchyma. By about six weeks flukes migrate to the bile duct and mature to become adults. These mature adult flukes can lay up to 20 000 eggs per day. These eggs are carried to the duodenum through bile and later passed in the stool.
- **Pathogenesis**: Pathogenesis depends on the number of metacercariae ingested: the larger the number, the more severe will be the clinical signs. Migration of immature flukes in the liver leads to traumatic hepatitis, destruction of parenchyma, and massive hemorrhage. In its chronic form hepatic fibrosis and cholangitis are the

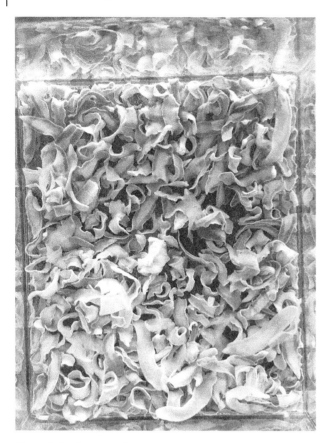

Figure 6.1 Gross specimen of adult liver fluke recovered from a goat.

principal pathological changes observed. Sometime acute fasciolosis can lead to infectious necrotic hepatitis or "black disease" caused by *Clostridium novyi*, which is an anaerobic organism that can proliferate in necrotic hepatic parenchyma.

- **Clinical signs**: Acute fasciolosis, mainly because of immature flukes, is common in goats and sheep but seldom reported in cattle. Chronic fasciolosis is due to adult flukes, and occurs in goats, cattle, and sheep. Animals affected with immature flukes exhibit signs of hepatitis and cholangitis, which can be have other potential causes as well. An animal with adult flukes will exhibit clinical signs of anemia, bottle jaw, loss of appetite, weight loss, and weakness. These signs develop gradually after adult flukes become established in the bile duct.

- **Diagnosis**: Diagnosis is by clinical signs, identification of eggs in the stool, and postmortem examination. Liver fluke eggs are operculated, yellowish to green in color, measuring about $80 \times 140\,\mu m$. Adult flukes lay egg in the biliary tract, and these are carried to and stored in the gallbladder. Eggs are released only when the gallbladder is emptied. Hence a negative fecal examination result is always not conclusive, and the fecal examination should be repeated. In acute fasciolosis the affected liver is increased, will be fragile, and extensive bleeding is noticed because of migration of immature flukes in the liver parenchyma. In chronic fasciolosis the bile duct is thickened and calcified, which can obstruct normal bile flow. Because of calcification of bile duct, the liver appears like a pipe-stem liver. Enzyme-linked immunosorbent assay (ELISA) and a passive hemagglutination test can also be used to identify antibodies against *Fasciola* spp.

- **Treatment and control**: Triclabendazole is an effective benzimidazole derivative that acts against both adult worms and immature flukes. Diamphenethide is the drug of choice for acute fasciolosis. Control of snails and effective treatment of affected animals are very important to control fasciolosis. To control snails and reduce

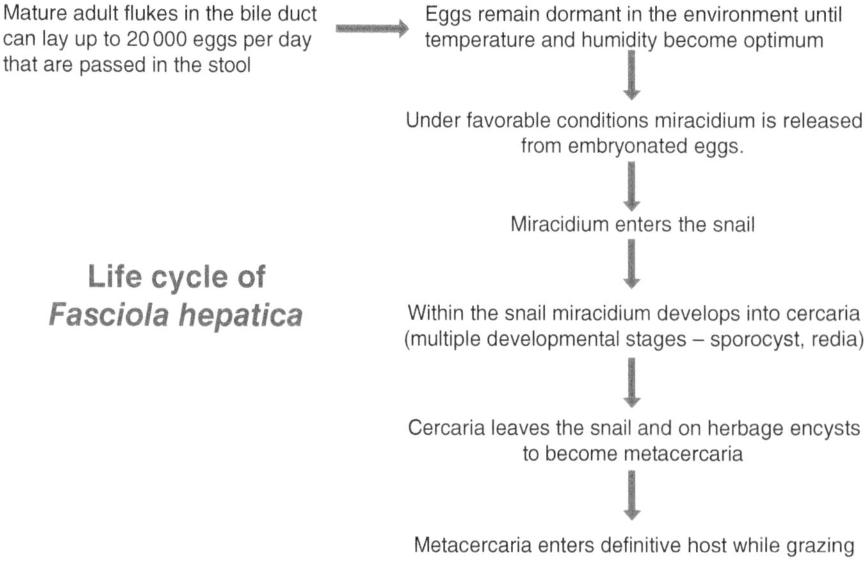

Figure 6.2 Life cycle of *Fasciola* spp.

Life cycle of *Fasciola hepatica*

Mature adult flukes in the bile duct can lay up to 20 000 eggs per day that are passed in the stool

→ Eggs remain dormant in the environment until temperature and humidity become optimum

↓

Under favorable conditions miracidium is released from embryonated eggs.

↓

Miracidium enters the snail

↓

Within the snail miracidium develops into cercaria (multiple developmental stages – sporocyst, redia)

↓

Cercaria leaves the snail and on herbage encysts to become metacercaria

↓

Metacercaria enters definitive host while grazing

the metacercaria load, ensure adequate drainage at pasture and all water points that could facilitate snail survival should be closed.

To reduce fluke infestation, rotational grazing should be adopted, and during the rest phase of pasture the larvae count will be reduced. Alternative grazing with cattle, sheep, and goats is not very useful because these flukes infest all these species. Natural enemies such as fish (Cichlidae), frogs, turtles, waterfowl, ducks, and geese can be used to control snails by biological means. However, the biological method of control is not particularly feasible because these natural enemies also predate other than snails.

Chemicals such as methiocarb, metaldehyde, and ferric tthylenediaminetetraacetic acid (EDTA) can be used as bait to control snails, but should be used with caution. Routine deworming of susceptible flocks is also important. Triclabendazole and rafoxanide can be used to control fluke infestation in goats. Triclabendazole is a narrow-spectrum flukicide and is effective against both adult and immature flukes. Rafoxanide is a medium-spectrum anthelmintic, effective against adult flukes and gastrointestinal roundworms.

6.1.2 Dicrocoeliosis in Goats

- **Etiology and parasite description**: Dicrocoeliosis in goats is caused by *Dicrocoelium dendriticum* (Zajac and Conboy 2012). *D. dendriticum* flukes are much smaller than liver flukes; they have a flat body and are oval in shape. Like liver flukes they are hermaphrodites, and their digestive system is blind with no external segmentation. The adult fluke measures about 10 mm in length and 2 mm in width. Lancet flukes have two suckers, an oral sucker and a ventral sucker, both placed in the anterior part.
- **Synonyms**: Small liver flukes or lancet flukes.

- **Predilection site**: *D. dendriticum* flukes are found in the bile ducts and gallbladder of various domestic and wildlife species.
- **Host and susceptibility**: Dicrocoeliosis affects sheep, cattle, pigs, and goats. Goats are comparatively less susceptible to it than sheep
- **Geographic distribution**: Though the disease occurs worldwide, the condition is quite common in hilly regions like the Himachal Pradesh and Northern Himalayan areas of India.
- **Life cycle and pathogenesis**: The life cycle of *D. dendriticum* flukes is complex; they require two intermediate hosts to complete it (Figure 6.3). A land snail, such as *Macrochlamys cassida*, *Zebrina detrital*, or *Coinella lubrica*, acts as the first intermediate host and the brown ant, *Formica fusca*, acts as the second intermediate host. The definitive host gets the infection by ingestion of metacercariae from infected ants along with herbage. In the definitive host metacercariae excyst and develop into adult worms in the liver. Adult worms reproduce by hermaphroditism or cross-insemination and eggs are released into stool. Released eggs do not hatch till they are swallowed by the first intermediate host; that is, land snails. In the snails, the eggs hatch into sporocysts, develop, and then become cercariae. The cercariae are released from the snail as mucoid slime balls. Cercariae are ingested by ants and develop into metacercariae over a period of two months.
- **Clinical signs**: Clinical signs depend on the migration of *D. dendriticum* young flukes, which migrate directly up the biliary duct system of the liver without penetrating the gut wall, liver capsule, or liver parenchyma as in fasciolosis. Generally no clinical signs are observed in mild infections, but in case of heavy infection signs such as anemia, edema, and emaciation are noticed. Unlike liver fluke infection, fatalities are very rare in dicrocoeliosis.

Figure 6.3 Life cycle of *Dicrocoelium* spp.

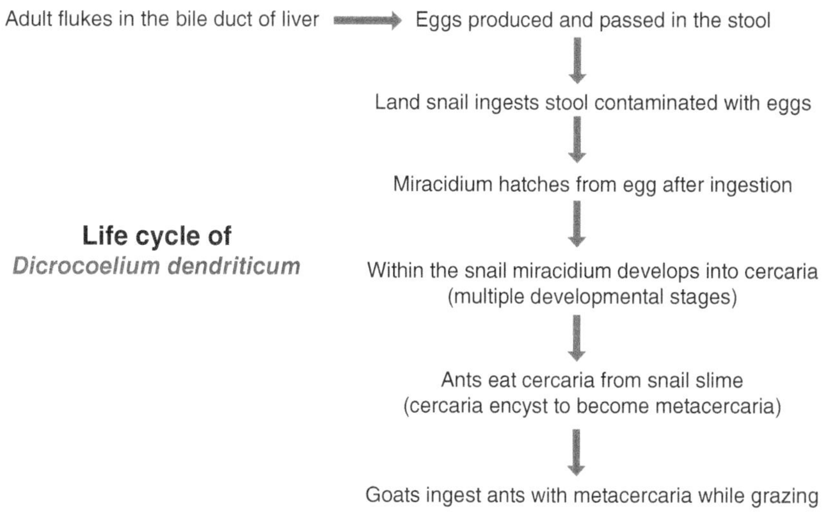

Adult flukes in the bile duct of liver ⟹ Eggs produced and passed in the stool

⬇

Land snail ingests stool contaminated with eggs

⬇

Miracidium hatches from egg after ingestion

⬇

Life cycle of *Dicrocoelium dendriticum*

Within the snail miracidium develops into cercaria (multiple developmental stages)

⬇

Ants eat cercaria from snail slime (cercaria encyst to become metacercaria)

⬇

Goats ingest ants with metacercaria while grazing

- **Diagnosis**: Often dicrocoeliosis is clinically undetected or undiagnosed, because of the subclinical nature of the infection. Diagnosis is mainly by identifying eggs at fecal examination and by recovering adult worms during postmortem examination of an affected animal. Like with liver flukes, negative fecal reports are not conclusive because emptying of the gall bladder is necessary to find eggs in the fecal sample. The eggs are oval in shape, measuring about 25 × 40 μm, brownish in color, and contain miracidium larvae.
- **Treatment and control**: Thiabendazole, fenbendazole, netobimin, and praziquantel are effective in the management of dicrocoeliosis. Control of snails and pasture management are very important to prevent dicrocoeliosis in goats. Albendazole (15 mg/kg body weight), praziquantel (20 mg/kg), and triclabendazole (20 mg/kg) can be used to control lancet flukes. In practice it is not possible to control or eliminate ants to keep the lancet fluke infection low.

6.1.3 Paramphistomiasis in Goats

- **Etiology and parasite description**: Many genera of paramphistomes affect goats and sheep, but the most common species are *Paramphistomum cervi*, *Cotylophoron*, *Calicophoron*, and *Gigantocotyle*. The adult paramphistome parasites are grayish to reddish in color and small in size, measuring 1.5 cm in length and 0.5 cm in width; they are pear shaped with two suckers (Constable et al. 2012).
- **Synonyms**: Stomach flukes or rumen flukes.
- **Predilection sites**: The predilection site of adult *Paramphistomum* flukes is the rumen. Immature flukes are recovered from the duodenum and jejunum.
- **Host and susceptibility**: Paramphistomes are known to infect goats, cattle, sheep, and wild ruminants. Rumen fluke infection is not reported in dogs, cats, or poultry.
- **Geographic distribution**: Paramphistomes occur worldwide, especially in humid regions. *P. cervi* is commonly seen in temperate regions of the world, whereas *Cotylophoron*, *Calicophoron*, and *Gigantocotyle* are seen in tropical and subtropical regions.
- **Life cycle and pathogenesis**: The life cycle is indirect. Planorbid or bulinid snails acts as the intermediate host. Paramphistome eggs are passed in the stool and miracidia hatch in the water and infect the snails (Figure 6.4). The life cycle of *D. dendriticum* in the snail is the same as that of *F. hepatica*, where cercariae released from the snail encyst on herbage. In the goat, the young flukes excyst and remain in the small intestine for 3–6 weeks before migrating forward through the reticulum to the rumen. Paramphistomes usually do not cause overt disease, but large numbers may be encountered. Immature flukes congregate in the duodenum and jejunum and these immature flukes attach to small intestinal mucosa via a large posterior sucker, leading to severe enteritis

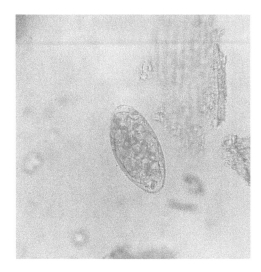

Figure 6.4 Clear, operculated eggs of paramphistome in goat fecal sample (40×).

and hemorrhage (Figure 6.5). The severity of disease depends on how deep the immature flukes have burrowed into the small intestinal mucosa.
- **Clinical signs**: Adult flukes are less harmful, but young flukes are very harmful. The affected animal exhibits diarrhea, anorexia, unthriftiness, anemia, loss of weight, and polydipsia.
- **Diagnosis**: Diagnosis is by identification of large, clear, operculated eggs in the fecal sample. In acute infections eggs will not be identified in feces. Sometimes immature flukes are seen in feces.
- **Treatment and control**: Oxyclozanide at a dose of 15 mg/kg body weight is effective against adult rumen flukes. Control of planorbid or bulinid snails is very important to prevent the occurrence of paramphistomiasis in goats. Oxyclozanide and niclosamide can be used to control paramphistomiasis in goats.

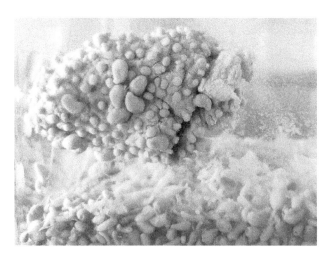

Figure 6.5 Adult paramphistomes recovered from goat rumen.

Oxyclozanide is effective against adult flukes and niclosamide is effective only against immature rumen flukes, not against adults.

6.2 Common Tapeworm Diseases of Goats

6.2.1 Monieziasis

- **Etiology and parasite description**: Monieziasis in goats and sheep is caused by *Moniezia expansa*, which are flat, ribbon-like worms (Fox et al. 2002). *M. expansa* is the longest worm, measuring 1.5 cm in width and up to 10 m in length. They do not have digestive, circulatory, or respiratory systems. Their body is made up of proglottids. Each proglottid has both male and female reproductive organs and once proglottids are filled with eggs, they detach from the body and are seen in feces of the definitive host. The boundary between the two proglottids is studded with a row of interproglottid glands, arranged in a rosette pattern around depressions in the posterior surface in *M. expansa*.
- **Synonyms**: Double-pored tapeworm and sheep tapeworm.
- **Predilection site**: The small intestine is the site of predilection in the definitive host.
- **Host and susceptibility**: Sheep, goats, cattle, and other ungulates are susceptible to monieziasis.
- **Geographic distribution**: Monieziasis occurs worldwide.
- **Life cycle and pathogenesis**: The life cycle of *Monezia* species is indirect. Sheep, goats, and cattle act as the final host, whereas oribatid mites or beetle mites act as the intermediate host. Adult *Monezia* worms lay eggs in the intestinal tract of goats and are passed in stool (Figure 6.6). Sometime gravid segments of *Monezia* worms are passed in stool. Eggs present in feces are ingested by oribatid mites; within the oribatid mites cysticercoids develop and the definitive host gets infected while grazing pasture contaminated with oribatid mites.
- **Clinical signs**: Monieziasis in goats and sheep is often a very mild infection, but it can be dangerous to younger animals in massive infections. Diarrhea, reduced weight gain, and intestinal obstruction are the common clinical signs.
- **Diagnosis**: Diagnosis of monieziasis is mainly by observing mature segments of worms in stool, which look like cooked rice grain, or by identifying characteristic triangular-shaped eggs in the fecal sample by the flotation method. On postmortem examination a large number of adult worms can be seen in the intestine.
- **Treatment and control**: Niclosamide, fenbendazole, and albendazole are effective in the management of monieziasis in goats, but praziquantel is the best choice. Regular deworming is the preferred method to control monieziasis, rather than control of the oribatid mite that is not feasible in practice.

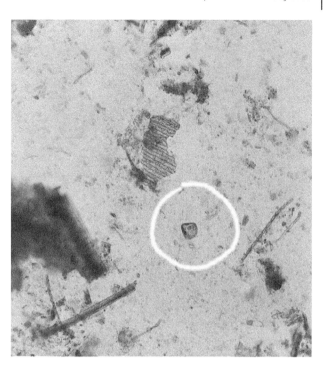

Figure 6.6 Triangular-shaped *Moniezia* spp. egg (circled) in goat fecal sample.

6.2.2 *Avitellina* Species

- **Etiology and parasite description**: Many *Avitellina* species are identified in goats and important *Avitellina* species are listed in Table 6.1. The body of the adult *Avitellina* is made up of proglottids, each of which has its own reproductive organs of both sexes (Figure 6.7). Mature proglottids filled with eggs detach from the body and are seen in the feces. These gravid segments are easily visible to the naked eye (Zachary 2016). The adult worm measures about 3 m in length and 3 mm

Table 6.1 *Avitellina* species of goats.

Species of parasite	Definitive hosts	Intermediate host
Avitellina centripunctata sensulatu (including Avitellina goughi, Avitellina lahorea, Avitellina sudanea)	Sheep (primarily), goats, cattle, buffalo, zebu, camels, other ruminants	Punctoribates, Scheloribates, Trichoribates
Avitellina bangaonensis	Cattle, goats	Oribatids and/or psocids
Avitellina chalmersi	Sheep, goats	Oribatids and/or psocids
Avitellina tatia	Goats	Oribatids and/or psocids
Avitellina woodland	Sheep, goats	Oribatids

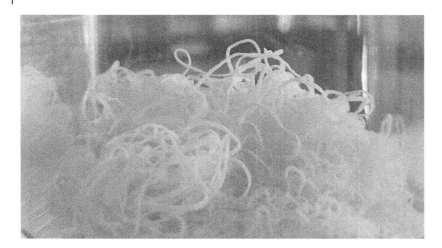

Figure 6.7 Adult *Avitellina* species tapeworms.

in width; these worms do not have respiratory, digestive, and circulatory systems. As the segmentations are not distinct, the worms look like ribbons.

- **Synonyms**: Infection caused by *Avitellina* spp. is called avitelliniasis or avitellinosis.
- **Predilection site**: The small intestine is the predilection site of adult *Avitellina* tapeworms in their final hosts. **Host and susceptibility**: Goats, cattle, and sheep are susceptible. *Avitellina centripunctata* tapeworms are not known to affect dogs, horses, cats, or poultry.
- **Geographic distribution**: *Avitellina* spp. are reported in Africa, Asia, and Europe, and are common in arid regions.
- **Life cycle and pathogenesis**: The life cycle is indirect, where oribatids and/or *Psocoptera* (dark lice, dust lice, and bark lice) act as intermediate hosts. The definitive host gets the infection by ingesting an intermediate host carrying infective cysticercoids while grazing in the pasture.
- **Clinical signs**: Most *Avitellina* infections are very mild and do not produce any clinical signs. Even with massive infection the animal remains asymptomatic, but the presence of *Avitellina* spp. worms affects productivity and immunity because they compete for essential nutrients.
- **Diagnosis**: Diagnosis is by identification of gravid segments in stool that look like rice grains or by detection of eggs in feces. The eggs are oval in shape, measuring about 20 × 45 μm, and they are embryonated.
- **Treatment and control**: Narrow-spectrum anthelmintics like niclosamide (75–150 mg/kg body weight), praziquantel (15 mg/kg), and butanamide (25–50 mg/kg), and broad-spectrum anthelmintics like oxibendazole (5 mg/kg), fenbendazole (5 mg/kg), albendazole (10 mg/kg), and cambendazole (20 mg/kg) can be used in the treatment of avitellinosis. To control avitellinosis, regular deworming and control of lice are necessary.

6.2.3 *Stilesia globipunctata*

- **Etiology and parasite description**: *Stilesia hepatica* and *Stilesia globipunctata* adult parasites are about 60 cm in length and 3 mm in width. The female worm has a dumbbell-shaped uterus (Soulsby 1982). The proglottids are short and have both male and female reproductive organs.
- **Synonym**: *S. hepatica* is also known as the liver tapeworm.
- **Predilection site**: The site of predilection of *S. hepatica* is the bile duct and for *S. globipunctata* it is the small intestine, especially at the junction of the duodenum and jejunum.
- **Host and susceptibility**: Goats, sheep, and cattle are the final hosts. *S. hepatica* infections are not reported in poultry, horses, dogs, cats, or swine.
- **Geographic distribution**: The condition is reported in Asia, tropical and southern Africa, and North and South America.
- **Life cycle and pathogenesis**: The life cycle is not fully understood. Oribatid mites/psocids acts as intermediate hosts. Immature worms are highly pathogenic, and heavy infections of *S. hepatica* lead to bile duct occlusion and cirrhosis, whereas *S. globipunctata* forms nodules in the intestine of the host.
- **Clinical signs**: The clinical signs are often non-specific and most of the time affected animals are asymptomatic.
- **Diagnosis**: Diagnosis is by identification of gravid segments or oval-shaped, rather small (16 × 25 mm) eggs in the fecal sample. As clinical signs are non-specific, most of the time diagnosis occurs at the time of meat inspection or during postmortem examination.
- **Treatment and control**: Praziquantel and fenbendazole are very effective in the management of *Stilesia* infections in goats, but the dose should be on the high side. Control is by regular deworming with these medications.

6.3 Common Roundworm Infections of Goats

6.3.1 Trichuriasis

- **Etiology and parasite description**: *Trichuris ovis*, *Trichuris discolor*, and *Trichuris globulosa* belongs to family *Trichuridae*. *Trichuris* worms have a unique shape that looks like a whip with its handle, which is why these worms are known as whipworms (Taylor et al. 2007). They measure about 3–8 cm in length and the color varies between whitish and yellow. These worms do not have excretory or circulatory systems, but they have a digestive system with two openings. Their body is covered with cuticle, which is tough and flexible.
- **Synonym**: Whipworms.
- **Predilection site**: *Trichuris* worms are found in the caecum and colon of the definitive host.
- **Host and susceptibility**: Sheep, goats, cattle, and other ruminants are susceptible. *Trichuris* worms are more prevalent in goats than in sheep.
- **Geographic distribution**: In animals the disease is reported in Australia, Europe, Asia, and North and South America. In humans trichuriasis is reported throughout the world and it is common in children and in poor sanitation areas.
- **Life cycle and pathogenesis**: The life cycle of *Trichuris ovis* is direct. After ingestion of an embryonated egg, larvae released into the intestine burrow into the wall of caecum and the proximal colon (Figure 6.8). In the intestinal wall larvae develop into mature adult male and female worms. After copulation, these adult worms release eggs into the lumen, which are later passed in feces. Affected animals suffer from hemorrhagic colitis and diphtheritic caecitis, which can lead to ulcerative and necrotic lesions in the intestinal wall.
- **Clinical signs**: *Trichuris* spp. are relatively harmless. The infected animal exhibits diarrhea with blood, signs of anemia, jaundice, poor appetite, weight loss, and dehydration.
- **Diagnosis**: Clinical signs are not pathognomonic, hence the diagnosis is made by demonstration of the characteristic barrel-shaped eggs with conspicuous plugs at both ends in feces (Figure 6.9). They measure about 40×70 μm and are brownish-yellow in color. The eggs are highly resistant to dry and cold conditions, and can remain infective for several years in the soil.

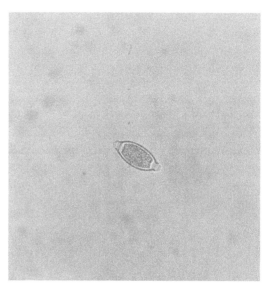

Figure 6.9 Barrel-shaped *Trichuris* eggs with conspicuous plugs at both ends (40×).

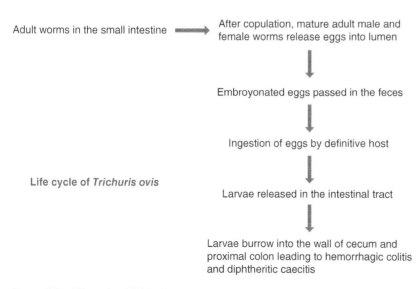

Adult worms in the small intestine ⟶ After copulation, mature adult male and female worms release eggs into lumen

↓

Embroyonated eggs passed in the feces

↓

Ingestion of eggs by definitive host

↓

Life cycle of *Trichuris ovis*

Larvae released in the intestinal tract

↓

Larvae burrow into the wall of cecum and proximal colon leading to hemorrhagic colitis and diphtheritic caecitis

Figure 6.8 Life cycle of *Trichuris* spp.

- **Treatment and control**: Fenbendazole (5–20 mg/kg body weight) or oxfendazole (2.5 mg/kg) is effective against both adult worms (89–99% efficacy) and immature parasites (62–100% efficacy).

6.3.2 Strongyle Infections

Among all strongyles, *Haemonchus contortus* and *Trichostrongylus* spp. are the most important and prevalent strongyles in goats (Anderson and Rings 2009).

6.3.2.1 Haemonchosis

- **Etiology and parasite description**: *H. contortus* worms are reddish in color, measuring about 1–3 cm in length. The body is covered with flexible, transparent, and rough membrane called cuticle. They have a tubular digestive system with a dorsal lancet to cut host gut tissue. As the worms are transparent, when the gut is filled with red blood the uterus of a female worm looks like a small barber's pole.
- **Synonyms**: Barber pole worm, twisted wireworm, and large stomach worm.
- **Predilection site**: Abomasum.
- **Host and susceptibility**: *H. contortus* is the most economically significant parasite of cattle, sheep, goats, and other wild animals. *H. contortus* mainly affects sheep and goats, and to a lesser extent cattle, whereas *H. placei* affects mainly cattle but is also seen in sheep and goats.
- **Geographic distribution**: The disease occurs worldwide, but is most common in tropical and subtropical regions.
- **Life cycle and pathogenesis**: *Haemonchus* spp. life cycle is simple. It takes approximately 21 days to complete the entire life cycle (Figure 6.10). Infective L3 larvae are ingested by the goat while grazing on pasture. L3 develop into adults in the abomasum and produce eggs that are passed in stool. These eggs will hatch within six days and undergo molts to become L3 larvae. These L3 larvae can survive up to 180 days on pasture.

- **Clinical signs**: *H. contortus* is a blood-sucking parasite. It has been estimated that a single adult worm can consume about 0.05 ml of blood per day, which can lead severe anemia, protein loss, and death in goats. Failure to thrive and weight loss are the major clinical signs observed. Adults can survive several months in goats, and as the worm load increases within the host signs such as anemia, hypoproteinemia, submandibular edema (bottle jaw), weakness, and collapse will develop. Unlike with many other gastrointestinal parasites, haemonchosis does not cause diarrhea.
- **Diagnosis**: Diagnosis of haemonchosis is mainly based on clinical signs and identification of eggs by the fecal flotation method. As anemia is the main clinical problem, examination of mucus membranes is one of the best ways for diagnosing and monitoring the treatment apart from hematological examination. The McMaster's technique is useful to calculate the number of eggs per gram of feces.
- **Treatment and control**: Benzimidazoles, imidazothiazoles, macrocyclic lactones, closantel, and monepantel can be used to treat haemonchosis, but the major challenge in treatment is anthelminthic resistance. Pasture management is very important to control haemonchosis because infective larvae can survive for long periods of time on pasture. A rotational grazing system helps to reduce the infective larvae load in the pasture. Routine monitoring for anemia through the FAMACHA conjunctival color index and fecal worm/egg counts are the key to controlling haemonchosis. In the FAMACHA method, the color of the conjunctival mucus membrane is classified into five categories, depending on the parasite load, and the effectiveness of a dewormer can be assessed (Table 6.2).

6.3.2.2 Trichostrongylosis

- **Etiology and parasite description**: *Trichostrongylus axei*, *T. colubriformis*, *T. vitrines*, and *T. rugatus* are the most common *Trichostrongylus* species found in small ruminants (Urquhart et al. 1996). *Trichostrongylus*

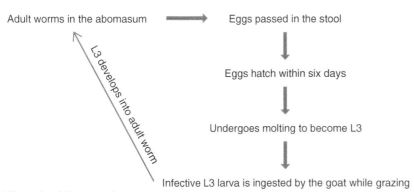

Figure 6.10 Life cycle of *Haemonchus* spp.

Life cycle of *Haemonchus contortus*

Table 6.2 FAMACHA score card.

FAMACHA score	Mucus membrane color	Interpretation	Treatment
1	Red	Non-anemic	No
2	Red-pink	Non-anemic	No
3	Pink	Mildly anemic	?
4	Pink-white	Anemic	Yes
5	White	Severely anemic	Yes

worms are brownish-red in color and measure about 5–10 mm in length. They have an outer cuticle with a tubular digestive system. Male worms have a pair of spicules for attachment during copulation.

- **Synonym**: Trichostongyles are also known as black scour worms, because the diarrhea in trichostrongylosis is often dark in color. Trichostongyles are also known as hair worms. *T. axei* is known as the stomach hairworm and *T. colubriformis* is known as the bankrupt worm.
- **Predilection site**: The small intestine is the site of predilection for *T. colubriformis*, *T vitrines*, and *T rugatus*. For *T. axei* the site of predilection is the abomasum or stomach.
- **Host and susceptibility**: Cattle, sheep, goats, and other ruminants are susceptible.
- **Geographic distribution**: The disease is reported worldwide.
- **Life cycle and pathogenesis**: The life cycle is direct. Eggs are passed through the feces of infected goats, and under favorable environmental conditions rhabditiform larvae hatch from the eggs. The rhabditiform larva undergoes two molts and becomes an infective filariform (L3) larva. A susceptible host ingests L3, the larva reaches the small intestine, and matures into an egg-laying adult worm within 18–21 days in the definitive host. The larva burrows superficially into crypts of mucosa, leading to extensive duodenal mucosal damage.
- **Clinical signs**: The animal exhibits signs of generalized enteritis including hemorrhage and edema due to the loss of plasma proteins into gut lumen. Trichostrongylosis is commonly found as a mixed infection with other gastrointestinal parasites.
- **Diagnosis**: The diagnosis of *Trichostrongylus* spp. is by identification of eggs in a fecal sample along with recovery of adult trichostongyles from the abomasum or small intestine. The eggs are thin shelled, ovoid in shape, measuring about 40 × 80 μm, and they are embryonated when shed.
- **Treatment and control**: Pyrantel pamoate, fenbendazole, mebendazole, ivermectin, moxidectin, and albendazole are

effective in the management of trichostrongylosis. As it occurs as a mixed infection with other gastrointestinal parasites such as *Haemonchus*, *Ostertagia*, and *Cooperia*, use of a broad-spectrum anthelmintic is advised. To avoid pasture contamination, either a rotational or alternate grazing methodology should be followed.

6.3.3 Strongyloidiasis or Strongyloidosis

- **Etiology and parasite description**: Strongyloides worms belong to the Rhabditoidea superfamily, which are small, slender nematodes of the small intestine. Strongyloidiasis in goats is due to *Strongyloides papillosus*, which affects cattle and sheep as well (Figures 6.11 and 6.12). *Strongyloides* worms are very small and thin,

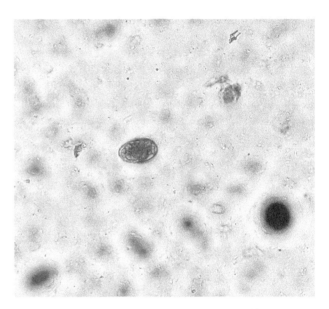

Figure 6.11 Strongyle egg in goat fecal sample (10×).

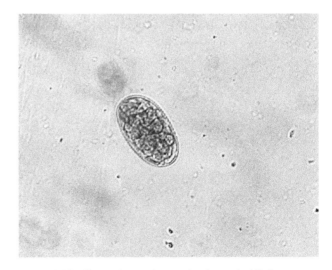

Figure 6.12 Strongyle egg in goat fecal sample (40×).

and their body is covered with cuticle with no signs of clear segmentation. Male worms are shorter than female worms. These worms have a very long esophagus that is almost one-third of the total body length.

- **Synonyms**: Threadworms or pinworms.
- **Predilection site**: The site of predilection of adult *Strongyloides* in goats, sheep, horses, cattle, and pigs is the small intestine, but migrating larvae can be found in lung, skin, blood, and other visceral organs.
- **Host and susceptibility**: Goats, sheep, and cattle are susceptible.
- **Geographic distribution**: The disease occurs worldwide.
- **Life cycle and pathogenesis**: *S. papillosus* has both heterogenic and homogenic life cycles. Only female worms are parasitic; they produce eggs by parthenogenesis. First-stage larvae or larvated eggs are passed in feces, and undergo rapid development into infective third-stage larvae. In the homogenic or intrahost life cycle, L3-stage larvae enter the host percutaneously or through the oral mucosa, then migrate to the duodenum, where they mature into parthenogenic egg-producing adult females. In the heterogenic or free-living life cycle, L3-stage larvae can mature to adult male and female worms in the environment, which reproduce in the external environment to generate infective L3.
- **Clinical signs**: Young goats up to 12 months of age are found to be more susceptible to strongyloidiasis. Major clinical signs include transient diarrhea, misshapen elongated fecal pellets terminally, dehydration, anorexia, cachexia, gnashing of teeth, foaming at the mouth, anemia, and nervous signs. Migrating larvae can damage the lung parenchyma, which leads to secondary bacterial infection and respiratory distress. Migrating larvae in the skin produce dermatitis and pruritus, especially in the limbs.
- **Diagnosis**: On postmortem the pathological changes noticed are enteritis, status spongiosus in the brain, hepatosis leading to rupture of the liver, nephrosis, pulmonary edema, interstitial pneumonia, and pneumonia. Diagnosis is by detection of eggs in a fecal sample; these are ellipsoidal in shape, thin shelled, measuring $25 \times 50\,\mu m$, and contains fully developed larvae when laid.
- **Treatment and control**: Broad-spectrum anthelmintics such as albendazole, fenbendazole, mebendazole, levamisole, and pyrantel are effective against adult worms and larvae in the gut, but not effective against migrating larvae. Ivermectin and moxidectin are effective against adult worms, and dormant and migrating larvae.

6.3.4 Ostertagiasis

- **Etiology and parasite description**: Ostertagiasis in goats is caused by *Teladorsagia circumcincta* (previously known as *Ostertagia circumcincta*), *Teladorsagia pinnata* (previously known as *Ostertagia pinnata*), and *Teladorsagia trifurcata* (previously known as *Ostertagia trifurcate*). *Ostertagia* worms are very small, measuring up to 12 mm in length, and brown in color. The body of these worms is covered with tough and flexible cuticle. They have a tubular digestive system with a couple of openings.
- **Synonym**: Brown stomach worm.
- **Predilection site**: Abomasum.
- **Host and susceptibility**: Goats, sheep, and cattle are susceptible. *Ostertagia* worms are not known to affect cats, pigs, or dogs.
- **Geographic distribution**: The disease occurs worldwide, and is more common in areas with cool and temperate weather.
- **Life cycle and pathogenesis**: *O. circumcincta* is highly pathogenic for kids and lambs, especially in cool and temperate parts of the world. Like *H. contortus*, *O. circumcincta* has a direct life cycle and attaches to the abomasal mucosa to ingest blood. *O. circumcincta* worms are much smaller and uniformly brown compared to *H. contortus* worms. *O. circumcincta* eggs are passed in feces, the eggs hatch, and larvae develop into the L3 stage and migrate into pasture. When a susceptible host ingests L3, the L3 mature to adult parasites in the abomasal glands. During this maturation phase within the abomasal glands, the larvae induce a type I hypersensitivity reaction leading to hyperplasia and hypertrophy of abomasal glands. In heavily infected goats/kids, the abomasum appears like Morocco leather or has a cobblestone appearance because of enlargement of the gastric glands.
- **Clinical signs**: Ostertagiasis occurs in two forms. Type I ostertagiasis, which is also known as summer ostertagiasis, is common in young animals. These young animals get the infection for the first time during their first grazing period. Type II ostertagiasis, which is also called winter ostertagiasis, is common in adult animals where dormant/inactive larvae become active. In both types of ostertagiasis the larval stage of the parasite is highly pathogenic. Burrowing larvae damage the abomasal wall, leading to abomasitis, improper digestion, and malabsorption. Signs observed in ostertagiasis-affected animals are anemia, diarrhea, loss of appetite, unthriftiness, improper mentation, and dehydration. Hypoproteinemia leads to ascites and submandibular edema, which is known as bottle jaw.
- **Diagnosis**: Diagnosis of ostertagiasis is based on clinical signs, season, and fecal egg counts. The eggs are slightly asymmetric, thin shelled, ovoid in shape, measuring about $45 \times 85\,\mu m$, and contain 16–32 blastomeres. As the disease is common during the late summer/early autumn season, during this period any goat/kid exhibiting signs such as diarrhea or weight loss should be subjected for fecal examination to rule out ostertagiasis. Infiltration of

mononuclear inflammatory cells and eosinophils in the lamina propria of the abomasum are the characteristic findings on histopathological examination of the abomasum. The serum pepsinogen level will be increased in animals suffering with ostertagiasis.

- **Treatment and control**: Ostertagiasis in goats can be best managed with levamisole, ivermectin, moxidectin, doramectin, and fenbendazole. Morbidity is high and mortality is low in type I, but in type II mortality is very high and morbidity is low.

6.3.5 Oesophagostomiasis

- **Etiology and parasite description**: *Oesophagostomum radiatum*, *O. columbianum*, and *O. multifoliatum* are the common species reported to cause oesophagostomiasis in goats. They belong to the family Strongyloidae, genus *Oesophagostomum*. Adult *Oesophagostomum* worms measure about 15–20 mm in length and have a prominent cephalic vesicle on the head.
- **Synonym**: *Oesophagostomum* spp. worms are known as nodular worms because they produce characteristic nodules in the large intestine of their respective hosts.
- **Predilection site**: The large intestine.
- **Host and susceptibility**: Goats, cattle, sheep, pigs, and antelopes.
- **Geographic distribution**: The disease occurs worldwide.
- **Life cycle and pathogenesis**: The life cycle of all *Oesophagostomum* species is direct. The adult female lays eggs in the definitive host's large intestine and these eggs will be passed in stool. L1 is released and within a week in a favorable environment develops into infective L3 larvae. After ingestion of L3 larvae by the susceptible host, the larvae penetrate into the large intestinal mucosa and form nodules. After about a week, the larvae abandon the nodule and move to the colon to complete development into adults and start laying eggs. After entry of infective larvae into a susceptible host, it takes about 5–6 weeks to find the first eggs in feces. Some of the larvae can also migrate into the abdominal cavity or the liver through the gut mucosa.
- **Clinical signs**: Most of the time oesophagostomiasis occurs as a mixed infection with other gastrointestinal worms such as *Haemonchus*, *Cooperia*, *Ostertagia*, or *Nematodirus*.
- **Diagnosis**: Disease is confirmed by identification of thin-shelled ovoid eggs measuring 40–60 × 70–100 μm in a fecal sample. These eggs contain cells depending on the *Oesophagostomum* species. Finding an adult worm during postmortem or surgeries provides a definitive diagnosis.
- **Treatment and control**: Broad-spectral anthelmintics such as fenbendazole, morantel, moxidectin, ivermectin,

and albendazole are effective against oesophagostomiasis. To control oesophagostomiasis manure/dung should be disposed of properly, because parasitic larvae develop in the manure in one week. Overcrowding of goats should be avoided.

6.3.6 Cooperiasis or Cooperiosis

- **Etiology and parasite description**: Cooperiasis in goats is caused by *Cooperia curticei*, *C. punctata*, and *C. oncophora*. They belong to the class Secernentea and the superfamily Trichostrongyloidea. The worms are red in color, measuring about 10 mm in length. They have characteristic transverse striations and longitudinal ridges.
- **Synonym**: Small intestinal worms.
- **Predilection site**: The small intestine.
- **Host and susceptibility**: Cattle, sheep, goats, and other ruminants are susceptible. Kids less than 1 year old are more susceptible. These worms are not known to affect dogs, pigs, or cats.
- **Geographic distribution**: *Cooperia* species are commonly found in warm and humid regions.
- **Life cycle and pathogenesis**: The life cycle of *Cooperia* species is direct. Adult female worms lay eggs in the small intestine of goats and is passed in stool. In the environment L1 is released from the eggs and molts to become an infective L3. The prepatent period is very short, about 2–3 weeks.
- **Clinical signs**: The presence of adult *Cooperia* worms in the intestine leads to signs such as diarrhea, gastrointestinal hemorrhage, anemia, malnutrition, weight loss, and depression.
- **Diagnosis**: Diagnosis is based on identification of eggs in a fecal sample. *Cooperia* spp. eggs are elliptical in shape and consist of a segmented ovum and a double-layered covering.
- **Treatment and control**: Fenbendazole, oxfendazole, levamisole, doramectin, ivermectin, and moxidectin are effective on larvae and adult worms. It is very difficult to control cooperiasis because *Cooperia* larvae can survive up to 12 months on pasture.

6.3.7 *Nematodirus* in Goats

- **Etiology and parasite description**: *Nematodirus battus*, *Nematodirus filicollis*, *Nematodirus spathiger*, and *Nematodirus abnormalis* are the species reported to infect goats. They belong to the phylum Nematoda, class Secernentea, and superfamily Trichostrongyloidea. Worms are white in color, measuring 1–2.5 cm in length. The body of the worms is covered with flexible, tough cuticle, males are shorter than females, and they have a tubular digestive system.

- **Synonym**: Also known as thin-necked worms or thread-necked worms, because they have a swollen head followed by a thin neck.
- **Predilection site**: The small intestine is the site of predilection of adult worms.
- **Host and susceptibility**: Cattle, sheep, goats, and other ruminants are susceptible. Lambs are more susceptible.
- **Geographic distribution**: The disease is found worldwide, especially in temperate regions.
- **Life cycle and pathogenesis**: The life cycle of *Nematodirus* spp. is direct, where adult females lay eggs in the intestine that are passed in stool. Unlike other nematodes, after shedding the larvae remain within the egg until they become infective L3. The eggs of *Nematodirus* spp. are elliptical in shape and contain an embryo of about eight cells when passed. Compared to adult worms, the larvae are very harmful to goats: they lead to diarrhea and dehydration even before eggs are identified in stool.
- **Clinical signs**: *Nematodirus* worms are not harmful, but the larvae are pathogenic. Chronic infection leads to weight loss, poor productivity, and loss of appetite. In acute infections diarrhea, dehydration, and sudden death are observed.
- **Diagnosis**: Diagnosis is mainly by clinical signs and identifying eggs in stool. The eggs are largest among the gastrointestinal nematodes of ruminants, measuring about $70–120 \times 130–230\,\mu m$. The eggs are thick shelled and brown in color, ovoid in shape, and contains 4–8 blastomeres when they are passed in stool.
- **Treatment and control**: Benzimidazoles, levamisole, and macrolides are effective against both larval-stage and adult worms. Rotational grazing is useful in reducing the larval load in pasture.

6.3.8 Chabertiasis or Chabertiosis

- **Etiology and parasite description**: *Chabertia ovina* worms are 1–2 cm long, females are larger than males, and males have large copulatory bursa and two spicules for attachment during copulation. A characteristic feature of these worms is a large cup-shaped mouth capsule, without teeth.
- **Synonym**: Large-mouthed large worm.
- **Predilection site**: The large intestine (adult worms are localized in the colon of the definitive host).
- **Host and susceptibility**: Goats and sheep are susceptible, and it is sometimes seen in cattle.
- **Geographic distribution**: Chabertiasis is found worldwide and is common in temperate regions.
- **Life cycle and pathogenesis**: The life cycle of *C. ovina* is direct and the prepatent period is about seven weeks. The adult female lays eggs in the intestinal tract of the goat and is passed in stool. L1 is released in the environment molts to become L3. These infective L3 are ingested by the definitive host while grazing on pasture.
- **Clinical signs**: Neither adults nor larvae suck blood in the host, but rather lead to the formation of ulcers at the site of attachment and also alter the gut lining, resulting in malabsorption. Animals affected with *C. ovina* exhibit signs such as diarrhea, anemia, weakness, and weight loss.
- **Diagnosis**: Diagnosis is by clinical signs and identification of *C. ovina* eggs in a fecal sample. *C. ovina* eggs are oval in shape, measure $50 \times 90\,\mu m$, and contain more than 16 cells/blastomeres when laid.
- **Treatment and control**: Broad-spectrum anthelminthic drugs such as benzimidazoles, tetrahydropyrimidines, and macrolides are effective in the treatment of chabertiosis. To control the disease, pasture contamination with infective larvae should be reduced.

6.3.9 Capillariasis in Goats

- **Etiology and parasite description**: Approximately 300 species of parasites of genus *Capillaria* comes under the phylum Nematoda, order Trichurida, and family *Trichinellidae*. *Capillaria bovis* and *Capillaria longipes* are known to affect sheep, goats, and cattle. *Capillaria* comes from the Latin *capillus*, meaning head hair. *Capillaria* worms are very small, thin, and hair-like. These worms do not have excretory organs or a circulatory system, but they do have nervous and tubular digestive systems.
- **Synonym**: Hairworms. The disease caused by these worms is called capillariasis, not capillariosis.
- **Predilection site**: The site of predilection varies with the species. The site of predilection for *C. bovis* and *C. longipes* is the small intestine. For *C. aerophila* it is the respiratory tract, for *C. hepatica* the liver, and for *C. philippinensis* the intestinal tract.
- **Host and susceptibility**: Sheep, goats, cattle, dogs, cats, humans, other livestock species, and poultry are susceptible.
- **Geographic distribution**: Capillariasis occurs worldwide, but its abundance and occurrence depend on the availability of host species and distribution of parasite species.
- **Life cycle and pathogenesis**: Some of the species in this genus require an intermediate host to complete their life cycle (e.g. *C. bovis*, *C. aerophila*, *C. philippinensis*) and some do not (e.g. *C. hepatica*). Not much is known about their pathogenicity, but they cause little or no harm in ruminant species.
- **Clinical signs**: The prevalence of capillariasis in goats is often low. Signs are non-specific and occur mostly because of other associated gastrointestinal parasites.

- **Diagnosis**: Diagnosis is by identification of eggs in stool. The eggs look like *Trichuris* spp. eggs and are colorless, barrel-shaped, and have lateral striations. Various authors identified *Capillaria* eggs in goat fecal samples, but prevalence was very low and most of the time capillariasis was a mixed infection.
- **Treatment and control**: Fenbendazole, mebendazole, and ivermectin are known to be effective against *Capillaria* infection. To control capillariasis there should be strict treatment of all in-contact animals, considering them as infected. Regular deworming with ivermectin or fenbendazole is effective in controlling capillariasis.

6.3.10 Bunostomosis

- **Etiology and parasite description**: *Bunostomum trigonocephalum* belongs to the phylum Nematoda, class Chromadorea, order Rhabditida, suborder Strongylida, family Ancylostomatidae, and genus *Bunostomum*. The worms are grayish white in color and measure about 1–3 cm in length. Their mouth capsule is funnel-shaped and they have two cutting plates that help in attachment to the host gut mucosa.
- **Synonym**: Hookworm.
- **Predilection site**: The small intestine.
- **Host and susceptibility**: Goats and sheep are susceptible.
- **Geographic distribution**: The disease is found worldwide, and is common in warm and humid weather.
- **Life cycle and pathogenesis**: The life cycle is direct. The definitive host acquires the infection through ingestion or penetration through the skin. These adult hookworms are mainly parasitized in the small intestine of the definitive host, leading to anemia and hypoproteinemia, especially in young animals.
- **Clinical signs**: Adult *Bunostomum* worms have a large and strong mouth capsule that can damage the intestinal wall and blood vessels, and leads to huge blood loss. Classic signs of *Bunostomum* infection are blood-mixed diarrhea, weight loss, reduced appetite, anemia, bottle jaw, weakness, and dehydration.
- **Diagnosis**: Diagnosis is based on clinical signs and identification of adult worms in the small intestine or by identifying eggs in a fecal sample. The eggs are irregular and ovoid in shape, measuring about 55 × 95 μm, with 4–8 blastomeres.
- **Treatment and control**: Macrocyclic lactones, benzimidazoles, and levamisole are effective against both larval-stage and adult worms. Closantel and nitroxinil are effective against adult worms, and help in control of larvae.

6.4 General Aspects of Preventing Parasitic Disease in Goats

Parasitic infestation is the biggest problem to goat farmers. To control or prevent parasitic infestation no technique is 100% effective, so we need to depend on multiple techniques to achieve our goal.

6.4.1 Pasture Management

Pasture management is a very important aspect of controlling internal worms, because goats get infection by ingesting larvae/eggs present on forage/pasture. Normally larvae can crawl up to 1–2 in. from the ground, so goats should be allowed to graze when the pasture height is more than 6–10 in. Goats should not be allowed to feed near manure pits, which increase the chance of picking up larvae. Changing the feeding fields/pastures between seasons or moving to safe pastures within the same season reduces the worm load in goats. Pasture should be cultivated annually and forage crops can be used to prepare hay/silage.

6.4.2 Animal Management

While selecting animals, always select healthy parasite- and disease-free animals. Provide good and balanced nutrition. Keep vaccination and deworming up to date; deworming should be done once every three months to reduce the parasitic burden. Eliminate or cull animals that need repeated treatment or animals with a persistently high fecal egg count. Avoid overcrowding, mixed grazing, or alternate grazing with other host species, and mixed grazing with animals of different age groups.

6.4.3 General Management

Feeders and waterers should always be clean and free of fecal contamination. Animal sheds should be clean and keep separate facilities for day and night. Always check the weight of animals before deworming to avoid underdosing and monitor their growth. Tannins can be used to reduce internal parasites, egg output, and hatchability, and act as a source of bypass protein; at the same time tannins can reduce digestibility and in turn lead to poor productivity.

6.5 Anthelmintics

Dose rates for goats cannot be directly taken from dose rates of sheep, cattle, or pigs. Higher doses of anthelmintics are required for goats than for sheep; generally 1.5–2 times the sheep dose is required for goats (Table 6.3).

Table 6.3 Commonly used anthelmintics and their doses.

Anthelmintics	Dose for goats
Fenbendazole	Roundworms – 5 mg/kg orally *Dicrocoelium dendriticum* – 100 mg/kg; or 25 mg/kg/d for 5 days orally Adults: *Fasciola hepatica* – 150 mg/kg; or 30 mg/kg/d for 5 days orally *Moniezia* spp. – 5–15 mg/kg orally
Albendazole	Roundworms – 7.5 mg/kg orally Dictyocaulus filarial – 3.8 mg/kg orally Adults: *Fasciola hepatica* – 15 mg/kg orally *Fascioloides magna* – 15 mg/kg orally
Ivermectin	0.4 mg/kg orally
Moxidectin	0.4 mg/kg orally
Oxyclozanide	10–15 mg/kg orally
Triclabendazole	10–15 mg/kg orally
	Tapeworms – 10–15 mg/kg orally *Coenurus cerebralis* – 50–100 mg/kg/d for 2–5 days orally *Moniezia* spp. – 3.75 mg/kg orally
Levamisole	7.5–12 mg/kg orally (levamisole is toxic to goats, not recommended for debilitated animals and in the last three weeks of pregnancy)

Multiple-Choice Questions

1 In goats heavily infected with ostertagiasis, what does the abomasum resemble?
   A Morocco leather
   B Dry paper
   C Nodular
   D Cotton candy

2 Is the life cycle of all *Oesophagostomum* species direct or indirect?
   A Indirect
   B Direct
   C Both direct and indirect
   D None of the above

3 How many eggs per day can mature adult flukes lay?
   A 20 000
   B 40 000
   C 60 000
   D 80 000

4 What is the cause of dicrocoeliosis in goats?
   A *F. hepatica*
   B *D. dendriticum*
   C *F. gigantica*
   D *P. cervi*

5 How susceptible are goats to dicrocoeliosis compared to sheep?
   A Equally
   B Less
   C More
   D Highly

6 What are *Moniezia expansa* eggs present in feces ingested by?
   A Oribatid mites
   B Lizards
   C Ants
   D Snails

7 At what stage are *Stilesia globipunctata* worms highly pathogenic and form nodules in the intestine of the host?
   A Mature
   B Immature
   C Both
   D Adult

8 What is *Haemonchus contortus* also known as?
   A Barber worm
   B Pole worm
   C Lancet fluke
   D Barber pole worm

9 Which species of worms is commonly known as the thin-necked worm?
  A *Avitellina* sp.
  B *Nematodirus* sp.
  C *Haemonchus* sp.
  D *Fasciola* sp.

10 What does *Chabertia ovina* form at the site of attachment that alter the gut lining and lead to malabsorption?
  A Nodules
  B Tumors
  C Ulcers
  D Cysts

References

Anderson, D.E. and Rings, M. (2009). *Food Animal Practice, Current Veterinary Therapy series*. St. Louis, MO: Elsevier.

Barger, A.M. and MacNeill, A.L. (2015). *Clinical Pathology and Laboratory Techniques for Veterinary Technicians*. Hoboken, NJ: Wiley.

Constable, P.D., Hinchcliff, K., Done, S.H. et al. (2012). *Veterinary Medicine: A Textbook of the Diseases of Cattle, Sheep, Pigs, Goats, and Horses*. St. Louis, MO: Elsevier.

Fox, J.G., Anderson, L.C., Loew, F.M. et al. (2002). *Laboratory Animal Medicine*. St. Louis, MO: Elsevier.

Soulsby, E.J.L. (1982). *Helminths, Arthropods and Protozoa of Domesticated Animals*. London: Baillière Tindall/Blackwell Science.

Taylor, M.A., Coop, R.L., and Wall, R.L. (2007). *Veterinary Parasitology*. Oxford: Blackwell.

Urquhart, G.M., Armour, J., Duncan, J.L. et al. (1996). *Veterinary Parasitology*. Oxford: Blackwell Science.

Zachary, J. (2016). *Pathologic Basis of Veterinary Disease Expert Consult*. St. Louis, MO: Mosby/Elsevier Health Sciences.

Zajac, A.M. and Conboy, G.A. (2012). *Veterinary Clinical Parasitology*. Hoboken, NJ: Wiley Blackwell.

7

Mycoplasma, Rickettsia, and Chlamydia Diseases of Goats

Ranjani Rajasekaran[1,2], Hridya Susan Varughese[3,4], Padmanath Krishnan[2,5], and Panikkaparambil Shilpa[6]

[1] Department of Veterinary Microbiology, Veterinary College and Research Institute, Theni, Tamil Nadu, India
[2] Tamil Nadu Veterinary and Animal Sciences University, Chennai, Tamil Nadu, India
[3] Department of Veterinary Microbiology, Veterinary College, Hebbal, Bangalore, Karnataka, India
[4] Karnataka Veterinary Animal and Fisheries Sciences University, Bidar, Karnataka, India
[5] Veterinary Clinical Complex, Veterinary College and Research Institute, Theni, Tamil Nadu, India
[6] Veterinary Surgeon, Veterinary Dispensary, Vilayur, Palakkad, Kerala, India

7.1 Mycoplasma

Mycoplasma (Greek *mykes*, "fungus," and *plasma*, "formed") was first identified in cattle in 1898 and was called pleuropneumonia-like organisms (PPLO) for almost five decades. During the 1950s, it assumed the name *Mycoplasma*. The taxonomy of *Mycoplasma* was unclear until the early 1960s, after which it was designated within the bacteria domain. It is a unique bacterium, because it lacks a cell wall, which is a major characteristic of bacterial organisms. It is the smallest bacterium (0.3–0.8 μm in size) identified so far. There are over 100 species of *Mycoplasma* reported across the world and it is regarded as an important bacterial pathogen of livestock globally. In goats, *Mycoplasma* primarily causes respiratory and reproductive diseases. The diseases it causes in goats are listed in Table 7.1. The details of former and current taxonomic names of *Mycoplasma* are provided in Table 7.2.

7.1.1 Contagious Caprine Pleuropneumonia

Synonyms: abu-nini, bou-frida, pleuropneumonie contagieuse caprine.

7.1.1.1 History
The first report of contagious caprine pleuropneumonia (CCPP) was described in Algeria in 1873, where goats showed disease involvement only in one lung. Similarly in 1881, on an Angora goat farm in Bedford, UK, an outbreak showing unilateral pleuropneumonia was reported. It was highly contagious in nature with a 70% mortality rate. The incidence of this outbreak was traced back to infected goats

that were imported from Turkey to England and South Africa. Ever since then, CCPP has been reported from several parts of Africa and Asia and is currently endemic in Asia, Africa, the Middle East, and Eastern Europe.

7.1.1.2 Etiology
The causative organism for CCPP is *Mycoplasma capricolum* subsp. *capripneumoniae* (*Mccp*). It was first isolated in Kenya as *Mycoplasma* strain F38 (MacOwan and Minette 1977).

Mccp is the smallest fastidious bacteria at a size of 0.3 μm. It consists of a triple-layered membrane and is devoid of a rigid cell wall. It is phylogenetically related to Gram-positive bacteria with low G + C content.

Mycoplasma affecting ruminants have been classified into three sub-clusters: *Mycoplasma mycoides*, *M. capricolum*, and *M. leachii*, under the major *M. mycoides* cluster. Listed within the *M. mycoides* sub-cluster are *M. mycoides* subsp. *mycoides* small-colony (*MmmSC*), recently renamed *Mycoplasma mycoides mycoides* (*Mmm*); *M. mycoides* subsp. *capri* (*Mmc*); and *M. mycoides* subsp. *mycoides* large-colony (*MmmLC*), currently reclassified as *Mmc* (Figure 7.1). *M. capricolum* subsp. *capricolum* (*Mcc*) and *Mccp* are grouped within the *M. capricolum* sub-cluster, whereas *Mycoplasma* sp. bovine group 7 of leach (MBG7) is grouped within the *M. leachii* sub-cluster. All these six *Mycoplasma* sp. are closely related and are difficult to differentiate on grounds of serological, biochemical, genomic, and antigenic characteristics. This led to uncertainty in the past about identifying the definite *Mycoplasma* sp. causing CCPP. Prior to the identification of *Mccp* as the causative organism of CCPP, *Mmc* and *MmmLC* were regarded as the etiological agents of CCPP.

Principles of Goat Disease and Prevention, First Edition. Edited by Tanmoy Rana.
© 2024 John Wiley & Sons, Inc. Published 2024 by John Wiley & Sons, Inc.

Table 7.1 List of diseases caused by *Mycoplasma* spp. in goats.

Mycoplasma species	Disease
Mycoplasma capricolum subsp. *capripneumoniae*	Contagious caprine pleuropneumonia (CCPP)
Mycoplasma agalactiae	Contagious agalactia (CA)
Mycoplasma mycoides subsp. *capri*	
M. capricolum subsp. *capricolum*	
Mycoplasma putrefaciens	
Mycoplasma ovipneumoniae	Mastitis, arthritis, keratoconjunctivitis, pneumonia, and septicemia (MAKePS)
Mycoplasma arginini	
Mycoplasma conjunctivae (In addition to these organisms)	
M. ovis	Anemia

Isolation of *Mccp* remains difficult to date and only 20 countries across the world have successfully isolated *Mccp*. However, with the advent of molecular diagnostic techniques, identification of *Mccp* directly from clinical samples has become effortless. Amplification of 16s rRNA by polymerase chain reaction (PCR) combined with *Pst*I restriction enzyme analysis was reported to be useful in the identification and differentiation of *Mccp* from other *Mycoplasma* spp. (Table 7.3).

CCPP is an Office International des Epizooties (OIE)-listed communicable notifiable disease. According to the OIE, a report of CCPP should be documented only if the animal shows postmortem lesions of pleuropneumonia restricted to lung and pleura, without enlargement of interlobular septa of the lung, and the diagnosis is supported by laboratory isolation or serological tests of *Mccp*.

7.1.1.3 Host Susceptibility

Goats are the primary host for CCPP. Incidence of CCPP in sheep as a result of close contact with infected goats has also been reported. The affected sheep showed respiratory disease. Other than affecting domestic ruminants, CCPP was reported in wild goats, Nubian ibex, Laristan mouflon, and gerenuk that were housed in animal breeding parks in Qatar; and in free-ranging gazelles and other deer species in the United Arab Emirates when they came into contact with CCPP-affected goats. In addition, CCPP was also reported in Arabian oryx and Tibetan antelopes, and was suspected in markhors (Ostrowski et al. 2011).

As wild ungulates are also susceptible to CCPP, it has been speculated that reintroduction of animals from captive breeding into the wild might infect other wild ungulates living in their natural habitats.

To date, there are no reports of CCPP in humans and hence it is not of zoonotic importance.

7.1.1.4 Transmission

CCPP is mainly transmitted through direct contact, when *Mccp*-laden microdroplets expelled from infected goats through coughing are inhaled by susceptible goats. The shorter the distance (up to 50 m) between infected and susceptible animals, the higher the chances of transmission of the disease within a short time.

In intensive breeding, the spread of CCPP is more due to overcrowding and confined spaces. In extensive breeding practices, common watering and grazing points become the sites of transmission of CCPP.

The survival time of *Mccp* in the environment is 3 days in tropical areas and 2 weeks in temperate areas, and it is 10 years in pleural fluid obtained from an infected goat. *Mccp* as a fragile bacterium cannot withstand higher temperatures, and is inactivated within 60 minutes at 56 °C and within 2 minutes at 60 °C, hence indirect

Table 7.2 Current and former taxonomic names of *Mycoplasma*, *Rickettsia*, and *Chlamydia* organisms affecting goats.

Former name	Current name	Disease caused
Mycoplasma strain F38	*Mycoplasma capricolum* subsp. *capripneumoniae* (Mccp)	Contagious caprine pleuropneumonia
Eperythrozoon ovis	*Mycoplasma ovis*	Hemolytic anemia
Cowdria ruminatium and *Rickettsia ruminatium*	*Ehrlichia ruminatium*	Heartwater disease
Ehrlichia phagocytophilum	*Anaplasma phagocytophilum*	Anaplasmosis
Chlamydia psittaci immunotype-1 and *Chlamydophila abortus*	*Chlamydia abortus*	Enzootic abortion
C. psittaci immunotype-2	*Chlamydia pecorum*	Chlamydial polyarthritis

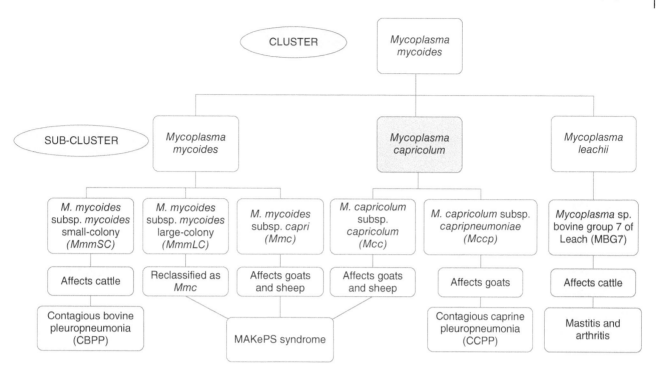

Figure 7.1 Details of *Mycoplasma mycoides* cluster. *Source:* Courtesy of Ranjani Rajasekaran (co-author). Created using www.mindthegraph.com online software.

Table 7.3 Genes targeted for polymerase chain reaction (PCR) identification of *Mycoplasma*, *Rickettsia*, and *Chlamydia* diseases of goats.

Disease	Causative	Gene/region targeted
Contagious caprine pleuropneumonia	*Mycoplasma capricolum* subspecies *capripneumoniae* (*Mccp*)	16s rRNA combined with *Pst*I restriction enzyme analysis
Contagious agalactia	To differentiate *Mycoplasma mycoides* subsp. *capri* and *M. capricolum* subsp. *capricolum*	restriction fragment length polymorphism (RFLP) on *IpdA* gene
Anemia caused by *Mycoplasma* sp.	*Candidatus Mycoplasma haemovis*	16S rRNA
Heartwater disease	*Ehrlichia ruminatium*	pCS20 and map-1
Anaplasmosis	*Anaplasma ovis*	Major surface protein 1
Enzootic abortion	*Chlamydia abortus*	16S–23S rRNA along with RFLP

transmission of CCPP through fomites, vectors, and other objects is unfeasible.

The spread of CCPP is higher during cold and rainy weather, and elevated environmental temperature and relative humidity favor the survival and replication of *Mccp* in goats.

Infected goats can remain asymptomatic carriers and latent chronic carriers. Shedding of *Mccp* can occur during sudden climatic changes due to stress.

The duration of latency is expected to be 7 days and the site of latency is unclear. The latent and chronic status of *Mccp* in goats causes persistence of the disease. The transmission of CCPP in goats is depicted in Figure 7.2.

The morbidity and mortality rates of CCPP are 100% and 80%, respectively. Morbidity has been reported to be higher in disease-free regions and lower in endemic regions. The mortality rate is affected by age, breed, region, endemicity, and weather conditions. It has also been reported that the mortality rate is lower in endemic regions.

7.1.1.5 Pathogenesis

The pathogenesis of CCPP in goats involves:

- Inhalation of oronasal or ocular secretions from infected goats.
- Adhesion of *Mccp* to the ciliated respiratory epithelium.
- Colonization and multiplication of *Mccp* in the epithelial cells causing ciliostasis.

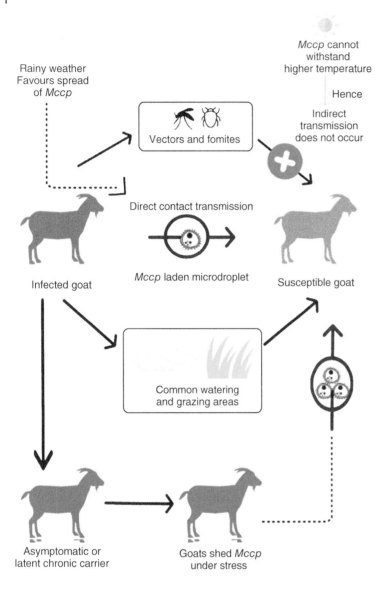

Figure 7.2 Transmission of contagious caprine pleuropneumonia in goats. *Source:* Courtesy of Ranjani Rajasekaran (co-author). Created using www. mindthegraph.com online software.

- Production of hydrogen superoxide and superoxide radicals in the adhered epithelial cell.
- Destruction of the epithelial cells causing loss of cilia.
- Dissemination of infection causes inflammation and oxidative stress.

Mccp does not produce toxins or invasins for adhesion. The predilection site of *Mccp* is the mucosal surface.

Antigenic structures including surface antigens and cytoplasmic antigens along with galactan present in the capsule of *Mccp* induce secretion of cytokines: tumor necrosis factor (TNF)-α, interleukins, and interferon-γ.

The incubation period of CCPP is 10 days and sometimes may be as long as 3–4 weeks. In naïve goats, CCPP causes death within 2 days.

7.1.1.6 Clinical Signs

Peracute CCPP occurs in naïve goats. No respiratory signs are observed as sudden death occurs within 2 days of infection.

In acute CCPP, onset of fever (41–42 °C) along with inability to walk are observed as the initial clinical signs. Abducted limbs and an extended neck are observed. Respiratory signs include tachypnea, bouts of violent painful coughs, and bilateral mucopurulent nasal discharge that is straw colored initially and later changes to rust-colored, thick mucoid or purulent discharge. Open-mouthed breathing along with excessive frothy salivation is also observed. Septicemia, anorexia, weight loss, and decrease in production are found. In the terminal stages, goats become exercise intolerant and reluctant to move, followed by death.

In the subacute or chronic forms, a prominent cough is observed, especially after exercise.

Peracute and acute forms of CCPP are observed in susceptible goats and the chronic form of CCPP is observed in endemic regions.

7.1.1.7 Lesions

Postmortem lesions are limited to the thoracic cavity. Unilateral hepatization of the lungs, adhesion of pleura and lung, and accumulation of straw-colored fluid in the pleural cavity are observed. Port wine–colored lungs with pea-sized yellow nodules are observed. The pleural exudate becomes solidified and covers the lung like a gelatinous covering. Fibrinous mucous plugs in the trachea and enlargement of bronchial and mediastinal lymph nodes are also seed. The interlobular septa is thickened in wild ruminants, which is absent in domesticated goats.

Histopathological examination of lung tissue shows sero-fibrinous fluid infiltrates and neutrophil cells in alveoli, bronchioles, interstitial septae, and sub-pleural connective tissue. Intralobular and interlobular edema are also observed. Hyperplasia of type II pneumocytes, congested septal capillaries, and alveolar lumen consisting of neutrophils and lymphocytes are seen as well.

7.1.1.8 Diagnosis

The preliminary diagnosis includes direct examination of pleural fluid or tissue suspensions under a dark-field microscope that shows branching filamentous structures, and staining of smears made from lung tissues using the May–Grünwald–Giemsa method under light microscopy.

Amplification of 16s rRNA along with *Pst*I restriction enzyme analysis directly from clinical samples including pleural fluid and lung tissues is an easy choice for diagnosis of CCPP. A gel precipitin test can detect antigenic polysaccharide released by *Mccp*, which gets immunoprecipitated with a specific monoclonal antibody (mAb), WM-25.

Isolation of *Mccp* is the confirmatory test for CCPP. Samples of choice for isolation include pleural fluid and lung tissue, obtained preferably between normal and affected regions. Samples should be kept cool during transport. The medium of choice for culture of *Mccp* is "viande foie goat." Broth cultures and plates are incubated at 37 °C in anaerobic conditions. Appearance of a "fried-egg" colony after a few passages with colonies of 3 mm diameter are confirmatory of *Mccp*.

Serological tests include the growth inhibition test (GIT), complement fixation test (CFT), latex agglutination test (LAT), and competitive enzyme-linked immunosorbent assay (c-ELISA) with a specific mAb:

- GIT uses WM-25–specific mAb in the disc growth inhibition method and differentiated *Mccp* from other species of the *M. mycoides* cluster.
- CFT is not recommended due to cross-reaction among the species of the *M. mycoides* cluster.
- LAT involves agglutination of *Mccp*-specific polysaccharide-sensitized latex beads with a suspected whole blood sample. Cross-reaction is observed with *Mcc* and *M. leachii*.
- c-ELISA is specific and sensitive for detection using mAb 4/52.

7.1.2 Zoonosis

No zoonotic potential of CCPP has been reported so far.

7.1.2.1 Treatment and Control Strategy

- Antibiotics such as tetracyclines, tylosin, fluoroquinolones, and the macrolide family can be used.
- Vaccination of 3-month-old kids with inactivated CCPP vaccine suspended in saponin provides protection for over 1 year.
- Proper control measures including quarantine of newly purchased or imported goats, slaughter of infected goats, and proper cleaning and disinfection of farms will reduce the incidence of CCPP.
- Screening of captive animals for CCPP prior to reintroduction into the wild and screening of wild animals during transport from one zoo to another should also be considered.

7.1.3 Contagious Agalactia

7.1.3.1 History

The disease was known as *mal di sito* ("disease of the place") when it was first reported in Italy in 1816 and got the name contagious agalactia (CA) in 1857. The term "agalactia" is a misnomer as the disease is not restricted to lactating does, and is not limited to the udder or mammary glands.

The etiological agent of CA was initially termed *Anulomyces agalaxie,* after which the name *Mycoplasma agalactiae (Ma)* was coined. *Ma* was also known as a "filterable but not visible" microorganism, similar to the causative of bovine pleuropneumonia.

CA is an economically important disease. Once introduced into a region, it becomes persistent in that particular region. The disease is prevalent in regions where the small ruminant dairy population is high, especially in the Middle East, Southern Europe, Asia, and North Africa. Numerous outbreaks from Spain, France, Italy, Iran, and Mongolia and sporadic outbreaks in the USA and Canada have been reported.

Table 7.4 Differentiating features of *Mycoplasma* spp. causing contagious agalactiae.

Feature	*Ma*	*Mcc*	*Mmc*	*Mp*
Geographic distribution	Spain, France, Italy, Iran, Mongolia	North Africa	Wide distribution – present on all continents	Western France
Gene cluster	*Mycoplasma bovis*	*Mycoplasma capricolum*		Closely related to *Mycoplasma mycoides* cluster
Host susceptibility	Both sheep and goats	Primarily affects goats		
Clinical form of disease	Acute or chronic	Hyperacute or subacute		No data available
Clinical signs				
Mastitis	+	+	+	+
Rotten milk smell
Arthritis	+	+	+	+
Keratoconjunctivitis	+	+	+	−
Pneumonia	−	+	+	−
Mortality	Low	High		
Morbidity	>70%	>80%		
Biofilm production	Abundant	Comparatively lower		Abundant

7.1.3.2 Etiology

CA is mainly caused by *Ma*. The other *Mycoplasma* spp. that are involved in causing CA include *Mmc*, *Mcc*, and *Mycoplasma putrefaciens* (*Mp*). The differentiating features of these four organisms are provided in Table 7.4.

About 90% of CA occurrence in goats is attributed to *Ma*. *Mcc* is prevalent widely in North Africa and *Mp* in western France.

7.1.3.3 Host Susceptibility

Lactating females and young animals are primarily affected. *Ma* affects both sheep and goats, whereas *Mmc*, *Mcc*, and *Mp* affect goats primarily.

Ma has been isolated from the wild ruminants Iberian ibex, Alpine ibex, Pyrenean ibex, and chamois, and also in bulls from eyes, ears, and brain spinal fluid. *Mmc* has been reported in Alpine ibex and captive Vaal rhebok. *Mcc* has been reported in Alpine and Pyrenean ibex, captive Vaal rhebok, captive Dall's sheep, wild markhor, and in apparently healthy cattle. *Mp* has been reported in healthy and affected milking goats. In roe deer and red deer, antibodies to *Ma* have been reported. In South American camelids like llamas, alpacas, and vicunas, antibodies to *Mcc* and *Mmc* have been reported.

7.1.3.4 Transmission

Infection occurs primarily through ingestion or inhalation of the secretions or excretions of infected goats. Inhalation of nasal and ocular secretions and ingestion of excretions

like urine and feces from infected goats lead to infection. Aerosol transmission over a short distance may also occur.

Mycoplasma is shed through milk and colostrum, and hence nursing kids might acquire infection from infected dams. Milk might remain infectious for several months to years.

Venereal transmission might occur through shedding of *Mycoplasma* through semen. Fomite transmission through contaminated feeding and watering troughs, milking machines, and bedding materials also occurs. The external ear canal of infected goats harbors CA-causing organisms, which are transmitted through ear mites.

Biofilm production for *Ma* and *Mp* is abundant and hence their survival in the environment is comparatively less fragile. Asymptomatic carriers can shed *Mycoplasma* for several months to years.

7.1.3.5 Pathogenesis

The incubation period is 1–8 weeks. The entry of CA-causing agents occurs through oral, respiratory, or mammary routes. The mucosa of the small intestine, respiratory tract, and alveoli of mammary glands are the predilection sites.

On entering the blood circulation, the organisms reach the mammary gland, eyes, lymph nodes, joints, and tendons, causing mastitis, agalactia, keratoconjunctivitis, and pneumonia (MAKePS syndrome). The inflammation in mammary gland inflammation is catarrhal or parenchymatous mastitis, which leads to atrophy and agalactia.

7.1.3.6 Clinical Symptoms

CA occurs in acute, subacute, and chronic forms. The acute form of CA is associated with *Ma* infection causing fever, and occasionally death. The subacute form of CA causes MAKePS syndrome, which is the major clinical sign. However, all the signs will not be present in a single goat. Other signs such as weakness, pyrexia, and anorexia will be mild and unnoticeable.

Mastitis occur in lactating does. The udder becomes hot and swollen; the milk is discolored with a yellowish tinge. The consistency of the milk can either be watery, granular, or clotted. Due to catarrhal or parenchymatous mastitis, the mammary gland becomes atrophied causing permanent damage to the udder. Agalactia can be observed. In CA caused by *Mp*, the milk smells rotten.

Arthritis or polyarthritis occurs mainly in carpal and tarsal joints. Swelling of these joints causes lameness and leads to recumbency slowly.

Keratoconjunctivitis can occur either for a short span of time or as a chronic infection, leading to blindness of one or both eyes. So far, *Mp* has not been reported to cause keratoconjunctivitis.

Pneumonia is generally not associated with CA; however, severe pneumonia forms have been reported in young goats. Septicemia has been reported in nursing lambs and kids. In addition, meningitis, abortion, congenital polyarthritis, genital lesions such as vulvovaginitis, salpingitis, metritis, balanoposthitis, and testicular degeneration have been reported in goats infected with CA. Abortion has been reported to occur in the first third of pregnancy and *Ma* has been isolated from placenta, liver, and spleen of the fetus. In the chronic form of CA, subclinical mastitis is exhibited.

Asymptomatically, these organisms can survive in infected goats for several months to years. Mortality is 100% in young animals and 40–50% in adults; and morbidity is 50–90%.

7.1.3.7 Lesions

Postmortem lesions include catarrhal mastitis, enlargement of mammary lymph nodes, periarticular edema, acute synovitis with hemorrhagic or turbid joint fluid, serous or mucopurulent conjunctivitis or keratitis, corneal ulceration, septicemia, bronchopneumonia, generalized peritonitis, and genital lesions including vulvovaginitis, cystic catarrhal metritis, and/or salpingitis in females, and balanoposthitis or testicular degeneration in males. Inflammation of the interstitial tissues of the udder and later secondary acinar involvement, fibrosis, and parenchymatous udder atrophy can also be observed. On experimental infection, acute diffuse interstitial pneumonia, arthritis, and multifocal necrotic purulent splenitis were the observed histopathological findings.

7.1.3.8 Diagnosis

- Samples of choice include the following:
  - Mastitis in lactating does – milk.
  - Arthritis – joint fluid.
  - Keratoconjunctivitis – eye swab.
  - Blood during acute disease phase.
  - Dead animals – lungs, lymph nodes, mammary gland, and pleural/pericardial fluid.
  - In milk, excretion of *Mycoplasma* will be more during the clinical phase after which it becomes intermittent, so multiple sampling (individual/pooled) at various points of time is required.
  - In joint fluid and eye swab, the load of *Mycoplasma* might be lower.
  - Ear canal swab samples are not recommended, as *Mycoplasma* inhabit the ear canal of healthy goats too.
  - Multiple samples from several goats are required.
  - Samples should be transported immediately in a cool condition. A transport medium with thallium acetate will reduce bacterial contamination of the samples.
- **Isolation**: *Ma*, *Mmc*, *Mcc*, and *Mp* have been reported to be isolated easily in most *Mycoplasma* media. Organic acids like pyruvate or isopropanol as well as sterol are required for the growth of *Ma*. Growth is slow in solid media and fast in liquid media. Hence, samples are initially cultivated in liquid-enrichment media for 2–3 days, following which cultivation on solid media is done. The colonies of *Ma* show a "film and spot" appearance in 4–7 days, producing a typical fried-egg appearance with dark centers.
- **Biochemical tests**: Sensitivity to digitonin differentiates *Mycoplasma* from *Acholeplasma*. *Mp* produces a putrefied odor in broth and solid media. In casein and coagulated serum, proteolysis can be observed with *Mcc* and *Mmc*.
- **Serological tests**: GIT, film inhibition test (FIT), indirect fluorescent antibody (IFA), dot immunoblotting, ELISA, and CFT can be performed. FIT is more suitable for diagnosis of *Ma*. ELISA along with immunoblotting is reported to be a sensitive test.
- **Molecular tests**: PCR, real-time PCR, and multiplex real-time PCR are used for diagnosis. Individual PCR is for *Mcc*, *Mmc*, and *Mp*; multiplex PCR for *Ma*, *Mcc*, and *Mmc*; and restriction fragment length polymorphism (RFLP) on the *lpdA* gene to differentiate *Mmc* and *Mcc* have been described (Table 7.3). Loop-mediated isothermal amplification (LAMP) can be used as a pen-side test for detection of *Ma*. Denaturing gradient gel electrophoresis (DGGE), a PCR-based method, is also used for identification of the causative agents of CA.
- Differential diagnosis involves:
  - Mastitis – staphylococcal and streptococcal infection.
  - Arthritis – caprine arthritis encephalitis virus.

– Keratoconjunctivitis – *Mycoplasma conjunctivae.*
– Pneumonia – *Pasteurellaceae*, parainfluenza, Visna-Maëdi, peste des petits ruminants (PPR), CCPP, and *Mycoplasma ovipneumoniae.*

7.1.3.9 Zoonosis

A report of *Mcc* from a human was isolated after they exhibited symptoms of recurrent fever, septicemia, and suspected meningitis.

7.1.3.10 Treatment and Control Strategy

Ma is genetically resistant to erythromycin. Fluoroquinolones, macrolides, and tetracyclines are used for treatment. Early and repeated treatment is required for successful recovery; however, bacterial clearance from the infected goats cannot be ensured.

Prevention and control involve vaccination, culling, and therapeutic treatment.

To date, no licensed vaccine for CA is available. Autogenous vaccines that are produced locally during one outbreak will be effective to prevent future outbreaks. Inactivated vaccines provide short-term immunity and do not prevent infection, but rather minimize the severity of the disease. Live attenuated vaccines are effective with long-term immunity, but their use is not recommended, especially in lactating does.

7.1.4 MAKePS Syndrome

Mastitis is caused primarily by *Ma*, *Mcc*, *Mmc*, and *Mp*. In addition, *Mycoplasma arginini* is associated with causing mastitis in goats. Inflammation of mammary glands,

enlargement of supramammary lymph nodes, atrophy, and agalactia can be observed. Abortion is also reported.

Arthritis is caused by *Ma*, *Mcc*, and *Mp*. An elevated temperature along with swollen joints can be observed in affected kids and goats. Pneumonia may or may not occur. Purulent or fibro-purulent arthritis can be observed during postmortem. Treatment involves administration of tylosin.

Keratoconjunctivitis is caused by *M. conjunctivae*. Lacrimation, conjunctival hyperemia, pannus, neovascularization, and iritis can be observed. *M. ovipneumoniae* and *M. arginini* also cause keratoconjunctivitis.

Pneumonia is caused by *Mccp*, *Mcc*, *Mmc* and *Ma*: *M. ovipneumoniae*, *M. conjunctivae*, and *M. arginini*. *Mp* has not been reported to be involved in respiratory disease. *M. ovipneumoniae* was first described in 1972 as causing severe pneumonia in kids and adult goats leading to death. A mild respiratory form of *M. ovipneumoniae* infection in kids is known as coughing syndrome. *M. arginini* is usually found along with *M. ovipneumoniae* infection. In kids, *M. arginini* causes pyrexia, circulating monocytes and neutrophils, and blood fibrinogen. MAKePS syndrome and the *Mycoplasma* spp. involved in causing it are depicted in Figure 7.3.

7.1.5 Hemotropic *Mycoplasma*

Hemotropic *Mycoplasma* (hemoplasma) are emerging or reemerging pathogens of zoonotic importance. Hemoplasmas affecting goats include *M. ovis* and *Candidatus Mycoplasma haemovis* (*C.M. haemovis*).

M. ovis, formerly known as *Eperythrozoon ovis*, causes hemoplasmosis in goats. It is transmitted through

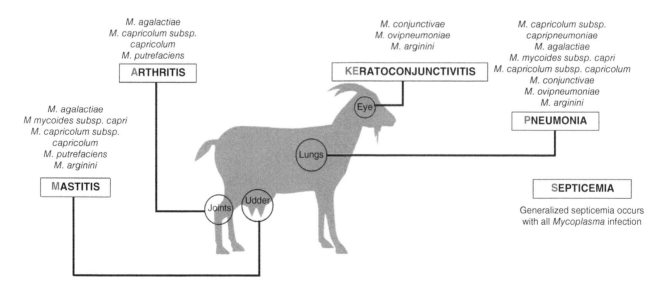

Figure 7.3 *Mycoplasma* spp. involved in MAKePS syndrome. *Source:* Courtesy of Ranjani Rajasekaran (co-author). Created using www.mindthegraph.com online software.

Table 7.5 Arthropod vectors involved in the transmission of *Mycoplasma* and *Rickettsia* diseases of goats.

Causative	Arthropod vector
Candidatus Mycoplasma haemovis	Ticks – *Rhipicephalus bursa* and *Haemaphysalis plubeum* Mosquitoes – *Aedes camptorhynchus* and *Culex annulirostris*
Ehrlichia ruminatium	*Ambylomma variegatum* (tropical bont tick), *Ambylomma hebraeum*, *Ambylomma lepidum, Amblyomma gemma, Amblyomma astrion*, and *Amblyomma pomposum* ticks
Anaplasma phagocytophilum	*Ixodes ricinus, Ixodes scapularis*, and *Ixodes pacifus* ticks
Anaplasma ovis	*Dermacentor* sp. ticks

mechanical vectors including lice, fleas, and mosquitoes. Young goats are severely affected, while adult goats acquire immunity on exposure. The organism affects red blood cells, and hence extravascular hemolysis followed by reticuloendothelial destruction is observed. Diagnosis involves blood smear examination using Giemsa, Romanowsky, or acridine orange stain, and PCR. Oxytetracycline can be used for treatment.

C.M. haemovis was first reported in sheep in Hungary in 2009 as a co-infection with *M. ovis* causing severe anemia. Later, *C.M. haemovis* was reported in goats, which have been shown to be persistent carriers of this organism. Transmission of this disease occurs through arthropods including ticks, namely *Rhipicephalus bursa* and *Haemaphysalis plubeum*, and mosquitoes, namely *Aedes camptorhynchus* and *Culex annulirostris* (Table 7.5). *C.M. haemovis* can be diagnosed through PCR based on 16S rRNA (Table 7.3). Further research on this organism is ongoing.

7.2 Rickettsia

In the order of Rickettsiales there are currently two families, namely Anaplasmataceae and Rickettsiaceae. The organisms that cause disease in goats include *Ehrlichia ruminatium* causing heartwater disease; *Anaplasma phagocytophilum* and *Anaplasma ovis* causing anaplasmosis are classified in the family of Anaplasmataceae. *Coxiella burnetii* causing Q-fever, earlier classified in the family of Rickettsiaceae, has now been reclassified to the family Coxiellaceae of order Legionellales. The details of the former and current taxonomic names of *Rickettsia* are provided in Table 7.2.

7.2.1 Heartwater Disease

7.2.1.1 History
The first report of heartwater was documented in South Africa in 1838 as a fatal disease in sheep and was called "a type of Nintas." In the late 1900s, this disease was identified as a tick-borne non-contagious rickettsial disease.

The disease is endemic in Africa, around the region of the Sahara desert, and in the islands of the Caribbean and Madagascar.

7.2.1.2 Etiology
The causative agent is *E. ruminatium,* formerly known as *Rickettsia ruminantium* and *Cowdria ruminantium. E. ruminatium* is a Gram-negative, small pleomorphic, obligate intracellular organism, particularly intracytoplasmic and not intranuclear.

7.2.1.3 Host Susceptibility
Sheep and goats, cattle, water buffalo, and wild ungulates are susceptible. Experimental infection of various wild animals caused the disease.

7.2.1.4 Transmission
Transmission is through ticks of the genus *Amblyomma*. The major species of *Amblyomma* transmitting heartwater disease is *A. variegatum*, also called as tropical bont tick, which is predominant in Africa and the Caribbean. Other *Amblyomma* species include *Amblyomma hebraeum*, *A. lepidum, A. gemma, Amblyomma astrion*, and *Amblyomma pomposum* (Table 7.5). Laboratory demonstration of transmission of *E. ruminatium* was confirmed in *A. sparsum, A. cohaerans, Amblyomma marmoreum, A. tholloni, A. maculatum* (Gulf Coast tick), *Amblyomma mixtum*, and *Amblyomma dissimile* tick species.

Ticks obtain *E. ruminantium* by feeding on infected goats. Infected goats remain carriers for 2–12 months. Transstadial transmission of *E. ruminatium* occurs in these ticks and transovarial transmission is not reported. Vertical transmission of *E. ruminantium* through colostrum and iatrogenic transmission has also been reported.

7.2.1.5 Pathogenesis
The incubation period is 14 days. Ticks that obtained *E. ruminatium* from an infected goat are replicated and amplified in the intestinal epithelium of the ticks, which transmit the organism to a susceptible goat through either salivary or regurgitated gut contents while feeding.

On entering the host *E. ruminatium* replicates in the regional lymph nodes, enters the bloodstream, and invades the endothelial cells. The organism gets localized as vacuole clusters in the cytoplasm of vascular endothelial cells.

E. ruminatium occurs in three different stages of growth while replicating in the host: elementary, intermediate, and reticulated bodies. The elementary bodies are infectious, and the reticulated bodies are in the proliferative stage.

7.2.1.6 Clinical Symptoms
Clinical forms of the disease include peracute, acute, subacute, and mild forms:

- The peracute form involves sudden death preceded by fever, convulsions, severe respiratory distress, hyperesthesia, and lacrimation. This form is quite rare and is often seen in native goats in Africa.
- The acute form of disease is the most common. Clinical signs include pyrexia, anorexia, diarrhea, respiratory distress that can lead to dyspnea, and nervous involvement. Neurological involvement is less severe in goats. Death occurs within a week of infection. Prior to death, the body temperature reduces abruptly to a sub-normal level. This form is seen in both non-native and indigenous goats in Africa.
- The subacute form is not frequently reported. In this form, prolonged pyrexia, cough, and mild nervous involvement are observed. The affected goats either recover or die within two weeks of infection. Pregnant goats are prone to abortion. This form is mostly observed in kids and partially immune goats.
- The mild form of this disease is called heartwater fever. Goats with natural resistance to *E. ruminatium* suffer a brief fever that is unnoticeable. Affected goats recover within a week.

7.2.1.7 Lesions
Hydropericardium is the major postmortem lesion of heartwater disease, along with hydrothorax, edema of the mediastinal and bronchial lymph nodes, pulmonary edema, and serous or frothy fluid oozing out from cut surfaces of the lung as a result of increased vascular permeability. The presence of froth in trachea and bronchi explains death by asphyxia. Straw-colored to reddish fluid in the pericardium, petechiae on the epicardium and endocardium, intestinal congestion, moderate splenomegaly, nephritic pale kidneys, and congested liver with fatty degeneration and congestion of the brain have also been observed.

Histopathological findings include alveolar and interstitial edema of the lungs, and multifocal and lymphocytic interstitial nephritis can be observed.

7.2.1.8 Diagnosis
Clinical samples to be collected include blood smear (live and dead goat), brain (cerebrum, cerebellum, or hippocampus), lung, kidney, spleen, and heart tissues. *Amblyomma* ticks can be collected in 70% alcohol for detection of *E. ruminantium* using molecular methods.

Staining can be done using eosin and methylene blue or Giemsa stain. In the brain tissues, *E. ruminantium* can be observed as clumps inside capillary endothelial cells, as reddish-purple to blue coccoid to pleomorphic organisms. Close to the nucleus, *E. ruminantium* is ring shaped or horseshoe shaped.

Nucleic acid detection in blood or tissues through nested and real-time PCR based on pCS20 and map-1 region (Table 7.3), LAMP, immunoperoxidase tests on formalin-fixed brain tissues, and serological tests including indirect immunofluorescence, ELISA, and western blotting can also be done.

7.2.1.9 Zoonotic Potential
E. ruminatium was detected by PCR in adult humans and children affected with human ehrlichiosis in 2005 and 2015, respectively.

7.2.1.10 Treatment
Tetracycline and supportive treatment can be given. Vaccination with live moderately virulent *E. ruminantium* to 1-week-old kids, followed by antibiotic treatment when fever develops, are reported to be effective. Control of ticks can reduce the spread of this disease.

7.2.2 Anaplasmosis

7.2.2.1 History
Anaplasma was initially identified as a parasitic and was later reclassified as a bacterial pathogen. In 1910, anaplasmosis was first described as "yellow bag" or "gall sickness" when the animals developed jaundice.

7.2.2.2 Etiology
Anaplasmosis in goats is a tick-borne rickettsial infection caused by *A. ovis*. *A. phagocytophilum* and *A. marginale*, which affect dogs and cattle, respectively, have also been reported to infect goats.

Anaplasma spp. are Gram-negative obligate intracellular bacteria affecting the red blood cells of host species.

7.2.2.3 Host Susceptibility
Goats, sheep, and cattle are highly susceptible.

7.2.2.4 Transmission
Anaplasmosis is transmitted through vectors like *Ixodes ricinus*, *Ixodes scapularis*, and *Ixodes pacifus* tick for *A. phagocytophilum* and *Dermacentor* sp. for *A. ovis* (Table 7.5). Ticks obtain the organism from infected goats

while feeding and transmit it to a susceptible goat through saliva. Iatrogenic transmission is also possible.

7.2.2.5 Pathogenesis

The incubation period is 1–2 weeks. Anaplasmosis is a mild or subclinical infection in goats generally, although sometimes a severe form can also be noticed.

Ticks harboring the elementary bodies of *Anaplasma* spp. on feeding a susceptible goat infect the goat. The elementary body is the infective stage, and it enters the host cell by phagocytosis. The phagosome is formed, where the organism replicates to form multiple elementary bodies packed tightly to form clusters. These clusters are called initial bodies, which then form microcolonies called morulae. Morulae are released into the bloodstream either by apoptosis or exocytosis to infect new cells (Figure 7.4). The organism disseminates to bone marrow and spleen, and primarily attacks neutrophils and eosinophils, and later monocytes and lymphocytes. Cytoplasmic vacuoles of polymorphonuclear cells serve as the site of survival and multiplication of *Anaplasma* spp.

The course of anaplasmosis in goats can be categorized in four phases: incubation, developmental, convalescent, and carrier phases. The first stage lasts for about 1–3 months. In the second stage, anemia develops and reticulocytes can be detected in peripheral blood. This stage lasts for 4–9 days. In the third stage, resolution of anemia can be seen, and finally in the fourth stage *A. ovis* is completely removed from the peripheral blood. However, goats remain carriers for an indefinite period.

Spread of anaplasmosis can be observed due to stress, which includes high environmental temperature, low nutrition, tick infestation, body condition, vaccination, and long-distance transportation.

7.2.2.6 Clinical Symptoms
- Fever, fatigue, and respiratory distress.
- Anorexia, loss of weight, and icteric mucous membrane.
- Hemolytic anemia and hemoglobinuria.

7.2.2.7 Lesions

Postmortem lesions include watery unclotted blood, pale or icteric mucous membrane, pale and edematous lungs, hepatomegaly with icteric appearance, splenomegaly with reddish-brown pulp, distended gall bladder with yellowish-brown appearance, and accumulation of straw-colored fluid in body cavities. Histopathological lesions include bone marrow hyperplasia and extramedullary hematopoiesis in the spleen and in other organs.

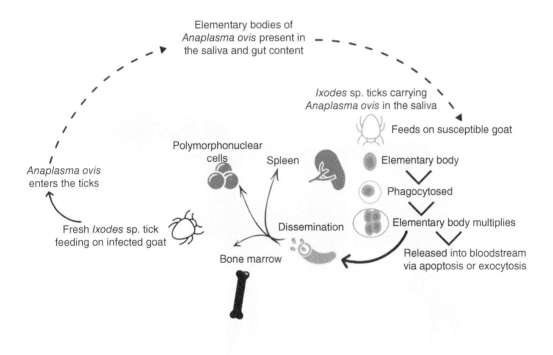

Figure 7.4 Transmission and pathogenesis of *Anaplasma ovis*. *Source:* Courtesy of Ranjani Rajasekaran (co-author). Created using www.mindthegraph.com online software.

7.2.2.8 Diagnosis

- Demonstration of *A. ovis* in peripheral blood smear using Giemsa stain. It appears as small, purple intraerythrocytic inclusions.
- Detection of antibody titer using ELISA, IFA, and CFT. IFA is mostly used in epidemiological studies as it is economical.
- cELISA using mAb ANAF16C1 to identify major surface protein(MSP)-5 antigen. The MSP-5 antigen is conserved and differentiated for the various *Anaplasma* spp. described so far. cELISA is highly sensitive and specific.
- PCR to confirm presence of *A. ovis* in blood or other tissues based on MSP-1 (Table 7.3). It can also be used to differentiate among the various *Anaplasma* spp. It is a reliable and sensitive test.

- The gold-standard test for diagnosis and confirmation of anaplasmosis involves both microscopic examination and cELISA.

7.2.2.9 Zoonotic Potential

A. ovis has been reported to infect human beings and is considered as an emerging zoonotic disease.

7.2.2.10 Treatment

Long-acting tetracyclines can be administered. Anti-tick injections remove tick infestations both internally and externally. Control of ticks in the surrounding environment reduces the spread.

7.3 Chlamydia

Chlamydial infections in goats is attributed to *Chlamydia abortus* that causes enzootic abortion and *Chlamydia pecorum* that causes polyarthritis. The details of the former and current taxonomic names of *Rickettsia* are provided in Table 7.2.

7.3.1 Enzootic Abortion

7.3.1.1 History

Enzootic abortion was first described in Scotland in 1936.

7.3.1.2 Etiology

C. abortus is the causative organism, formerly known as *Chlamydia psittaci* immunotype-1 and *C. abortus*. *C. abortus* are small Gram-negative, obligate intracellular, non-motile bacteria with a cell wall possessing an outer membrane similar to Gram-negative bacteria, but they lack peptidoglycan, which differentiates these organisms from *Rickettsia*.

There are two developmental forms of *C. abortus*: elementary bodies and reticulate bodies. Elementary bodies are the infectious form that are present extracellularly, and on entry into the host cell differentiate into metabolically active reticulate bodies inside a membrane-bound endocytic vacuole. These reticulate bodies mature and again differentiate into mature infectious elementary bodies, which are released by either cell lysis or exocytosis to infect new host cells.

7.3.1.3 Host Susceptibility

Goats and sheep are susceptible, and both pregnant naïve goats and the fetus.

7.3.1.4 Transmission

Aborted contents including placenta and fetus, uterine secretions, vaginal discharge, and semen are the primary sources of infectious material. Nine days prior to abortion and two weeks after abortion, *C. abortus* is shed through uterine secretions. In carrier does, *C. abortus* is shed around the time of estrus. *C. abortus* is occasionally shed through milk and feces.

Ingestion of feed or water contaminated with infectious material from infected goats, inhalation of infected discharge directly through nasopharynx contact with the infected goat or from the environment, direct inoculation into the eye, and venereal transmission are the different modes of transmission of *C. abortus*. *C. abortus* can remain infectious in the environment for several days in cold temperatures and for several months in freezing temperatures.

7.3.1.5 Pathogenesis

The incubation period is two weeks. On contact with the infected material, the infectious elementary bodies enter the host cell and cause infection.

When an infected doe becomes pregnant, *C. abortus* spreads to the cotyledons, placenta, and fetus within 95 days of gestation. After infection through the vaginal route, naïve pregnant does will give birth to weak infected kids. Abortion in goats can occur at any stage of pregnancy.

Infected goats remain inapparent carriers with continuous shedding of *C. abortus*. However, their fertility remains unaffected in future pregnancies.

7.3.1.6 Clinical Symptoms

The primary clinical symptom is abortion, along with septicemia and pneumonia. Stillbirth, delivery of weak lambs, retained placenta, and metritis can also be observed. Vaginal bleeding two weeks before abortion and reddish-brown vaginal discharge for several days after abortion will be observed. Fever may also be seen.

7.3.1.7 Lesions

Postmortem lesions include necrotizing thickened placenta affecting cotyledons and intercotyledonary spaces, and autolyzed or well-preserved or mummified fetus. A leathery appearance of the placenta with dark reddish-brown cotyledons and red to brown intercotyledonary areas covered in creamy exudate can be noticed. In pregnant or aborted goats, petechiae are observed in the tongue, hooves, and buccal cavity of the fetus.

7.3.1.8 Diagnosis

Samples to be collected are aborted contents including placenta, cotyledons, aborted or stillborn fetal lung or liver, vaginal discharges, abomasal contents, feces, urine, semen, and ocular and nasal secretions.

Smears made from placenta, vaginal discharge, or fetal contents can be examined for the presence of elementary bodies using modified Ziehl–Neelsen stain. Red clumps of elementary bodies against a blue background of cellular debris can be observed. This should be differentiated from *C. burnetii* organisms. Pale green elementary bodies can be observed in dark-ground illumination.

Serological tests include ELISA and CFT. However, due to the shared antigenicity of lipopolysaccharide among *Chlamydia* spp., cross-reactivity can occur.

Immunostaining methods to detect antigens of *Chlamydia* include immunohistochemistry and immunofluorescence. Also, chlamydial antigens can be detected using antigen-capture ELISAs and FATs.

Molecular methods of identification include PCR, real-time PCR, and DNA microarray. Detection by PCR involves amplification of 16S-23S rRNA along with RFLP analysis (Table 7.3). Real-time PCR to detect *C. abortus* involves initial screening of *Chlamydiaceae* infection using the 23S rRNA gene, followed by outer membrane protein A (*ompA*) gene amplification specific for *C. abortus*. Real-time PCR and DNA microarray have been considered as valid diagnostic tests for detection of *C. abortus*. In order to differentiate between vaccinated and infected animals, PCR along with RFLP has been developed.

Isolation of *C. abortus* can be done in cell culture and embryonated chicken eggs. McCoy, Buffalo Green Monkey (BGM), or baby hamster kidney (BHK) cells can be used for cell culture isolation. Yolk sac inoculation of infected cotyledons, placental membranes, fetal lung or liver, or vaginal swabs done in 6–8-day-old embryonated chicken eggs causes death of the embryo with 4–13 days post inoculation. Smear examination of the yolk sac membrane reveals elementary bodies.

7.3.1.9 Zoonotic Potential

Placentitis, abortion, premature births, and life-threatening illnesses have been reported in pregnant women on infection with *C. abortus*.

7.3.1.10 Treatment

- Tetracyclines, macrolides, and fluoroquinolones are effective.
- Disposal of infected materials like placenta and fetus and disinfection of the area are recommended.
- Infected kids should be culled and aborted goats isolated for two weeks until shedding of *C. abortus* is absent.
- Goats in herds where infection was already present should be vaccinated. Immunity in infected goats will remain for three years, after which waning will occur.

7.3.2 Chlamydial Polyarthritis

C. pecorum, formerly known as *C. psittaci* immunotype 2, causes keratoconjunctivitis and polyarthritis in goats. It is present asymptomatically in the intestinal tract. It causes abortion, respiratory disease, orchitis, or mastitis. Weaned kids and young goats up to 10 months of age are susceptible. Swelling of joints and stiffness are the primary clinical symptoms. Fibrinous arthritis with no involvement of cartilage and no purulent appearance of joint fluid are observed during postmortem. Lethargy and acute fever can be observed. Histopathological lesions include fibrinosuppurative, and necrotizing enteritis in intestinal tissue and hepatitis in liver were reported in aborted goat fetuses.

Multiple-Choice Questions

1 Which is the current taxonomic name of *Mycoplasma* strain F38?
   A *Mycoplasma agalactiae*
   B *Mycoplasma ovipneumoniae*
   C *Mycoplasma capricolum* subsp. *capripneumoniae* (*Mccp*)
   D *Mycoplasma ovis*

2 Milk smells rotten in which causative agent of contagious agalactia?
   A *Mycoplasma agalactiae*
   B *M. mycoides* subsp. *capri*
   C *Mycoplasma capricolum* subsp. *capricolum*
   D *Mycoplasma putrefaciens*

3 For the growth of *Mycoplasma agalactiae,* which of the following is/are required?
  A Isopropanol
  B Sterol
  C Pyruvate
  D All the above

4 Pulmonary involvement is absent in which cause of contagious agalactia?
  A *Mycoplasma agalactiae*
  B *M. mycoides subsp. capri*
  C *Mycoplasma capricolum* subsp. *capricolum*
  D *Mycoplasma putrefaciens*

5 No invasins or toxins are produced by which *Mycoplasma* sp. for adhesion?
  A *Mycoplasma agalactiae*
  B *M. mycoides subsp. capri*
  C *Mycoplasma capricolum* subsp. *capripneumoniae*
  D *Mycoplasma putrefaciens*

6 Which of the following statements is/are correct?
  1 Hemotropic *Mycoplasmas* are also called hemoplasmas
  2 Hemotropic *Mycoplasmas* affecting goats include *M. ovis* only
  3 Hemotropic *Mycoplasmas* affecting goats are not transmitted by vectors
    A 1 is wrong, 2 and 3 are correct
    B 1, 2, and 3 are correct
    C 1 is correct, 2 and 3 are wrong
    D All statements are wrong

7 Which of the following statements is/are false about *Mccp*?
  1 *Mccp* is a fragile bacterium
  2 *Mccp* is resistant and does not get inactivated at higher temperatures
  3 Aerosol spread of *Mccp* is possible at shorter distances
  4 *Mccp* is spread through fomites and arthropod vectors
    A 1 only
    B 2 and 4
    C 1, 2, and 3
    D 1, 3, and 4

8 What is coughing syndrome?
  A A mild respiratory form of *M. ovipneumoniae* infection in kids
  B An infection caused by *M. putrefaciens* in adult goats
  C A pneumonia caused by *M. agalactiae*
  D A hemotropic mycoplasma causing pneumonia in goats

9 For diagnosis of contagious agalactia in goats, which of the following clinical samples is/are not recommended?
  A Milk
  B Swab from ear canal
  C Joint fluid
  D Blood

10 According to the OIE, contagious caprine pleuro-pneumonia can be documented in which of the following circumstances?
  1 Laboratory isolation of *Mccp* from suspected samples is successful
  2 Serological tests confirm the isolation of *Mccp*
  3 Lesions are confined to lung and pleura causing pleuropneumonia
  4 No enlargement of interlobular septa of lungs
    A Statements 1 and 2 are true
    B Statements 1, 2, and 3 are true
    C Statement 2 is true
    D All statements are true

11 How is *Ehrlichia ruminatium* transmitted?
  1 Vertical transmission
  2 Vector-borne transmission
  3 Transstadial transmission in ticks
  4 Transovarial transmission in ticks
    A 1, 2, and 3
    B 4 only
    C 2 only
    D 3 and 4 only

12 Which developmental stage of *Ehrlichia ruminatium* is infectious?
  A Elementary bodies
  B Intermediate bodies
  C Reticulate bodies
  D Both elementary and reticulate bodies

13 What is microscopic examination of a horseshoe- or ring-shaped appearance of an organism close to the nucleus suggestive of?
  A *Anaplasma ovis*
  B *Mycoplasmsa agalactiae*
  C *Ehrlichia ruminatium*
  D *Chlamydia pecorum*

14 What is the gold-standard test for confirmation of anaplasmosis in goats?
  A cELISA
  B PCR and cELISA
  C Indirect ELISA along with microscopic examination
  D cELISA along with microscopic examination

15 During *Chlamydia abortus* infection, when can pregnant goats abort?
A Third stage of pregnancy
B Any stage of pregnancy
C First third of pregnancy
D Abortion does not occur

16 Which of the following features of *Anaplasma ovis* infection in goats is/are true?
1 Presence of *Ixodes* sp. ticks in the environment
2 Yellowish-brown distended gall bladder
3 Purple-colored intraerythrocytic inclusion body in Giemsa-stained peripheral blood smear
4 Hydropericardium
A 1 and 2
B 2 and 4
C 3 and 4
D 1, 2, and 3

17 Which of the following is the primary postmortem lesion of heartwater disease?
A Hydropericardium along with hydrothorax
B Congested liver with fatty degeneration
C Unilateral pleuropneumonia
D Distended gall bladder

18 Elementary bodies of what against a blue background are confirmatory of *Chlamydia abortus* and what should they be differentiated from?
A Red clumps, *Anaplasma ovis*
B Purple clumps, *Ehrlichia ruminatium*
C Red clumps, *Coxiella burnetii*
D Green clumps, *Mycoplasma agalactiae*

19 What is the route of inoculation for isolation of *Chlamydia abortus* in embryonated chicken eggs?
A Chorio allantoic membrane
B Yolk sac
C Amnio allantoic fluid
D Intravenous route

20 What is swelling of joints in weaned kids and young goats suggestive of?
A *Chlamydia pecorum* infection
B *Chlamydia abortus* infection
C *Ehrlichia ruminatium*
D *Mycoplasma ovis*

References

MacOwan, K.J. and Minette, J.E. (1977). The role of *Mycoplasma* strain F38 in contagious caprine pleuropneumonia (CCCP) in Kenya. *Veterinary Record* 101 (19): 380–381. https://doi.org/10.1136/vr.101.19.380.

Ostrowski, S., Thiaucourt, F., Amirbekov, M. et al. (2011). Fatal outbreak of *Mycoplasma capricolum* pneumonia in endangered markhors. *Emerging Infectious Diseases* 17 (12): 2338–2341. https://doi.org/10.3201/eid1712.110187.

Further Readings

Mycoplasma

Chaber, A.L., Lignereux, L., Qassimi, A. et al. (2014). Fatal transmission of contagious caprine pleuropneumonia to an Arabian oryx (*Oryx leucoryx*). *Veterinary Microbiology* 173 (1–2): 156–159. https://doi.org/10.1016/j.vetmic.2014.07.003.

Dereje, T. and Teshale, S. (2021). Contagious caprine pleuropneumonia: A review. *Journal of Veterinary Medicine and Animal Health* 13 (3): 132–143. doi: 10.5897/JVMAH2020.0906.

Fischer, A., Shapiro, B., Muriuki, C. et al. (2012). The origin of the "Mycoplasma mycoides cluster" coincides with domestication of ruminants. *PLoS One* 7 (4): e36150. https://doi.org/10.1371/journal.pone.0036150.

Galon, E.M.S., Moumouni, P.F.A., Ybanez, R.H.D. et al. (2019). Molecular evidence of hemotropic mycoplasmas in goats from Cebu, Philippines. *Journal of Veterinary Medical Science* 81 (6): 869–873. https://doi.org/10.1292/jvms.19-0042.

Gebremedhin, S.G., Basore, B.A., and Beta, A.M. (2020). Contagious caprine pleuropneumonia, A review. *Advances in Biological Research* 14 (3): 136–142. https://doi.org/10.5829/idosi.abr.2020.136.142.

Hutcheon, D. (1881). Contagious pleuro-pneumonia in angora goats. *Veterinary Journal and Annals of Comparative Pathology* 13 (9): 171–180. https://doi.org/10.1016/S2543-3377(17)43153-0.

IDRC•CRDI (2016). *Contagious Caprine Pleuropneumonia*, Disease monograph series 3. Ottawa: International Development Research Centre https://idl-bnc-idrc. dspacedirect.org/handle/10625/58278.

Matthews, J.G. (2016). Lameness in kids. In: *Diseases of the Goat* (ed. J. Matthews), 109–110. Chichester: Wiley https://doi.org/10.1002/9781119073543.

Nicholas, R. and Churchward, C. (2012). Contagious caprine pleuropneumonia: new aspects of an old disease. *Transboundary and Emerging Diseases* 59 (3): 189–196. https://doi. org/10.1111/j.1865-1682.2011.01262.x.

OIE (World Organization for Animal Health) (2018). Contagious agalactia. In: *Manual of Diagnostic Tests and Vaccines for Terrestrial Animals*. Paris: OIE, ch. 3.7.3. http://www.woah.org/fileadmin/Home/fr/Health_standards/tahm/3.07.03_CONT_AGALACT.pdf.

OIE (World Organization for Animal Health) (2021). Contagious caprine pleuropneumonia. In: *Manual of Diagnostic Tests and Vaccines for Terrestrial Animals*. Paris: OIE, ch. 3.7.4. http://www.woah.org/fileadmin/Home/fr/Health_standards/tahm/3.07.04_CCPP.pdf.

Samiullah, S. (2013). Contagious caprine pleuropneumonia and its current picture in Pakistan: a review. *Veterinárni Medicina* 58 (8): 389–398. https://doi.org/10.17221/6977-VETMED.

Wang, X., Cui, Y., Zhang, Y. et al. (2017). Molecular characterization of hemotropic mycoplasmas (*Mycoplasma ovis* and "Candidatus Mycoplasma haemovis") in sheep and goats in China. *BMC Veterinary Research* 13 (1): 1–8. https://doi.org/10.1186/s12917-017-1062-z.

Yatoo, M.I., Parray, O.R., Bashir, S.T. et al. (2019). Contagious caprine pleuropneumonia – a comprehensive review. *Veterinary Quarterly* 39 (1): 1–25. https://doi.org/10.108 0/01652176.2019.1580826.

Rickettsia

CVBD (2023). Anaplasmosis. Greenfield, IN: Elanco. https://cvbd.elanco.com/diseases/tick-borne-diseases/anaplasmosis.

Deem, S.L. (1998). A review of heartwater and the threat of introduction of *Cowdria ruminantium* and *Amblyomma* spp. ticks to the American mainland. *Journal of Zoo and Wildlife Medicine* 29 (2): 109–113. http://www.jstor.org/stable/20095732.

Matthews, J.G. (2016). Anaemia. In: *Diseases of the Goat* (ed. J. Matthews), 280–281. Chichester: Wiley https://doi.org/10.1002/9781119073543.

OIE (World Organization for Animal Health) (2018). Heartwater. In: *Manual of Diagnostic Tests and Vaccines for Terrestrial Animals*. Paris, OIE, ch. 2.1.9. http://www.woah.org/fileadmin/Home/eng/Health_standards/tahm/2.01.09_HEARTWATER.pdf.

Spickler, A.R. (2015). Heartwater. Ames, IA: Center for Food Security and Public Health. http://www.cfsph.iastate.edu/Factsheets/pdfs/heartwater.pdf

Underwood, W.J., Blauwiekel, R., Delano, M.L. et al. (2015). Biology and diseases of ruminants (sheep, goats, and cattle). In: *Laboratory Animal Medicine*, 3e (ed. J.G. Fox, L.C. Anderson, G.M. Otto, et al.), 623–694. Cambridge, MA: Academic Press http://doi.org/10.1016/B978-0-12-409527-4.00015-8.

Chlamydia

Matthews, J.G. (2016). Eye disease. In: *Diseases of the Goat* (ed. J. Matthews), 297. Chichester: Wiley https://doi.org/10.1002/9781119073543.

Menzies, A.I. (2007). Abortion in sheep: diagnosis and control. In: *Current Therapy in Large Animal Theriogenology*, 2e (ed. R.S. Youngquist and W.R. Threlfall), 667–680. Philadelphia, PA: W.B. Saunders https://doi.org/10.1016/B978-072169323-1.50093-3.

OIE (World Organization for Animal Health) (2018). Enzootic abortion of ewes. In: *Manual of Diagnostic Tests and Vaccines for Terrestrial Animals*. Paris: OIE, ch. 3.8.5. http://www.woah.org/fileadmin/Home/fr/Health_standards/tahm/3.08.05_ENZ_ABOR.pdf.

8

Bacterial Diseases of Goats

Vipin Maurya

Department of Livestock Production Management, Faculty of Veterinary & Animal Sciences, Institute of Agricultural Sciences, Banaras Hindu University, Mirzapur, Uttar Pradesh, India

Intensive production systems are on trend for increasing profits. Such intensification in small ruminant farming has led to a rise in disease outbreaks. Bacteria are among the disease-causing pathogens as well as various other microbes, viruses, and so on that cause severe diseases in goats, leading to heavy economic losses to farmers (decreased production, productivity, loss of life, and costs involved in managing the outbreak). Numerous influences like increased herd intensity, poor ventilation in sheds, poor sanitation, and poor management practices can predispose goats to bacterial diseases, which may lead to heavy mortality. Some of the important bacterial diseases of goats are discussed in detail in this chapter. Figure 8.1 illustrates the organs and tissues affected by various bacterial diseases.

8.1 Anthrax

Anthrax is an often fatal zoonotic disease, characterized by septicemia, splenomegaly, and sudden death of the infected animal, with oozing of blood from natural orifices (Hamborsky et al. 2015).

8.1.1 Etiology

The disease is caused by *Bacillus anthracis*, a large, Gram-positive, spore-forming, capsulated, non-motile, aerobic, rod-shaped bacterium (Misgie et al. 2015).

The disease spreads through contaminated feed, water, pasture, or through the byproducts obtained from an affected animal. The disease in goats is usually peracute (it kills the animal in 2–6 hours) or in the acute form, which takes up to 48 hours for death (Popoff 2020).

B. anthracis is considered a bioterrorism agent. It not only affects sheep and goats but cattle, buffalo, equines, swine, and even humans. When endospores enter through abraded skin, the cutaneous form of anthrax (malignant pustules) advances. The pulmonary form (wool sorters' disease) trails the inhalation route and the intestinal form is due to ingestion of infective material.

8.1.2 Clinical Features

Peracute cases of anthrax are characterized by staggering, dyspnea, hyperthermia, trembling, convulsions, and a rapidly fatal course leading to sudden mortality. Acute cases exhibit excitement followed by lethargy, stupor, respiratory or cardiac distress, high fever, staggering, seizures, and death. Ruminal stasis, hemorrhagic mucosae, milk production reducing drastically, bloody discharge from the natural orifices, and abortion may also be noticed.

8.1.3 Pathological Features

Necropsy of anthrax-suspected corpses is not recommended due to the risk of environmental contamination with the endospores. Important features of anthrax in goats include dark, tarry, thick blood from natural orifices that fails to clot; the non-appearance of rigor mortis; and quick decomposition of the carcass due to high body temperature. Septicemic lesions, enteritis, ulcers, epicardial and endocardial hemorrhages may be seen along with ecchymosis, edema, and reddish effusions under the serosa of several tissues/organs.

8.1.4 Diagnosis

Clinical symptoms are distinctly indicative of anthrax, which is confirmed by demonstration of the causative organism in blood smears. Air-dried, fixed smears stained

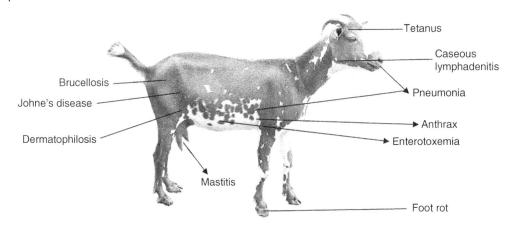

Figure 8.1 Organs/tissues affected by various bacterial diseases. Tetanus ➜ nervous system; pasteurellosis/pneumonia, contagious caprine pleuropneumonia ➜ respiratory system; enterotoxemia, colibacillosis, salmonellosis ➜ intestines; brucellosis ➜ reproductive tract; foot rot ➜ laminae of the foot and skin–horn junction; dermatophilosis ➜ skin; mastitis ➜ udders/teats; Johne's disease ➜ corrugation of intestine; caseous lymphadenitis ➜ lymph nodes.

with polychrome methylene blue (M'Fadyean stain) or Giemsa should be used. Ascoli's thermoprecipitation test may also be used for diagnosis; this test was developed to supply rapid retrospective evidence of anthrax infection in an animal product. The chromatographic test, a simple, rapid, reliable, and sensitive test based on monoclonal antibodies, can also be used for diagnosis.

8.1.5 Treatment

Treatment of the peracute condition is futile due to sudden death. Antisera of anthrax may help if injected in the early stages along with parenteral antibiotics like tetracyclines at 5 mg/kg body weight. Higher doses of combination antibiotics, such as penicillin–streptomycin, can be recommended.

8.1.6 Preventive Measures

- Annual vaccination should take place with live attenuated or avirulent spore vaccines.
- Strict biosecurity measures should be maintained with regular disinfection of farm premises.
- In case of an outbreak, affected animals should be isolated and strict quarantine measures should be imposed, followed by vaccination of the unaffected animals.
- The infected premises should be sanitized using strong disinfectants, for instance 5% sodium hydroxide or formalin.
- Proper disposal of carcasses and the infected materials should be done by either deep burial or incineration. A 2–2.5 m deep pit should be dug to dispose of carcasses,

litter, and leftover feed. The pit should be covered with quicklime/disinfectants to prevent spore formation.
- Attires and fomites should be disinfected by soaking in 10% formaldehyde. If gamma-irradiation facilities are available, they must be used to avoid human infection.

8.2 Pneumonia

Inflammation of the lungs of goats by infectious and noninfectious agents is characterized by respiratory distress or occasionally toxemia. Pneumonia is one of the most common respiratory problems in small ruminants and leads to increased production costs due to expensive treatments. The mortality rate is high both in kids and adults (Matthews and Wiley 2016).

8.2.1 Etiology

Pasteurella spp. (*Pasteurella multocida*, *Mannheimia haemolytica*, etc.) are causative of pneumonia.

P. multocida and *M. haemolytica* are found in the upper respiratory tract of goats. *M. haemolytica* are subdivided in two groups, A and T. Type A is more prevalent and is associated with a severe form of pneumonia, though several types of bacteria may be isolated from the same pneumonic lesions. *Corynebacterium pyogenes*, *Staphylococcus aureus*, *Proteus mirabilis*, *Pseudomonas aeruginosa*, *Streptococcus* spp., and *Escherichia coli* are some other bacteria that may be isolated from pneumonic lungs. Along with bacteria, *Mycoplasma* may also be responsible for pneumonia in goats (Yatoo et al. 2019) (Figure 8.2).

Figure 8.2 Pathogenesis of pneumonia in goats.

Bacterial pneumonia/any respiratory infections ⮕ Transmission ⮕ inhalation of infective aerosols ⮕ establishment of *P. haemolytica*/pathogenic bacteria in respiratory system
> ➤ Bacterial fimbriae facilitate attachment on the mucosa
> ➤ Proteolytic enzymes disrupts the mucosal barrier
> ➤ Impairing the functions of the respiratory tract
> ➤ Thus further facilitating colonization
> ➤ Cytotoxin cause lysis of respiratory tract cells.

8.2.2 Clinical Features

There are acute, subacute, and chronic forms of pasteurellosis. The acute form is characterized by respiratory distress, mucous discharge from the nostril, anorexia (reduced feed intake), dyspnea, cough, severe lacrimation, despair, and pyrexia. Kids are more susceptible than adults and death may occur without any clinical signs. Subacute and chronic cases are characterized by unthriftiness, rhinitis, or pharyngitis.

8.2.3 Pathological Features

Hemorrhage, congestion, emphysema, and reddish/grayish hepatization of the lung tissue can be grossly observed. The lungs are predominantly the affected organs. Pleuritis, frothing in the trachea, and lymph node enlargement, especially bronchial and mediastinal, are important features. In subacute and chronic cases, pulmonary abscess and adhesive fibrinous pleuritis and pericarditis may be seen.

Abundance of Gram-negative bacteria around the necrosed lesions, abscessation, thrombosis of lymphatic and blood vessels, and fibroplasia of the affected tissue may be noticed at histopathology.

8.2.4 Diagnosis

Epidemiology and clinical and pathological findings are suggestive of the disease. Isolation of Gram-negative small coccobacilli from the lung lesions, lymph nodes, pleural exudates, and so on using methylene blue may be confirmatory for *Pasteurella* spp. infections. It may show bipolar staining and may also be confirmed by culturing on sheep blood or MacConkey agar. Pneumonia caused by other bacteria, mycoplasma, or virus can be confirmed by various bacteriological/microbial/biochemical tests.

8.2.5 Treatment

Oxytetracycline at 20 mg/kg body weight if given parenterally can reduce the bacterial load. Supportive treatment to control pneumonia, cough, and fever is required according to the situation. Further tetracyclines may be repeated after

3–5 days to avoid relapse. Penicillins may also be used in a combination of sulfadimidine, ampicillin, and trimethoprim-sulfonamide.

8.2.6 Preventive Measures

Isolation and treatment of the affected animals are the best preventive measures in bacterial pneumonia. Vaccines are not effective due to the diversity of etiological agent and serotypes. Circumvention of influencing factors, such as overcrowding, stress, or inclement meteorological conditions, can decrease the incidence.

8.3 Brucellosis

Brucellosis is characterized by abortion in late pregnancy and a subsequent high rate of infertility (Figure 8.3) (Corbel 1997).

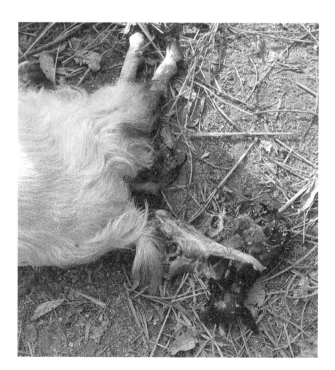

Figure 8.3 Abortion of goat because of brucellosis.

8.3.1 Etiology

Brucella melitensis is a Gram-negative coccobacillary rod, non-motile, facultative-intracellular bacterium capable of surviving and replicating in phagocytic leukocytes and epithelial cells. Caprines may be susceptible to infection by *Brucella abortus*, if they come into direct contact with infected cattle. Epididymitis in rams may be caused by *Brucella ovis*. *B. melitensis* is zoonotic and causes undulant fever or Malta fever in humans, characterized by intermittent fever, restlessness, fatigue, nocturnal hyperhidrosis, and skeletal pain.

Replication of *Brucella* spp. in regional lymph nodes followed by circulation in the blood in macrophages, in neutrophils, and free in the plasma causes lymphadenitis, followed by bacteremia, a lymphoplasmacytic and histiocytic interstitial mastitis, and lymphofollicular proliferation. Gravid uterus, mammary tissue, and lymph nodes are the target organs. The exotoxin produced causes vasculitis and other lesions, resulting in placental trophoblasts and maternal epithelium separation, which may cause fetal mortality and thereby abortion. In the mammary gland, inflammatory foci involve several alveoli or entire lobules. The virulence of the bacteria, resistance, the immune system of the host, and reproductive status are factors affecting the intensity of infection.

8.3.2 Clinical Features

Depression, hyperthermia, body-weight loss, diarrhea, and enlargement of supramammary lymph nodes are some common signs of brucellosis. Abortion in the third trimester of pregnancy, involving about 60% of the pregnant does in the herd, is a characteristic sign of *Brucella* spp. There may be mastitis, decreased milk production, and increased numbers of leukocytes in the milk, as well as the birth of emaciated kids. Neonatal deaths are common in *B. abortus* infection.

In males, epididymitis, orchitis, hygromas, osteoarthritis, lameness, and infertility may be seen. Scrotal swelling, orchitis, epididymis, and testicular atrophy in rams are common in *B. ovis* infection.

8.3.3 Diagnosis

The clinical signs may be indicative as well as the history of the animal and whether the area is endemic for brucellosis. Final confirmation can be achieved by isolating the bacteria from the milk of an infected animal (milk ring test, MRT), placenta, vagina, and abomasum of the aborted fetus by modified Ziehl–Neelsen stain or the Koster method.

Serological procedures such as a serum agglutination test, Rose Bengal plate test, enzyme-linked immunosorbent assays (ELISA), agar gel immunodiffusion, and complement fixation test are apt for the diagnosis. The Coombs test, whey complement fixation test, and MRT detect the infection in milk.

8.3.4 Treatment

Generally, infected goats ought to be culled to reduce the infection sources.

8.3.5 Prevention

- Screening animals on a regular basis.
- Restricted movement of animals and people between herds.
- Procurement of sound animals with known health and reproductive records.
- Pasteurization of milk to reduce the incidence of the disease in humans.
- Incineration of infected materials and disinfection of contaminated premises.
- A test and slaughter policy should be adopted by the government.
- Vaccination with a live attenuated *B. melitensis* Rev 1 strain vaccine may be judiciously used (it may cause abortion if used in pregnant does; formalin-killed adjuvant vaccine may be advised in pregnancy).
- Vaccination of kids and lambs at 3–8 months, while adults should be vaccinated two months before breeding.

8.4 Blackquarter (Blackleg)

8.4.1 Epidemiology

Blackquarter is an acute, highly communicable, inflammatory, and fatal bacterial disease of ruminants caused by *Clostridium chauvoei*, a Gram-positive, spore-forming, and rod-shaped bacterium (Karthik and Manimuthu 2021).

The organism is harbored in various organs, but onset of clinical disease is manifested when the tissues become favorable for spore formation and the immune system of animals is compromised. Contaminated fodder, soil, and water bodies are the major sources of infection. Infection is mainly by ingestion of contaminated food or water.

The spores reach the muscles and other tissues via the lymphatic and circulatory systems. The latent spores proliferate and produce toxins (α, β, γ, δ) when conditions are favorable. The α-toxin leads to necrotizing myositis and absorption of the toxin by the muscles leads to toxemia and death. The nuclei of cells are disrupted by the β-toxin and other metabolites cause abrasions in the myocardium.

8.4.2 Clinical Features

Important clinical signs and symptoms are:

- Hyperthermia, anorexia.
- Depression and dullness.
- Tachycardia and difficult breathing (dyspnea).
- Lameness in the affected leg (muscles become edematous and spongy).
- Stiff gait and hot, painful swelling.
- Crepitation swelling over hip, back, and shoulder.
- Swelling is hot and painful in early stages, then in later stages becomes cold and painless.
- Recumbency (prostration) followed by death within 12–48 hours.

8.4.3 Pathological Features

Decomposition, putrefaction, and bloating of the carcass begin immediately after death. Exudation of blood-stained fluid from the nostrils; the presence of fluid, gas, and air bubbles in the body cavities; and reddish or blackish discoloration of affected muscles with a rancid odor are generally observed pathological features.

8.4.4 Diagnosis

History and clinical and pathological features may assist in diagnosing blackquarter. Confirmation of the disease can be done by making smears from oozing fluid from the affected areas and isolation of Gram-positive rods with spores. A bacterial culture test on sheep blood agar will detect small, rough grayish colonies with a clear hemolytic zone. Colonies of most clostridia resemble each other and can be differentiated by Gram stain or fluorescent antibody test. The latter test uses a fluorochrome-labeled *C. chauvoei* antiserum.

8.4.5 Treatment

Penicillin at 10 000 IU/kg body weight intravenously aids in recovery in the early stages. Delayed-release penicillin preparations can also be administered for an effective response.

8.4.6 Prevention

- Quarantine of goats during outbreak.
- Deep burial or burning of carcasses.
- Vaccination annually by polyvalent clostridial preparations.
- Vaccination of pregnant animals a month before kidding, which stimulates antibody production that passively protects the newborn kids.

8.5 Tetanus

8.5.1 Epidemiology

Goats are highly susceptible to tetanus, an infectious disease caused by toxins produced by *Clostridium tetani*, characterized by neuropathy, spasms, tremors, and tetany with high fatality (Laishevtsev 2020). *C. tetani* is a Gram-positive bacillus, motile, anaerobic, rod shaped (up to 2.5 μm in length), and spore forming (spherical spores at the end giving a typical "drumstick" appearance).

The spores of *C. tetani* gain entry via wounds but remain in the dormant stage. A disease outbreak may occur when suitable conditions for the production of toxins prevail. Wounds or cuts during vaccination, castration, docking, shearing, or other surgical processes that facilitate entry of the bacteria may lead to tetanus, if proper attention is not paid.

Proliferation of dormant *C. tetani* spores following trauma and necrosis of tissues creates anaerobic conditions favoring the production of toxins. The tetanospasmin (the neurotoxin produced) blocks the inhibitory neural impulses at motor neurons, leading to constant spasticity of muscles and hyperesthesia. There may be asphyxia, cardiac arrest, and death if spasms occur in the respiratory muscles.

8.5.2 Clinical Features

Signs of tetanus are muscle stiffness, prolapse of the third eyelid, wobbly/unsteady gait, drooping eyelids, altered voice, erect ears and tail followed by trismus, inability to move due to stiffness of the limbs, and abnormal flexion of joints (Figure 8.4).

8.5.3 Diagnosis

A history of recent surgery or trauma and clinical signs are indicative of tetanus. Muscular spasms, prolapse of the third eyelid, and tetany are characteristic features of the disease, which may be confirmed by demonstration of *C. tetani* in smears or culture from the affected parts.

8.5.4 Treatment

Infected animals should be treated with tetanus antitoxin. Penicillin and other antibiotics alone or in combination

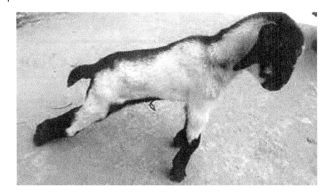

Figure 8.4 Tetany in a kid. Tetany of the masseter muscles causes drooling of saliva and inability to eat or drink. Death occurs from asphyxiation secondary to respiratory paralysis. Spasms cause retention of urine, opisthotonos, curvature of the spine, and tail bending. It is a quickly fatal disease: animals struggle and may die within 4–5 days from expression of clinical signs.

reduce the chances of proliferation of *C. tetani* and toxin production. Anti-inflammatory drugs should also be given for supportive treatment. To prevent the further spread of toxins, an antitoxin injection near the wound locally may be recommended. Muscle relaxants such as chlorpromazine or acepromazine are recommended. A calm, spacious area with soft bedding may be made available to avoid injury. Intravenous or stomach tube feeding may be necessary.

8.5.5 Prevention

The disease can be controlled with proper feeding, management, immunization, and avoidance of penetrating wounds. Trauma to animals should be avoided during handling, surgical procedures, disbudding, dehorning, and castration if there is a wound, then preventing it from contamination by strict hygienic practices. Vaccination (tetanus toxoid) and booster vaccination of the animals should be done to prevent outbreaks and confer lifelong immunity. Vaccination of expecting females 2 months prior and then 2–3 weeks before kidding stimulates antibody production for passive defense of the newborns.

8.6 Caseous Lymphadenitis

8.6.1 Epidemiology

Caseous lymphadenitis is a chronic disease of goats and sheep characterized by chronic suppurative lymphadenitis and abscessation of peripheral lymph nodes caused by *Corynebacterium pseudotuberculosis*, a Gram-positive facultative anaerobic, pleomorphic bacterium that is

pyogenic and leads to thick-walled abscess formation (Fontaine and Baird 2008). The severe economic consequences of this disease are due to mortality, condemnation of the affected carcass, decreased hide quality, loss of sales for breeding animals, and premature culling. Insects or ticks are responsible for the transmission of the disease. Wounds may become an entry point for the bacteria to cause infection.

C. pseudotuberculosis via the blood vascular and lymphatic system reaches the regional lymph nodes. The organism produces a hemolysin and a toxic wall factor, with phospholipase activity that acts on the sphingomyelin of red blood cells and endothelial cell membranes, which leads to hemolysis and increased vascular permeability, hence a higher likelihood of infection. The bacteria are protected from phagocytosis via lysosomes by the toxic wall factor, thus enabling it to survive within phagolysosomes.

8.6.2 Clinical Features

Signs and symptoms include enlargement of the skin and peripheral lymph nodes. Abscessation of the retropharyngeal, submandibular/mandibular, prescapular, parotid, precrural, prefemoral, popliteal lymph nodes, and internal organs is observed. These nodes and subcutaneous tissues are enlarged with thick, cheesy pus (pale green in color), and may rupture during rough handling or shearing/dipping. The incubation time of the disease varies between 1 and 5 months. Active abscesses result in progressive weight loss, poor productivity with decreased fertility, weakness, collapse, mastitis, coughing or respiratory distress, depending on the location of internal abscessation.

8.6.3 Pathological Features

Suppuration of the affected lymph nodes, with an onion-like appearance on cross-section, is due to the stages of necrosis and capsule formation of the abscess. *C. pseudotuberculosis* can be demonstrated from the lesions. Infection of the lungs is associated with interstitial fibrosis.

8.6.4 Diagnosis

History, clinical signs, and pathological characters may be indicative, but confirmation can be obtained by demonstration of the causative organism in smears made from pus. Serological tests like the hemolysis inhibition test, an ELISA test, or an agar gel immunoprecipitation test may be undertaken.

8.6.5 Treatment

Antibiotic treatment is long term and does not cure the disease. Surgical removal of abscesses remains the most effective treatment, but does not cure the infection. Hence treatment is futile and expensive, but supportive treatment along with antibiotics (intralesional and/or systemic) may be provided to high-value stocks.

8.6.6 Prevention

The disease can be controlled by:

- Biosecurity measures.
- Elimination of infection through culling of affected animals from the herd/flock.
- Vaccination.
- Disinfection of equipment used for production procedures (castration, ear tagging, etc.).
- Exclusion of hazards that could potentially cause trauma.
- Prepurchase examination for wounds,
- Quarantine before introduction of new stock.

8.7 Foot Rot

Foot rot is an aggressive progression of foot scald, an infectious disease of legs/feet marked by interdigital necrobacillosis (Winkelmann and Sue 2017).

8.7.1 Etiology

Dichelobacter nodosus, formerly *Bacteroides nodosus*, is a Gram-negative, obligate anaerobe of the family Cardiobacteriaceae. It has polar fimbriae and is the causative agent of ovine foot rot as well as interdigital dermatitis. Along with *D. nodosus*, other aerobic/anaerobic bacteria may also be responsible for foot-rot lesions.

The disease is associated with production losses and sometimes mortality due to starvation. Pasture/bedding may be contaminated by exudation of feet, leading to infection as the organism enters via penetration of broken skin. Nematodes, insects, and mites aid the entry of the causative bacteria through the skin.

In India, high relative humidity/rainfall areas and intensively managed herds are predisposed to foot rot. Poor sanitation, hygiene, a hot and humid climate, overcrowding, and poor health management favor its rapid spread. The synergism of organisms (*D. nodosus* and *Fusobacterium necrophorum*) produces proteolytic enzymes potentiating infiltration, establishment, progress, and proliferation in the tissues, causing severe tissue destruction.

8.7.2 Clinical Features

Limping/staggering of the feet, foot scald (skin inflammation between the toes), and moist, swollen, hyperemic, and macerated interdigital skin are a few of the symptoms seen in goats. There is erosion of the tissue between the sole of the toe and the hard outer hoof along with pus and a bad odor (rotten cheese). Hyperthermia, anorexia, reduced weight gain, decreased milk, with hoof deformity and decreased reproductive capabilities, may also be observed in a few cases.

8.7.3 Pathological Features

Inflammation of the periople (skin–horn junction), interdigital necrosis, ulceration, necrosis of the sensitive laminae of the foot, and accumulation of pus in the joint cavity are important pathological findings.

8.7.4 Diagnosis

Clinical symptoms are generally sufficient for the diagnosis. However, confirmation may be had by demonstration of *D. nodosus* in pus smears and scrapings taken from the edge of the lesions.

8.7.5 Treatment

Systemic antibiotics (procaine penicillin, florfenicol, or oxytetracycline) in high doses given intramuscularly can be effective. In severe cases where joint or other deep structures of one claw are affected, amputation of the claw may be required. Chloramphenicol, tylosin, clindamycin, or nitrofurazone parenteral and topical preparations may be recommended depending on the gravity of the disease. A solution of copper sulfate/zinc sulfate or 7% iodine solution directly on the feet may also be helpful. Isolation of the affected animals and regular hoof trimming facilitate recovery.

8.7.6 Prevention

Foot baths with 5% $CuSO_4$, 10% $ZnSO_4$, and 6–10% formalin can help to control foot scald and foot rot. They also minimize the culling percentage. Maintenance of good hygiene conditions, biosecurity checkpoints in the herd, and avoidance of predisposing factors like muddy conditions, ectoparasites, traumatic objects, or high humidity may aid in reducing the incidence. Oil-adjuvant vaccine of *D. nodosus* can be used in intensive production units.

8.8 Dermatophilosis (Streptothricosis)

Dermatophilosis is exudative dermatitis, crustiness, and exudations at the base of the hair or wool fibers, leading to folliculitis, matting, and thick scab formation, affecting a wide range of animals (domestic as well as wild). Goats are more susceptible than sheep (Msami et al. 2001).

8.8.1 Etiology

The causative agent is *Dermatophilus congolensis*, a Gram-positive, non-acid-fast, facultative anaerobe that is dimorphic in nature, with filamentous hyphae and motile zoospores.

Trauma, contusions, damage to the skin, cuts, scratches, or surgical wounds favor the transmission of the etiological agent. Arthropods like *Amblyomma* spp. ticks also predispose animals to dermatophilosis. The prevalence is higher during the rainy season. The organisms penetrate into the epidermis and subsequently spreads, causing acute infection in the immunocompromised host. In chronic cases, infected hair follicles and scabs are sites responsible for epidermal invasion, which cornifies and scab formation occurs.

8.8.2 Clinical Features

The disease is characterized by exudative, proliferative, or hyperkeratotic dermatitis, loss of hair, and scab and crust formation on the skin. The area beneath the scabs is yellowish-reddish or hemorrhagic and hair-matting exudate may be seen. *D. congolensis* may cause proliferative dermatitis leading to dome-shaped crusts on the anterior part of the legs. Mutilation in skin/hide, reduced meat and milk production, culling or death of the affected animals lead to huge economic losses to owners.

8.8.3 Pathological Features

Enlargement of lymph nodes, exudative dermatitis, ulcers, fibrosis of the liver, enlarged thickened bile ducts full of trematodes, and pneumonia may be seen at necropsy.

8.8.4 Diagnosis

Epidemiological and clinical features are suggestive of the disease. For confirmation, skin scrapings containing crusts and purulent exudate may be used to isolate Gram-positive organisms in impression smears made from the undersurface of the scabs. Giemsa and Gram stain can be used for making smears. A fluorescent antibody test or ELISA may also be used for serological study.

8.8.5 Treatment

Systemic and topical antibiotics, along with good herd management practices, play a vital role in the treatment of dermatophilosis. A wide range of antimicrobials are capable of tackling the etiological agent, including chloramphenicol, streptomycin, amoxicillin, erythromycin, penicillins, ampicillin, and tetracyclines.

8.8.6 Prevention

Strict isolation and culling of the infected animals, controlling ectoparasites by dipping or spraying with insecticides, avoidance of injury to animals, use of topical agents such as $CuSO_4$ and $ZnSO_4$, and biosecurity measures may break the infective cycle and control the disease to a greater extent.

8.9 Malignant Edema (Gas Gangrene)

Malignant edema is a fatal wound infection in grazing animals characterized by hyperthermia, toxemia, edema, and necrotizing infection of subcutaneous tissues (OIE 2014).

8.9.1 Etiology

Several clostridial bacteria may be responsible for the disease, primarily *Clostridium septicum*, *C. chauvoei*, *Clostridium perfringens*, *C. norvyi*, and *Clostridium sordellii*.

C. septicum spores present in soil and intestinal contents of animals may persist without infecting the host for a longer period. Wounds/trauma due to castration, docking, cuts, bruises, insanitary vaccination, and kidding may lead to activation of dormant spores. Contamination of such deep wounds/tissue with the spores infects the animals.

8.9.2 Clinical Features

High fever, edema in tissues, tachycardia, respiratory distress, muscle tremors, erythema, and anorexia are the signs observed in gas gangrene. Emphysema and frothy exudation from the wound may occur. These signs develop 8–12 hours after infection. There may be weakness; depression; muscle stiffness; swelling of the vulva, perineal region, and pelvic tissues; tremors; and lameness. This is a fatal disease and death may occur 2–4 days post infection.

8.9.3 Pathological Features

The major findings are blood-stained and gelatinous subcutaneous and intermuscular connective tissue edema, gangrene of the skin, and emphysema. There is extensive necrosis of the infected muscles with serosanguineous exudate that contains gas accumulates. Severe pulmonary congestion and hemorrhages may be observed along with a foul rancid/putrid odor.

8.9.4 Diagnosis

The presumptive diagnosis is based on history, clinical signs, and necropsy features. Confirmation of gas gangrene can be done by isolation of the etiological agent from the affected tissues in smears. A positive Gram stain (rods) and fine-needle aspiration may also confirm the clostridial infection. The samples from affected tissues should be submitted to the laboratory for anaerobic culture/polymerase chain reaction (PCR) assay/positive culture.

8.9.5 Treatment

Generally, treatment is not possible due to the acuteness of the disease and sudden death of the infected animals. However, long-acting penicillins or broad-spectrum antibiotics may suppress proliferation of the bacteria and toxins. Surgical drainage of the wounds and washing with H_2O_2 may be helpful along with supportive treatment.

8.9.6 Prevention

- Immunization of animals and strict hygiene measures.
- Asepsis maintenance during surgical procedures.
- Avoidance of wounds to decrease the transmission and incidence of the disease.
- Regular disinfection of premises.
- Vaccination (specific or polyvalent formalized bacterins and toxoids against the clostridial species involved in gas gangrene).
- Proper carcass disposal.

8.10 Enterotoxemia

8.10.1 Etiology

Clostridium perfringens types B, C, and D are major etiological agents of various histotoxic and enteric diseases causing different types of illness in animals. Intestines of animals, pastures, or a soil/water reservoir generally harbor *C. perfringens*, a Gram-positive, spore-forming, anaerobic bacterium. Ingestion of contaminated food or water with fecal matter of infected animals leads to the disease in an immunocompromised host. Type B is responsible for lamb dysentery and enterotoxemia, type C for acute enteritis. Type D causes a toxemic disease known as pulpy kidney

disease (PKD) by toxins produced by in the intestines. Goats are less commonly affected by PKD; however, lambs and kids are more susceptible (Karthik et al. 2017).

8.10.2 Clinical Signs

Enterotoxemia with sudden death in kids without any premonitory signs is a feature of peracute disease. Despair, dullness, anorexia, abdominal pain, cramps, bloody diarrhea, bleating, and recumbency are characteristics of acute disease. Death may occur within 1–2 days from the onset of the disease. Tenesmus, sluggish movements, depression, abdominal pain, and blood-stained diarrhea may be noticed in subacute and chronic cases.

8.10.3 Pathological Features

Acute and subacute cases of enterotoxemia by *C. perfringens* types B and C may develop hemorrhagic enteritis or mucosal ulcers, and there may be bloodstained serosanguinous fluid in the intestines and peritoneal cavity. Peritoneal effusion and peritonitis may also be seen as a result of ulcerated intestines.

C. perfringens type D (PKD) is characterized by hemorrhages under the skin, heart, and kidney; straw-colored fluid in the pericardial sac with floating strands of protein; and hemorrhages may be observed in the epicardium, endocardium, intestinal mucosa, or abomasum, with jelly-like clots in the small intestines. The kidneys become dark and jelly-like with a mottled appearance and putrefy rapidly (PKD).

8.10.4 Diagnosis

Enterotoxemia can be diagnosed by clinical and pathological features; however, examination of the gut contents for epsilon toxin demonstration must be done as early as possible after mortality, as the carcass decomposes rapidly. Confirmation can be of the etiological agent via Gram-stained smears from affected portions of the small intestine correlated with the clinical signs. Bacterial isolation and typing, as well as toxin determination in intestinal contents, can also be carried out. Other diagnostic tests include ELISA, mouse neutralization test, counter-immunofluorescence, passive hemagglutination, and radial immunodiffusion.

8.10.5 Treatment

Generally, the treatment is futile, but in the early stages of the disease antibiotics, non-steroidal anti-inflammatory drugs, and a combination of hyperimmune serum with sulfadimidine are effective in goats. Use of a suitable antibiotic can also be done after an antibiotic sensitivity test. Chelating agents may be used to neutralize the toxins.

8.10.6 Prevention

Outbreaks of the disease may be prevented by vaccination of animals prior to anticipated changes in diet. Proper and timely vaccination of animals against all the strains of the clostridial organism is the key to controlling the disease. Vaccination (alum-precipitated, formalin-killed whole culture toxoid against *C. perfringens* type D) accompanied by reduction of feed intake aids in control. Scientific and proper management practices, biosecurity checkpoints, and good hygiene on the farm reduce the chances of transmission. Avoidance of excessive carbohydrates in feed, feed volume reduction, and exercise may help in preventing enterotoxemia.

8.11 Colibacillosis

Colibacillosis is a common diarrheal illness of kids resulting in morbidity and mortality due to poor management practices, hygiene, and nutrition. Pathogenic strains of *E. coli* (gram-negative bacillus) are responsible for causing colibacillosis, which is manifested by septicemia or enteritis. Fecal contamination of pasture, fodder, bedding, or premises is the primary cause of infection.

8.11.1 Pathogenesis

Septicemia (colisepticemia) and enteric colibacillosis are two forms of the disease. Invasive strains of *E. coli* possess specific virulence factors that cause colisepticemia. When the favorable condition arises, bacteria produce endotoxins resulting in bronchoconstriction, pulmonary hypertension, and pulmonary edema, and cause tissue damage.

Enterotoxigenic strains of *E. coli* cause enteric colibacillosis. The bacteria proliferate and colonize the villi of intestines, producing enterotoxins and leading to impaired absorption, resulting in electrolyte imbalance, dehydration, acidosis, cardiovascular failure, and death.

8.11.2 Clinical and Pathological Features

Kids and lambs are more susceptible to septicemic colibacillosis. There may be sudden death without any premonitory signs. Acute cases show stiff gait or recumbency, despair, hyperthermia, hyperesthesia, and tetanic convulsions. Enteric colibacillosis is characterized by hemorrhagic or mucoid diarrhea with fever, depression,

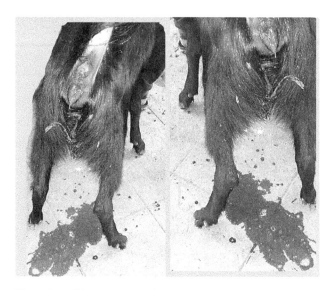
Figure 8.5 Diarrheic goat with pasty feces.

and abdominal pain (Figure 8.5). Polyarthritis, anorexia, or meningitis may be observed in chronic cases.

Petechial hemorrhages, enteritis, gastritis, and fibrinous exudation in serous cavities are seen on necropsy. Widespread hemorrhages in the intestinal mucosa are a common feature in colibacillosis.

8.11.3 Diagnosis

Epidemiology, history, clinical signs, hematology, serum biochemistry, and pathological features may aid in diagnosis. Confirmatory diagnosis can be done by isolation of *E. coli* from ill animals. Bacteria can be demonstrated in smears from the intestinal mucosa and demonstration of specific toxins may support the diagnosis. The organisms can also be cultured from heart blood, intestinal contents, urine, milk, and vaginal exudates.

8.11.4 Treatment

Keeping in view the diversity of *E. coli*, drug sensitivity testing is recommended before starting any treatment. A trimethoprim-sulfonamide combination (15–25 mg/kg body weight) and kanamycin (20 mg/kg) given parenterally and colistin administered at a rate of 1–2 g/kg in drinking water have been found to be effective in the treatment of the disease. Other antibiotics such as oxytetracycline, neomycin, chloramphenicol, and sulfadimidine are also used.

8.11.5 Prevention

Vaccination of dams 2–4 weeks before parturition to stimulate the production of specific antibodies is recommended in order to provide passive protection through colostrum in kids. Formalin-killed whole-cell vaccines may be injected as immunization and prevention.

Maintenance of improved sanitation, hygiene, avoidance of overcrowding, proper farm management practices (colostrum feeding, exercise and housing with adequate ventilation, and sunlight in the buildings) can reduce transmission of the disease.

8.12 Salmonellosis

In ovines and caprines, salmonellosis is manifested by the development of two distinct syndromes: an acute to subacute septicemic disease with enteritis and diarrhea, and abortion. *Salmonella dublin*, *Salmonella typhimurium,* and *Salmonella anatum* are some of the species responsible for salmonellosis in sheep and goats. *S. abortusovis* leads to abortion, while septicemic syndrome is caused by *S. typhimurium* and is precipitated by stress.

Salmonella spp. affect most animal species along with humans and is of zoonotic importance. The carrier animals contaminate the environment via shedding the enteric organisms in feces, resulting in a clinical disease or carrier state, if an animal acquires the infection through contaminated food, water, and pastures. Animal salmonellosis is the principal reservoir for human salmonellosis.

8.12.1 Clinical Features

Enteric salmonellosis is characterized by foul-smelling diarrhea/dysentery (blood clots, fibrin casts, or mucus may also be seen), abdominal pain, dehydration, hyperthermia, anorexia, listlessness, tenesmus depression, dyspnea, and weakness followed by death. Bacteria damage the lining of the intestines and makes the host more prone to enteritis, colitis, and further proliferation of the etiological agent. Newborn kids are more susceptible and develop severe enteritis, and may die if proper care and treatment are not provided.

Salmonella in goats has been reported to cause abortions. Does and ewes often die after abortion and lambs born alive may die subsequently. *S. dublin* is most common causative bacteria in goats.

8.12.2 Pathological Features

There is muco-hemorrhagic enteritis along with petechiae on villus and submucosal regions. Necrotic enteritis with mucoid and blood-tinged diarrhoeic feces is observed in *S. typhimurium* infection. The mesenteric lymph nodes are enlarged, edematous, and hemorrhagic. There is also enlargement and fatty degeneration of the liver, thickening of the gall bladder wall, and the presence of blood-stained fluid in the serous cavities. The histopathological picture is characterized by necrosis, edema, congestion, and infiltration of the lamina propria and submucosa of the caecum, colon, and small intestine with neutrophils, lymphocytes, plasma cells, and macrophages.

8.12.3 Diagnosis

Epidemiological, clinical, and pathological features may be indicative of the disease. Confirmation can be done by isolation of the etiological organism and serotyping. Selective media (MacConkey agar, brilliant green agar, and xylose-lysine deoxycholate medium) may aid in *Salmonella* spp. isolation. Direct slide agglutination test and specific antisera for the determination of O, H, and Vi antigens is also sometimes conducted. Samples from intestines may be analyzed by PCR test, nucleic acid-based assays, immunological techniques, and electrical conductance and impedance for high accuracy. The immunological techniques for detecting *Salmonella* include immune agglutination, immunoprecipitation, immunocapture, ELISA, enzyme-linked immunofluorescent assays S, and immunodiffusion.

8.12.4 Treatment

Fluid therapy along with antimicrobial and supportive treatment is effective in reducing mortality. The organism is highly sensitive to ciprofloxacin, spiramycin, and gentamicin, and moderately sensitive to oxytetracycline, streptomycin, sulfadimidine, and amoxicillin; combination antibiotics are also effective. A combination of oral and parenteral therapy is critical in the treatment of clinical salmonellosis. However, oral antibiotics can alter the gut flora and fauna and increase host susceptibility to the disease.

8.12.5 Prevention

Salmonellosis can be controlled by following strict biosecurity measures, proper disinfection and regular sanitation of the farm, proper farm management practices, maintaining good hygiene, avoiding fecal contamination of feed/water, strict isolation and care of infected animals, and reducing the use of common equipment between groups, as well as sanitization and disinfection on a regular basis. Farm personnel should practice good personal hygiene. Rodents and birds should be controlled on the premises to protect feed from contamination. Prevention of herd stresses, such as environmental stress and overcrowding, is also important.

8.13 Botulism

8.13.1 Epidemiology

Botulism is a rare disease in goats that occurs due to ingestion of toxins in food from decomposing carcasses, decaying grass, hay, grain, or spoiled silage or any vegetative matter, which may result in fatal motor paralysis caused by the neurotoxin produced by *Clostridium botulinum*. Seven antigenically distinct types of *C. botulinum* – A, B, C_1, D, E, F, and G – may cause the disease (Harish et al. 2006).

In the absence of oxygen, the Gram-positive, spore-forming anaerobic bacterium contaminates wounds or damaged tissues and produces toxins. Deficiencies of phosphorus and protein are predisposing factors.

8.13.2 Clinical Features

Weakness, debility, twisted necks/torticollis, arching of the back, salivation, serous nasal discharges, recumbency, and difficulty in chewing and swallowing are some of the signs exhibited by animals at various stages of the disease. Flaccid muscle paralysis, progressive motor paralysis, disturbed vision, progressive paresis, and abdominal respiration are observed in the terminal stages.

8.13.3 Diagnosis

Epidemiology, history of starvation, pica, or osteophagia, and clinical signs may be helpful in diagnosis. Toxin (botulism toxin) determination in intestines of carcass and suspicious feed/fodder and other samples may confirm the disease.

8.13.4 Treatment

Treatment is generally futile and not recommended; however, hyperimmune serum along with the antitoxin and supportive care may show some recovery. Good nursing, stomach lavage, and supportive intravenous or stomach tube feeding are also helpful.

8.13.5 Prevention

- Removal of contaminated feed and fodder.
- Provision of balanced feed to avoid deficiencies.
- Careful and apt carcass disposal.
- Prevent pasture and water-body contamination.
- Following proper vaccination/immunization with region-specific type toxoid (polyvalent toxoid containing type A, B, C, and D strains is commercially available) are the key points in controlling the disease.

8.14 Infectious Necrotic Hepatitis

Black disease or infectious necrotic hepatitis (INH) is an acute septicemic disease of farm animals, especially cattle and sheep, but it may be seen in goats. The disease is lethal in nature and the etiological agent is *Clostridium novyi* type B. Spores of *C. novyi* type B after ingestion from soil reach the liver via portal circulation. Following liver damage by migrating parasites/liver flukes (fasciolosis), this provides a favorable environment for the proliferation of the clostridial spores and production of lethal α-toxins, resulting in necrotizing hepatitis and hence clinical manifestations.

8.14.1 Clinical Features

Sudden onset of disease and abrupt death are features of peracute and acute cases. Signs in the animals that survive are depression, hyperthermia, rapid and shallow respiration, ruminal stasis, hyperesthesia, incoordination of muscles, and recumbency. Edematous and crepitant swellings develop in the body parts (hip, shoulder, chest, back, neck, etc.).

Rapid putrefaction after mortality with blood-stained froth from natural orifices, hemorrhagic subcutaneous edema in various regions, and congestion and cyanosis of the subcutaneous tissue resulting in blackening of the skin are observed at necropsy. There is evidence of recent infestation of liver flukes, and the liver appears dark brown with characteristic necrotic areas, surrounded by a bright red zone of congestion.

8.14.2 Diagnosis

Epidemiological data, history, clinical features, and gross and microscopic changes can be aids in diagnosis. *C. novyi* type B may be cultured from pieces of the necrotic liver or demonstrated in impression smears made from the edges of the necrotic lesion for confirmatory diagnosis. Histologically, the presence of a central zone of necrosis containing polymorphonuclear cells from an infected liver is a pathognomonic lesion. Demonstration of toxins in peritoneal fluid or in the liver, fluorescent antibody test, and ultrasonographic examination may also be undertaken for diagnosis of infectious necrotic hepatitis.

8.14.3 Prevention

- Following proper immunization of animals (multivalent vaccine containing prevailing antigens in endemic areas) may reduce mortality during outbreaks.
- Control of liver flukes/parasites and snails.

- Proper carcass disposal to avoid contamination with spores.
- Disinfection and sanitization of the premises.

8.15 Johne's Disease

Johne's disease (JD) is a chronic wasting disease characterized by weight loss, reduced production, and intermittent diarrhea that affects the small intestines of various species of animals.

8.15.1 Etiology

Mycobacterium avium subsp. *paratuberculosis* is the etiological agent, which is a Gram-positive, fastidious, facultative obligate intracellular bacterium, rod-shaped, acid-fast, non-spore-forming, and dependent on mycobactin for its replication. Kids are more susceptible, though adult goats are also affected. Infection is acquired by ingestion of contaminated milk, pasture, or water, or direct contact. Environmental contamination is by infected or suspected animals that shed bacteria in the feces.

8.15.2 Clinical Signs

The causative agent alters/thickens the intestinal wall, resulting in malabsorption, weakness, emaciation, pasty feces or diarrhea, and rapid weight loss. It is a chronic wasting disease with progressive granulomatous enteritis. Intestines of infected animals show a characteristic corrugated appearance at necropsy.

8.15.3 Diagnosis

The epidemiology, history, and clinical symptoms are suggestive of the disease. Suspects can be confirmed by intradermal skin testing using Johnin purified protein derivative (PPD). Acid-fast bacilli can be demonstrated from fecal samples, intestinal scrapings, or aspirates from ileal and ileocecal lymph nodes. Interferon-γ assay can assess the cellular immunity. Bacteria can be isolated from intestine, lymph node, and feces by culture method and PCR can be done for confirmation.

8.15.4 Treatment

Treating animals with antimycobacterial agents is futile. Due to the chronic nature of JD, identification of the disease in its early stages is difficult, hence it is recommended to test newly purchased animals before arrival on the farm.

8.15.5 Prevention

Following strict biosecurity measures and culling all infected animals after a positive test are key to preventing JD. Milk from suspected animals should not be fed to neonates. It is better to change the pastureland, as the bacteria may survive for longer in pasture. Proper disinfection of the farm premises should be done on a regular basis.

8.16 Mastitis

Mastitis is an important disease of small ruminants characterized by inflammation of the mammary glands, decreased yield and quality of the milk produced, and reduction in body weight of kids, with multiple causative agents and factors. *S. aureus* and *Streptococcus agalactiae* are common organisms isolated from goats suffering from mastitis. *C. pyogenes, Brucella* spp., and *Klebsiella* spp. may also be responsible. Other than bacteria, *Mycobacterium* spp., *Listeria* spp., *Mycoplasma agalactiae*, *Candida albicans*, *Actinobacillus* spp., and *Actinomyces* spp. alone or in association with bacteria may also cause mastitis.

Physical injury, stress, unhygienic conditions in sheds, poor health or hygiene of animals and workers, and unskilled and poor milking methods are the factors responsible for a predisposition to mastitis on a farm. The organism gains entry to udders via encountering contaminated feces, feed, fodder, or fomites. After entry through the teat canal, the bacteria colonize and multiply in the mammary tissue, causing inflammation and damage to the mammary tissue (Figure 8.6).

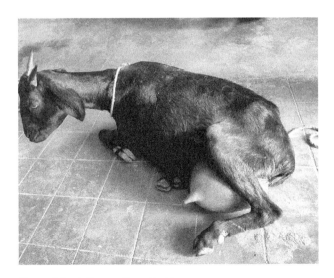

Figure 8.6 Inflammation of udder.

Table 8.1 Bacterial diseases of goats.

Disease	Etiology	Symptoms	Treatment	Prevention
Anthrax	*Bacillus anthracis*	Sudden fever and death Dark-colored, bloody discharge from natural orifices such as nose, anus, and vagina	No treatment is effective	Vaccination once a year in affected areas Disposal of carcass by either burying or burning Not opening up the carcass as the germs spread through air
Blackquarter	*Clostridium chauvoei*	Stiff gait, hot painful swelling of the affected muscles	Penicillin	Annual vaccination Quarantine measures Proper disposal of carcass
Brucellosis	*Brucella melitensis*	Abortion during late pregnancy, infertility, scrotal swelling in male, joint swelling	Culling of infected animals	Disposal of dead fetus and placenta Use gloves while handling infected items as the disease affects human beings
Enterotoxemia	*Clostridium perfringens* types B and C	Sudden death in young growing kids Mucous diarrhea may also be seen during death	Penicillins Oxytetracyclines Chloramphenicol	Vaccinate animals once a year before onset of monsoon Do not feed on young grass
Pneumonia	*Pasteurella* spp. (*Pasteurella haemolytica, Pasteurella multocida*)	Fever, respiratory distress, mucous discharge from nostril, reduced feed intake, weight gain, cough	Oxytetracycline	Clean water Well-ventilated housing
Foot rot	*Dichelobacter nodosus* (*Bacteroides nodosus*)	Wound in foot region	Penicillin–streptomycin	Keep animal in dry, clean housing
Mastitis	*Mycoplasma agalactiae, Candida albicans, Mycobacterium* spp., *Listeria* spp., *Actinobacillus* spp., *Actinomyces* spp.	Swelling of udder, change in milk	Penicillin Streptomycin Oxytretracycline Gentamycin	Clean shed Wash udder with disinfectant solution
Caseous lymphadenitis	*Corynebacterium pseudotuberculosis*	Abscessation of lymph nodes	Penicillin	Elimination of source of infection
Tetanus	*Clostridium tetani*	Muscle stiffness, tremors, prolapse of third eyelid Muscular tetany, drooling of saliva	Tetanus Antitoxin Penicillin	Prevention of wound contamination Tetanus antitoxin Tetanus toxoid vaccination

8.16.1 Clinical Features

The majority of cases are subclinical with reduced milk yield, flakes in milk, decreased production, and gradual weight loss. Restlessness, hyperthermia, raised pulse and respiratory rates, and enlarged, hot, painful, and inflamed mammary glands may be observed in acute staphylococcal mastitis. Blood-stained clotting or serum in the milk is evident.

Enlargement of the supramammary lymph nodes, swelling, redness of mammary glands that are enlarged, inflamed, and hard with blocked teat orifices, abscesses, and necrosis of the mammary tissues may be seen at necropsy.

8.16.2 Diagnosis

History, clinical signs (abnormalities in milk/inflamed udder), pathological lesions, and farm hygiene may indicate mastitis. Isolation of the etiological agents from pus or milk secretions may confirm the disease. The California mastitis test (CMT), strip cup test, somatic cell count, and inflammatory cell count or culturing milk in the laboratory can also aid in diagnosis.

8.16.3 Treatment

Intramammary infusions or parenteral administration of antibiotics (erythromycin, trimethoprim, penicillins, gentamicin, florfenicol, oxytetracycline, sulfa, or tylosin) in systemic cases may manage the condition. For serious cases, intensive therapies to combat septicemia (intravenous fluids, antibiotics, and anti-inflammatories) may be used along with a systemic and intramammary antibiotic combination. Culture and antibacterial sensitivity testing are recommended before the use of drugs.

In severe cases hemi-mastectomy or mastectomy may be performed.

8.16.4 Prevention

Culling the infected animals from the herd; regular disinfection and sanitization of sheds, equipment, and the farm as a whole; and maintenance of good herd and milking hygiene along with proper farm management practices may prevent mastitis.

8.16.5 Common Control Measures for Various Bacterial Diseases of Goats

- Avoid overcrowding in an intensive system.
- Proper housing and ventilation.
- Routine deworming and vaccination.
- Balanced nutritive ration.
- Proper drainage and sprinkling of copper sulfate near water bodies will help to control fluke infection.
- Avoid early-morning and late-evening grazing.
- Keep the shed clean and provide clean, good-quality drinking water.
- Regular disinfection of farm premises.
- Isolation of infected animals from healthy ones.
- Proper quarantine measures when purchasing new animals.
- Proper disposal of dead animals.
- Test and cull policy.
- Health and hygiene of workers.
- Restriction of visitors during epidemic.
- Biosecurity checkpoints and measures.
- Rotational grazing to control infection.

A summary of bacterial diseases of goats is provided in Table 8.1.

Multiple-Choice Questions

1 The milk ring test in milk/colostrum aids in detecting which disease?
   A Anthrax
   B Brucellosis
   C Salmonellosis
   D Caseous lymphadenitis

2 Crepitating swelling is a characteristic feature of which bacterial disease?
   A Anthrax
   B Foot rot
   C Blackquarter
   D Caseous lymphadenitis

3 Which disease can be prevented by the ATS vaccine?
   A Anthrax
   B Tetanus
   C Enterotoxemia
   D Foot rot

4 What does *Dichelobacter nodosus* cause?
   A Mastitis
   B Tetanus
   C Blackquarter
   D Foot rot

5 A carcass should never be opened at postmortem if it is suspected of what disease?
A Pneumonia
B Anthrax
C Botulism
D Johne's disease

6 Which etiological agent causes Johne's disease?
A *Pasteurella* spp.
B *Mycobacterium avium*
C *Clostridium perfringens*
D *Clostridium chauvoei*

7 Caseous abscesses in peripheral lymph nodes are a characteristic feature of which disease?
A Anthrax
B Foot rot
C Blackquarter
D Caseous lymphadenitis

8 What is pulpy kidney disease caused by?
A *Clostridium perfringens*
B *Escherichia coli*
C *Salmonella dublin*
D *Pasteurella* spp.

9 Which form of anthrax is known a wool sorters' disease?
A Pulmonary form
B Intestinal form
C Cutaneous form
D Cardiac form

10 What is bacterial pneumonia in caprines caused by?
A *Clostridium chauvoei*
B *Pasteurella* spp.
C *Mycobacterium avium*
D *Salmonella typhimurium*

References

Corbel, M.J. (1997). Brucellosis: an overview. *Emerging Infectious Diseases* 3: 213–221.

Fontaine, M.C. and Baird, G.J. (2008). Caseous lymphadenitis. *Small Ruminant Research* 76: 42–48.

Hamborsky, J., Kroger, A., and Wolfe, S. (2015). *Epidemiology and Prevention of Vaccine Preventable Diseases*, 13e. Washington, DC: Centers for Disease Control and Prevention.

Harish, B.R., Chandranaik, B.M., Bhanuprakash, R.A. et al. (2006). Clostridium tetaniinfection in goats. *Intas Polivet* 7: 72–74.

Karthik, K. and Manimuthu, P. (2021). Bacterial diseases of goat and its preventive measures. In: S. Kukovics (ed.), *Goat Science: Environment, Health and Economy*. London: IntechOpen, ch. 13. http://dx.doi.org/10.5772/intechopen.97434.

Karthik, K., Manimaran, K., Bharathi, R., and Shoba, K. (2017). Report of enterotoxaemia in goat kids. *Advances in Animal and Veterinary Sciences* 5 (7): 289–292.

Laishevtsev, A.I. (2020). Mannheimiosis of cattle, sheep and goats. *IOP Conference Series: Earth and Environmental Science* 548: 072038.

Matthews, J. (2016). *Diseases of the Goat*, 4e. Chichester: Wiley.

Misgie, F., Atnaf, A., and Surafel, K. (2015). A review on anthrax and its public health and economic importance. *Academic Journal of Animal Diseases* 4 (3): 196–204.

Msami, H.M., Khaschabi, D., Schöpf, K. et al. (2001). *Dermatophilus congolensis* infection in goats in Tanzania. *Tropical Animal Health and Production* 33 (5): 367–377.

OIE (World Organisation for Animal Health) (2014). Contagious caprine pleuropneumonia. In: *Manual of Diagnostic Tests and Vaccines for Terrestrial Animals*. Paris: OIE, ch. 2.7.5.

Popoff, M.R. (2020). Tetanus in animals. *Journal of Veterinary Diagnostic Investigation* 32 (2): 184–191.

Winkelmann, J. and Sue, A. (2017). *Sheep and Goat Diseases: Veterinary Book for Farmers and Smallholders*, 4e. Great Easton: 5m Publishing.

Yatoo, M.I., Parraya, O.R., Bashir, S.T. et al. (2019). Contagious caprine pleuropneumonia – a comprehensive review. *Veterinary Quarterly* 39 (1): 1–25.

9

Fungal Diseases of Goats

Pardeep Sharma[1] and Tanmoy Rana[2]

[1] *Department of Veterinary Medicine, DGCN College of Veterinary and Animal Sciences, CSK Himachal Pradesh Krishi Vishvavidyalaya, Palampur, Himachal Pradesh, India*
[2] *Department of Veterinary Clinical Complex, West Bengal University of Animal & Fishery Sciences, Kolkata, West Bengal, India*

9.1 Fundamentals of Fungal Diseases of Goats

Goats are ruminant herbivores of a particular genus of mammals belonging to the most important large Bovidae family. These animals play a significant role in contributing to the economy of poor and marginal farmers throughout the globe, especially in Southeast Asian, African, and European countries. The goats are named the "poor man's cow" and are important and valuable assets of farmers due to their potential role in contributing milk, meat, and wool production. These small ruminants have high potential to replicate as well as grow rapidly (Chakrabarti 1984). However, they are highly prone to various diseases, which could be manifested through various etiological factors, among which fungi are one of the most important causative factors in producing diseases in the goat.

Various fungal diseases cause morbidity and mortality with a huge concern for economic losses. Ringworm, mycotic mastitis, aspergillosis, and pythiosis are the most common fungal diseases affecting goats (Table 9.1). Environmental indices are responsible for causing the spread of disease in warm and humid seasons. Various pathogenic fungi can produce mycotoxins in low humidity and thereby create favorable conditions for bacterial growth. During animal feed-making procedures, grains and silage may be responsible for induction of the contamination of fungal toxins. Mycotoxin-contaminated feed when consumed can lead to contamination of food products of animals through utilization of milk or meat and thereby be of great concern for animal and human health. These diseases can be directly spread through contact with animals, their excreta, and contaminated food products.

9.2 Dermatophytosis in the Goat: Ringworm, Tinea

Ringworm is a very significant fungal disease recorded worldwide. The most isolated causal organisms include *Trichophyton verrucosum* and *Trichophyton mentagrophytes*. Generally, dermatophytosis is transmitted directly or indirectly through contact with contaminated equipment as well as environmental indices. Documentary evidence suggests that the fungi play a significant role in invading the skin and hair fibers, thereby causing breaks in the hair (Pal 2001). It is also said to cause hair loss because of the breakdown of the hair shaft. Malnourished young goats reared in damp housing or dark, damp barns are those who suffer most. Debilitated goats are the worst sufferers of these diseases. Unhealthy management practices and stopping shearing and washing procedures are also predisposing factors to cause fungal diseases of goats.

9.2.1 Etiology

Dermatophytes include *Microsporum*, *Epidermophyton*, and *Trichosporum*.

9.2.2 Epidemiology

The infection spreads primarily through direct contact between animals, with the clinically infected animal becoming the main source of infection. The spores of ringworm fungi survive for many months and in some cases years in the farm environment and may be transmitted either by fomites or by an asymptomatic carrier to a susceptible host.

Table 9.1 Fungal infections of goats.

Disease	Causative agents	Mode of transmission	Geographical distribution	Pathogenesis	Line of treatment	References
Dermatophytosis/ringworm	*Trichophyton verrucosum Trichophyton mentagrophytes*	Direct or indirect transmission, anthropophilic or zoophilic or geophilic	Worldwide	Perforation of the hair structure Consumption of contents of keratin through secretion of keratinase enzyme	Systemic antibiotics, topical therapy, antifungal drug, orally and topically	Pal (2001)
Candidiasis	*Candida albicans*	Penetration of the skin via puncture or absorption (through scratches, cuts, abrasions, dermatitis, or other lesions)	Worldwide	Epidermal proliferation and T-lymphocyte immune responses, inflammatory responses	Fluconazole	Sudhakara et al. (2018)
Cryptococcosis	*Cryptococcus neoformans*	Inhalation of spores or contamination of wounds. In avian droppings	Worldwide	Disease in immunocompromised goats, rhinitis, meningitis, encephalitis, and pneumonia	Fluconazole (2.5–10 mg/kg/d) or itraconazole (10 mg/kg/d)	Chapman et al. (1990)
Malasseziosis	*Malassezia* spp.	Contact directly or indirectly, droplet, airborne, vector and aerosols, anal (feco-oral) secretions, tears, saliva, vertical transmission	Worldwide	Cutaneous inflammation, immune suppressive mechanisms, enlargement of the ceruminous glands	Ketoconazole at 5–10 mg/kg body weight Itraconazole at 5–10 mg/kg body weight	Pin (2004)
Rhodotorulosis	*Rhodotorula glutinis* and *Rhodotorula minuta*	Direct transmission from infected animals, droplets, open wounds	Worldwide	Lung infections and otitis, skin infections	Initiation of antifungal agents, povidone iodine	Nagahama et al. (2006)
Pneumocystosis	Opportunistic fungal pathogen *Pneumocystis carinii* Class Fungus (Ascomycota), family Pneumocystidaceae, order Pneumocystidales	Direct contact Airborne routes (aerosol)	Worldwide	Fatal pneumonia in immunosuppressed hosts Abomasal and intestinal hemorrhage coupled with immune dysfunction	Pentamidine isethionate Trimethoprim sulfamethoxazole Atovaquone Trimetrexate	Fatima (2021)
Aspergillosis	*Aspergillus fumigatus, Aspergillus niger*	Inhalation of airborne conidia, through contaminated materials	Worldwide	Mycotic abortion, mycotic mastitis, and mycotic pneumonia	Voriconazole and/or isavuconazole, liposomal amphotericin B, posaconazole, long-term oral itraconazole or voriconazole	Mandal and Gupta (1993)
Microsporidiosis	Emerging opportunistic fungal pathogens *Enterocytozoon bieneusi* and *Enteromorpha intestinalis* Class Enterocytozoon. family Enterocytozoonidae, order Chytridiopsida	Water sources	Worldwide	Infects the intestinal epithelial cells Lesions in kidneys Diarrhea	Fenbendazole	Al-Herrawy and Gad (2016)
Pythiosis	*Pythium insidiosum*	Cutaneous, inhalation, ingestion, or dermal exposure to spores via minor trauma or insect bites	Worldwide	Inflammation, pneumonia, granulomatous rhinitis, ulcerative cutaneous lesions in skin, metastasis in lungs and lymph nodes	Long-term itraconazole	Carmo et al. (2015)

Disease	Causative agent	Source/Transmission	Distribution	Clinical signs	Treatment	Reference
Coccidiomycosis	*Coccidiodes immitis*	Inhaling spores, airborne in dust	Worldwide	Upper respiratory tract, invasion into lungs, hypersensitivity, inflammation, pneumonia	Intravenous amphotericin B, fluconazole, and itraconazole	Plummer et al. (2012)
Conidiobolomycosis	*Conidiodobolus coronatus*	Soil, decaying vegetation, insects	Central America, equatorial Africa, India	Subcutaneous infection or rhinofacial, nasopharyngeal infection	Long-term itraconazole	Carmo et al. (2020)
Pneumocystosis	*P. carinii*	Direct contact and airborne routes	Worldwide	Fatal pneumonia in immunosuppressed goats, rhinitis, inflammation	Trimethoprim + sulfamethoxazole at 15–20 mg/kg body weight/d	McConnell et al. (1971)
Scopulariopsis	Dematiaceous fungi *Scopulariopsis brevicaulis* and *Scopulariopsis brumptii* Class Sordariomycetes, family Microascaceae, order Microascales	Soil, air, in plant litter, paper, wood, dung, and animal remains	Worldwide	Hair loss and skin changes	Itraconazole D-biotin	Ozturk et al. (2009)
Sporotrichosis	*Sporotrichosis schenckii*	Soil and on plant matter, fungal spores in environment	India, Europe, USA	Skin and subcutaneous, inflammation, hypersensitivity	Itraconazole, liposomal amphotericin B, supersaturated potassium iodide	Pereira et al. (2015)
Keratinophilic fungi	*T. mentagrophytes, T. verrucosum, Microsporum nanum, Arthroderma cuniculi, Ar. curreyi, Acremonium kiliense, Alternaria alternata, Aspergillus flavus, A. versicolor, Cladosporium carrionii, Chrysosporium tropicum, Ch. anamorph, Acremonium kiliense, Aphanoascus fulvuscens, Paecilomyces lilacinus, Scopulariopsis brevicaulis,* and others	Hair, wool, cloven hooves, and horns of goats and sheep Contaminated working areas and dwelling places Wet and dirty surfaces	Worldwide	Infections of the skin like club fungus, athlete's foot, *Tinea* infection of some keratinized surfaces, and ringworm of the hair and nails	Fluconazole, ketoconazole, miconazole	
Facial eczema (pithomycotoxicosis, photodermatitis)	*Pithomyces chartarum* Class Dothideomycetes, family Pleosporaceae, order Pleosporales	Presence of mycotoxin sporidesmin in forage grasses	Subtropical countries and other localities with warmer climates such as New Zealand, UK, Netherlands, rest of Europe	Facial eczema Drooping ears and swollen eyes Skin lesions	Feeding cattle zinc or by using benzimidazole fungicides on pastures	Pinto et al. (2005)
Protothecosis	*Prototheca zopfii, Prototheca cutis, Prototheca blaschkeae,* and *Prototheca wickerhamii*	Nasal, oral, and ear	Worldwide	Cutaneous infections, rhinitis, inspiratory dyspnea and stertor, dermatitis, life-threatening sepsis	Tetracycline, amphotericin B (intravenous and intraperitoneal) Antifungals such as ketoconazole, itraconazole, fluconazole, conventional amphotericin B, and liposomal amphotericin B	Riet-Correa et al. (2021)

A natural outbreak will generally affect only younger animals, though older animals that have not previously had contact with the dermatophyte can also easily be affected due to lack of natural immunity.

9.2.3 Transmission

Transmission is through direct contact with other infected animals or infected equipment.

9.2.4 Pathogenesis

Dermatophytes principally attack the keratinized layer of skin, hair, and nails, autolyze the fibrous structure, break the hair, and thus produce alopecia. Dermatophytes do not invade living tissues. They produce skin lesions through elaboration or excretion of toxins or allergens. These agents affect malpighian and basal layers and thus induce increased proliferation of rete cells of the Malpighian layers. These also act on the vascular component, leading to effusion of serum. The capillary dilatation and hyperemia along with serous edema cause spongiosis of the epithelium and thus interfere with the regular process of keratinization there by parakeratosis. Toxins damage the hair follicles and thus alopecia develops.

The signs of inflammatory reaction happen at the site of invasion when the host parasite equilibrium is disturbed. Scale and encrustation occur. The hair loss is not complete until the follicles are destroyed by secondary bacterial infection. Fungus invades the growing hair as it meets their metabolic needs. Growing hair contains carbohydrate, nitrogenous substances, and nucleoprotein derivatives in addition to keratin. There are three types of hair attachment: ectothrix, endothrix, and favic. Mycelium can be found in all three types. Dermatophytes are strict anaerobes and fungi die out under the crust in the center of most lesions, leaving an active lesion on the periphery and thus forming a characteristic patch of ringworm. Secondary bacterial infection may produce microabscesses in the superficial epidermis together with suppurative folliculitis. Prolonged use of systemic corticoids to alleviate itching may produce severe lesions known as tinea incognito.

9.2.5 Factors That Influence Susceptibility to Dermatophyte Infection

- Age of the animal – young animals are far more susceptible to infection.
- Crowding together with young animals.
- Factors that decrease resistance to infection.
- Poor nutrition.
- Concurrent infection.
- Previous use of immunosuppressive drugs.

9.2.6 Clinical Signs

The number and size of affected sites vary, but the head and neck area are most susceptible. The primary changes that are observed clinically are severe alopecia, scaling, and crusting of skin. Lesions are characteristically grayish white and have an ash-like surface. Their outline is circular, and they are slightly raised due to the accumulation of many layers of scales and the swelling of tissue beneath due to a moderate inflammatory reaction (Figures 9.1 and 9.2).

In most cases the infection is self-limiting, with the duration of infection ranging from 1–4 months followed by spontaneous regression.

Alopecia and circular lesions on eyelids, face, head, and non-wooled areas of legs and widespread lesions may be found under wool when lambs are sheared. Matting of hair also occurs.

9.2.7 Diagnosis

- **Wood's lamp examination**: Certain strains of *Microsporum canis* and *Microsporum audouinii* produce fluorescence, a positive yellow-green color when examined under a Wood's lamp. This fluorescence is due to tryptophan metabolites produced by the fungi that have invaded actively growing hair. Fluorescence is not present in scales and crust in culture of the dermatophyte.
- **Culture examination** on brain heart infusion or Sabouraud dextrose agar (SDA), or dermatophyte test medium.
- **Direct examination of skin scraping** on a 20% KOH mount reveals an ectothrix pattern of invasion of wool with arthospores.
- **Special fungal stain** like Gömöri methamine silver (GMS) technique or periodic acid–Schiff (PAS) technique.
- **Skin test**: Like in tuberculosis, the fungal antigen (0.1 ml) can be given subcutaneously, with the reaction noted after 24–48 hours.

9.2.8 Treatment

At first, goats are isolated and treated aggressively as early as possible. In healthy animals the disease is self-limiting.

Whitfield's ointment (thiabendazole) can be applied topically directly on the lesion. Clip the hair, clean the area, and use a wire brush to remove the crusted area, followed by topical application of 2% solution of tincture of iodine for 2–3 weeks.

The lesions, once removed, should be collected and burned to prevent contamination of other areas. Topical antifungal applications are to be continued for up to

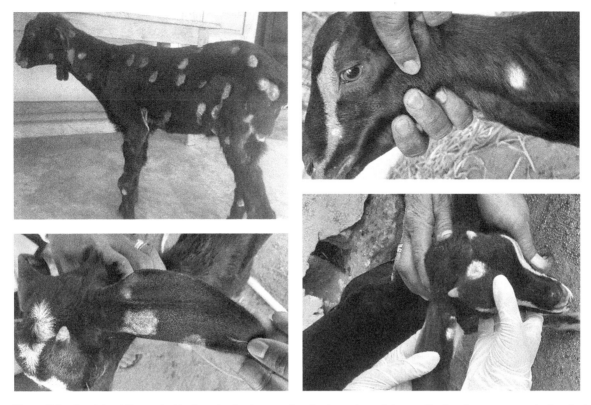

Figure 9.1   Grayish-white crusted lesions, in circular or extensive irregular patches, on the head, ears, nose, and other body parts.

Figure 9.2   (a, b) Fungal infections in goats. (c) Skin scrapings collected from fungal lesions. (d) Fungus under the microscope.

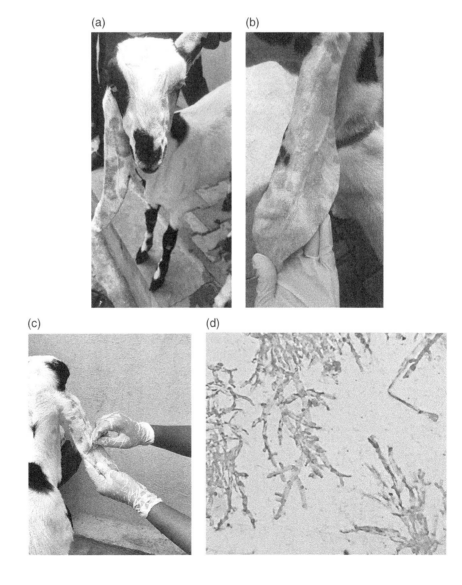

(a)

(b)

(c)

(d)

6 weeks. All equipment needs to be disinfected, as well as the area used for shelter and feeding zones daily. A systemic antibiotic like penicillin G or florfenicol is to be applied for prevention of secondary bacterial infections if the fungus has invaded deeper than the skin only.

In some cases, a systemic antifungal drug should be applied whenever necessary, with the understanding that there is a long withdrawal time for antifungal drugs. It should also be noted that fungus infection in goat is also contagious to humans.

9.2.9 Prevention

- Remove spores from the environment.
- Prevent recurrent infection.
- Limit contamination by treating affected goats.
- Reduce the number of animals in a specific area to decrease daily contact with each other.
- Keep the area where animals often lay down clean.
- Disinfection should be done with bleach 1 : 10 in water.
- Farm premises must be disinfected between batches of animals and wooden surfaces need to be treated with creosote (tar-based wood paint).
- Animals should be handled with gloves.
- Bought-in animals should be screened for skin lesions on arrival and separated and treated until all lesions have gone, because sores may still present.

9.2.10 Zoonotic Aspect

Dermatophytes can spread to people, especially young children, and be quite uncomfortable. Because the disease is highly contagious, infected cattle are prohibited from sales, shows, and interstate travel.

9.3 Diseases Caused by Yeast

9.3.1 Candidiasis/Thrush/Moniliasis

Candidiasis is a fungal disease affecting the mucus membranes and skin and may cause infection of any organ or system or systemic infection. The disease is distributed globally in goats and is characterized by yeast species of the genus *Candida*, especially *Candida albicans* (Sudhakara et al. 2018).

C. albicans is a polymorphic fungus that grows in both yeast and filamentous forms.

It is also an opportunistic pathogen and is one of the major etiological agents of mucosal and systemic fungal infection.

In susceptible individuals systemic *C. albicans* infections are thought to arise from organisms in the gastrointestinal tract. As filamentous forms predominate at sites of primary epithelial cells, *C. albicans* reach the bloodstream and subsequently spread.

9.3.1.1 Predisposing Factors
- Immunosuppression due to long-term corticosteroid therapy.
- Disruption of mucosal membrane.
- Use of antimicrobial therapy for a long time.
- Excessive use of disinfectant.

9.3.1.2 Clinical Signs
- Single and multiple raised circular white masses covered with scales.
- Marked keratinous thickening of mucosa of tongue and esophagus.
- Foul-smelling black discharge.
- Early signs may look like yeast.
- Pain when applying pressure.
- Limping.
- Mastitis.

Pathological examination revealed extensive suppurative mycotic mastitis characterized by diffuse enlargement of milk acini, which were highly infiltrated with neutrophils, macrophages, and lymphocytes, and giant cells phagocytizing some fungal elements were detected. *C. albicans* pseudo hyphae were seen in the affected lesions.

9.3.1.3 Diagnosis
- Microscopic and cultural examination of clinical material and serological tests.
- Scraping and biopsy of specimen from mucocutaneous lesion (samples are collected from affected area, e.g. skin, vaginal discharge, sputum, blood, milk, tissues, etc.).
- Direct microscopic examination of 10% KOH preparation or stained films by Gram, PAS, etc.
- Culture on SDA incubated at 37 and 25 °C for 3–5 days.
- Germ tube test – a suspension of suspected colony in 0.5 ml serum, incubate for 2–4 hours at 37 °C, and examine microscopically for the development of germ tubes, which extend the cell without septum or constriction.
- Skin test – *C. albicans* is removed from the skin surface by neutrophils. The fungal hyphae on reaching the stratum corneum activate C5 (complement) and produce chemotactic factors, leading to neutrophilic infiltration.
- Animal inoculation – *C. albicans* is pathogenic to mice and rabbit. For this 1 ml of 15 ml saline suspension of the organism is to be injected intravenously to the rabbit. The animal will die in 4–5 days with abscess formation on the kidneys. In the case of mice, 1 ml of saline suspension of the organism is to be injected intraperitoneally.

The mice will die within 4–5 days with abscessation of the kidneys. A smear or section prepared with Gram stain will look like short budding cells.

9.3.1.4 Treatment
Because *Candida* spp. may remain as commensals in animals, the predisposing factors that induce the disease should be taken care of by:

- Various azole formations.
- Nystatin ointment.
- Topical application of amphotericin B or 1% iodine/$CuSO_4$.

9.3.1.5 Prevention and Control
- The affected animal should be segregated.
- Clean water should be provided without contamination with yeast.
- Good food without mold should be provided.
- Maintain aseptic conditions.
- Antimicrobial should be used judiciously.
- Maintain hygienic conditions and strict biosecurity.
- Nystatin can be used for control and prophylactic treatment.

9.3.2 Cryptococcosis in Goats

Cryptococcosis, one of the important systemic fungal diseases, causes problems in eyes, respiratory tract (especially the nasal cavity), skin, and nervous system (brain) in goats. *Cryptococcus* spp. play a major role in causing mastitis and pneumonia in immunocompromised goats. In addition, saprophytic and opportunistic fungal pathogens *Cryptococcus neoformans* and *Cryptococcus gattii* are prevalent in the environment, soil, fowl manure, and tissues as a yeast form. Transmission of *Cryptococcus* spp. occurs through inhalation of basidiospores, ingestion of desiccated yeast cells, or contamination of wounds. The most noticeable signs are sneezing, depression, snorting, weight loss, disorientation, diminished appetite, lethargy, seizures, nasal discharge, eye problems, change in behavior, and moving difficulties. Azole drugs including itraconazole, ketoconazole, amphotericin B (with or without flucytosine), fluconazole, and glucocorticoids are the most common antifungal drugs used for treatment. Surgical procedures are needed to remove an unwanted subcutaneous or internal mass followed by antifungal therapy (Chapman et al. 1990).

9.3.3 Malasseziosis in Goats

Malassezia dermatitis or otitis is a very common mycotic disease caused by some *Malassezia* species, including *M. slooffiae*, *M. restricta*, *M. globosa*, *M. sympodialis*, *M. furfur*, and *M. pachydermatis*. In addition, *M. pachydermatis* is the most important fungus that causes diseases in goats and belongs to the zoophilic yeast, division Basidiomycota. *Malassezia* spp. are yeasts with a lipophilic nature belonging to the normal cutaneous or mucosal microbiota of goats and they are normally seen in very low numbers in the external ear canals, in perianal regions, in perioral areas, and also in moist skin folds of goats (Eguchi-Coe et al. 2011).

Malassezia species are demarcated as opportunistic pathogens that play a major role in the development of various diseases, including seborrheic dermatitis and otitis externa in goats. Malasseziosis is prevalent in goats suffering from various skin allergies, immunosuppressive diseases, endocrinopathies (hypothyroidism, Cushing's disease), and other skin diseases. The infection may spread due to hypersensitivity to the yeast and accelerated growth of the organism (Pin 2004). Malnourished and debilitated goats suffer from *Malassezia* dermatitis mostly. The most important lesions are non-painful, non-pruritic to mildly pruritic, and are also characterized by hyperpigmentation, greasiness, erythema, yellow waxy crusts and scale, lichenification, follicular orthokeratotic hyperkeratosis, and mild lymphocytic perivascular dermatitis. Lesions are typically multifocal and observed in the trunk and back region, and may become generalized in a time-dependent manner. *Malassezia* are a generally thermotolerant species in the summer season.

9.3.3.1 Cause: *Malassezia pachydermatis*
Malassezia yeasts belong to the normal cutaneous or mucosal microbiota of many warm-blooded vertebrates. They are recognized as opportunistic pathogens that play a significant role in the development of different human and animal diseases such as otitis externa or seborrheic dermatitis.

9.3.3.2 Distribution
The disease has been reported from almost all states in India.

9.3.3.3 Predisposing Factors
- Cutaneous hypersensitivity including atopic dermatitis.
- Pyoderma.
- Ectoparasitic skin disease, particularly hypothyroidism.
- Endocrine disorders, particularly hypothyroidism.
- Treatment with glucocorticoids.

9.3.3.4 Pathogenesis
The *Malassezia* organism produces lipases that can liberate acids and zymogens in the yeast cell wall that activate complement, resulting in cutaneous inflammation. This opportunistic pathogen produces skin infection

depending on host factors and immune suppressive mechanisms, and produces skin infections either independently or as a sequel to other diseases like hypothyroidism, dermatomycosis, demodicosis, hypoandrogenism, Sertoli cell tumor, food allergy, or flea-bite hypersensitivity. Metabolic products of the organism irritate the ear canal and change the microbial flora. It also produces proteolytic enzymes damaging the ear canal epithelium, which leads to hyperplasia with enlargement of the ceruminous glands.

9.3.3.5 Clinical Signs
- Dermatological examination shows generalized greasy seborrheic dermatosis and alopecia that spare the head and extremities of the limbs.
- Alopecia with dry seborrhea.
- Mild pruritis, hyperkeratosis, and plugging of hair follicles.
- Severe enteritis associated with weight loss.

9.3.3.6 Diagnosis
- **Direct microscopic examination**: Cotton swab smears, skin scrapings, direct impression smears, and acetate tape impressions are routinely used to identify *M. pachydermatis* cytologically. Smears are fixed then stained with a modified Wright's stain or ink. The tape is not fixed, and stained with modified Wright's stain or ink.
- The stained tape is then applied to a glass slide with the adhesive side down. The slide is examined under oil immersion, looking for unipolar budding yeast that are described as peanut-, footprint- or bottle-shaped organisms.
- **Isolation on SDA**: *Malassezia* comprises 14 species, of which 13 show an absolute requirement for long-chain fatty acids. These "lipid-dependent" yeasts are therefore seldom isolated in the laboratory unless specific nutrients are provided in the medium. The species *M. pachydermatis* is the only lipophilic yeast that can be isolated in regular media like SDA.
- **PCR or restriction endonuclease analyses**: This usually involves amplification and subsequent restriction of portions of the highly variable ribosomal RNA gene that are potentially applicable for routine laboratory use.

9.3.3.7 Treatment
- Topical and oral antifungal agents such as ketoconazole and fluconazole.
- Seborrheic dermatitis treated with topical steroids.
- Systemic therapy:
  – Ketoconazole at 5–10 mg/kg body weight.
  – Itraconazole at 5–10 mg/kg body weight.
- Antifungal dips.

9.3.4 Rhodotorulosis in the Goat

Rhodotorula species are attributed as being opportunistic pathogens that can colonize and infect susceptible goats. These species are ubiquitous saprophytic yeasts in nature and grow in different ecosystems with unfavorable conditions (Wirth and Goldani 2012). Malnourished, debilitated, and immunocompromised goats mostly suffer. Documentary evidence suggested that *Rhodotorula glutinis* and *Rhodotorula minuta* are mostly found in goat milk (Nagahama et al. 2006) and cause mastitis. In addition, *Rhodotorula rubra* (*R. mucilaginosa*) is the species most frequently associated with infection in goats. These *Rhodotorula* species are commonly obtained from various water sources, the environment, and also food substances. The genus *Rhodotorula* has eight species, out of which *R. mucilaginosa*, *R. glutinis*, and *R. minuta* were reported to cause disease in small ruminants (Wirth and Goldani 2012). These species play a key role in causing lung and skin infections in goats. Itraconazole, voriconazole, posaconazole, fluconazole, amphotericin B, ketoconazole, and flucytosine are the main antifungal drugs for the treatment of goats (Refai et al. 2017).

9.3.5 Phaeohyphomycosis

Phaeohyphomycosis is an infection caused by a well-known black yeast, *Cladosporium cladosporioides*, from class Dothideomycetes, order Capnodiales, and family Davidiellaceae. These species are ubiquitous in nature and obtained from environmental origins such as air, water, soil, and plant materials. The saprobic spore-forming dematiaceous fungi cause opportunistic allergic infections through invasion into wounds on the skin (Fatima 2021).

C. cladosporioides is responsible for causing cutaneous and pulmonary phaeohyphomycosis by attacking the lungs and thereby causing respiratory troubles, sneezing, anorexia, fever, and death. Necropsy findings reveal severe hemorrhages in lungs, lymph nodes, heart, abomasum, and kidneys. The fungus also causes thrombosis and vasculitis, suggesting hematogenous dissemination.

Free-living fungus *Peyronellaea glomerata* causes verrucas, abscesses, papulonodules, cysts, hyperkeratotic or ulcerated plaques, pyogranuloma, or non-healing ulcers or sinuses, papules, and aural plaques on the ears. The disease appears to be self-limiting and is treated with surgical intervention by excision of local lesions, followed by application of antifungals including ketoconazole, fluconazole, liposomal amphotericin B, posaconazole, itraconazole, and terbinafine.

9.4 Diseases Caused by Molds

9.4.1 Aspergillosis in Goats

Aspergillus fumigatus and *Aspergillus niger* have been reported to be causative agents of opportunistic infections in goats. These cause poor growth, mycotic abortion, mycotic mastitis, and mycotic pneumonia in goats (Mandal and Gupta 1993).

9.4.1.1 Diagnosis

- **Isolation of fungi**: *Aspergillus* spp. grow rapidly within 48 hours in SDA and blood agar media.
- **Serology**: Agar gel immunodiffusion (AGID), complement fixation, and enzyme-linked immunosorbent assay (ELISA) techniques.

9.4.1.2 Histopathology

- Presence of fungal hyphae.
- Exhibited high sensitivity.
- Presence of mucosal ulceration and inflammation with an abundance of lymphocytes and plasma cells.

9.4.1.3 Cytological Identification

Cytology identifies the presence of fungus in urine, synovial fluid, blood, lymph node, intervertebral disk material, or bone.

9.4.1.4 Molecular Identification

Sequencing of genes, such as actin, calmodulin, internal transcribed spacer (ITS), rodlet A (rodA), and/or β-tubulin (βtub), has been used to distinguish *A. fumigatus* from related species. This can be done by:

- Multilocus sequence typing.
- Random amplified polymorphic DNA.
- Restriction fragment length polymorphisms.
- Microsphere-based Luminex assay.

9.4.2 Facial Eczema (Pithomycotoxicosis/Photodermatitis)

9.4.2.1 Cause: *Pithomyces chartarum*

Facial eczema (pithomycotoxicosis) is a photosensitization of ruminants grazing pasture, but its cause is a toxin produced by a largely saprophytic fungus, *Pithomyces chartarum*, growing on litter at the base of the pasture and sporing profusely under warm, moist conditions in late summer and autumn (Pinto et al. 2005).

As the fungus spores it produces the toxin sporidesmin which, when eaten by the goat, causes liver injury with inflammation and blockage of the bile ducts. Phylloerythrin, a photodynamic pigment that breaks down chlorophyll, is no longer excreted but circulates in the blood, causing lesions of unpigmented skin when the affected animal is exposed to sunlight.

9.4.2.2 Clinical Signs

- Red skin that turns black and crusty before peeling off. Other signs are jaundice and inflammation causing swelling of teats, ears, face, and vulva.
- Drooping ears and swollen eyes, so the sheep may be effectively blind.
- The goats shake their heads and rub their eyes on fence posts and gates, which causes sores and bleeding.
- Their lesions are often attacked by blow flies.
- Badly affected animals stop eating and typically die very quickly

9.4.2.3 Diagnosis

- By clinical signs.
- *P. chartarum* was characterized by hand-grenade spores.
- Careful pathological examination of demonstration of a large population of sporidesmin producing *P. chartarum*.
- On postmortem the goats have an abnormal hard, misshapen liver.

9.4.2.4 Treatment

- Zinc supplements reacts with sporidesmin to create mercaptide so that poison can be eliminated from the body.
- Itraconazole at 4 mg/kg body weight.
- Ketoconazole at 10 mg/kg body weight.

9.4.2.5 Control

Facial eczema can be controlled by avoiding toxic pasture, detected by *P. chartarum* spore counts on herbage. *P. chartarum* pasture populations can also be produced by spray application of substituted thiabendazole fungicides.

Breeding resistant animals by selection after sporedesmin challenge is the best long-term control method at present.

9.4.3 Pythiosis in Goats

Pythium, a genus of parasitic oomycotes, is more prevalent in tropic and subtropic regions. *Pythium insidiosum* plays a major role in causing fast-growing clinical conditions leading to death. It is more prevalent in the summer season and develops from open wounds with eosinophilic granulomatous inflammation. Pneumonia, granulomatous rhinitis, ulcerative cutaneous lesions on the skin, and metastasis in lungs and lymph nodes also develop (Carmo et al. 2015).

- **Diagnosis**: Wet mounts.
- **Histopathology**: Eosinophilic inflammatory reaction.
- **Serology**: Complement fixation test, immunodiffusion (ID) test, ELISA, immunoperoxidase assay, nested PCR assay.

9.4.4 Conidiobolomycosis in Goats

Conidiobolomycosis is a zygomycosis caused by fungi of the class Zygomycetes, order Entomophthorales, which affects goats.

9.4.4.1 Cause

Conidiodobolus coronatus occurs mainly as a subcutaneous, rhinofacial, or nasopharyngeal infection (Carmo et al. 2020). *Conidiodobolus* spp. are found mainly in soil, decaying vegetation, and insects of tropical and subtropical regions. The disease is distributed in Central America, Equatorial Africa, and India.

9.4.4.2 Signs

- Serous nasal discharge, dyspnea, and dermatitis in limbs and ears.
- Enlargement of anterior or posterior nasal cavity.
- The rhinopharyngeal form is the most common, causing unilateral exophthalmos depression, progressive emaciation, and serosanguinous nasal discharge.
- Tachycardia.
- Unilateral exophthalmia with increased ocular globe volume and hypopyon corneal ulceration.
- Nervous signs.
- Granulomatous necrotic tissue in the ethmoidal region extending through the turbinate bones into the brain and into soft tissues of the nose, with dissemination to the lungs and lymph nodes.

9.4.4.3 Microscopic Findings

- Meningitis, cortex necrosis, and encephalitis with the presence of eosinophilic Splendore-Hoeppli substances.
- The main hematological alteration was neutrophilia.
- Cerebrospinal fluid analysis showed the presence of fibrin reticules and pleocytosis.
- Histopathology.
- Lungs revealed Splendore-Hoeppli–like material and hyperplasia of alveolar and bronchiolar epithelium.
- Renal lesions were suggestive of amyloidosis.
- Longitudinal section of the head revealed the presence of a nodular mass with a friable consistency and a white yellowish coloration.

9.4.4.4 Diagnosis

- Direct microscopy is done with blades made by the Gram technique and KOH, and displays large non-septate hyphae.
- Culture is done by inoculation on potato dextrose agar, Sabouraud chloramphenicol agar, or dichloran Rose Bengal chloramphenicol agar, which are selective agar for pathogenic fungi.
- Fluorescent antibody and agglutination test.
- PCR.

9.4.4.5 Treatment

Long-term itraconazole treatment is recommended.

9.4.5 Pneumocystosis in Goats

Pneumocystis carinii, an opportunistic fungal pathogen, plays a key role in causing fatal pneumonia in immunosuppressed goats. *P. carinii* is either a protozoan or a fungus on the basis of its taxonomy. It is a well-structured thick-walled cyst with the thin-walled trophozoite, as well as a sporozoite in an intracystic structure.

Transmission is by direct contact and airborne routes. Interspecies transmission does not happen in immunodeficient hosts (McConnell et al. 1971).

9.4.6 Microsporidiosis in Goats

Microsporidia, currently considered as emerging opportunistic fungal pathogens, are unicellular, obligate intracellular parasite eukaryotes. *Enterocytozoon bieneusi* generally occurs in fecal samples and the intestinal tissue of goats. Microsporidiosis is generally treated with albendazole and fumagillin (Al-Herrawy and Gad 2016).

9.4.7 Scopulariopsis Goats

The genus *Scopulariopsis*, an opportunistic pathogen, contains both hyaline and dematiaceous molds. These play a key role in causing superficial tissue infections with non-dermatophytic onychomycoses. They are commonly found in air, plant debris, soil, moist indoor environments, and on paper. They are responsible for developing brain abscesses, peritonitis, endophthalmitis, otomycosis, endocarditis, pneumonia, and keratitis followed by eye trauma. *Scopulariopsis flava*, *Microascus niger*, *Microascus manginii*, *Scopulariopsis brumptii*, *Microascus cinereus*, *Microascus cirrosus*, and *Microascus trigonosporus* are causative agents for developing diseases (Ozturk et al. 2009).

9.4.8 Sporotrichosis

This is also known as rose handler disease, rose gardener disease, and rose thorn disease.

9.4.8.1 Etiology

This is caused by *Sporotrichosis schenckii*, which is a dimorphic fungus. It is a contagious, suppurative granulomatous disease of skin and subcutaneous tissue. The disease may be characterized by nodules and ulcers. The agent is commonly found on decaying vegetation and has been isolated many times from soil.

9.4.8.2 Epidemiology

Sporotrichosis occurs in India, Europe, and the USA, and in sheep, goats, cattle, dogs, horses, foxes, and camels.

9.4.8.3 Mode of Transmission

The organisms gain entry through trauma to skin, which may be through scratches from thorns or splinters. A hot and humid atmosphere favors the growth of the organism. It is an occupational hazard to persons who are engaged in agriculture and horticulture practices.

9.4.8.4 Zoonotic Aspect

Sporotrichosis is a universal mycosis that occurs all over the world, but it is endemic in regions with tropical and subtropical climates. It is an emergent disease and, over the past two decades, the incidence of zoonotic sporotrichosis has been on the rise.

9.4.8.5 Pathogenesis

The infection spreads through contaminated cutaneous wounds, then reaches underlying tissues. Initially the lesion begins as suppurative inflammation of the skin and as the disease progresses, ulceration and necrosis of the superficial layer of the skin become marked (Pereira et al. 2015). The organisms then invade the tissues and lymphatics and thereby reach regional lymph nodes and produce lymphadenitis. Thus, granuloma on the skin, lymph nodes, and subcutis are produced.

9.4.8.6 Clinical Findings

Sporotrichosis occur in three forms:

- **Lymphocutaneous**: This form is infectious and is limited to the subcutaneous and adjacent lymphatics. It is mostly seen in goats. Multiple nodules appear on the lymph channel like nodular cords. The nodules become ulcerated and deep lesions are produced, which have a tendency to retard healing.
- **Cutaneous**: This form is without the involvement of the lymphatics system. It is characterized by the development of multiple nodules on the skin that ulcerate and drain with pus. The lesions are mostly located at the extremities, especially at the fetlock joint region.
- **Disseminated/systemic**: This form is characterized by infection disseminated to different parts of the body. This may involve bones and internal organs.

9.4.8.7 Lesions

The lesions occur as ulcerative necrotic nodules. The primary lesion comprises granuloma. There are granulomatous changes with a purulent center surrounded by a wide band of epithelioid granulation tissue containing giant cells and lymphocytes. Cellular infiltration is via macrophages, epithelioid cells, multinucleated giant cells, and lymphocytes.

9.4.8.8 Diagnosis

- Demonstration of the organism in exudates. Stained smear of exudate may reveal a small number of Gram-positive spores.
- PAS stain can be used to demonstrate the organism, which may be oval, round, or cigar shaped.
- Culture on SDA.
- The tube agglutination test is effective in detecting visceral form of the disease.
- The latex slide agglutination test along with the ID test are most reliable and most specific.
- Animal inoculation can be done in rat and mice. Intraperitoneal inoculation will produce disseminated lesions from which fungus can be isolated.

9.4.8.9 Treatment

- Itraconazole at 10 mg/kg body weight is the drug of choice.
- Potassium iodide (orally) and sodium iodide at 1 g/40 kg body weight as a 10% solution through the intravenous route is recommended.
- Amphotericin B at 4 mg/kg body weight.
- Oral administration of griseofulvin is reported to have satisfactory results.

9.4.8.10 Control

- Isolation and segregation of infected animals.
- Prompt treatment of cuts, wounds, and abrasions with tincture of iodine.
- Treatment of equipment and sheds with antifungal agents.

9.4.9 Coccidiomycosis

This is also known as Posada's disease, valley fever, desert rheumatism, California disease, valley bumps, and coccidioidal granuloma.

9.4.9.1 Cause

The disease is caused by *Coccidiodes immitis*, a dimorphic fungus with white fluffy mold, in a non-building spherical form (Plummer et al. 2012).

It is a mildly severe disease of the upper respiratory tract that occurs in three forms: acute; chronic or severe disseminating; and fatal.

9.4.9.2 Epidemiology

- Affect almost all species including sheep and goats.
- Infection by inhalation.
- Usually occurs in arid zones.

9.4.9.3 Clinical Findings
- Coughing (dry), shortness of breath.
- Poor appetite, intermittent diarrhea, loss of weight.
- Lameness, enlarged joints, muscle atrophy.
- Involvement of bronchial and mediastinal lymph nodes.
- Specific symptoms are absent.

9.4.9.4 Necropsy Finding
Pyogranulomatous lesions are present. In the center is caseous necrosis or liquefaction, but calcification is rare.

9.4.9.5 Diagnosis
- Clinical signs.
- Necropsy.
- Histopathology – spherules, refractile walls containing endospores.
- Latex agglutination Agar gel diffusion test.
- Complement fixation test.

9.4.9.6 Treatment
No complete or satisfactory treatment is available. Amphotericin B and itraconazole can be used.

9.5 Diseases Caused by Multiple Agents

9.5.1 Mycotic Mastitis in Goats

9.5.1.1 Cause: *Aspergillus* spp.
Mycotic mastitis occurs as sporadic cases or sometimes as outbreaks.

9.5.1.2 Mode of Transmission
Fungal mastitis occurs in epizootic or enzootic proportions. The spread of the fungi depends on the fungal character transmission mechanism. The fungal characteristics concerned are:

- The fungal potential to lodge in the mammary gland.
- The capability of the fungi to survive in the mammary gland.
- The ability of the fungi to withstand cleaning and disinfection.
- The ability of the fungi to resist antifungal antibiotic therapy.

9.5.1.3 Pathogenesis
The pathogenesis varies with the involvement of infecting organisms. After gaining entry the fungus gets established in mammary tissues and sets up inflammatory changes. *Aspergillus* spp. produce densely fibrosed granulomatous changes in the mammary glands (Carmo et al. 2020).

9.5.1.4 Clinical Signs
It is very difficult to distinguish fungal from bacterial mastitis from the standpoint of clinical considerations, which are:

- Purulent mammary secretion, progressive induration of the affected glands, slight fever.
- Swollen, painful udder not allowing lambs to suck.
- Anorexia and weight loss.
- Variable-sized grayish-white nodules in the affected udder.
- Reduced milk yield or permanent stoppage of milk yield.
- Fungal mastitis does not respond to antibacterial therapy.

9.5.1.5 Microscopic
A granulomatous reaction occurs with well-developed multiple granulomas in the infected udders. Marked infiltration of lymphocytes, macrophages, extensive fibrosis, and hyphae and spores of *A. fumigatus* could be demonstrated in sections of the infected udder.

9.5.1.6 Lesions
In acute cases there is dissolution of acinar epithelium, but a chronic case will show diffused granulomatous foci in mammary tissues and lymph nodes. A well-marked cellular reaction with neutrophilic, eosinophilic, and histiocytic cells along with epithelial cells is noted. There is destruction of all glandular structure except the fibrous framework of the gland, and aggregation of large giant cells in collagenized fibrous tissues.

9.5.1.7 Diagnosis
- History of the case as being nonresponsive to antibiotics.
- Indirect immunofluorescent labeling, which gave a strong and uniform reaction with polyclonal and monoclonal antibodies to *A. fumigatus*.
- Zygomycotic hyphae can also be identified using immunohistochemistry in granulomatous lesions at terminal swellings of *Aspergillus* hyphae.
- Microscopic detection of fungal agents:
  - The suspected milk sample should be centrifuged at 12 000 rpm at 4 °C for 10 minutes. Smears from the sediment should be made on a clean glass slide. The slide should be stained with 0.5% gentian violet or Grocott silver methanamine method or with lactophenol cotton blue (LCPB) and examined under the microscope. A fungal element or yeast-like bodies can be detected.
  - A loopful of the suspected milk sample should be inoculated in SDA slants containing streptomycin and penicillin or chloramphenicol. The slants should be incubated at 37 °C. The culture showing growth should be identified based on macroscopic and microscopic morphology of the organisms. Characteristics of the fungi on different media like corn meal-tween agar or eosin methylene

blue agar Levine should be noted. The identification may be made by staining with LCPB. The biochemical characterization can be studied, such as Reynold and brand effect, sugar fermentation reaction using glucose, maltose, lactose, and sucrose, as well urease activity.

9.5.1.8 Treatment
Fungal mastitis is resistant to antibiotics. Antifungal preparations may be used:

- Potassium iodide orally at a dose of 8–10 g for 7 days.
- Sodium iodide (10%) solution intravenously.
- Iodine in oil as an infusion.
- Merthiolate solution as an infusion.
- Miconazole (400 mg) intravenously following thiabendazole orally for 3 days.
- Fluconazole at 5 mg/kg body weight.
- Natamycin, amphotericin B, nystatin, maxxitol, or chlorpheniramine maleate.

9.5.1.9 Control
- Awareness should be created among dairy personnel about the probability of a problem with mastitis.
- Identification of the affected herd should be made promptly.
- Following detection, immediate treatment should be rendered with appropriate drugs.
- Hygiene of the udder should be maintained by cleaning with water and using teat dips (iodophor solution).
- Feeds with fungal contamination should not be fed.
- Milking should be done at regular intervals.
- The hands of the milkers should be thoroughly clean.
- Dairy utensils should be cleaned effectively.
- Indiscriminate use of antibiotics as an udder infusion should be discouraged (if possible, antibiotics should be used after a sensitivity test).
- Udders should be treated in the dry period. Composition of the teat dip may be:
  - Iodine 1% or chlorine 4%.
  - Sodium hydroxide 0.08% + sodium carbonate 0.3% + sodium chloride 0.217%.

9.5.2 Mycotic Abortion in Goats

Mycotic abortion may be caused by:

- *M. canis* (Pal 2001).
- *A. fumigatus.*
- *C. albicans.*

9.5.3 Mycotic Pneumonia in Goats

Pneumonia is inflammation of the pulmonary parenchyma accompanied by inflammation of the bronchioles and possibly the pleura. The most important fungi attributed as causing mycotic pneumonia in goats (Pawaiya et al. 2015) are:

- *Aspergillus* spp.
- *Emmonsia crescens.*
- *Mortierella wolfii.*
- *R. rubra.*
- *P. carinii.*
- *C. neoformans.*
- *C. albicans.*

9.5.4 Aspergillosis

9.5.4.1 Epidemiology
C. neoformans is a yeast-like fungus with worldwide distribution. It causes diseases in both animals and humans. The organism occurs as a saprophyte in nature, usually in soil contaminated with pigeon and chicken manure, and is considered an opportunist pathogen.

9.5.4.2 Clinical Signs
- Respiratory distress.
- Dyspnea.
- Mild fever.
- Noisy respiration.
- Nasal discharge.
- Cough.
- Increase in respiration rate.
- Abnormal sounds on auscultation.
- Mucopurulent discharge.

9.5.4.3 Diagnosis
Diagnosis is by stains including GMS and hematoxylin and eosin (H&E) stain. The capsule and fungus cell exhibited marked Asian Blue and PAS staining, respectively.

Histopathology of the lungs showed areas of parenchymal necrosis, containing blastoconidia with a slightly basophilic central cell, surrounded by an unstained capsule.

9.5.4.4 Treatment
Treatment is by amphotericin B with fluorinated pyrimidine analog flucytosine followed by triazole, fluconazole, ketoconazole, and anti-inflammatory drugs.

9.5.4.5 Prevention
- Avoid exposure to dust, especially at the site of habitats of bats and birds.
- Remove sick or affected animals from the herd and place them in isolation.
- Pay attention to proper ventilation, housing, and nutrition.
- Avoid crowding and isolate purchased goats or those stressed by traveling or showing.

9.6 Diseases Caused by Algae: Protothecosis in Goats

Prototheca spp. are very important achlorophyllous, ovoid to globose, microscopic, unicellular algae with a hyaline refractile cellulose wall surrounding a granular cytoplasm. *Prototheca zopfii*, *Prototheca cutis*, *Prototheca blaschkeae*, and *Prototheca wickerhamii* are species causing the infection in goats (Riet-Correa et al. 2021). Ulcerated pyogranulomatous necrotizing multifocal nodules are found in the nasal vestibule, mucocutaneous regions, lip and nasal skin, and on the border of the right ear. Normally, prototheca are found in acidic streams, lake waters, soil, potato skin, mud, marine waters, sludges from milking machines, dung, soil, feces, and sewage channels.

Diagnosis is via samples taken from secretions and tissues from mastitis-infected animals. Isolation and identification of *Prototheca* spp. can be done in suitable mycological media. Light microscopy, fluorescence microscopy using Fungiqual, indirect ELISA, AGID test, antigen, and hyperimmune serum can be implicated as diagnostic tools for *Prototheca* strains.

9.7 Keratinophilic Fungi

Keratinophilic filamentous fungi are hyphomycetes and are generally colonizing on keratinous substrates. Hyphomycetes include dermatophytes and a great diversity of nondermatophyte filamentous fungi. Keratolytic fungi can play a key role in decomposing α-keratins, insoluble fibrous proteins. These are prevalent as cornfield debris in the soil.

Keratinophilic fungi, especially dermatophytes, decompose the residue of keratin and act as a potential source of human and animal infections by direct contact. They also cause various cutaneous mycoses (Ali-Shtayeh et al. 1988).

9.8 Mycotoxins in Feed and Milk of Sheep and Goats

The following mycotoxins are reported in goats:

- Aflatoxins, mainly aflatoxin B1 (AFB1) and M1 (AFM1).
- Zearalenone.
- Ochratoxin A.
- T-2 toxin.
- Cyclopiazonic acid.
- Fuminosin B1.

The presence of toxigenic species in samples of feed for lactating goats indicates a potential risk of contamination of dairy products, if they are exposed to environmental conditions favorable to fungal growth and mycotoxin production (Layton et al. 2009).

9.9 Conclusion

Maintenance of proper hygiene procedures, biosecurity measures, proper selection of animals, animal surveillance, animal welfare, and proper grazing systems are very important to prevent and control fungal diseases in goats.

Multiple-Choice Questions

1 What is the most common fungal pathogen recovered from a respiratory tract infection?
   A *Histoplasma capsulatum*
   B *Aspergillus niger*
   C *Trichophyton rubrum*
   D *Malassezia furfur*

2 What are the most common laboratory culture media for fungi?
   A Sabouraud dextrose agar
   B Brain heart infusion agar
   C Thayer Martin medium
   D a and b

3 Which antifungal medicine is most effective for the treatment of rashes in athlete's foot or ringworm fungal infection?
   A Optochin
   B Bacitracin and zinc
   C Clotrimazole
   D Tobramycin

4 What is histoplasmosis caused by?
   A Protozoa
   B Fungus
   C Bacteria
   D Virus

5 Which of the following is used in routine microscopic laboratory methods of identifying fungal specimens?
A 70% KOH mount
B 50% H$_2$O$_2$
C 10% KOH
D Formalin

6 In the 1920s Sir Alexander Fleming was able to discover an antibiotic from which mold?
A *Aspergillus* spp.
B *Mucor* spp.
C *Fusarium* spp.
D *Penicillium* spp.

7 What is a fungal disease that affects the internal organs and spreads through the body called?

A Mycoses
B Systemic mycoses
C Mycotoxicosis
D Superficial mycoses

8 Which of the following is the sun ray fungus?
A Actinomyces irraeli
B Chromoblastomycosis
C *Streptomyces griseus*
D Cryptococcosis

9 Who was mycorrhiza first observed by?
A Funk
B Frank
C Crick
D Fisher

References

Al-Herrawy, A.Z. and Gad, M.A. (2016). Microsporidial spores in fecal samples of some domesticated animals living in Giza, Egypt. *Iranian Journal of Parasitology* 11 (2): 195–203.

Ali-Shtayeh, M.S., Arda, H.M., Hassouna, M. et al. (1988). Keratinophilic fungi on the hair of goats from the West Bank of Jordan. *Mycopathologia* 104: 103–108. https://doi.org/10.1007/BF00436935.

do Carmo, P.M.S., Portela, R.A., Silva, T.R. et al. (2015). Cutaneous pythiosis in a goat. *Journal of Comparative Pathology* 152 (2–3): 103–105. https://doi.org/10.1016/j.jcpa.2014.11.005.

do Carmo, P.M.S., Uzal, F.A., Pedroso, P.M.O., and Riet-Correa, F. (2020). Conidiobolomycosis, cryptococcosis, and aspergillosis in sheep and goats: a review. *Journal of Veterinary Diagnostic Investigation* 32 (6): 826–834. https://doi.org/10.1177/1040638720958338.

Chakrabarti, A. (1984). *Textbook of Clinical Veterinary Medicine*. New Delhi: Kalyani Publishers.

Chapman, H.M., Robinson, W.F., Bolton, J.R., and Robertson, J.P. (1990). *Cryptococcus neoformans* infection in goats. *Australian Veterinary Journal* 67 (7): 263–265. https://doi.org/10.1111/j.1751-0813.1990.tb07783.x.

Eguchi-Coe, Y., Valentine, B.A., Gorman, E., and Villarroel, A. (2011). Putative Malassezia dermatitis in six goats. *Veterinary Dermatology* 22 (6): 497–501. https://doi.org/10.1111/j.1365-3164.2011.00980.x. E.

Fatima, D. (2021). Ovine fungal diseases. In: *Fungal Diseases in Animals* (ed. A. Gupta and N.P. Singh), 63–71. Cham: Springer.

Layton, R.C., Purdy, C.W., Jumper, C.A., and Straus, D.C. (2009). Detection of macrocyclic trichothecene mycotoxin in a caprine (goat) tracheal instillation model. *Toxicology and Industrial Health* 25 (9–10): 693–701. https://doi.org/10.1177/0748233709348275.

Mandal, P.C. and Gupta, P.P. (1993). Experimental aspergillosis in goats: clinical, haematological and mycological studies. *Zentralblatt für Veterinärmedizin. Reihe B* 40 (4): 283–286.

McConnell, E.E., Basson, P.A., and Pienaar, J.G. (1971). Pneumocystosis in a domestic goat. *Onderstepoort Journal of Veterinary Research* 38 (2): 117–126.

Nagahama, T., Hamamoto, M., and Horikoshi, K. (2006). Rhodotorula pacifica sp. nov., a novel yeast species from sediment collected on the deep-sea floor of the north-west Pacific Ocean. *International Journal of Systematic and Evolutionary Microbiology* 56 (1): 295–299.

Ozturk, D., Adanir, R., and Turutoglu, H. (2009). Superficial skin infection with *Scopulariopsis brevicaulis* in two goats. A case report. *Bulletin of the Veterinary Institute in Pulawy* 53: 361–363.

Pal, M. (2001). Dermatophytosis in a goat and its handler due to *Microsporm canis*. *Indian Journal of Animal Sciences* 71: 138–140.

Pawaiya, R.V.S., Shivasharanappa, N., Sharma, N. et al. (2015). Patho-morphological study of a spontaneous case of mycotic pneumonia in sheep. *Indian Journal of Veterinary Pathology* 39 (1): 78–80.

Pereira, S.A., Gremião, I.D.F., and Menezes, R.C. (2015). Sporotrichosis in animals: zoonotic transmission. In: *Sporotrichosis* (ed. I.Z. Carlos), 83–102. Cham: Springer.

Pin, D. (2004). Seborrhoeic dermatitis in a goat due to *Malassezia pachydermatis*. *Veterinary Dermatology* 15 (1): 53–56.

Pinto, P.C., Santos, V.M., Dinis, J. et al. (2005). Pithomycotoxicosis (facial eczema) in ruminants in the Azores. *Veterinary Record* 157 (25): 805–810.

Plummer, P.J., Plummer, C.L., and Stil, K.M. (2012). Diseases of the respiratory system. In: *Sheep and Goat Medicine*, 2e (ed. D.G. Pugh and A.N. Baird), 107–128. St. Louis, MO: Elsevier.

Refai, M.K., El-Naggar, A.L., and El-Mokhtar, N.M. (2017). *Monograph on Fungal Diseases of Sheep & Goats: A Guide for Postgraduate Students in Developing Countries*. Cairo: Cairo University.

Riet-Correa, F., Carmo, P.M.S.D., and Uzal, F.A. (2021). Prototabecosis and chlorellosis in sheep and goats: a review. *Journal of Veterinary Diagnostic Investigation* 33 (2): 283–287. https://doi.org/10.1177/1040638720978781.

Sudhakara, R.B., Sivajothi, S., and Deepika, K. (2018). Successful management of fungal mastitis in goats – a report of three cases. *Approaches in Poultry, Dairy & Veterinary Sciences* 3 (5): APDV.000575. https://doi.org/10.31031/APDV.2018.03.000575.

Wirth, F. and Goldani, L.Z. (2012). Epidemiology of Rhodotorula: an emerging pathogen. *Interdisciplinary Perspectives on Infectious Diseases* 2012: 465717. https://doi.org/10.1155/2012/465717.

10

Viral Diseases of Goats

Abha Tikoo, Savleen Kour, and Rajesh Agrawal

Faculty of Veterinary Sciences & Animal Husbandry, Sher-e-Kashmir University of Agricultural Sciences and Technology-Jammu, Ranbir Singh Pura, UT Jammu & Kashmir, India

10.1 Peste des Petits Ruminants

Also known as goat plague or kata, peste des petits ruminants (PPR) is caused by the morbilli virus (*Paramyxoviridae*) from the order Mononegavirales alongside other important viral pathogens such as measles virus (MV) and canine distemper virus (CDV) (Parida et al. 2016) (Figure 10.1). A total of four lineages have been found: lineages 1 and 2 in West Africa, lineage 3 in East Africa, southern India, and Arab countries; and lineage 4 in the Middle East and Asian subcontinent (Radiostitis et al. 2007). A natural form of the infection is present in wild sheep and deer, with higher innate resistance in Sahelian goats and sheep (Radiostitis et al. 2007). Goats and sheep are the primary hosts, whereas there are some reports of outbreaks in camels (Roger et al. 2001; Khalafalla et al. 2010; Kwiatek et al. 2011), cattle (Sen et al. 2014; Abubakar et al. 2015), buffalo (Govindarajan et al. 1997), and pigs (Nawathe and Taylor 1979). Cattle and pigs are not thought to be capable of excreting virus in their body secretions, thus they do not contribute in the epidemiology of the disease.

The virus spreads through infected animals when introduced to a new herd or during transportation for trade or migration. An infection that spreads in a mild form can later lead to a severe, virulent form when it spreads to a naïve population with high susceptibility (Couacy-Hymann et al. 2007). Recovered animals show lifelong immunity with no carrier state (Hamdy et al. 1976). In India, the first ever case of PPR was recorded in Tamil Nadu and it later became an epidemic in the northern region of country (Singh et al. 2004). The acute form of disease is seen in goats, whereas in sheep the subacute form is commonly seen.

The incubation period of PPR is typically 4–6 days, although it may range between 3 and 10 days. Systems involved in PPR are alimentary, respiratory, and lymph nodes. Initially a fever of 104 °F (40 °C) on the fourth day of incubation with serous ocular and nasal discharge is seen. In later stages, there is mucopurulent discharge and matting of eyelid and nostrils. Necrotic erosions of oral mucosa, lips, and the buccal cavity form diphtheritic plaques along with halitosis and swelling of the lips and muzzle. Erosions are also seen in the vulva and prepuce. The alimentary form is seen after the fourth day of incubation with diarrhea containing mucus or blood tinged. Lymphoid involvement (necrosis) is not as marked as in rinderpest (cattle plague). Respiratory signs are developed/hastened by concurrent infection with a secondary bacterial infection such as *Pasturella* sp. or collibacillosis, which causes labored breathing with a productive cough (Parida et al. 2016). Death is generally due to dehydration and diarrhea (Radiostitis; 10th edition). The case fatality rate is high and morbidity may reach 100% in the acute form (Parida et al. 2016).

A seroprevalence study of PPR in small ruminants in the northern region of India showed 44.05% overall, with 57.32%, 55.2%, 65.69%, 37.09%, 32.73%, and 29.35% antibodies of PPR virus in goats and sheep in Haryana, Punjab, Uttar Pradesh, Himachal Pradesh, Jammu & Kashmir, and Uttarakhand states, respectively (Balamurugan et al. 2020). In order to control the disease, a highly sensitive and specific diagnostic test along with a potent vaccine for the mass population are important prerequisites. In India, three live attenuated vaccines are available: Sungri 96, Arasur 87, and Coimbatore 97. Sungri 96 (developed by IVRI, Mukhteshwar, Uttarakhand, India) and Coimbatore 97 (TANUVAS, Chennai, India) is a goat isolate vaccine, whereas Arasur 87 (TANUVAS) is a sheep-origin vaccine. These vaccines are used for mass populations of both sheep and goats to contemplate a PPR control program

(a)　　　　　　　　　(b)　　　　　　　　(c)

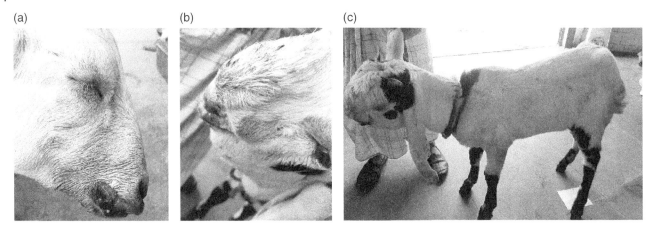

Figure 10.1　(a) Mouth lesions, (b) and nasal discharge, and (c) dullness and depression of peste des petits ruminants in the goat.

(Saravanan et al. 2010). These vaccines contain 10^3 tissue culture infective dose 50 (TCID50) of cell-cultured attenuated PPR virus. They are administered via the subcutaneous route and provide protection for >4 years (Singh et al. 2009). Kids/lambs born from a vaccinated dam must not be vaccinated in the first three months of life as maternal antibodies interfere with the functioning of the vaccine (Ata et al. 1989).

10.2　Goat Pox

Goat pox is a highly contagious systemic viral disease and is considered the most severe pox disease among domestic animals (Sharma et al. 2021) (Figure 10.2). It is characterized by skin eruptions, generalized papules/nodules, and rarely vesicles on non-wool areas of the body, systemic signs like fever, and involvement of respiratory and alimentary systems, causing death (OIE 2013). The etiological agent responsible for pox disease is the epitheliotropic DNA pox virus of genus *Capripoxvirus* (CaPV; family Poxviridae). The sheep pox virus (SPV) and goat pox virus (GPV) show similarity antigenically and physiochemically

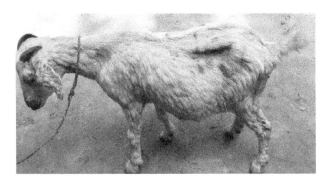

Figure 10.2　Pox lesions in the goat.

(OIE 2013). These viruses are host specific: SPV and GPV infect sheep and goats, respectively (Tulman et al. 2002), but host specificity varies from isolate to isolate in restricted geographic locations due to gene adaptation in SPV and GPV (Kitching et al. 1987).

Sheep pox and goat pox are enzootic in some parts of Africa and Asia, including the Indian subcontinent (Venkatesan et al. 2010). In India, outbreaks of sheep pox in goats were evident during 2008 (Bhanuprakash et al. 2010). A recent outbreak occurred in 2016 in Assam, which was confirmed by identification and phylogenetic analysis of GPV (Bora et al. 2021). In Mizoram, infection with GPV has been reported in the wild ruminant the red serow (*Capricornis rubidus*) (Dutta et al. 2019).

CaPV is highly stable in ambient environmental conditions and can survive for prolonged periods of time (Davies 1981). Morbidity may reach 100% and the mortality rate ranges from 50% in adults to 100% in young animals (Bhanuprakash et al. 2010). SPV and GPTV affect animal of all ages, breeds, and sexes. In sheep pox, exotic (Merino) and some European breeds show higher susceptibility than indigenous breeds.

Sheep pox and goat pox have no zoonoses (Ebissa and Waktole 2020). The mode of transmission is mainly through the aerosol route via contact with an infected animal or fomites (Webbs et al. 1980). The virus can live in oronasal secretions for weeks and for months in scabs that have fallen off the infected animal (Tsegaye et al. 2013). Experimentally, *Stomoxys* flies have been used for transmission of GPV and SPV (Kitching and Mellor 1986). The incubation period of sheep pox is 4–9 days and that of goat pox is 4–15 days. Since the virus is epitheliotropic, it gets localized in local tissue after entry and on the seventh day the virus titer reaches its peak. The virus spreads to regional lymph nodes 3–4 days post primary viremia, affecting lung, spleen, and liver. Skin lesions are evident after 7–15 days of virus inoculation with the development of serum antibodies and a decrease in virus titer. With the development of skin lesions, the occurrence of conjunctivitis, rhinitis, and superficial enlargement of lymph nodes, in particular suprascapular lymph nodes, are seen within 24 hours. There are five stages of lesions formed in skin: macule, papule (0.5–1.5 cm in diameter, usually devoid of fluid), vesicle, pustule, and finally scab formation (Bowden et al. 2008).

SPV and GPV share similar clinical signs (Kitching and Taylor 1985). Pox lesions can be either benign or malignant, and an affected lamb may die without any observable pox lesions. The malignant form is commonly seen in lambs, characterized by high fever (104–106 °F, 40–41 °C), dyspnea, mucopurulent nasal discharge, ocular discharge, conjunctivitis, blepharitis, and pox lesions on unwooled skin. In the benign form, adult sheep and goats are affected with pox lesions found particularly under the tail, and on the perineum, vulva, and nostrils. A nodular form, called "stone pox," has been recorded, present all over the thickness of the skin, which eventually becomes necrotic. Soon after necrosis, the nodules break off and shed from the underlying skin, leaving ulcerative lesions and scabs that heal within 3–4 weeks. Secondary complications like abortion and acute respiratory distress due to pneumonia are common in adults (Hamdi et al. 2021).

CaPV is a large, enveloped, and double-stranded DNA virus. The comparison of the full genome sequence of their isolates showed 96% similarity between GPV, SPPV, and lumpy skin disease (LSD) virus (Tulman et al. 2002). Therefore, diagnostic assays for differentiation between the field and vaccine strains are required for epidemiological investigation (Tuppurainen et al. 2014).

Species-specific molecular assays using G-protein coupled chemokine receptor (GPCR) or 30 kDa RNA polymerase subunit (RPO30) genes have been utilized (Le Goff et al. 2009; Lamien et al. 2011). GPCR sequencing provides an aid for differentiation between field and vaccine strains (Le Goff et al. 2009). Detection of SPV through reverse transcription polymerase chain reaction (RT-PCR) has been described by Haegeman et al. (2016) and Chibssa et al. (2018). For CaPV group diagnosis, serological tests include enzyme-linked immunosorbent assay (ELISA), fluorescent antibody test (FAT), indirect fluorescent antibody, serum/virus neutralization, and agar gel immuno diffusion test (Babiuk et al. 2009). In 2017, the first ever ELISA kit for detection of antibodies against CaPV was developed (ID Screen® Capripox Double Antigen Multi-species, IDvet, Guichanville, France), enabling sero-surveillance in the field (Tuppurainen et al. 2021).

Control and eradication of SPV and GPV require slaughter of infected animals, a quarantine system, monitoring of movements among flocks, and a vaccination schedule (Hamdi et al. 2021). Vaccination is considered the best method for controlling the spread of infection among flocks (Tuppurainen et al. 2021). Several strains are used for manufacturing vaccines, named on the basis of the place of isolation. A list of available vaccines is given in Table 10.1.

Live attenuated vaccines are mostly used against CaPV infection. In East Africa KSGP O 240 and KSGP O 180 are commonly used, whereas in Africa and the Middle East, the

Table 10.1 Commonly used vaccines against sheep pox virus (SPV), goat pox virus (GPV), and lumpy skin disease (LPD) virus.

Isolate	Origin	Cells	References
SPV RM65	Sheep	Sheep kidney cells	Ramyar and Hessami (1967)
SPV Romania	Sheep	Lamb kidney cells	Précausta et al. (1979)
SPV Bakirkoy	Sheep	Calf kidney cells	Martin et al. (1973)
SPV Rumania Fanar	Sheep	Lamb testis	Penkova et al. (1974)
SPV Perego	Sheep	Lamb and calf kidney	Mateva and Stojchev (1975)
SPV Ranipet	Sheep	Sheep thyroid cells	Anandan et al. (1972)
GPV Gorgan	Goat	Kid kidney cortex cells	Abbas et al. (2010)
GPV Uttarkashi	Goat	Primary lamb testis cells and Vero cells	Hosamani et al. (2004)
GPV Mysore	Goat	Primary lamb testis cells	Dubey and Sawhney (1978)
GPV Kedong	Sheep	Lamb testis cells	Capstick et al. (1959)
GPV Isiolo	Sheep	Lamb testis cells	Capstick et al. (1959)
LSD Neethling	Cattle	Lamb kidney cells and chorio-allantoic membrane	Van Rooyen et al. (1969)

Romania strain is used to protect sheep (Yogisharadhya et al. 2011). The protections conferred by CaPV vaccine vary among sheep, goats, and cattle. GPV Uttarkashi (Hosamani et al. 2004) and Mysore (Dubey and Sawhney 1978) are considered safe and protective for goats only, whereas GPV Gorgan is considered safe and partially protective for sheep and cattle (Hedayati et al. 2008). Similarly, SPV RM65 is protective for sheep (Ben-Gera et al. 2015) and SPV Romania provides partial protection to goats and cattle (Hamdi et al. 2020). After vaccination, the titer reaches its highest peak 15–21 days post vaccination (Tuppurainen et al. 2021). According to the recommendations of the OIE (2013), the titer of virus in the CaPV vaccine should range from $10^{2.5}$ to $10^{3.5}$ TCID50. The duration of immunity ranges between 12 months and 2 years and annual vaccination is recommended (Kitching 2003). The commercially available ELISA kit (ID Screen Capripox Double Antigen Multi-species) validates that it can detect antibody titer up to 7 months after vaccination. It was believed that calves, lambs, and kids born from immunized or naturally infected mothers have antibodies for 3–6 months (Weiss 1968). However, more recently published data has shown that calves were not protected by maternal antibodies after 3 months of age (Agianniotaki et al. 2018).

10.3 Foot and Mouth Disease

Foot and mouth disease (FMD) is a highly contagious transboundary disease that affects domesticated animals in Africa, parts of South America, the Middle East, and Asia (Figure 10.3). The causative agent, foot and mouth disease virus (FMDV), is a small, non-enveloped picornavirus (genus *Aphthovirus*) that has seven serotypes (Alexandersen et al. 2002). FMDV exists as seven distinct serotypes: O, A, C, Asia 1, Southern African territory 1 (SAT1), SAT2, and SAT3. In India, incidence of FMD is reported throughout the country with the prevalence of FMDV serotypes O, A, and Asia 1 (Thomson 2002).

There is a paucity of information on the role of goats in FMD epidemiology and transmission. The route by which most ruminants are likely to encounter FMDV in field conditions is via the respiratory tract. Experimental infection of sheep reported that FMDV could be readily detected at two time points after aerosol exposure to the virus – first, between 30 minutes and 22 hours, attributable to virus trapped in the wool during initial exposure to the virus; and secondly between 2 and 7 days, attributable to limited replication in the respiratory tract. Control of movement for two weeks after infection was therefore recommended as a means of preventing disease spread (Sellers et al. 1977). FMD-infected sheep and goats transmitted the subclinical infection to cattle, buffalo, sheep, and goats.

Lameness and agalactia (Nazliglu 1972) are the most common signs in goats infected with FMDV, and outbreaks have been recorded in which pyrexia, nasal discharge, and salivation are seen (Pay 1988; Shukla et al. 1974). Mouth lesions are more likely to occur in goats (Olah et al. 1976). Mortality is often seen in lambs and kids in the absence of any clinical signs and is generally the result of myocarditis or myocardial lesions (Geering 1967; Pay 1988). Goats experimentally infected by the intra-dermo-lingual route did not exhibit clinical signs of FMD and goats inoculated by the coronary band route showed clinical signs of FMD such as inappetence, panting, pyrexia ($\geq 40\,°C$), lameness, and vesicles on the foot and in the mouth at 2–5 days post

(a)   (b)

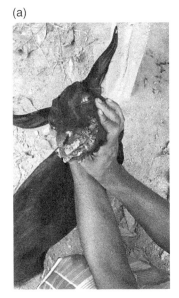 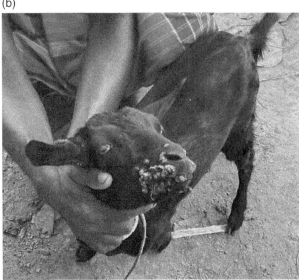

Figure 10.3 (a, b) Mouth lesions of foot and mouth disease in the goat.

inoculation. Goats inoculated by both intra-dermo-lingual and coronary band routes also showed FMD clinical signs at 3 days post inoculation (Muthukrishnan et al. 2020). The unchallenged control sheep and goats did not show any FMD clinical signs.

In sheep and goats FMD is usually mild, with minor clinical signs, if any, and superficial lesions. After contact with FMDV, cattle, sheep, and goats may become persistently infected. An FMDV carrier is defined as an animal from which virus can be recovered for more than 28 days post infection. The duration of persistent FMDV infections in cattle can be up to 3.5 years; in sheep, 9 months; and in goats, 4 months. Tissues from the pharyngeal areas have been shown to be important during both acute and persistent FMDV infections (Donaldson et al. 2019).

Efforts directed at the eradication and prevention of FMD centering on stamping-out policies are controversial, and the prevention and control of the disease using vaccines have become areas of extreme interest. Traditionally, FMD vaccines have been developed and evaluated mainly based on cattle. The World Organisation for Animal Health (OIE) has standardized experimental methods using vaccinated bovine serum for vaccine-matching tests, but experimental methods for goats and pigs have not been standardized. Inactivated FMD vaccines are commonly produced as gel or oil adjuvants, depending on the serotype. Gel vaccines are used only in cattle or small ruminants and are not suitable for pigs due to their short duration of immunity (Park 2013). Dairy goats were inoculated with ED +AL-adjuvanted vaccine (Emulsigen-D and aluminum hydroxide gel) and challenged 28 days after vaccination. The viral neutralization test (VNT) showed that high titers of antibodies were detected in three vaccinated goats starting 7 days after vaccination, and the titers continuously increased until days 21–28. The dairy goats were

challenged with the FMDV on day 28 after vaccination, after which viremia and virus secretion were observed until day 8 post challenge. High levels of viremia were observed until 7 days after challenge in the unvaccinated group. However, the virus was not detected in the serum samples from the vaccinated group, indicating protection against FMD (Park et al. 2014).

10.4 Caprine Arthritis and Encephalitis

Caprine arthritis encephalitis (CAE) and maedi–visna virus (MVV) disease is a worldwide infectious disease of goats caused by small ruminant lentiviruses (SRLV) (Figure 10.4). Early phylogenetic studies suggested that SRLV can be divided into five genetic groups, A–E. Genotypes C and D as well subtypes A5–A7 circulate only in goats; subtype A2 circulates only in sheep; while subtypes A1, A3, A4, A6, B1, and B2 have been found in both species (Giacobini and Bertolotti 2021). In goats, SRLV have a long incubation time and symptoms may be evident in only 10% of goats from a SRLV-infected herd (Olech et al. 2012). CAE is a chronic devastating disease of goats caused by a lentivirus that is characterized by significant economic loss (Gregory et al. 2009). It may lead to a negative impact on milk production and increases the risk of mastitis development (Leitner et al. 2010).

Caprine arthritis encephalitis virus (CAEV) infection is manifested as polyarthritis in adult goats and encephalitis in kids. However, other clinical signs of the disease include swelling of the joint capsule, which subsequently leads to lameness. Signs of mastitis, synovitis, reduced growth rate, and pneumonia have also been reported in cases of MVV infection. The classic sign of CAE is central nervous system (CNS) dysfunction, including ataxia, paresis, and progressive

(a)

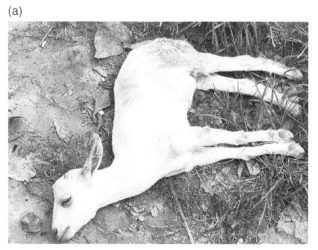

(b)

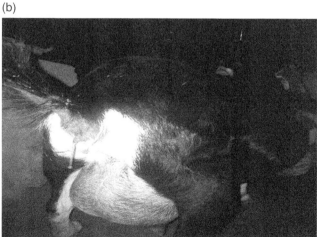

Figure 10.4 (a, b) Arthritis, wasting, and starting abortion of goats suffering from caprine encephalitis.

paralysis. CAEV transcripts, in the absence of inflammatory lesions, have been reported in the renal tubular epithelium of goats naturally infected with CAEV (in situ hybridization). In sheep and goats, inflammatory renal lesions associated with the deposition of MVV antigen and amplifiable proviral SRLV DNA have been reported in animals naturally infected with SRLV. Multiple pale, wedge-shaped regions within the renal cortex and medulla of both kidneys were interpreted as infarcts (Murphy et al. 2021). On histological examination, all of these animals had multifocal areas of necrosis and malacia in both the brain and spinal cord, accompanied by marked infiltration of macrophages and lymphocytes (Zink et al. 1990). The virus is transmitted both vertically by ingestion of milk and horizontally by direct contact with infected animals (Faez et al. 2017). CAEV can also be transmitted to sheep in farms where goats and sheep are raised together; hence indicating interspecies transmission.

SRLV can be divided into six sequence clades (I–VI) as defined by early phylogenetic studies. The Icelandic visna virus and other closely related members of MVV virus strains belong to clade I, while the North American lentivirus isolated from sheep belongs to clade II. Clades III and IV contain the French and Norwegian SRLV, while clade V contains both Swiss and French CAEV strains. Finally, the French SRLV belongs to clade VI (Ghanem et al. 2009).

Diagnosis of CAE involves a combination of clinical manifestation, postmortem examination, and histopathological findings. However, serology is considered one of the easiest and most efficient ways to diagnose infections caused by CAEV. In practice, the most common serological tests adopted for the diagnosis of CAEV infection is ELISA and agar gel immunodiffusion (AGID) (Waseem et al. 2015). However, ELISA is the preferred test due to the low sensitivity associated with AGID.

SRLV do not infect T cells and the infected animals remain immunocompetent throughout the infection. Monocytes are the principal cellular targets of SRLV, and virus replication in these cells is restricted until their maturation to macrophages in tissues. In spite of their resistance to SRLV infection, CD4+ T cells have been shown to be crucial in MVV infection. The effect of inducing a CAEV-specific T-helper-cell response on virus replication in vivo was tested in immunized goats with a CAEV synthetic peptide capable of priming a strong CD4+ T-cell response and subsequently challenged with CAEV. The peptide used was a part of the Gag structural protein of CAEV, which shows a strong structural and sequence homology with the homologous peptide of HIV and other retroviruses. The synthetic peptide is known to encompass an immunodominant helper T-cell epitope of CAEV. The measurement of interferon-γ and interleukin-4 gene expression showed that these cytokines were reliable markers of an ongoing immune response. In contrast, granulocyte–macrophage colony-stimulating factor appeared to be a key cytokine that might support virus replication in the early phase of infection. The observation of a potential T-cell-mediated enhancement of virus replication supports other recent findings showing that lentivirus-specific T cells can be detrimental to the host, suggesting caution in designing vaccine candidates (Nenci et al. 2007).

10.5 Rabies

Rabies is an acute, progressive, and fatal viral encephalitis caused by neurotropic RNA virus of the family Rhabdoviridae, genus *Lyssa* virus, affecting all mammals (Rupprecht et al. 2002). In goats, rabies has been considered an infrequent disease and one of the most difficult to diagnose clinically because of diversity in presentation. Some of the non-specific signs are fever, dehydration, discrete proprioceptive ataxia, somnolence, apathy, opisthotonus, and medullary signs (recumbence and paddling movement). In goats, the furious form appears more commonly and aggressive behavior may occur in the majority, with excessive salivation, bleating, and paralysis in a few cases. The clinical course is usually between 1 and 5 days and always results in death (Mayhew 2009).

Cerebrospinal fluid is always an integral component of the evaluation of ruminants presenting nervous signs of rabies (Stokol et al. 2009). Mononuclear pleocytosis is typically associated with rabies viral infection, particularly of lymphocytes. Non-suppurative meningoencephalitis is the main microscopic CNS lesion observed in all species, with variations in anatomic distribution. Also, the brainstem shows perivascular lymphocytic cuffing in white matter, and Babes' nodules and necrotic neurons at the rostral colliculus. In Gasser's ganglia, neuronophagia and mild mononuclear ganglioneuritis are observed (Allen et al. 2013).

Even in the absence of Negri bodies, the direct fluorescent antibody test (dFAT) and mouse inoculation test (MIT) are considered gold standard for diagnosis. Additionally, Negri bodies' presence and number appear to be inversely proportional to the degree of inflammation (Cantile and Youssef 2016). Ruminants are considered highly susceptible to rabies infection and may show minor CNS inflammatory changes and a few or absent Negri bodies, especially in euthanized animals (Mayhew 2009). Clinical reports of rabies in goats are rare, and sometimes they are accompanied by atypical clinical-pathological presentations. The definitive diagnosis of paralytic rabies is obtained through the association of epidemiological, clinical, laboratory, and pathological findings (histology and immunohistochemistry) and gold-standard confirmatory tests (dFAT and MIT) (Moreira et al. 2018).

Multiple-Choice Questions

1 A natural form of PPR infection is present in which animals?
   A Wild sheep
   B Wild deer
   C Sahelian goat
   D a and b

2 PPR involves which system(s)?
   A Cardiac system
   B Alimentary system
   C Respiratory system
   D b and c

3 PPR-affected goats display which common clinical sign(s)?
   A Mucopurulent discharge
   B Matting of eyelids and nostrils
   C Necrotic lesions on oral mucosa and lips forming diphtheritic plaques
   D All of the above

4 Which live attenuated vaccine is available in India for PPR?
   A Sungri 96
   B Raksha-triovac
   C Raksha-ovac
   D None of the above

5 What is the morbidity and mortality rate of pox virus infection in young goats?
   A 20%
   B 50%
   C 100%
   D <5%

6 The malignant form of goat pox virus infection is seen in which animals?
   A Lambs
   B Adult ewes
   C Adult rams
   D All of the above

7 What test is available for the detection of antibodies against CaPV?
   A ELISA
   B RT-PCR
   C Virus neutralization tests
   D All of the above

8 Which goat pox virus vaccination is considered safe for goats only?
   A GPV Utterkashi
   B GPV Mysore
   C Both a and b
   D GPV Gorgan

9 What are the most common signs of FMD in goats?
   A Lameness, S. agalactiae
   B Pyrexia, nasal discharge, and salivation
   C Both a and b
   D Myocarditis

10 How long do persistent FMDV infections in goats last?
   A 3.5 years
   B 9 months
   C 4 months
   D 30 days

11 Dairy goats are challenged 28 days after which vaccination?
   A Emulsigen-D and aluminum hydroxide gel
   B Inactivated FMD vaccine
   C Raksha-triovac
   D None of the above

12 What are the manifestations of CAEV infection in adult goats and kids, respectively?
   A Encephalitis and polyarthritis
   B Polyarthritis and encephalitis
   C Polyarthritis and diarrhea
   D Encephalitis and dysentery

13 Multiple regions of which kind within the renal cortex and medulla of both kidneys are interpreted as infarcts in CAE infection?
   A Whitish, oval-shaped regions
   B Pale, oval-shaped regions
   C Pale, wedge-shaped regions
   D Whitish, wedge-shaped regions

14 In CAE, interspecies transmission occurs between which animals?
   A Cattle and goats
   B Goats and pigs
   C Sheep and cattle
   D Sheep and goats

References

Abbas, F., Khan, F.A., Hussain, A. et al. (2010). Production of goat pox virus vaccine from a live attenuated goat pox virus strain. *Journal of Animal and Plant Sciences* 20: 315–317.

Abubakar, M., Manzoor, S., and Ali, Q. (2015). Evaluating the role of vaccine to combat peste des petits ruminants outbreaks in endemic disease situation. *Journal of Animal Science and Technology* 57 (1): 1–5.

Agianniotaki, E.I., Babiuk, S., Katsoulos, P.D. et al. (2018). Colostrum transfer of neutralizing antibodies against lumpy skin disease virus from vaccinated cows to their calves. *Transboundary and Emerging Diseases* 65 (6): 2043–2048.

Alexandersen, S., Zhang, Z., and Donaldson, A.I. (2002). Aspects of the persistence of foot-and-mouth disease virus in animals—the carrier problem. *Emerging Microbes & Infections* 4: 1099–1110.

Allen, A.L., Goupil, B.A., and Valentine, B.A. (2013). A retrospective study of brain lesions in goats submitted to three veterinary diagnostic laboratories. *Journal of Veterinary Diagnostic Investigation* 25 (4): 482–489.

Anandan, R., Sundara Rajan, S., Kannamani, G., and Jayaraman, M.S. (1972). Studies on live and inactivated sheep pox vaccines. *Cheiron* 1: 42–55.

Ata, F.A., al Sumry, H.S., King, G.J. et al. (1989). Duration of maternal immunity to peste des petits ruminants. *Veterinary Record* 124: 590–591.

Babiuk, S., Wallace, D.B., Smith, S.J. et al. (2009). Detection of antibodies against capripoxviruses using an inactivated sheeppox virus ELISA. *Transboundary and Emerging Diseases* 56 (4): 132–141.

Balamurugan, V., Varghese, B., Kumar, K.V. et al. (2020). Seroprevalence study of peste des petits ruminants in sheep and goats in the northern region of India. *Veterinary World Journal* 13 (8): 1573.

Ben-Gera, J., Klement, E., Khinich, E. et al. (2015). Comparison of the efficacy of Neethling lumpy skin disease virus and x10RM65 sheep-pox live attenuated vaccines for the prevention of lumpy skin disease–the results of a randomized controlled field study. *Vaccine* 33 (38): 4837–4842.

Bhanuprakash, V., Venkatesan, G., Balamurugan, V. et al. (2010). Pox outbreaks in sheep and goats at Makhdoom (Uttar Pradesh), India: evidence of sheeppox virus infection in goats. *Transboundary and Emerging Diseases* 57 (5): 375–382.

Bora, D.P., Venkatesan, G., Arya, S. et al. (2021). Molecular evidence and sequence analysis of goatpox virus isolates from Assam, India: an emerging viral disease of goats. *Proceedings of the National Academy of Sciences, India Section B: Biological Sciences* 91 (3): 607–614.

Bowden, T.R., Babiuk, S.L., Parkyn, G.R. et al. (2008). Capripoxvirus tissue tropism and shedding: a quantitative study in experimentally infected sheep and goats. *Virology Journal* 371 (2): 380–393.

Cantile, C. and Youssef, S. (2016). Nervous system. In: *Jubb, Kennedy, and Palmer's Pathology of Domestic Animals*, 6e (ed. M.G. Maxie), 251–406. St. Louis, MO: Saunders Elsevier.

Capstick, P.B., Prydie, J., Coackley, W., and Burdin, M.L. (1959). Protection of cattle against "Neethling" type virus of lumpy skin disease. *Veterinary Record* 71: 422.

Chibssa, T.R., Grabherr, R., Loitsch, A. et al. (2018). A gel-based PCR method to differentiate sheeppox virus field isolates from vaccine strains. *Virology Journal* 15 (1): 1–7.

Couacy-Hymann, E., Bodjo, C., Danho, T. et al. (2007). Evaluation of the virulence of some strains of peste-des-petits-ruminants virus (PPRV) in experimentally infected West African dwarf goats. *Veterinary Journal* 173 (1): 178–183.

Davies, F.G. (1981). Sheep and goat pox. In: *Virus Diseases of Food Animals*, 2e (ed. E.P.J. Gibbs), 733–749. London: Academic Press.

Donaldson, A. (2019). Clinical signs of foot-and-mouth disease. In: *Foot and Mouth Disease* (ed. F. Sobrino and E. Domingo), 93–102. Boca Raton, FL: CRC Press.

Dubey, S.C. and Sawhney, A.V. (1978). Live and inactivated tissue culture vaccine against goat pox [India]. Short communication. *Indian Veterinary Journal* 55 (11): 926–927.

Dutta, T.K., Roychoudhury, P., Kawlni, L. et al. (2019). An outbreak of goatpox virus infection in wild red serow (*Capricornis rubidus*) in Mizoram, India. *Transboundary and Emerging Diseases* 66 (1): 181–185.

Ebissa, T. and Waktole, H. (2020). Current status of sheep and goat pox diseases in Ethiopia. *Researcher* 12 (1): 19–35. https://doi.org/10.7537/marsrsj120120.04.

Faez, F.A.J., Innocent, D.P., Yusuf, A. et al. (2017). A suspected clinical case of Caprine arthritis encephalitis (CAE) in a sheep. *Journal of Veterinary Science and Animal Husbandry* 2: 15–17.

Geering, W.A. (1967). Foot and mouth disease in sheep. *Australian Veterinary Journal* 43: 485–489.

Ghanem, Y.M., El-Khodery, S.A., Saad, A.A. et al. (2009). Prevalence and risk factors of caprine arthritis encephalitis virus infection (CAEV) in Northern Somalia. *Small Ruminant Research* 85 (2–3): 142–148.

Giacobini, M. and Bertolotti, L. (2021). Caprine arthritis encephalitis virus disease modelling review. *Animals* 11 (5): 1457.

Govindarajan, R., Koteeswaran, A., Venugopalan, A.T. et al. (1997). Isolation of pestes des petits ruminants virus from an outbreak in Indian buffalo (Bubalus bubalis). *Veterinary Record Open* 141 (22): 573–574.

Gregory, L., Birgel Junior, E.H., Lara, M.C.C.S.H. et al. (2009). Clinical features of indurative mastitis caused by caprine arthritis encephalitis virus. *Brazilian Journal of Veterinary Pathology* 2 (2): 64–68.

Haegeman, A., Zro, K., Sammin, D. et al. (2016). Investigation of a possible link between vaccination and the 2010 sheep pox epizootic in Morocco. *Transboundary and Emerging Diseases* 63 (6): e278–e287.

Hamdi, J., Bamouh, Z., Jazouli, M. et al. (2020). Experimental evaluation of the cross-protection between Sheeppox and bovine Lumpy skin vaccines. *Scientific Reports* 10 (1): 1–9.

Hamdi, J., Bamouh, Z., Jazouli, M. et al. (2021). Experimental infection of indigenous North African goats with goatpox virus. *Acta Veterinaria Scandinavica* 63 (1): 1–9.

Hamdy, F.M., Dardiri, A.H., Nduaka, O. et al. (1976). Etiology of the stomatitis pneumoenteritis complex in Nigerian dwarf goats. *Canadian Journal of Comparative Medicine* 40 (3): 276.

Hedayati, Z., Varshuei, H.R., Aqa Ebrahimiyan, M. et al. (2008). Study of safety and immunogenicity of goat pox vaccine against sheep pox in susceptible sheep. Karaj, Iran: Razi Vaccine and Serum Research Institute.

Hosamani, M., Nandi, S., Mondal, B. et al. (2004). A Vero cell-attenuated Goatpox virus provides protection against virulent virus challenge. *Acta Virologica* 48 (1): 15–21.

Khalafalla, A.I., Saeed, I.K., Ali, Y.H. et al. (2010). An outbreak of peste des petits ruminants (PPR) in camels in the Sudan. *Acta Tropica* 116 (2): 161–165.

Kitching, R.P. (2003). Vaccines for lumpy skin disease, sheep pox and goat pox. *Developmental Biology* 114: 161–167.

Kitching, R.P. and Mellor, P.S. (1986). Insect transmission of capripoxvirus. *Research in Veterinary Science* 40 (2): 255–258.

Kitching, R.P. and Taylor, W.P. (1985). Clinical and antigenic relationship between isolates of sheep and goat pox viruses. *Tropical Animal Health and Production* 17: 64–74.

Kitching, R.P., Hammond, J.M., and Taylor, W.P. (1987). A single vaccine for the control of capripox infection in sheep and goats. *Research in Veterinary Science* 42 (1): 53–60.

Kwiatek, O., Ali, Y.H., Saeed, I.K. et al. (2011). Asian lineage of peste des petits ruminants virus, Africa. *Emerging Infectious Diseases* 17 (7): 1223.

Le Goff, C., Lamien, C.E., Fakhfakh, E. et al. (2009). Capripoxvirus G-protein-coupled chemokine receptor: a host-range gene suitable for virus animal origin discrimination. *Journal of General Virology* 90 (8): 1967–1977.

Leitner, G., Krifucks, O., Weisblit, L. et al. (2010). The effect of caprine arthritis encephalitis virus infection on production in goats. *Veterinary Journal* 183 (3): 328–331.

Martin, W.B., Ergin, H., and Köylü, A. (1973). Tests in sheep of attenuated sheep pox vaccines. *Research in Veterinary Science* 14 (1): 53–62.

Mateva, V. and Stojchev, S. (1975). Adaptation and cultivation of the virus of sheep pox strain Perego in tissue cultures, and evaluation of its immunogenic properties. *Veterinary Science* 12 (10): 18–23.

Mayhew, I.G.J. (2009). Infectious, inflammatory and immune diseases. In: *Large Animal Neurology*, 2e (ed. I.G.J. Mayhew), 225–293. Singapore: Wiley-Blackwell.

Moreira, I.L., de Sousa, D.E.R., Ferreira-Junior, J.A. et al. (2018). Paralytic rabies in a goat. *BMC Veterinary Research* 14 (1): 1–5.

Murphy, B.G., Castillo, D., Mete, A. et al. (2021). Caprine arthritis encephalitis virus is associated with renal lesions. *Viruses* 13 (6): 1051.

Muthukrishnan, M., Singanallur Balasubramanian, N., and Villuppanoor Alwar, S. (2020). Experimental infection of foot and mouth disease in indian sheep and goats. *Frontiers in Veterinary Science* 7: 356.

Nawathe, D.R. and Taylor, W.P. (1979). Experimental infection of domestic pigs with the virus of peste des petits ruminants. *Tropical Animal Health and Production* 11 (1): 120–122.

Nazliglu, M. (1972). Foot and mouth disease in sheep and goats. *Bulletin – Office International des épizooties* 77: 1281–1284.

OIE (2013). Sheep pox and goat pox. Paris: OIE. www.woah. org/fileadmin/Home/eng/Animal_Health_in_the_World/ docs/pdf/Disease_cards/SHEEP_GOAT_POX.pdf.

Olah, M., Pavlovic, R., and Panjevic, D. (1976). Clinical picture and differential diagnosis of foot and mouth disease in sheep and goats. *Veterinarski Glasnik* 30: 239–245.

Olech, M., Rachid, A., Croisé, B. et al. (2012). Genetic and antigenic characterization of small ruminant lentiviruses circulating in Poland. *Virus Research* 163: 528–536.

Parida, S., Muniraju, M., Altan, E. et al. (2016). Emergence of PPR and its threat to Europe. *Small Ruminant Research* 142: 16–21.

Park, J.H. (2013). Requirements for improved vaccines against foot-and-mouth disease epidemics. *Clinical and Experimental Vaccine Research* 2: 8–18.

Park, M.E., Lee, S.Y., Kim, R.H. et al. (2014). Enhanced immune responses of foot-and-mouth disease vaccine using new oil/gel adjuvant mixtures in pigs and goats. *Vaccine* 32 (40): 5221–5227.

Penkova, V.M., Jassim, F.A., Thompson, J.R., and Al-Doori, T.M. (1974). The propagation of an attenuated sheep pox virus and its use as a vaccine. *Bulletin de l'Office International des Epizooties* 81: 329–339.

Précausta, P., Kato, F., and Vellut, G. (1979). A new freeze-dried living virus vaccine against sheep-pox. *Comparative Immunology, Microbiology & Infectious Diseases* 1 (4): 305–319.

Radostits, O.M., Gay, C.C., Hinchcliff, K.W. et al. (2007). A textbook of the diseases of cattle, horses, sheep, pigs and goats. *Veterinary Medicine* 10: 2045–2050.

Ramyar, H. and Hessami, M. (1967). Development of an attenuated live virus vaccine against sheep pox. *Zentralblatt für Veterinärmedizin Reihe.* 14 (6): 516–519.

Roger, F., Guebre Yesus, M., Libeau, G. et al. (2001). Detection of antibodies of rinderpest and peste des petits ruminants viruses (Paramyxoviridae, Morbillivirus) during a new epizootic disease in Ethiopian camels (*Camelus dromedarius*). *Révue de Médecine Vétérinaire* 152 (3): 265–268.

Rupprecht, C.E., Hanlon, C.A., and Hemachudha, T. (2002). Rabies re-examined. *Lancet Infectious Diseases* 2 (6): 327–343.

Saravanan, P., Sen, A., Balamurugan, V. et al. (2010). Comparative efficacy of peste des petits ruminants (PPR) vaccines. *Biologicals* 38 (4): 479–485.

Sellers, R.F., Herniman, K.A.J., and Gumm, I.D. (1977). The airborne dispersal of foot-and-mouth disease virus from vaccinated and recovered pigs, cattle and sheep after exposure to infection. *Research in Veterinary Science* 23: 70–75.

Sen, A., Saravanan, P., Balamurugan, V. et al. (2014). Detection of subclinical peste des petits ruminants virus infection in experimental cattle. *VirusDisease* 25 (3): 408–411.

Sharma, S., Nawab Nashiruddullah, A.T., Roychoudhury, P., and Ahmed, J.A. (2021). Identification and comparative phylogeny of sheep and goat pox isolates from Jammu, India. *Indian Journal of Animal Research* 55 (6): 710–715.

Shukla, R.R., Valdya, T.N., and Joshi, D.D. (1974). Studies on the diseases of domesticated animals and birds in Nepal. VI observations of the epidemiology of an outbreak of foot-and-mouth disease at a government livestock farm, Khumaltar. *Bulletin of Veterinary Research and Animal Husbandry* 3: 10–15.

Singh, R.P., Saravanan, P., Sreenivasa, B.P. et al. (2004). Prevalence and distribution of peste des petits ruminants virus infection in small ruminants in India. *Revue Scientifique et Technique* 23 (3): 807–819.

Singh, R.K., Balamurugan, V., Bhanuprakash, V. et al. (2009). Possible control and eradication of peste des petits ruminants from India: technical aspects. *Veterinaria Italiana* 45 (3): 449–462.

Stokol, T., Divers, T.J., Arrigan, J.W., and McDonough, S.P. (2009). Cerebrospinal fluid findings in cattle with central nervous system disorders: a retrospective study of 102 cases (1990–2008). *Veterinary Clinical Pathology* 38 (1): 103–112.

Thomson, G. (2002). Foot and mouth disease: facing the new dilemmas. *Revue Scientifique et Technique (International Office of Epizootics)* 21 (3): 425–428.

Tsegaye, D., Belay, B., and Haile, A. (2013). Prevalence of major goat diseases and mortality of goat in Daro-Labu District of West Hararghe, Eastern Ethiopia. *Journal of Scientific and Innovative Research* 2 (3): 665–672.

Tulman, E.R., Afonso, C.L., Lu, Z. et al. (2002). The genomes of sheeppox and goatpox viruses. *Journal of Virology* 76 (12): 6054–6061.

Tuppurainen, E.S., Pearson, C.R., Bachanek-Bankowska, K. et al. (2014). Characterization of sheep pox virus vaccine for cattle against lumpy skin disease virus. *Antiviral Research* 109: 1–6.

Tuppurainen, E.S., Lamien, C.E., and Diallo, A. (2021). Capripox (lumpy skin disease, sheep pox, and goat pox). In: *Veterinary Vaccines: Principles and Applications* (ed. S. Metwally, A. El Idrissi, and G. Viljoen), 383–397. Chichester: Wiley.

Van Rooyen, P.J., Munz, E.K., and Weiss, K.E. (1969). The optimal conditions for the multiplication of Neethling-type lumpy skin disease virus in embryonated eggs. *Onderstepoort Journal of Veterinary Research* 36 (2): 165–174.

Webbs, G., Jennings, D.M., Redding, A.J., and Mellor, P.S. (1980). Sheep and goat pox, transmission of capripox viruses by various flies indicated the need for a reassessment of the methods of controlling this disease. Annual report. Pirbright, UK: Institute for Animal Health.

Weiss, K.E. (1968). Lumpy skin disease virus. In: *Cytomegaloviruses. Rinderpest Virus. Lumpy Skin Disease Virus* (ed. J.B. Hanshaw, W. Plowright, and K.E. Weiss), 111–131. Berlin: Springer.

Yogisharadhya, R., Bhanuprakash, V., Hosamani, M. et al. (2011). Comparative efficacy of live replicating sheeppox vaccine strains in Ovines. *Biologicals* 39 (6): 417–423.

Zink, M.C., Yager, J.A., and Myers, J.D. (1990). Pathogenesis of caprine arthritis encephalitis virus. Cellular localization of viral transcripts in tissues of infected goats. *American Journal of Pathology* 136 (4): 843.

11

Transboundary, Emerging, and Exotic Diseases of Goats

Subir Singh

Department of Veterinary Medicine and Public Health, Faculty of Animal Science, Veterinary Science and Fisheries, Agriculture and Forestry University, Rampur, Chitwan, Nepal

Transboundary animal diseases (TADs) are defined as those epidemic diseases that are highly contagious or transmissible and have the potential for very rapid spread, irrespective of national borders, causing serious socio-economic and possibly public health consequences. These diseases, which cause high morbidity and mortality in susceptible animal populations, constitute a constant threat to the livelihood of livestock farmers and may also have a significant detrimental effect on national economies. In simpler words, TADs are greatly contagious epidemic diseases that can spread very rapidly, irrespective of national borders. They cause high rates of death and disease in animals, thereby having serious socioeconomic and sometimes public health consequences, while constituting a steady threat to the livelihoods of livestock farmers. The Food and Agriculture Organization (FAO) of the United Nations defines TADs as "Those diseases with an essential impact on the economy, trade and/or food security of a group of countries, which can be easily spread to other countries, reaching epidemic proportions and that require control and eradication cooperation between different nations" (FAO 1997). TADs represent a serious threat and with rapidly increasing globalization, an associated risk of movement of TADs is emerging.

With an economic impact on international trade, TADs are of two major types: emerging diseases and zoonoses. The World Organisation for Animal Health (WOAH, founded as OIE) defines *emerging diseases* as "Those that are able to expand its epidemiological spectrum, appearing in a not endemic geographic area, affecting new susceptible species; or referring to a completely unknown pathogen which is detected for the first time." *Zoonoses* are "Any diseases or infections which are naturally transmissible from animals to humans" (WOAH 2022). When a zoonotic disease is not well addressed by national or international public or animal health services, it is known as a *neglected zoonosis*. Such a definition should include *emerging infectious diseases* (EIDs), most of which will likely be zoonoses, but of uncertain impact. So, EIDs are defined as infectious diseases that have newly appeared in a population or have existed but are rapidly increasing in incidence or geographic range. Similarly, *exotic diseases* are infectious diseases that normally do not occur in the region, either because they have never been present there or because they were eradicated and then kept out by government control measures.

Many countries use the term exotic or foreign animal disease to designate those diseases that would have a disastrous consequence if they were to enter their territory, either because of the direct losses to the domestic population suffering the disease or the required counter-epizootic measures, loss in trade, or possibly the potential zoonotic spillover. From a United Nations point of view, the preferred term is TADs, as nothing is per se exotic or foreign in the global theater (Lubroth and Balogh 2009).

The most common TADs (FAO/OIE 2004; Otte et al. 2004) in this category are provided in Table 11.1.

FAO's Emergency Prevention System for animal health focuses on 12–14 diseases of a transboundary nature: Foot-and-Mouth Disease (FMD), Rinderpest, Contagious Bovine Pleuropneumonia, Sheep and Goat pox, Peste des Petits Ruminants (PPR), highly pathogenic Avian Influenza, Rift Valley fever (RVF), Newcastle disease, African and Classical Swine Fever, Equine Encephalitides, and under certain circumstances Rabies and Brucellosis. The links between wildlife and livestock are seamless and knowledge on management issues is imperative for the future practitioner in understanding disease ecology. The key aspect to detection and containment of TADs and EIDs is to have all actors within the production and marketing chain linked with veterinary systems.

The impact of animal diseases on health and human welfare is being increasingly considered. Some 60% of

Table 11.1 Major transboundary animal diseases.

Disease	Animal affected	Regions with major incidence
Foot and mouth disease	Cattle, buffalo, sheep, goats, and pigs	Parts of Africa, Middle East, and Asia
Peste des petits ruminants	Sheep and goats	Africa, Middle East, and Asia
Classical swine fever	Pigs	South and Southeast Asia
African swine fever	Pigs	Sub-Saharan Africa, West Africa, parts of Europe and Latin America, Asia
Bluetongue	Sheep, cattle	Australia, USA, Africa, Middle East, Asia, and Europe
Rift Valley fever	Sheep, cattle, and goats	Africa
Contagious bovine pleuropneumonia	Cattle	Eastern, Southern and West Africa, parts of Asia
Lumpy skin disease	Cattle	Africa and Asia
Sheep and goat pox	Sheep and goats	South Asia, China, Middle East, Africa
Bovine spongiform encephalopathy (BSE)	Cattle	UK and other parts of Europe
Venezuelan equine encephalomyelitis	Equines	Central American and South American countries
Newcastle disease	Poultry	Asia and Africa
Highly pathogenic avian influenza	Poultry	Asia, Europe, and Africa
Hendra virus infection	Horses	Australia
Nipah virus infection	Pig	Malaysia and Singapore

emerging diseases that affect humans are zoonoses, most of them (about 75%) originating from wildlife. Many of those diseases are common to productive domestic animals, due to the multiple interrelationships and the ability of many microorganisms to mutate and to colonize new hosts. Therefore, the direct impacts of TADs on agriculture and public health constitute a serious limitation to exporting living animals and their products, as well as to international trade. Moreover, they seriously compromise food security and cause a high socioeconomic impact on agricultural exporting nations (Cartín-Rojas 2012).

The potential consequences of TADs are of such magnitude that their occurrence may also have a significant detrimental effect on national economies. TADs have the potential to (Islam 2016):

- Threaten food security through serious loss of animal protein and/or loss of draught animal power for cropping.
- Increase poverty levels, particularly in poor communities that have a high incidence of dependence on livestock farming for sustenance.
- Cause major production losses for livestock products such as meat, milk and other dairy products, wool and other fibers, and skins and hides, thereby reducing farm incomes. They may also restrict opportunities for upgrading the production potential of local livestock industries by making it difficult to utilize exotic high-producing breeds that tend to be very susceptible to the TAD.
- Add significantly to the cost of livestock production through the necessity to apply costly disease control measures.
- Seriously disrupt or inhibit trade in livestock and livestock products either within a country or internationally. Their occurrence may thereby cause major losses in national export income in significant livestock-producing countries.
- Cause public health consequences in the case of those TADs that can be transmitted to humans (i.e. zoonoses).
- Cause environmental consequences through die-offs in wildlife populations in some cases.
- Cause pain and suffering for affected animals.

Similarly, WOAH maintains a list of more than 130 diseases that qualify as "transboundary" and are therefore worthy of regulatory control. Of these 130, about 25 are of concern for goats (Corrie Brown 2011). Of that number, there are four that have the greatest capacity for entering a new region and creating economic havoc. These four – PPR, FMD, goat pox, and RVF – are the ones discussed in this chapter.

Each of these diseases will be reviewed, with a brief summary of the pertinent features of the disease and the current methods used to control it.

11.1 Peste des Petits Ruminants

PPR is a highly contagious TAD affecting mainly goats and sheep, as well as dromedaries, and has severe negative socioeconomic impacts on the income of livestock farmers and, in particular, the livelihoods and food security of the most vulnerable rural communities, notably of women (WOAH 2022). PPR is an acute or subacute viral disease caused by a morbillivirus closely related to the rinderpest virus (RPV), which affects goats, sheep, and some wild relatives of domesticated small ruminants, as well as camels, and is characterized by fever, necrotic stomatitis, gastroenteritis, severe pneumonia, and sometimes death (Saliki 2022). It was first reported in Ivory Coast in 1942. The disease shows severe morbidity and mortality rates, and has a high economic impact in areas of Africa, the Middle East, and Asia, where small ruminants contribute to guaranteeing livelihoods. Globally, over one billion small ruminants are exposed to the risk of PPR. The socioeconomic consequences of the disease are often dramatic. PPR has a direct impact on the food security and livelihoods of the poorest populations and hinders rural development in the countries affected.

PPR is listed as a notifiable disease by WOAH, all of whose member countries are obliged to report cases and outbreaks to it, according to the Terrestrial Animal Health Code (WOAH 2022e). WOAH and FAO, in their joint strategy for control and eradication of PPR, have set the goal of eradicating the disease by 2030.

11.1.1 Etiology and Epidemiology

The causative agent, PPR virus (PPRV), is an enveloped RNA virus belonging to the genus *Morbillivirus* of the family Paramyxoviridae (subfamily Paramyxovirinae) under the order Mononegavirales (Gibbs et al. 1979) with other members of the genus, which include RPV, measles virus (MV), canine distemper virus (CDV), phocine distemper virus (PDV), and dolphin and porpoise morbillivirus (DMV) (Barrett et al. 1993). The virus is a pleomorphic

particle with a lipoprotein membrane enveloping a ribonucleoprotein core, which contains the RNA genome. The genome is a negative-sense single-stranded RNA, approximately 16 kilo bases (kb) long, with negative polarity (Chard et al. 2008). The causal virus preferentially replicates in lymphoid tissues and epithelial tissue of the gastrointestinal (GI) and respiratory tracts, where it produces characteristic lesions.

PPR has been reported in virtually all parts of the African continent, except for the southern tip; the Middle East; and the entire Indian subcontinent. In the last 15 years, PPR has rapidly expanded within Africa and to large parts of Central Asia, South Asia, and East Asia (including China) (Figure 11.1). After its identification 75 years ago in the Ivory Coast, it reached South Asia in 1987 (when it was diagnosed in India) and now has become a panzootic.

Because PPRV and the now-eradicated RPV are crossprotective, it is possible that the recent rapid expansion of PPRV within endemic zones and into new regions may be because of the disappearance of the cross-protection previously afforded by natural rinderpest infection of small ruminants and/or the use hitherto of rinderpest vaccine to prevent small ruminant infection with PPRV in certain endemic areas. Based on this theory, PPRV has the potential to cause severe epidemics, or even pandemics, in more small ruminant populations in an increasingly expanding area of the developing world. The spread of the disease to a number of new countries in Africa and Asia with the

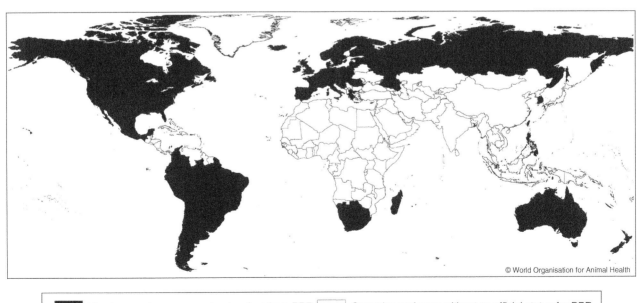

© World Organisation for Animal Health

■ Members and zone recognised as free from PPR ☐ Countries and zone without an official status for PPR

Figure 11.1 World Organisation for Animal Health members' official peste des petits ruminants (PPR) status map. Last update May 2022. *Source:* Peste des petits ruminants, 2022 © World Organisation for Animal Health.

involvement of various lineages of PPRV is a cause of global concern, especially the recent introduction of the Asian lineage to some African countries and the presence of PPR in Europe through western Turkey (Albina et al. 2013). The transboundary nature of this disease is one of the main constraints on augmenting the productivity of small ruminants in enzootic regions, including parts of Africa, the Middle East, and parts of Asia.

At a local level, an epidemic may eliminate the entire goat or sheep population of an affected village. Between epidemics, PPR can assume an endemic profile. Mortality and morbidity rates vary within an infected country, presumably due to two factors: the varying immune status of the affected populations and varying levels of viral virulence.

PPR evolves in two epidemiological forms, one epizootic, the other enzootic:

- **Epizootic form**: When PPR hits previously disease-free areas where animals have had no prior exposure to the virus, the disease is epizootic. Its clinical expression is most often acute, with mortality and morbidity rates that are a function of the susceptibility of the species and breed, but can reach 90–100%.
- **Enzootic form**: In numerous countries in Africa, the Middle East, and Asia, PPR is present in an enzootic form with a low mortality rate (20% or less) and variable but high seroprevalence rates, which can exceed 50%. In these areas, the virus circulates quietly, its clinical expression unapparent, but it remains ready to clinically manifest itself as soon as the population of susceptible small ruminants is sufficiently large, or when animals are in poor health, environmental conditions are favorable, or social, cultural, or economic practices increase the risk of virus transmission. The disease then expresses itself in epizootic outbreaks that appear with a cyclical and/or seasonal frequency.

11.1.2 Transmission

Transmission is by close contact, and confinement seems to favor outbreaks. Secretions and excretions of sick animals are the sources of infection. Transmission can occur during the incubation period. It is generally accepted that there is no carrier state. The common husbandry system whereby goats roam freely in urban areas contributes to the spread and maintenance of the virus. There are also numerous instances of livestock dealers being associated with the spread of infection, especially during religious festivals when the high demand for animals increases the trade in infected stock.

Several species of gazelle, oryx, and white-tailed deer are fully susceptible; these and other wild small ruminants

may play a role in the epidemiology of the disease, but few epidemiological data are available for PPR in wild small ruminants. Cattle, buffalo, and pigs can become naturally or experimentally infected with PPRV, but these species are dead-end hosts, because they do not exhibit any clinical disease and do not transmit the virus to other in-contact animals of any species.

11.1.3 Clinical Findings

Clinically, the disease resembles rinderpest in cattle and is characterized by high fever (pyrexia), conjunctivitis, oculonasal discharges, necrotizing and erosive stomatitis, diarrhea (Taylor 1984), and bronchopneumonia, followed by either death of the animal or recovery from the disease (Gibbs et al. 1979). PPR is also described as a "stomatitis pneumoenteritis complex," which reflects how the virus affects the mucous membranes of an animal's digestive and respiratory systems.

PPR can take four forms depending on the susceptibility of the species, breed, and animal infected. All four forms (acute, peracute, subacute, and subclinical) can be present within the same herd. No clinical signs suggesting PPR are specific to the disease. They can all be confused with other diseases.

11.1.3.1 Acute Form
This is the form observed most frequently.

- After a 5–6-day incubation period, the disease manifests itself with a sudden rise in body temperature to 40–41.3 °C (104–106 °F). The animal is listless, refuses to eat, has a dry muzzle and dull coat, and its hair stands erect. The animal withdraws from the herd and has difficulty moving. The mucous membranes of the mouth and eyes become congested.
- One or two days after the onset of fever, lacrimation and discharge appear. At first the nasal discharge is serous (clear and watery); later, it becomes mucopurulent and gives a putrid odor to the breath. The eyelids gum together and the obstructed nostrils render breathing difficult (Figure 11.2). Occasionally a productive cough characteristic of bronchopneumonia signals the presence of a secondary bacterial infection. Bronchopneumonia, characterized by coughing, may develop at late stages of the disease. Necrotic stomatitis affects the lower lip and gum and the gumline of the incisor teeth; in more severe cases, it may involve the dental pad, palate, cheeks and papillae, and tongue. Diarrhea may be profuse and accompanied by dehydration and emaciation; hypothermia and death follow, usually after 5–10 days. Morbidity and mortality rates are higher in young animals than in adults.

(a)

(b)

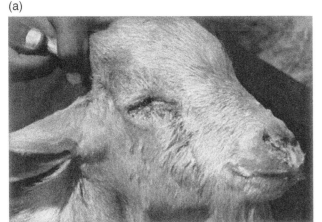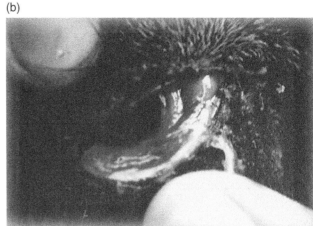

Figure 11.2   (a) Eyelids gummed together and nostrils blocked by purulent discharge in a goat suffering an advanced stage of peste des petits ruminants (PPR). (b) Inflammation of the ocular mucosa and purulent discharge in a goat infected with PPR.

- Four or five days after the appearance of the first clinical signs, the temperature drops, followed by the onset of occasionally bloody diarrhea and oral lesions. These become covered by a necrotic, whitish, pulpy tissue (with a mushy consistency), which emits a nauseating odor when the animal opens its mouth. In females, pus and erosive lesions are visible on the vulvo-vaginal mucous membranes. At this stage, pregnant animals abort.
- Death follows in 70–80% of cases, on average 10 days after the onset of the first clinical signs, in animals often in a state of hypothermia. When an animal recovers, convalescence is rapid and generally takes no more than one week.

11.1.3.2   Peracute Form

This is observed most often in young goats over 4 months old that are no longer protected by maternal antibodies.

- Incubation lasts about three days. The disease begins with the same clinical signs: a high fever (40–42 °C) followed by congestion of mucosa manifested by watery eyes and serous discharge. However, it evolves more rapidly.
- After five or six days, 100% of infected animals die even if they have shown no erosive lesions, diarrhea, or secondary bacterial infection.

11.1.3.3   Subacute Form

Despite the frequent occurrence of microbial complications, this is the least severe form of the disease. It is not fatal.

After a five-day incubation period, the disease causes a fever that remains moderate (39–40 °C) and lasts only one or two days. All of the other clinical signs are discreet and

may go unnoticed. Small amounts of discharge dry around the nostrils to form crusts that can steer the diagnosis toward another disease, contagious ecthyma.

11.1.3.4   Subclinical Form

Asymptomatic or unapparent, this form is often observed in sheep in the Sahel. In the absence of clinical signs, it is only revealed through serological investigations.

11.1.4   Lesions

Emaciation, conjunctivitis, and stomatitis are seen; necrotic lesions are observed inside the lower lip and on the adjacent gum, on the cheeks near the commissures, and on the ventral surface of the tongue. In severe cases, the lesions may extend to the hard palate and pharynx. The erosions are shallow, with a red, raw base, and later become pinkish white; they are bounded by healthy epithelium that provides a sharply demarcated margin. The rumen, reticulum, and omasum are rarely involved. The abomasum exhibits regularly outlined erosions that have red, raw floors and ooze blood.

Severe lesions are less common in the small intestines than in the mouth, abomasum, or large intestines. Streaks of hemorrhages, and less frequently erosions, may be present in the first portion of the duodenum and terminal ileum. Peyer's patches are severely affected; entire patches of lymphoid tissue may be sloughed. The large intestine is usually more severely affected, with lesions developing around the ileocecal valve and at the cecocolic junction and rectum. The latter exhibits streaks of congestion along the folds of the mucosa, resulting in the characteristic "zebra-striped" appearance.

Petechiae may appear in the turbinates, larynx, and trachea. Patches of bronchopneumonia may be present.

11.1.5 Diagnosis

A presumptive diagnosis is based on clinical, pathological, and epidemiological findings and may be confirmed by viral isolation and identification.

- **Clinical diagnosis**: Suspicion of PPR is based on a combination of several clinical signs that should alert livestock farmers, notably fever associated with nasal discharge and lacrimation, which appear suddenly in several small ruminants in a herd. However, these three elements are not enough to establish a diagnosis because they are not specific to PPR. They also are expressed in other pathologies of small ruminants present in PPR-enzootic areas such as contagious ecthyma and contagious caprine pleuropneumonia. A rigorous differential comparison of symptoms and the careful inspection of all animals in a herd are thus critical to assemble all of the clinical and lesional clues, which are not all always visible on a single individual. Depending on the breed, species, age, and immune status of the animals, the disease can take different clinical forms within the same herd. This poses additional difficulties for untrained farmers trying to identify the disease, especially if PPR is accompanied by confusing secondary infections such as respiratory pasteurellosis. The occurrence at the herd level of outside events considered to be risk factors must be taken into account and can reinforce the suspicion of PPR.
- **Postmortem diagnosis**: Postmortem examination of animals with the macroscopic observation of characteristic tissue lesions on digestive, respiratory, and lymphoid organs will confirm the provisional clinical diagnosis. Diagnosis will only be definitive following the laboratory examination of samples drawn from living animals (blood samples, swabs of nasal and ocular secretions, scraping of gingival mucosa) and dead animals (tissue fragments from lungs, intestines, lymph nodes, and spleen) to discover the direct or indirect presence of the virus.
- **Laboratory diagnosis**: Simple, rapid, and reliable laboratory methods have been developed over the past 30 years and are routinely used today to confirm the field diagnosis.
  - Indirect diagnostic methods are:
    - immuno-enzymatic tests or competitive enzyme-linked immunosorbent assay (ELISA), to detect antibodies in biological samples.
  - Direct diagnostic methods are:
    - Immuno-enzymatic tests, sandwich ELISA, and immunocapture ELISA, for the detection of antigens.
    - Reverse transcription polymerase chain reaction (RT-PCR) for detection of the virus genome.
    - Cell cultures for isolation of the virus.

Simple techniques such as agar-gel immunodiffusion have been used in developing countries for confirmation and reporting purposes. However, PPRV cross-reacts with RPV in these tests. Virus isolation is a definitive test, but is labor intensive, cumbersome, and takes a long time to complete. Currently, antigen capture ELISA and RT-PCR are the preferred laboratory tests for confirmation of the virus. For antibody detection (such as might be needed for epidemiological surveillance, confirmation of vaccine efficacy, or confirmation of the absence of the disease in a population), competitive ELISA and virus neutralization are the WOAH-recommended tests.

The specimens required are lymph nodes, tonsils, spleen, and whole lung for antigen or nucleic acid detection, and serum for antibody detection. The virus neutralization test may also be used to confirm an infection if paired serum samples from a surviving animal yield rising titers of $\geq$4-fold. PPR must be differentiated from other GI infections (e.g. GI parasites), respiratory infections (e.g. contagious caprine pleuropneumonia), and such other diseases as contagious ecthyma, heartwater, coccidiosis, and mineral poisoning.

11.1.6 Treatment and Control

There is no specific treatment for PPR, but treatment for bacterial and parasitic complications decreases mortality in affected flocks or herds. PPR has become a TAD. Although a highly effective vaccine has been available for 25 years, it continues to spread and expose previously disease-free countries in the South and North to the risk of virus incursion and disease emergence. Despite the existence of a highly effective vaccine, PPR is spreading geographically. Disease-free countries of the South and countries of the North are exposed to the risk of virus incursion and disease emergence. An attenuated PPR vaccine prepared in Vero cell culture is available and affords protection from natural disease for >1 year. The available homologous PPR vaccine would play an important role in that effort.

11.1.7 Eradication

Eradication is recommended when the disease appears in previously PPR-free countries. Currently a global initiative driven by FAO and WOAH exists to eradicate PPR by 2030. For this to be attainable, it is important to understand the specific epidemiological features of the disease and identify the socioeconomic factors that must be considered to stop the transmission of the disease.

To drive the PPR eradication effort on a global scale and effectively support countries in fighting the disease, FAO and WOAH established a Joint PPR Secretariat in March 2016, to oversee the implementation of the adopted PPR

Global Control and Eradication Strategy (PPR GCES). In October 2016, an initial PPR Global Eradication Programme (PPR GEP) for 2017–2021 was launched by FAO and WOAH to put the PPR GCES into action. The PPR GEP is a multicountry, multistage process that will decrease epidemiological risk levels and increase prevention and control.

11.2 Foot and Mouth Disease

FMD is a severe, highly contagious, acute viral disease of livestock that has a significant economic impact. The disease affects cattle, swine, sheep, goats, deer, camelids (such as camels, llamas, and alpacas), and other cloven-hoofed ruminants. Horses are not susceptible to infection with the foot and mouth disease virus (FMDV). Although FMD is rarely fatal in adult animals, it causes serious production losses and is a major constraint on international trade.

FMD is characterized by fever and fluid-filled blister-like (vesicles) sores and erosions on the tongue and lips, in the mouth, on the teats, and between the hooves, which may result in lameness, fever, and excessive salivation. FMD may be fatal in young stock. The disease causes severe production losses, and while the majority of affected animals recover, the disease often leaves them weakened and debilitated. It is a TAD that deeply affects the production of livestock and disrupts regional and international trade in animals and animal products.

FMDV mainly affects members of the order Artiodactyla (cloven-hooved mammals). Most species in this order are thought to be susceptible to some degree. Important livestock hosts include cattle, pigs, sheep, goats, water buffalo, and yaks. Wildlife species like wild boar, deer, and African buffalo are also susceptible to FMD. It is not readily transmissible to humans and is not a public health risk.

FMD is a WOAH-listed disease and must be reported to the organization, as indicated in the Terrestrial Animal Health Code (WOAH 2022). FMD is the first disease for which WOAH established an official status recognition as free of the disease, either in an entire country or in defined zones and compartments.

11.2.1 Etiology

The organism that causes FMD is an Aphthovirus of the family Picornaviridae. There are seven distinctive strains (A, O, C, SAT1, SAT2, SAT3, and Asia1) that are endemic in different countries worldwide. Each strain requires a specific vaccine to provide immunity to a vaccinated animal; that is, immunity to one serotype provides little to no protection against other serotypes.

All seven of the serotypes have been found in wildlife, although the latter does not play a significant role in the maintenance of the disease. To date, the only confirmed reservoir in wildlife is in African buffalo (*Syncerus caffer*).

FMDV can remain infective in the environment for several weeks and possibly longer in the presence of organic matter, such as soil, manure, and dried animal secretions, or on chemically inert materials, such as straw, hair, and leather. In carcasses that have undergone normal postslaughter acidification, the virus is inactivated within three days. However, it can remain viable for months in chilled lymph nodes, bone marrow, viscera, and residual blood clots. The virus may be shed in milk from infected animals up to four days before the onset of clinical signs and for up to three weeks afterwards.

11.2.2 Epidemiology and Transmission

FMD is one of the most contagious animal diseases known. Animals may be infectious before clinical signs develop. Intensively reared animals are more susceptible to the disease than are traditional breeds. The disease is rarely fatal in adult animals, but there is often high mortality in young animals due to myocarditis or, when the dam is infected by the disease, lack of milk. FMD is found in all excretions and secretions from infected animals, which excrete virus in fluid from ruptured vesicles, exhaled air, saliva, milk, semen, feces, urine, and so on. The main transmission method within herds or flocks is by direct contact or via respiratory particles and droplets. Notably, these animals breathe out a large amount of aerosolized virus, which can infect other animals via respiratory or oral routes. The virus may be present in milk and semen for up to four days before the animal shows clinical signs of disease.

The spread of FMD between properties and areas is often due to the movement of infected animals or via contaminated vehicles, equipment, people, and animal products. The significance of FMD is related to the ease with which the virus can spread through any or all of the following:

- Infected animals newly introduced into a herd (carrying virus in their saliva, milk, semen, etc.). Experimentally, FMD can be transmitted by insemination with infected semen. FMDV has been found in bull semen 4 days before, during, and up to at least 37 days of collection after the appearance of clinical signs. It has also been found in bovine semen stored at −50 °C for 320 days. FMDV has been found in pig semen and is likely to occur in sheep and goat semen. The virus enters semen as a result of viremia or lesions around the preputial orifice.
- Contaminated pens/buildings or contaminated animal transport vehicles.

- Contaminated materials such as hay, feed, water, milk, or biologics.
- Contaminated clothing, footwear, or equipment.
- Virus-infected meat or other contaminated animal products (if fed to animals when raw or improperly cooked).
- Infected aerosols (spread of virus from an infected property via air currents). Under certain weather conditions, infected aerosols can spread the virus over many kilometers by wind.

Animals that have recovered from infection may sometimes carry the virus and initiate new outbreaks of the disease. Cattle (indicator species) are highly susceptible to aerosol infection and readily display clinical signs. Sheep and goats (maintenance species) are equally susceptible to aerosol infection, but are less infectious and may not show obvious clinical signs. Pigs (amplifying species) are less susceptible to aerosol infection, but are potent amplifiers and excretors of the virus, especially in their breath. They serve as a significant source of virus to susceptible animals. Pigs frequently show obvious clinical signs. Some ruminants may remain long-term FMD carriers, but their role in starting new infections in susceptible animals has not been demonstrated.

FMD is endemic in several parts of Asia (Figure 11.3). Australia, Indonesia, Japan, New Zealand, Philippines, Singapore, New Caledonia, Brunei, and Vanuatu are currently free of the disease. However, FMD is a TAD that can occur sporadically in any areas currently free of infection.

11.2.3 Clinical Signs

The incubation period of FMD is highly variable and changes according to the virus strain, virus dose, transmission route, animal species involved, and conditions in which animals are kept. The incubation period is typically 2–14 days, whereas WOAH (2022) depicted a considerable incubation period of up to 14 days. Large numbers of animals in a group may be infected by FMDV simultaneously. However, they may display differing clinical signs depending on how long each individual animal has been infected.

FMD is clinically characterized by vesicles and erosions in the mouth and nostrils, on teats, and on skin between the claws and at the coronary band. A variety of other signs also appear in cattle, pigs, and sheep and goats. A range of clinical signs may indicate the presence of FMD in sheep and goats, where the disease is usually mild with few lesions; however, clinical signs can include pyrexia, lameness, and oral lesions (which are often mild), foot lesions along the coronary band or interdigital spaces, and lesions on the dental pad (although these may go unrecognized),

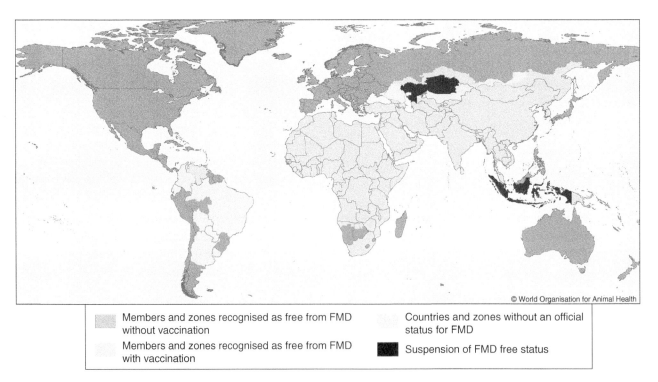

| | Members and zones recognised as free from FMD without vaccination | | Countries and zones without an official status for FMD |
| Members and zones recognised as free from FMD with vaccination | | Suspension of FMD free status |

Figure 11.3 World Organisation for Animal Health members' official foot and mouth disease (FMD) status map. Last update September 2022. *Source:* Foot and Mouth Disease (FMD), 2022 © World Organisation for Animal Health.

agalactia in milking sheep and goats, as well as death of young stock without clinical signs.

Clinical signs can range from mild or inapparent to severe: they are more severe in cattle and intensively reared pigs than in sheep and goats.

The typical clinical sign is the occurrence of blisters (or vesicles) on the nose, tongue, or lips, inside the oral cavity, between the toes, above the hooves, on the teats, and at pressure points on the skin. Ruptured blisters can result in extreme lameness and reluctance to move or eat. Usually, blisters heal within seven days (sometimes longer), but complications, such as secondary bacterial infection of open blisters, can also occur.

Other frequent symptoms are fever, depression, hypersalivation, loss of appetite, weight loss, growth retardation, and a drop in milk production, which can persist even after recovery. Chronically affected animals are reported to have an overall reduction of 80% in milk yield. The health of young calves, lambs, and piglets may be compromised by lack of milk if dams are infected.

Death can occur before the development of blisters due to a multifocal myocarditis. Myositis may also occur in other sites.

Severely affected animals can succumb to sudden, severe lameness affecting one or more feet. The mild or subclinical expression of the disease in sheep is a significant risk factor for the spread of the disease. The severity of clinical signs will depend on the strain of virus, the exposure dose, the age and species of animal, and the host immunity. Morbidity can reach 100% in susceptible populations. Mortality is generally low in adult animals (1–5%), but higher in young calves, lambs, and piglets (20% or higher).

11.2.4 Diagnosis

The disease may be suspected based on clinical signs. The clinical signs of FMD are similar to those of a number of other animal diseases. Confirmation of any suspected FMD case through laboratory tests is therefore a matter of urgency. Diseases that are clinically indistinguishable from FMD include:

- Vesicular stomatitis.
- Swine vesicular disease.
- Vesicular exanthema.

Other differential diagnoses include:

- Senecavirus A.
- Rinderpest (Eradicated in 2011 as WOAH declaration).
- Bluetongue.
- PPR.
- Mucosal disease.
- Bovine papular stomatitis.

- Bovine ulcerative mammalitis.
- Pseudocowpox.
- Bovine malignant catarrh.
- Contagious ecthyma ("scabby mouth").
- Infectious bovine rhinotracheitis/infectious pustular vulvovaginitis.
- Scalding, wetting, contact dermatitis, photosensitization.
- Mouth lesions in pigs from hot feed.
- Laminitis, hoof abscess, foot rot (e.g. from bad floors, new concrete, mud).

FMD can only be confirmed or ruled out through laboratory testing of samples taken from infected animals. Sample to be collected from FMD-suspected animals are vesicular fluid, epithelial tissue tags, pharyngeal scrapings, and sera.

Diagnosis of FMD is achieved by many techniques such as virus isolation, sandwich ELISA, multiplex PCR, indirect ELISA (differentiation between infected and vaccinated animals, DIVA), and real-time PCR. Laboratory diagnosis is usually performed by real-time RT-PCR assay. Virus isolation onto cell culture is considered the "gold-standard" technique for FMD diagnosis. Moreover, detecting antibodies against the non-structural proteins (NSPs) of FMD using indirect ELISA was successful for DIVA. Differentiation of the infected from the vaccinated animal is of great importance in the control program for FMD.

11.2.5 Treatment and Control

The control program depends mainly on vaccination, treatment, effective quarantine measures, disinfection, and hygiene and sanitation measures. Treatment protocols of small ruminants showing typical clinical symptoms of FMD are achieved by the use of antipyretic and analgesic medicine and a broad-spectrum long-acting antibiotic. The initial measures described in the Global Food and Mouth disease control strategy are the presence of early detection and warning systems and the implementation of effective surveillance in accordance with the guidelines detailed in the Terrestrial Animal Health Code (WOAH 2022). The implementation of the FMD control strategy varies from country to country and depends on the epidemiological situation of the disease. In general, it is essential for livestock owners and producers to maintain sound biosecurity practices to prevent the introduction and spread of the virus.

11.2.5.1 Vaccination
Depending on the FMD situation, vaccination strategies can be designed to achieve mass coverage or be targeted to specific animal sub-populations or zones. Vaccination

programs carried out in a target population should meet several critical criteria:

- Coverage should be at least 80%.
- Campaigns should be completed in the shortest possible time.
- Vaccination should be scheduled to allow for interference from maternal immunity.
- Vaccines should be administered in the correct dose and by the correct route.

The vaccines used should meet WOAH standards of potency and safety, and the strain or strains in the vaccine must antigenically match those circulating in the field. It is important to use inactivated virus vaccines, as inactivated virus does not have the ability to multiply in vaccinated animals. The use of live virus vaccines is not acceptable due to the danger of reversion to virulence. Vaccination can play a role in an effective control strategy for FMD, but the decision on whether or not to use vaccination lies with national authorities.

The inactivated FMDV vaccine has succeeded in reducing outbreaks worldwide. It gives protection for all ruminants against FMDV for one year. FMD has the ability to cause milk production losses in small ruminants. Recent diagnostic tools are urgently needed not only for the diagnosis, but also for following up programs to combat and control FMD (Mahmoud et al. 2019).

FMD is one of the world's most economically important viral diseases of livestock. The disease is estimated to circulate in 77% of the global livestock population, in Africa, the Middle East, and Asia, as well as in a limited area of South America. Countries that are currently free of FMD without vaccination remain under constant threat of an incursion. Some 75% of the costs attributed to FMD prevention and control are incurred by low-income and lower-middle-income countries. Africa and Eurasia are the regions that incur the largest costs, accounting for 50% and 33% of the total costs, respectively.

More than one billion small farmers around the world depend on livestock for their livelihoods; however, outbreaks of FMD inflict an estimated annual global loss of billions of dollars and pose a continuous risk of disease spread into disease-free areas. FMD prevention is based on the presence of early detection and warning systems and the implementation of effective surveillance, among other measures. In order to decrease the impact of FMD worldwide, FAO and WOAH (2012) developed a Global FMD Control Strategy that was endorsed in 2012 by representatives from more than 100 countries and international and regional partners in Bangkok, Thailand. The aim of the Global FMD Control Strategy is to reduce the global burden of FMD and the risk of reintroduction of the disease

into disease-free areas. To do so, a global approach for the control of FMD is needed. Some countries may also be aiming at eradicating the disease and other countries that have already been recognized as free from FMD at maintaining their status. The FMD Global Control Strategy is applied at a national level, while the progress is assessed at a regional level using roadmap platforms, which permit the formulation of harmonized programs and the exchange of information on virus circulation, vaccination, and other control initiatives.

11.3 Goat Pox

Goat pox is also an economically significant and contagious viral diseases of goats (as few strains are contagious to sheep) caused by the genus *Capripoxvirus* (CaPV) of the family Poxviridae. Currently, CaPV infection of small ruminants (sheep and goats) has been distributed widely and is prevalent in Central Africa, the Middle East, Europe, and Asia. This disease poses challenges to food production and distribution, affecting rural livelihoods in most African and Asian countries (Zewdie et al. 2021). All breeds of domestic and wild goats are affected, and most strains cause severe clinical disease.

WOAH has classified CaPV as a notifiable disease because of its rapid transboundary nature and extensive economic impact on the livestock industry (Hamdi et al. 2021).

11.3.1 Etiology

Goat pox is closely related to, but distinct from, sheep pox, although many authors lump the two diseases together. Most strains are host specific and cause severe clinical disease in either sheep or goats, while some strains have equal virulence in both species. Further complicating this is that recombination can occur between sheep and goat strains, which produce a spectrum with intermediate host preference and range of virulence. Sheep pox virus and goat pox virus are also closely related to lumpy skin disease virus (LSDV), which causes a similar disease in cattle (Kitching 2008), but there is no evidence that LSDV causes disease in sheep and goats.

Sources of virus are ulcerated papules on mucous membranes prior to necrosis, skin lesions with scabs (which contain large amounts of virus in association with the antibody, but infectivity is not known), saliva, nasal and ocular secretions, milk, urine, feces, semen, and embryos.

The virus can be inactivated by heating at 56 °C for 60 minutes, and is also susceptible to a highly alkaline or acid pH. Pox virus can be inactivated by the application of phenol (2%) for 15 minutes, as well as detergents. It is also sensitive to sunlight, but remains viable in wool/hair and dry scabs on skin for up to three months. Goat pox virus is hardy and has good survivability in the environment.

11.3.2 Epidemiology and Transmission

Goat pox occurs in most parts of Africa and Asia. The Americas and Europe are free of the disease. Capripox is endemic in Africa north of the Equator, the Middle East, Turkey, Iran, Iraq, Afghanistan, Pakistan, India, Nepal, parts of the People's Republic of China, and Bangladesh. The most recent outbreaks occurred in Vietnam in 2005, Mongolia in 2008 and 2009, and Azerbaijan in 2009. The first outbreak in Chinese Taipei occurred in 2008 and was eradicated by stamping out the disease and movement control.

The virus is introduced into the animal in a variety of ways, through ingestion or skin abrasions, and it moves throughout the body, settling in many areas, but predominantly in the skin and lungs. Transmission is usually by aerosol after close contact with severely affected animals that have ulcerated papules on the mucous membranes. There is no transmission in the prepapular stage, for example animals early in disease or those dying peracutely. There is reduced transmission once the papules have become necrotic and neutralizing antibody is produced (about one week after onset). Animals with mild localized infections also rarely transmit the disease. Infection may occur through other mucous membranes or abraded skin. Chronically infected carriers do not occur. Indirect transmission by contaminated implements, vehicles, or products (litter, fodder) does occur. Indirect transmission by insects (mechanical vectors) has been established (minor role).

11.3.3 Clinical Findings

The incubation period is 8–13 days. It may be as short as 4 days following experimental infection by intradermal inoculation or mechanical transmission by insects.

Morbidity in a herd varies widely, but can be considerable. Generally, the morbidity rate in endemic areas is 70–90%, whereas the mortality rate in endemic areas is 5–10%, but is highest in non-native breeds that have been introduced, in which case it may reach 100% (Garner et al. 2000). One to two weeks after being infected, animals will become febrile, and multiple reddened areas (macules) appear on the skin (Figure 11.4).

These macules progress to raised foci (papules) and then within a week begin oozing serosanguinous exudate and ulcerating. Eventually a total core of epidermis may fall out, leaving a gaping wound for other organisms to enter and wreak havoc. Skin lesions can be particularly severe around the lips, nares, and conjunctiva. Internally, a pneumonia centered on the terminal bronchioles can occur. Also, typical pox lesions may form on the serosal surfaces of multiple organs.

The lesions are skin lesions: congestion, hemorrhage, edema, vasculitis, and necrosis. All the layers of the epidermis, dermis, and sometimes musculature are involved, as well as lymph nodes draining infected areas that undergo enlargement (up to eight times normal size), lymphoid

(a)

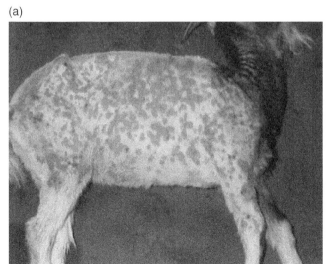

(b)

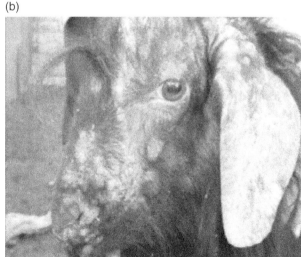

Figure 11.4   (a) Goat pox often begins as a macular rash over the surface of the body. (b) Pox lesions on the face and ears.

proliferation, edema, congestion, and hemorrhage. Pox lesions occur on mucous membranes of the eyes, mouth, nose, pharynx, epiglottis, and trachea, on the rumenal and abomasal mucosae, and on the muzzle, nares, vulva, prepuce, testicles, udder, and teats. Lesions may coalesce in severe cases. Lung lesions and severe and extensive pox lesions that are focal and uniformly distributed throughout the lungs, that face congestion, edema, focal areas of proliferation with necrosis, and lobular atelectasis. Enlargement, congestion, edema, and hemorrhages of mediastinal lymph nodes occur.

11.3.4 Diagnosis

Poxvirus infections can be suspected by clinical signs and lesions, whereas they can be confirmed in the laboratory using several diagnostic techniques. The *Orthopoxvirus* can usually be isolated in cell culture and by inoculation of embryonated eggs. Examination of clinical samples by negative-staining electron microscopy is frequently used to visualize virus particles. PCR and gene sequencing are widely used to further characterize virus isolates.

11.3.5 Clinical Diagnosis

Clinical signs vary from mild to severe, depending on host factors (e.g. age, breed, immunity) and viral factors (e.g. species predilection and virulence of viral strain). Inapparent infections also occur. Early clinical signs are rise in rectal temperature to above 40 °C, macules developing in 2–5 days (small circumscribed areas of hyperemia, most obvious on unpigmented skin), from which develop papules (hard swellings of between 0.5 and 1 cm in diameter), which may cover the body or be restricted to the groin, axilla, and perineum. Papules may be covered by fluid-filled vesicles, but this is rare. A flat hemorrhagic form of capripox has been observed in some breeds of European goat in which all the papules appear to coalesce over the body; this form is always fatal.

In the acute phase, within 24 hours after the appearance of generalized papules, affected animals develop rhinitis, conjunctivitis, and enlargement of all superficial lymph nodes, especially prescapular lymph nodes. Papules on the eyelids cause blepharitis of varying severity; papules on the mucous membranes of the eyes and nose ulcerate, creating mucopurulent discharge; mucosae of the mouth, anus, and prepuce or vagina become necrotic; and breathing may become labored and noisy due to pressure on the upper respiratory tract from the swollen retropharyngeal lymph nodes draining developing lung lesions.

When an animal survives the acute phase, papules become necrotic from vascular thrombosis and ischemic necrosis, and form scabs in the next 5–10 days, which persist for up to 6 weeks, leaving small scars. The skin lesions are susceptible to fly strike, secondary pneumonia is common, anorexia is unusual unless mouth lesions physically interfere with feeding, and abortion is rare.

11.3.6 Laboratory Diagnosis

Samples for virus isolation must be sent to the laboratory as soon as possible. They should be kept cold and shipped on gel packs. If these samples must be shipped long distances without refrigeration, glycerol (10%) can be added; tissue samples must be large enough that glycerol does not penetrate into the center of the tissue and destroy the virus.

Neutralizing antibodies can interfere with virus isolation and some antigen-detection tests; samples for these tests must be collected during the first week of illness. Samples for PCR can be taken after neutralizing antibodies have developed. Paired serum samples should be collected for serology:

- **Live animals**: Full skin thickness biopsies; vesicular fluid if available; scabs; skin scrapings; lymph node aspirates; whole blood collected into heparin or ethylenediaminetetraacetic acid (EDTA); paired sera.
- **Animals at necropsy**: skin lesions; lymph nodes; lung lesions; histology: full set of tissues, especially those with lesions.

The common laboratory diagnostic tests performed for goat pox disease are genome detection by PCR, virus identification by electron microscopy, virus isolation in cell culture, immunofluorescence staining techniques, agar gel immunodiffusion test (AGID), antigen-detection ELISA virus neutralization, indirect fluorescent antibody test, and western blotting.

11.3.7 Differential diagnosis

The clinical signs of severe sheep pox and goat pox are highly characteristic. However, in their mild form they can be confused with *Parapoxvirus* causing orf or urticaria from multiple insect bites. Other differential diagnoses are:

- Contagious ecthyma (contagious pustular dermatitis or orf).
- Insect bites.
- Bluetongue.
- PPR.
- Photosensitization.
- Dermatophilosis.
- Parasitic pneumonia.
- Caseous lymphadenitis.
- Mange.

11.3.8 Treatment, Prevention, and Control

There is no specific treatment. Early detection, farm biosecurity, vector control, and vaccinations are the key methods to control the disease. The sanitary prophylaxis is, if culling is not possible:

- Isolation of infected herds and sick animals for at least 45 days after recovery.
- Slaughtering of infected herd if possible.
- Proper disposal of cadavers and products – burning or burial is often used.
- Stringent cleaning and disinfection of farms and equipment.
- Quarantine of new animals before introduction into herds.
- Animal and vehicle movement controls within infected areas.

Vaccination may be considered when the disease has spread more widely.

11.3.9 Vaccination

Control of goat pox is usually affected through vaccination. Because sheep pox, goat pox, and LSD (the CaPV of cattle) are all so similar, a vaccine made of any of these three viruses will protect all three species against their own CaPV variant. Both inactivated and live vaccines are available. In regions of the world with extensive grazing and mixing of herds, 85% of the total population must be vaccinated to keep the virus from circulating. As discussed in the section on PPR, maintaining this level of protection is challenging.

Live and inactivated vaccines have been used for the control of capripox. All strains of CaPV so far examined share a major neutralization site and will cross-protect. There are several attenuated virus vaccines delivered by the subcutaneous or intradermal route; conferred immunity lasts up to two years. Inactivated vaccines give, at best, only short-term immunity. Currently, no recombinant vaccines for CaPV are commercially available. However, a new generation of capripox vaccines is being developed that uses the CaPV genome as a vector for the genes of other ruminant pathogens, for instance genes of rinderpest and PPR viruses.

Furthermore, awareness-raising campaigns for farmers to promote vaccine management and handling should be considered.

11.4 Rift Valley Fever

RVF is an acute or peracute disease of wild and domestic ruminants and humans caused by a *Phlebovirus* and transmitted by insect (mosquito) vectors or direct contact with organs or fluids of infected animals. The disease usually presents in an epizootic form over large areas of a country following heavy rains and sustained flooding, or linked to the construction of irrigation schemes and hydrological dams, which present suitable breeding sites for vector populations. The disease is characterized by high rates of abortion and neonatal mortality in domestic ruminants. In humans, it mainly develops as an influenza-like illness, sometimes with ophthalmic sequelae. The disease is prevalent throughout Eastern Africa, following the topography of the Great Rift Valley. In nature, it is only known in Africa and the Arabian Peninsula. However, vector distribution, climatic changes, and land usage dynamics may modify the temporal and spatial distribution of the infection.

11.4.1 Etiology, Hosts, and Transmission

RVF virus is a negative-sense, tri-segmented RNA virus within the order Bunyavirales, family Phenuiviridae, genus *Phlebovirus*. Only one serotype is recognized, but strains exist of variable virulence. The virus is destroyed by heat treatment at 56 °C for 120 minutes, and is inactivated at pH <6.8 and by lipid solvents. The virus can survive in 0.5% phenol solution at 4 °C for six months.

The most common hosts of the disease are cattle, sheep, goats, several rodents, as well as wild ruminants, buffalo, antelopes, and wildebeest. Humans are highly susceptible to infection, but represent dead-end hosts. No human-to-human infection has been reported. African monkeys and domestic carnivores present a transitory viremia, whereas camelids do not play a relevant role in hosting or transmitting the virus. Aedes mosquitoes may vertically transmit the virus to their offspring via eggs.

RVF virus regularly circulates in endemic areas between wild ruminants and hematophagous mosquitoes; the disease is usually inapparent in wild species of animals due to their lower susceptibility. Certain *Aedes* species act as reservoirs for RVF virus during interepidemic periods. Increased precipitation or flooding in dry areas leads to an explosive hatching of mosquito eggs, many of which harbor RVF virus. The longer the period between heavy precipitation events (usually from 5 to 25 years), the more individuals within the population will be naïve to infection, leading to explosive outbreaks of disease. Infected *Aedes* feed preferentially on domestic ruminants that act as an amplifier of RVF (a broad vector range of mosquitoes: *Aedes, Anopheles, Culex, Eretmapodites, Mansonia,* etc.), which coupled with increased circulating virus leads to expansion of disease as well as extrinsic incubation occurring in vectors. Sylvatic cycle and interepidemic maintenance occur in some areas. The duration of epizootic and interepizootic periods depends on the particularities of the area and animals concerned. Direct contamination occurs in humans when handling infected animals and meat, and mechanical transmission by various vectors has been demonstrated in laboratory studies.

Animals acquire the infection through the bite of an infected mosquito. Serological evidence of infection exists for a wide range of animal species, and it is likely that the virus is maintained in nature, only to emerge in epizootic (and/or epidemic) form after heavy rainfall that allows for an increase of the mosquito vector, corresponding infection of ruminants that develop high viremias, and subsequent further amplification within the vector populations and "spillover" to humans.

11.4.2 Clinical Findings

The pathogenesis of RVF occurs within a day or two of inoculation by an infected mosquito: goats will experience a viremia and may have fever. Younger animals will appear ill, and may become jaundiced due to the attack on the liver. In pregnant animals, the virus moves right through the placenta to attack and replicate in the fetal liver, causing death of the fetus and expulsion (abortion).

Severity of clinical disease varies by species: lambs, kids, puppies, kittens, mice, and hamsters are considered "extremely susceptible," with mortalities of 70–100%; sheep and calves are categorized as "highly susceptible," with mortality rates between 20% and 70%; in the "moderately susceptible" category are cattle, goats, African buffalo, domestic buffalo, Asian monkeys, and humans, with mortalities less than 10%; camels, equids, pigs, dogs, cats, African monkeys, baboons, rabbits, and guinea pigs are considered "resistant," with infection being inapparent; and birds, reptiles, and amphibians are not susceptible to RVF.

Signs of the disease tend to be non-specific; however, the presentation of numerous abortions and mortalities among young animals, together with influenza-like disease in humans, is indicative. Humans tend to be infected far later during the onset of an outbreak, due to direct contact with bodily fluids from infected animals or mosquito bites. However, if the outbreak happens in remote areas, humans may act as sentinels of infection with RVF virus.

In goats and sheep, clinical signs are quite similar. Newborn kids or those under 2 weeks of age (extremely susceptible) exhibit clinical signs as biphasic fever (40–42 °C) that subsides just prior to death; anorexia, in part due to disinclination to move; weakness; listlessness; abdominal pain; rapid, abdominal respiration prior to death; and death within 24–36 hours. Kids over 2 weeks of age (highly susceptible) and adult goats show peracute disease (sudden death with no appreciable signs), or acute disease (more often in adult goats) with fever (41–42 °C) lasting 24–96 hours, anorexia, weakness, listlessness and depression, increased respiratory rate, vomiting, bloody/fetid diarrhea, and mucopurulent nasal discharge; icterus may be evident in a few animals. In the case of pregnant goats, rates of "abortion storms" approach 100%.

Capable of infecting a large number of hosts, RVF causes the greatest damage in ruminants, especially sheep and goats. Disease in ruminants appears most frequently as abortion storms or deaths of neonates.

11.4.3 Lesions

The classic primary lesion is massive hepatic necrosis due to infection of hepatocytes. The common lesions are:

- Focal or generalized hepatic necrosis (white necrotic foci of about 1 mm in diameter).
- Congestion, enlargement, and discoloration of liver with subcapsular hemorrhages.
- Brown-yellowish color of liver in aborted fetuses.
- Widespread cutaneous hemorrhages, petechial to ecchymotic hemorrhages on parietal and visceral serosal membranes.
- Enlargement, edema, hemorrhages, and necrosis of lymph nodes.
- Congestion and cortical hemorrhages of kidneys and multifocal petechiation advancing to diffuse hemorrhages associated with gallbladder.
- Marked mesenteric and serosal inflammation and edema of digestive tract.
- Multifocal hemorrhagic enteritis.
- Icterus (low percentage except in calves).

11.4.4 Diagnosis

Diagnosis can be performed based on history, epidemiology, clinical signs, and lesions, as well as confirmation through laboratory tests.

Laboratory diagnosis can be performed for identification of the agent: virus isolation, immunostaining or PCR, antigen detection (through ELISA, histopathology with immunohistochemistry). Histopathological examination of the liver of affected animals will reveal characteristic cytopathology, and immunostaining will allow specific identification of RVF viral antigen in tissue. Serological test techniques include ELISA, AGID, hemagglutination inhibition, virus neutralization, plaque reduction neutralization (PRN), and neutralization in mice.

Samples for laboratory diagnosis can be heparinized or clotted blood, plasma or serum. Tissue samples of liver, spleen, kidney, lymph node, heart blood, and brain from dead animals or aborted fetuses should be submitted preserved in 10% buffered formalin and in glycerol/saline and transported at 4 °C. Liver or other tissue for histological examination may be placed in formol saline in the field for diagnostic purposes; this facilitates handling and transport in remote areas.

Differential diagnoses include:

- Bluetongue.
- Wesselsbron disease.
- Enterotoxemia of sheep.
- Ephemeral fever.
- Brucellosis.
- Vibriosis.
- Trichomonosis.
- Nairobi sheep disease.
- Heartwater.
- Ovine enzootic abortion.
- Toxic plants.
- Bacterial septicemias.
- Rinderpest and PPR.
- Anthrax.

11.4.5 Treatment, Prevention, and Control

There is no specific treatment for RVF.

Countermeasures for RVF exist, but none is completely adequate. Once a herd or flock of ruminants experiences disease, the virus is readily amplified and spreads extensively through mosquito vectors. Controlling an outbreak in animals requires rapid depopulation and stringent insect control. Various vaccine formulations are available for livestock, but each one has benefits and deficits, and none is approved for use in North America or Europe (Pepin et al. 2010).

Hides, skins, wool, and fiber are safe commodities, and meat from animals slaughtered in an approved slaughterhouse/abattoir, subject to ante- and postmortem inspection, and which has undergone a maturation process poses no risk of transmission of RVF virus. However, meat from animals from endemic areas must be accompanied by a veterinary certificate when exported, to attest to the listed conditions. Sanitary prophylaxis involves control of animal movements (extension of disease), controls at slaughterhouses (exposure to disease), draining of standing water to eliminate or reduce vectors, disinfestations of low-depression accumulations of water where mosquitoes may reproduce (in Africa known as "dambos"), use of methoprene spraying, or controlled burning. It is possible to forecast high-precipitation events up

to four months before that may lead to explosive outbreaks of RVF related to the increase in hatching of mosquito eggs. Thus, prophylactic measures such as monitoring risk factors and vector populations and assessment of livestock vaccination opportunity must be considered.

During widespread outbreaks, the focus should be on coordinating the efforts of stakeholders regarding human and animal health; promotion of education of personnel; control of animal movements; and clinical management of RVF cases. Medical prophylaxis is attenuated virus vaccine (Smithburn strain); one inoculation confers immunity lasting three years and is safe for all breeds of cattle, sheep, and goats. The vaccine may cause fetal abnormalities or abortion in pregnant animals and is pathogenic for humans. Another vaccine, Clone-13 live attenuated virus vaccine, is a natural attenuated strain, has no abortion or side effects seen in experimental trials, and is used as a single-injection regimen. Neither of these vaccines allows for differentiation of infected and vaccinated animals. An inactivated virus vaccine is also used that needs a booster 3–6 months after initial vaccination, followed by yearly boosters. This is used in outbreak situations and pregnant animals.

11.4.6 Zoonotic Importance

When RVF surfaces in an area, there is often a dramatic and expensive response, largely because of the concern about human infection. Failure to recognize an incursion can be costly as well. In 2000, RVF was transferred from East Africa to the Arabian Peninsula, a region where it had never occurred before, and there was considerable human morbidity and an alarming mortality rate of 14% (Madani et al. 2003; Nasher et al. 2000).

What makes RVF of such great concern is that it is a zoonotic threat, and although many humans are infected asymptomatically, there are also cases of severe liver disease, as well as other complications, mostly vascular in nature. The human case fatality rate with RVF is usually low, of the order of 1–5%, but it can on occasion be higher. For humans, TSI-GSD-200 inactivated human vaccine is used, although it is presently not available.

11.5 Control Strategy for Transboundary Animal Diseases

With increasing movement of human populations, livestock and livestock products, fish and fish products, and plants and plant products within and across countries, together with climate changes, the threat from TADs is intensifying. TADs are highly contagious and have the potential for rapid spread, irrespective of national borders, causing serious socioeconomic consequences (Otte et al. 2004). Traditionally, trade, traffic, and travel have been instruments of disease spread. Now, changing climate across the globe is adding to the problems. Climate change is creating a new ecological platform for the entry and establishment of pests and diseases from one geographic region to another (FAO 2008). Several new TADs have emerged, and old diseases reemerged, exhibiting increased chances for unexpected spread to new regions, often over great distances. Livestock TADs such as FMD have a direct economic impact by reducing agricultural and animal production (FAO/OIE 2004; Domenech et al. 2006). Apart from causing suffering and mortality in susceptible populations, the diseases adversely affect food safety, rural livelihoods, human health, and international trade. The effect on the national economy is felt by way of reduced access to international markets for agricultural products and higher costs involved with inspection, treatment, and compliance with international regulatory issues. Therefore, it is necessary to effectively manage TADs.

In developing countries, control of these diseases is a key pathway for poverty alleviation. It is advisable to have an effective quarantine system in place to prevent entry and establishment of TADs. As a second line of defense, a country must also have in place a suitable contingency plan to respond quickly to high-threat diseases. This could be achieved by timely application of scientific technology for rapid response. A disease outbreak in a neighboring country should always be taken as an immediate threat. Affected countries remain a threat to disease-free nations, and this is exemplified by recent incursions of FMD into FMD-free countries like Japan and Korea.

To better support livestock's contribution to alleviating poverty, hunger, and all forms of malnutrition, and to assist in reducing the threat from animal pathogens to human health, FAO and WOAH are partners in the Global Framework for the Progressive Control of Transboundary Animal Diseases (GF-TADs), a joint governance mechanism that they launched in 2004 to achieve coordinated prevention and control of TADs, and in particular to address their regional and global dimensions. This joint initiative, with the participation of the World Health Organization (WHO) in regard to zoonoses, to prevent, detect, and control priority TADs and, in particular, to address their national, regional, and global dimensions. Around the globe, GF-TADs is currently taking action on the global priority TADs FMD, PPR, and African swine fever, as well as participating in the Rinderpest Post-Eradication Programme (GF-TADs 2022).

The goals of GF-TADs are to safeguard its members from repeated incursions of infectious animal disease epidemics, to enhance safe trade in animals and animal products, and to improve food and nutrition security by reducing the damaging effects of TADs. To reach these long-term goals, the GF-TADs' strategy for 2021–2025 aims to enhance the control of TADs through the establishment of priority TADs strategies at the regional and sub-regional levels, by developing the capacity to prevent and control TADs, and by improving the sustainability of priority TADs strategies through multidisciplinary partners.

11.6 Conclusion

Attention to and control of TADs of goats could have very positive benefits for animal health in the developing world. Each of the four TADs presented here, PPR, FMD, goat pox, and RVF, presents prominent threats and complicated challenges.

Multiple-Choice Questions

1 African swine fever first occurred in which country?
   A Japan
   B China
   C USA
   D Norway

2 African swine fever is a devastating transboundary disease of which species?
   A Cattle
   B Goat
   C Horse
   D Pig

3 Lumpy skin disease is an emerging transboundary infectious disease of animals with what degree of morbidity and mortality?
   A High morbidity and low mortality
   B Low morbidity and high mortality
   C Low morbidity and low mortality
   D None of the above

4 Capripoxviruses are an emerging worldwide threat to which species?
   A Horse
   B Pig
   C Mule
   D Sheep

5 The Black Death was speculated to be which disease?
   A Leprosy
   B Rabies
   C Plague
   D None of the above

6 Which of the following *cannot* be transmitted via infectious droplets?
   A Influenza
   B Common cold
   C Rubella
   D None of the above

7 *Nipah henipavirus* is carried by what means?
   A Bat
   B Air
   C Water
   D None of the above

8 Creutzfeldt-Jakob disease (vCJD) can be contracted only in which way?
   A Consuming water tainted with *E. coli*
   B Consuming nerve tissues (brain and spine) of cattle infected with mad cow disease
   C Consuming shrimp infected with *E. coli*
   D None of the above

9 What does the bacterium *Yersinia pestis* cause?
   A Measles
   B Bubonic plague
   C Roseola
   D Rubella

10 What was the 1918 flu pandemic, also called Spanish flu, caused by?
   A Simian virus 5
   B Influenza C virus
   C H1N1 influenza A virus
   D SARS coronavirus 2

References

Albina, E., Kwiatek, O., Minet, C. et al. (2013). Peste des petits ruminants, the next eradicated animal disease? *Veterinary Microbiology* 165 (1–2): 38–44.

Barrett, T., Amarel-Doel, C., Kitching, R.P., and Gusev, A. (1993). Use of the polymerase chain reaction in differentiating rinderpest field virus and vaccine virus in the same animals. *Revue Scientifique et Technique* 12 (3): 865–872.

Cartín-Rojas, A. (2012). Transboundary animal diseases and international trade. In: *International Trade from Economic and Policy Perspective* (ed. V. Bobek). London: IntechOpen, ch. 7. https://doi.org/doi.org/10.5772/48151.

Chard, L.S., Bailey, D.S., Dash, P. et al. (2008). Full genome sequences of two virulent strains of peste-des-petits ruminants virus, the Côte d'Ivoire 1989 and Nigeria 1976 strains. *Virus Research* 136 (1–2): 192–197.

Corrie Brown, C. (2011). Transboundary diseases of goats. *Small Ruminant Research* 98: 21–25. https://doi.org/10.1016/j.smallrumres.2011.03.011.

Domenech, J., Lubroth, J., Eddi, C. et al. (2006). Regional and international approaches on prevention and control of animal transboundary and emerging diseases. *Annals of the New York Academy of Sciences* 1081 (1): 90–107. https://doi.org/10.1196/annals.1373.010.

FAO (1997). Prevention and control of transboundary animal diseases. Rome: FAO. https://www.fao.org/3/w3737e/W3737E00.htm#TOC.

FAO (2008). Expert meeting on climate related transboundary pests and diseases including relevant aquatic species. FAO headquarters, 25–27 February 2008. Rome: FAO. https://www.fao.org/fileadmin/user_upload/foodclimate/presentations/diseases/OptionsEM3.pdf.

FAO/OIE (2004). The global framework for the progressive control of trans-boundary animal diseases (GF-TADs). Paris/Rome: OIE/FAO. https://www.fao.org/3/ak136e/ak136e.pdf.

Garner, M., Sawarkar, S., Brett, E. et al. (2000). The extent and impact of sheep pox and goat pox in the state of

Maharashtra, India. *Tropical Animal Health and Production* 32 (4): 205–223.

GF-TADs (2022). GF-TADs and FMD. http://www.gf-tads.org/fmd/fmd/en.

Gibbs, P.J., Taylor, W.P., Lawman, M.J., and Bryant, J. (1979). Classification of peste des petits ruminants virus as the fourth member of the genus Morbillivirus. *Intervirology* 11 (5): 268–274.

Hamdi, J., Munyanduki, H., Omari Tadlaoui, K. et al. (2021). Capripoxvirus infections in ruminants: a review. *Microorganisms* 9 (5): 902.

Islam, M.A. (2016). Transboundary animal diseases: concerns and management strategies. *Res. Agric. Livest. Fish.* 3 (1): 121–126.

Kitching, P. (2008). Capripoxviruses. In: *Foreign Animal Diseases*, 7e (ed. C. Brown and A. Torres), 189–196. Boca Raton, FL: US Animal Health Association.

Lubroth, J. and Balogh, K.D. (2009). *Prevention/Control of Transboundary Diseases, Zoonoses and Emerging Infections*. Rome: Animal Health Service, Food and Agriculture Organisation of the United Nations (FAO).

Madani, T., Al-Mazrou, Y., Al-Jeffri, M. et al. (2003). Rift Valley fever epidemic in Saudi Arabia: epidemiological, clinical, and laboratory characteristics. *Clinical Infectious Diseases* 37: 1084–1092.

Mahmoud, M.A.E.F., Ghazy, A.A., and Shaapan, R.M. (2019). Diagnosis and control of foot and mouth disease (FMD) in dairy small ruminants; sheep and goats. *International Journal of Dairy Science* 14: 45–52. https://doi.org/10.3923/ijds.2019.45.52.

Nasher, A., Al Eriyani, M., Bourgy, A. et al. (2000). Outbreak of Rift Valley fever – Yemen, August–October 2000. *Morbidity and Mortality Weekly Report* 49: 1065–1066.

Otte, M.J., Nugent, R., and McLeod, A. (2004). Transboundary animal diseases: Assessment of socio-economic impacts and institutional responses. Livestock policy discussion paper No. 9. Rome: FAO. https://www.fao.org/3/ag273e/ag273e.pdf.

Pepin, M., Bouloy, M., Bird, B. et al. (2010). Rift Valley fever virus (Bunyaviridae: Phlebovirus): an update on pathogenesis, molecular epidemiology, vectors, diagnostics and prevention. *Veterinary Research* 41 (6): 61–70.

Saliki, J.T. (2022). Overview of peste des petits ruminants. In: *MSD Veterinary Manual*. Rahway, NJ: Merck https://www.msdvetmanual.com/generalized-conditions/peste-des-petits-ruminants/overview-of-peste-des-petits-ruminants.

Taylor, W.P. (1984). The distribution and epidemiology of peste des petits ruminants. *Preventive Veterinary Medicine* 2 (1–4): 157–166.

Torres, A., 2008. Foot-and-mouth disease. In: Brown, C., Torres, A. (Eds.), Foreign Animal Diseases. 7 US Animal Health Association, Boca Raton, FL, pp. 261–275

WOAH (2012). *Foot and mouth diseases (FMD)*. Bangkok: WOAH https://www.woah.org/app/uploads/2021/03/a-fmd-recommendations-bankok-2012.pdf.

WOAH (2022). Terrestrial Animal Health Code. Paris: WOAH. https://www.woah.org/en/what-we-do/standards/codes-and-manuals.

Zewdie, G., Derese, G., Getachew, B. et al. (2021). Review of sheep and goat pox disease: current updates on epidemiology, diagnosis, prevention and control measures in Ethiopia. *Animal Diseases* 1: 28. doi: 10.1186/s44149-021-00028-2.

12

Production Diseases of Goats

Gaurav Charaya[1], Jasleen Kaur[2], Chinmoy Maji[3], and Tanmoy Rana[4]

[1] *Department of Veterinary Medicine, College of Veterinary Sciences, Lala Lajpat Rai University of Veterinary and Animal Sciences, Hisar, Haryana, India*
[2] *Department of Veterinary Microbiology, College of Veterinary Sciences, Lala Lajpat Rai University of Veterinary and Animal Sciences, Hisar, Haryana, India*
[3] *North 24 Parganas Krishi Vigyan Kendra, West Bengal University of Animal & Fishery Sciences, Ashokenagar, West Bengal, India*
[4] *Department of Veterinary Clinical Complex, West Bengal University of Animal & Fishery Sciences, Kolkata, West Bengal, India*

Production diseases are those diseases that are caused by an imbalance between dietary input and output of production of certain nutrients in the body. In these diseases, output is more than input, which leads to depletion. This chapter discusses in detail the body condition score (BCS) and major production diseases of goats; that is, pregnancy toxemia, hypomagnesemia, tetany, and hypocalcemia (milk fever).

12.1 Body Condition Scoring in Goats and Its Significance in Relation to Production Diseases

The BCS relates to the availability of fat deposits, which is crucial for herders to assess the energy and nutritional status of a flock. It is determined by visual inspection and palpation of different body parts. Criteria for evaluation of BCS in goats are depicted in Table 12.1 and different body parts used as criteria are shown in Figure 12.1. BCS helps in assessing the health status of individual animals, as well as their management and welfare. It tells us the fat reserve present in goats irrespective of body size. Goats with a low BCS tend to have lower production and reproduction, whereas goats with a high BCS tend to be predisposed to production diseases because of a voluntary decrease in feed intake. Overconditioning at a flock/individual level can lead to fattening of does, which further increases the risk of developing pregnancy toxemia, especially in does carrying twins or triplets (Koyuncu and Altınçekiç 2013, p. 170). Regular screening of a flock for evaluation of BCS can help in optimization of the score within a range of 3–3.5, particularly in the breeding season. Flushing of goats by increasing the level of feed offered to the breeding does, mostly in the form of energy and

starting approximately one month prior to the introduction of the buck, should be done in flocks with BCS less than 3, whereas in the case of overfattened does low-energy food should be fed. It is ideal to keep the doe at the time of kidding as close to the optimum 3 BCS so as to have viable kids, adequate colostrum, and optimum milk production. In one study (Moeini et al. 2014, p. 91), Merghoze goats with a BCS of 3.0 had a better performance in terms of kidding rate and total kilogram weight of kids born per goat, while the kidding rate decreased in goats with a BCS of 3.5 or more.

12.2 Factors Affecting Nutritional Requirements in Goats

Multiple factors affect the nutritional requirements of goat and influence their metabolic state, predisposing them to several diseases:

- Body weight of animal (growth rate or weight gain).
- Sex.
- Body condition.
- Maintenance and activity levels.
- Stage of pregnancy, kidding rate, number of kids.
- Stage of lactation/milk production.
- Breed and utility: dairy, meat, or fiber.
- Weather/climate.

The body weight of animals has a direct influence on their nutrient requirements and an almost linear rise is seen with weight. Female and lactating animals require more nutrients compared to males. It depends on the activity, as animals reared in an intensive system require fewer nutrients than those who are grazed. The number of kids directly

Table 12.1 Criteria to evaluate the body condition score in goats.

	Visible features			Spinous process of lumbar vertebrae	Transition from spinous to transverse process	Transverse process	Sternum
Sr. No.	Physical appearance	Backbone	Thoracic cage				
1	Emaciated (poor health)	Highly visible	Clearly visible ribs	Very prominent	Severe noticeable dip	Clearly visible	Sternal fat easily grasped
2	Thin	Visible with continuous ridge	Ribs visible, little fat	Evident for about one-third to half of its length	Has noticeable dip	Difficult to see outline	Thumb and fingers can grab and pull sternal fat
3	Good	Not clear	Barely discernible, with even layer of fat	Difficult to grasp, transition has gentle slope	Has gentle slope	Faint outline visible for 1/4 of length	Sternal fat thick and broad, hardly perceptible
4	Fat	Not visible	Sleek appearance	Difficult to touch, runs in straight line	Rounded	Outline not visible	Tough to grasp
5	Obesity (fatty health)	Buried in fat	Excessive fat	Reference markings lost	Bulging	Impossible to grasp	Non-palpable

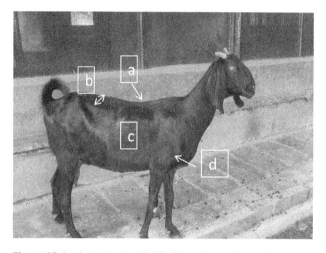

Figure 12.1 Assessment criteria for body condition score in a Beetal goat. (a) Backbone; (b) transition from spinous to transverse process; (c) rib cage; (d) sternum.

affects the requirement: as the number of kids increases, so does the nutrient requirement. In general, dairy breeds require more nutrients than reared for meat or fiber. A decreased plane of nutrition is evident in inclement weather.

12.3 Major Production Diseases Encountered in Goats

12.3.1 Pregnancy Toxemia in Ewes (Twin Kid Disease)

Pregnancy toxemia is a multifactorial disease characterized by nervous signs (convulsions and recumbency), dystocia,

and fetal mortality. The disease is seen mainly in late gestation, in goats with a BCS of 2 or with multiple fetuses.

12.3.1.1 Etiology
Increased energy demands in later pregnancy with a decreased plane of nutrition have been proposed as the most likely precipitating cause of pregnancy toxemia. In fact, in the latter part of pregnancy the demand increases rapidly, but feed intake cannot be increased because of decreased rumen size, leading to a decreased plane of nutrition. A metabolic state of hypoglycemia along with hyperketonemia results in ketonuria.

12.3.1.2 Epidemiology
The disease is seen more in pregnant ewes in the later part of pregnancy, especially in the last six weeks of gestation when there is a rapid rise in demand for metabolizable energy. Does carrying twins or triplets are most susceptible, as demand rise steeply and rumen space for feed is decreased. Animals overfed in early pregnancy are more prone to pregnancy toxemia, as a voluntary decrease is seen due to the decrease in rumen size because of high abdominal fat and increase in uterus size. In a recent study conducted in Brazil, 66 pregnant multiparous (third or fourth parturition) does were selected for determining the energy requirements for maintenance of dairy goats during pregnancy and their efficiency of use. Of these 66 does, 8 were selected for a baseline and the rest were randomly divided into three groups with a further three blocks. The conclusion of the study indicated that the female mobilizes body reserves to meet the energy demands of the pregnancy when the diet supplied does not meet those

Table 12.2 Changes in energy requirement in pregnant does of 70 kg with or without multiple kids.

	Total digestible nutrients (energy)	Dry matter intake
Maintenance	1.50 lb (53%)	2.82 lb
Late gestation, single kid	2.18 lb (53%)	4.11 lb
Last gestation, twins	2.46 lb (66%)	3.70 lb
Early lactation, single kid	2.02 lb (53%)	3.81 lb
Early lactation, twins	2.24 lb (53%)	4.25 lb

Source: Adapted from National Research Council, Nutrient Requirements of Small Ruminants, 2007.

requirements (Härter et al. 2017, p. 4181). A huge difference and increase in demand have been shown in a report by the National Research Council on the nutritional requirements of small ruminants and are shown in Table 12.2. As demonstrated, a 13% difference in energy requirement was reported with a difference in single kids or twins. At flock level, morbidity is seen to be around 5% and case mortality can reach 80% (Rook 2000, p. 293). From an epidemiological point of view, it is clear that a single case in a flock is said to be tip of an iceberg. Online tools for energy requirement calculation of the daily energy requirements for lactating goats can be used to determine the exact requirement (http://www.luresext.edu/sites/all/themes/hertz/html/me4pop.html), depending on the type of goat rearing being practiced and the body weight of the goat.

12.3.1.3 Types of Pregnancy Toxemia
On the basis of etiology, pregnancy toxemia can be classified into five types:

- **Primary pregnancy toxemia**: Mainly seen in does with a decrease in nutritional status caused by a short period of food deprivation, either due to lower availability of pasture or decreased grazing duration because of inclement weather.
- **Secondary pregnancy toxemia**: Due to intercurrent diseases (foot rot, haemonchus, or heavy parasitism) leading to anorexia and ultimately a decreased plane of nutrition.
- **Starvation pregnancy toxemia:** Due to starvation, feed deprivation, and bad management practices. This is more common in drought-prone areas and in goats with a poor BCS.
- **Stress-induced pregnancy toxemia:** Stress can be induced in goats subjected to strenuous exercise, long-distance walking, dipping, and change in environment, leading to release of cortisol and a hypoglycemic state.

- **Pregnancy toxemia associated with fatness**: Occurs in well-fed or overfed does in late pregnancy. If the animal is overfed in early pregnancy they are more prone to it as a voluntary decrease in nutrients takes place because of high abdominal fat decreasing the rumen size, or an increasing uterus size because of twins and triplets.

12.3.1.4 Pathogenesis
The exact pathophysiology of pregnancy toxemia is poorly understood in goats. Lack of energy and increasing demands from the fetus result in the creation of a negative energy balance leading to lipid mobilization, ketonemia, and increased cortisol production. Fetal development in the pregnant doe rises rapidly during the last six weeks. Encephalopathy is seen, which may be due to hypoglycemia. Usually, the disease is irreversible unless treated very early.

12.3.1.5 Clinical Signs
Severe clinical signs may be seen for a short duration, very infrequently, and they can be mixed. If the onset of disease occur earlier than day 140 of gestation, it will be more severe and with an increased risk of mortality. The major clinical signs observed are:

- Separation of some animals from the herd.
- Lack of interest in feeding and declining to move, but otherwise alert.
- Apparent blindness.
- Constipation (dry and scanty feces).
- Grinding of teeth.
- Depression.
- Drowsiness in later stages of the disease.

Nervous signs seen are:

- Tremors of head.
- Twitching of lips.
- Champing of jaw.
- Hypersalivation.
- Clonic contraction of cervical muscle (lateral deviation of head).
- Incoordination.
- Falling while walking.

After a convulsion episode fades, the animal may appear normal but is blind. Star gazing may be seen, and ketotic breath and fetal death are common and sometimes immediate.

12.3.1.6 Clinical Pathology
Hypoglycemia and ketonemia are the major alterations associated with pregnancy toxemia. In diseased recumbent does, hypoglycemia might not be present. Experimental induction of pregnancy toxemia in pregnant does by

fastening, as conducted in an experiment in Egypt, revealed a significant increase in β-hydroxybutyrate, cortisol, and insulin levels, while there were significant decreases in glucose, thyroid, and immunoglobulins (IgA, IgM, and IgG). Scientists working on the experiment determined correlations between the different key alterations and found that plasma glucose concentrations had significant negative correlations with β-hydroxybutyrate, cortisol, and insulin, while the correlations were significantly positive with immunoglobulins and thyroid hormone. Persistent elevated ketonemia can result in ketonuria, and goats can develop metabolic acidosis leading to renal failure. Dehydration and uremia develop, and liver function tests might show dysfunction (Hefnawy et al. 2010, pp. 1–4).

12.3.1.7 Diagnosis

Preliminary diagnosis of disease can be made on the basis of a history of the flock being affected and the appearance of clinical signs. On the basis of clinical pathology, hypoglycemia will be present. The normal serum level of glucose in goats is 30–50 mg%. While evaluating the glucose level, care must be taken as a normal level or hyperglycemia can be seen in advanced and recumbent animals. Cerebrospinal fluid (CSF) glucose levels are more accurate than blood, as they remain low even when serum glucose rebounds in advanced cases after fetal death. Urinalysis for the presence of ketone bodies can be done to determine ketonuria. The value of β-hydroxybutyrate can be evaluated using a ketometer; elevated values are consistent with the disease. Plasma cortisol is high in infected cases and can be estimated for research purposes. Postmortem changes in dead animals will reveal lesions showing fatty degeneration of the liver, degeneration of neurons, and necrosis in the central nervous system (CNS). A dead fetus may be seen in varying degrees of decomposition.

12.3.1.8 Differential Diagnosis

Pregnancy toxemia needs to be differentiated from hypocalcemia.

12.3.1.9 Treatment

For favorable results, early treatment needs to be given. Hypoglycemia can be treated by a single intravenous injection of 60–100 ml 50% dextrose, followed by balanced electrolyte solution with 5% dextrose. Along with this insulin are given 20–40 units protamine zinc insulin, intramuscularly, every other day. Once the animal is recumbent dextrose therapy can even lead to death, therefore simultaneous evaluation of the glucose level must be considered. Oral propylene glycol (60 ml twice a day for 3 days, or 100 ml/day). In the latter part of gestation and near to kidding, induction of parturition/cesarian in the early part of the disease may be helpful.

12.3.1.10 Prevention and Control Measures

The disease can be prevented by continuous monitoring of the herd and maintaining the flock within a range of 3–3.5 BCS on a scale of 1–5. Feeding good concentrate feed, and avoiding overfeeding and overfattening, are ideal to prevent pregnancy toxemia. Restrict stressful conditions as far as possible.

12.3.2 Hypomagnesemia Tetany (Grass Tetany, Grass Staggers, Lactation Tetany, Wheat Pasture Poisoning)

Hypomagnesemia tetany is a multifactorial, highly fatal condition directly or indirectly linked to deficiency of magnesium. The disease is characterized by tonic–clonic convulsions and tetany.

12.3.2.1 Etiology

Magnesium deficiency is the main etiological factor, which is attributable to multiple other factors. Magnesium is mainly present in bone and is not readily mobilized in adults (Martens and Schweigel 2001). Magnesium inside the body is absorbed through the ruminant forestomach and the balance between its availability and the demands determines the disease status. Dietary intake is the major input, whereas its usage inside the body and excretion through milk is the major output. Most of the time dietary input of magnesium is sufficient to meet requirement; in cases of dietary deficiency urinary excretion does not stop until a threshold is reached that leads to continuous drainage aggravating the condition. This excretion is under the control of parathyroid hormone (PTH). Drainage of magnesium in goat milk occurs at a rate of 14 mg/100 g of milk and on average, depending on the breed, a goat produces 2–5 kg of milk/day during a lactation period of 8–10 months. This drainage requires an adequate supply of magnesium throughout lactation, and therefore it is at the time of peak lactation with poor dietary supplementation that disease occurs. In kids, absorption of magnesium can occur from the intestine.

12.3.2.2 Factors Affecting Absorption of Magnesium

- Foraging on young, rapidly growing grasses can predispose the animal, as grasses at this stage are rich in potassium and low in sodium, which ultimately disrupts the functioning of sodium-dependent ATPase transportation across the ruminal wall. A potassium : magnesium ratio of 3 : 1 or less decreases absorption.
- Saliva plays a crucial role, as it contains a high sodium concentration, helping in absorption of magnesium. However, when deficiency of sodium occurs in the diet it

activates aldosterone, leading to replacement of potassium instead of sodium, further decreasing the absorption of magnesium.

- Feeding on grasses top-dressed with nitrogen, phosphorus, and potassium (NPK) fertilizers will result in excess ammonia being produced, which hinders absorption.
- Readily fermentable carbohydrates increase absorption as the volatile fatty acids (VFAs) produced provide the energy for active transportation of magnesium.
- An alkaline pH of the rumen decreases its absorption.
- Cereal crops of wheat, barley, and oats have a high potassium content.
- Decreased absorption is seen in animals suffering from diarrhea and gastroenteritis.

12.3.2.3 Epidemiology

Hypomagnesemia tetany is seen in goats grazed on forages grown on sandy, leached, and acidic soil, as they are magnesium deficient. Cold or inclement weather, transportation stress, and herd movement predispose goats to hypomagnesemia. Lactating does are more prone than non-lactating ones. Does carrying multiple fetuses are more affected than those carrying a single fetus. The disease is rarely seen in intensively reared goats as they are fed with concentrate (Figure 12.2).

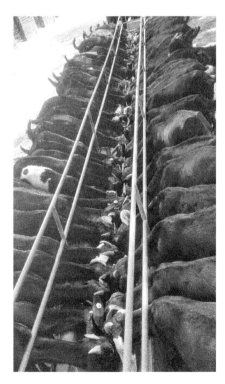

Figure 12.2 Regular feeding of concentrate to Beetal and Jakrana goats reared intensively without a single case report of hypomagnesemia in the last five years.

12.3.2.4 Pathogenesis

Magnesium is one of the major cations involved in the transmission of impulses and plays a crucial role as an adjuvant to enzymes. Magnesium influences four main things: activation of cholinesterase, release of acetylcholine, sensitivity of the motor plate, and threshold of the muscle membrane. Less availability of magnesium leads to irregular muscular impulses and muscular irritability results in nervous signs. The CSF function is more affected than the peripheral nerve function.

12.3.2.5 Clinical Signs

The disease is seen in three forms: acute, subacute, and chronic.

- In acute cases, initially the grazing animal stops eating suddenly, has unusual alertness, is uncomfortable, there is twitching of muscles and ears, severe hyperesthesia, and slight disturbances leading to continuous bellowing. Normal vitals are elevated because of severe muscle exertion.
- In subacute cases, onset is gradual with the animal becoming anorectic, uncomfortable, and hyperesthetic. Spasmodic urination, frequent defecation, muscular tremors, trismus, and tetany are seen. Sound around the animal will precipitate seizures.
- In chronic hypomagnesemia sudden death can occur in a few animals with non-diagnostic and non-typical signs.

12.3.2.6 Diagnosis

Tentative diagnosis can be done on the basis of clinical signs (nervous signs) and a history of grazing on lush grass. For final confirmation of the disease, serum levels of magnesium need to be estimated. The normal serum level of magnesium in goats is 0.90–1.26 mmol/l.

The CSF level of magnesium is more predictive than the serum level. Blood magnesium levels below 1.1 mg/dl coincide with clinical signs. The degree of decrease in level correlates with the severity of clinical signs.

12.3.2.7 Differential Diagnosis

- **Pregnancy toxemia**: Hypoglycemia will be present, which is not in hypomagnesemic tetany.
- **Rabies**: The clinical picture is different from hypomagnesemia as signs of frenzy will be present.

12.3.2.8 Treatment

In subacute cases, animals given early treatment respond well, but if treatment is delayed then recovery is transient and relapses may occur. The response varies from animal to animal and area to area. Treatment in goats is usually initiated by 50 ml intravenous therapy of a combination of calcium borogluconate (25%) and magnesium hypophosphate (5%) as a first dose followed by subcutaneous injection of a concentrated solution of a magnesium salt. Infusion of magnesium inside the body needs to be done cautiously, as there is a risk of cardiac arrest. Magnesium sulfate (20%) solution should be used as a second dose, although magnesium lactate or magnesium gluconate (15%) can be used. In emergency cases, use magnesium chloride at 30 g in 100 ml intrarectally.

12.3.2.9 Prevention and Control

- Management should consist of avoiding any type of stress, inclement type of weather, starvation, and unnecessary transport.
- Magnesium oxide should be given orally at 10 g/day/animal or magnesium phosphate at half the dose. As these magnesium salts are unpalatable they must be fed along with molasses.
- In those animals where there is a deficiency in the soil, magnesium oxide should be sprayed on the pasture at 30 kg/ha.
- When cases begin in a flock, give 7 g/day magnesium oxide orally to all animals to avoid further incidences at the farm.

12.3.3 Parturient Paresis (Milk Fever and Hypocalcemia)

Parturient paresis is a production disease of goats that occurs during the periparturient period, usually before and rarely after parturition. The etiology involves metabolic disturbance and is characterized by hypocalcemia, general muscular weakness, circulatory collapse, recumbency, shock, and ultimately death. A combination of tetany or flaccid paralysis or both is seen. The name "milk fever" is a mismoner, as the condition is non-febrile and no fever occurs during the disease, but on the other hand a subnormal temperature is seen in most cases.

12.3.3.1 Etiology

It is well known that hypocalcemia is the main cause of milk fever. Hypocalcemia occurs because of an increase in calcium requirements during the periparturient period. The requirement for calcium increases three weeks before parturition when mineralization of calcium in the fetal skeleton starts, particularly when twins or triplets are expected. Hence, the disease is mostly encountered before parturition and rarely after parturition. Drainage of calcium in colostrum (2 g/day) even exceeds the preparturient daily requirement of calcium associated with mineralization of the fetal skeleton (1.2 g/day), such that dairy animals are prone to suffer from milk fever in early lactation, as seen in cattle. However, goats kept for other purposes than milk production are rarely challenged with colostral

production and hence they generally suffer from the disease pre parturition. Dry-matter intake decreases as the doe approaches kidding and, because of the size of the uterus, the decrease is more in cases of twins. Decreased dry-matter intake means decreased calcium availability and at the same time the increased calcium demand for fetal skeleton development leads to deficiency. The normal serum level of calcium is 3.6–9.4 mg/dl (0.9–2.35 mmol/l). Levels below 5–6 mg/dl in animals make them dangerously predisposed to milk fever. This can be attributed to the fact that calcium gets drained in colostrum, so that colostrum contains a high level of calcium (2.3 g/kg) compared to milk, which contains 1.2 g/kg calcium. The levels of calcium in the ionized form are more important than those in the non-ionized (elemental) form.

There are three main precipitating factors of disease occurrence: high milk yield, low calcium absorption, and low calcium resorption; that is, mobilization of calcium from the body reserves (skeleton).

Several other factors are found to be associated with disease:

- **Feeding a high-calcium diet during pregnancy**: This leads to occurrence of the disease by inactivating the parathyroid gland. PTH is an important factor that regulates the body's calcium levels. Feeding excess calcium in the diet makes PTH quiescent. PTH plays a role in calcium metabolism by an increase in calcium absorption and resorption leading to an increase in calcium level. Because PTH is quiescent and there is an increase in the body's requirement for calcium after parturition, hypocalcemia occurs because a simultaneous increase in PTH level suddenly does not take place. Alongside this, heavy drainage of calcium in milk results in a decrease in the calcium level in the blood.
- **Prolonged dry period**: The body's demand of calcium is low in dry periods, hence inactivating PTH.
- **Deficiency of vitamin D3 (dihydrocholecalciferol)**: This is also one of the major factors in maintaining the balance of the calcium level in the blood, but the degree of association is less compared with that for PTH.
- **Oxalate in feed**: Some plants contain more oxalates than others. They chelate with calcium to form calcium oxalate, which leads to unavailability of free calcium. This is a minor factor in causation of the disease.
- **Hypophosphatemia**: This is associated with hypocalcemia, as the Ca : P ratio in the milk gets disturbed.
- **High estrogen level after kidding**: A high level of estrogen leads to decreased ionization of calcium and also a decrease in appetite or anorexia. It is also a minor factor.
- **Thyrocalcitonin**: This is formed by the thyroid gland and is responsible for decreasing the blood calcium level, thus influencing the development of disease.

- **Calcium cyclers**: These are cows or dairy animals in which there is periodical hypocalcemia that is subclinical in nature. It remains for one or two days and is normal for nine days, then the calcium level decreases again. It may have a minor association with the disease condition. Researchers say that the degree of ionization is related to calcium cyclers and some to the estrogen level (Gennari et al. 1990).

12.3.3.2 Epidemiology

The disease can occur from 6 weeks before to ten weeks after parturition. The incidence of milk fever generally increases alongside the increase in milk production. Pregnant pluriparous does are commonly predisposed to the condition, as they have larger feto-placental requirements before kidding. The disease is rarely encountered in goats raised for meat production because of less milk production and subsequent drainage of calcium. High-producing doe goats have an incidence of milk fever similar to dairy cattle. Grazing on forages rich in phosphorous can lead to inversion of the Ca : P ratio, leading to hypocalcemia, and grazing on poor pasture further increases the risk of disease. Winter climatic conditions also predispose does to hypocalcemia, as a state of vitamin D deficiency develops that ultimately leads to a decrease in calcium absorption from the gastrointestinal tract (GIT). Unlike cattle, individual animals are rarely affected and most cases in goats are seen as outbreaks and in flocks exposed to strenuous exercise. In general, 5% of animals in a flock can be affected, but the figure can reach 30%.

12.3.3.3 Pathogenesis

Calcium is responsible for the muscular tone of skeletal and smooth muscle. A low level of calcium leads to muscular atony, decreased GIT motility, decreased stroke volume, and decreased consciousness. This is seen because calcium is responsible for release of the neurotransmitter acetylcholine, which mediates the transmission of nerve impulses at the myoneural junction. In the initial phase of clinical illness, hyperesthesia is seen because of disruption of the membrane stability of peripheral nerves and muscle fibers, which leads to increased stimulation and conduction. This condition is soon followed by pronounced hypocalcemia and severe neuromuscular blockade, resulting in flaccid paralysis. Tetany and flaccid paralysis in does are reported to be severe compared to cattle. It is the interplay of calcium and magnesium levels that determines whether tetany or flaccid paralysis will occur. Pathogenesis with possible outcomes is explained in Figure 12.3.

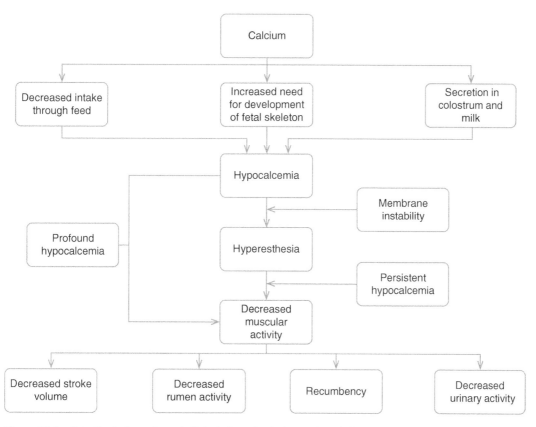

Figure 12.3 Flowchart of events and clinical signs due to hypocalcemia in goats.

12.3.3.4 Clinical Signs

Both preparturient and postparturient forms can occur, depending on the purpose for which the goat is reared. If does are raised purposefully and intensively for milk production, the postparturient form is seen, while the preparturient form is evident in does reared for kids. Disease onset is sudden and often follows within 24 hours of an abrupt change of feed, a sudden change in weather, or short periods of fasting imposed by shearing or transportation. During the early stages of the disease animals become isolated from the herd, have a temporary stiff gait with muscle tremors, and become hyperesthetic. Later they become hyposensitive, weak, and recumbent. Decrease in muscle contractions results in constipation and decreased rumen motility, which can lead to the development of bloat. As disease progression occurs, the affected animals can show symptoms of depression, which usually ends in coma. Goats suffering from milk fever typically have cold ears, whereas rectal temperature usually remains within the normal range.

12.3.3.5 Diagnosis

Diagnosis is mainly done on the basis of history, clinical signs, and clinical pathology. It is further confirmed by assessment of blood or serum calcium levels. Hypocalcemia is often classified as total serum calcium concentration <8 mg/dl or <4.4 mg/dl ionized calcium (normal value for serum calcium 8.8–12.2 mg/dl).

12.3.3.6 Differential Diagnosis

- **Pregnancy toxemia**: Hypocalcemia and pregnancy toxemia may co-exist. It is difficult to differentiate the two diseases at a farm level. They can only be differentiated by measuring concentrations of calcium and β-hydroxybutyrate in the blood of affected animals.
- **Ephemeral fever**: The disease is infectious in nature, involving fever for a short duration, whereas hypocalcemia is non-infectious with an absence of fever.
- **Injury to limbs due to obturator nerve or sciatic nerve injury or paralysis**: In these conditions the suffering animal is alert and conscious, whereas in hypocalcemia animals become comatose.
- **Coliform mastitis**: Fever is present in case of mastitis along with prevalent changes in the milk picture, which are absent in a case of hypocalcemia.
- **Septicemic metritis**: Fever is evident along with toxemic changes in the blood picture. There is discharge from the vagina in affected animals. These conditions are absent in a case of hypocalcemia.

12.3.3.7 Treatment

Several principles are followed for treatment and the most important is to give treatment as early as possible. Treating the case promptly can reduce the chances of mortality. Education of herders about the clinical signs they observe can bring a case to the notice of veterinarians.

Hypocalcemia responds immediately within five minutes in cases when no other concurrent illnesses exist. Intravenous administration of 30–60 ml of 20% borogluconate at body temperature can be done. Care must be taken to infuse the first dose strictly through the intravenous route. Always be on site to examine the animal during administration. Sometimes an unfavorable response to therapy is also observed, like cardiac arrythmia, but it should not be gross arrythmia; if it is, then stop and readminister very carefully. As soon as something adverse is seen, stop administration. The heart rate should be audible; if any sound is undesirable then stop the infusion and start again. If recovery does not occur, a second dose of 60 ml calcium borogluconate can be administered subcutaneously. A third dose of 50 ml if required can be repeated after 24 hours. The maximum dose administered to a doe should not exceed 170 ml (Brozos et al. 2011, p. 109). Causes of failure of therapy can be late therapy, insufficient dose, concurrent disease, and deficiency of other nutrients.

12.3.3.8 Prevention of Milk Fever

Milk fever can be prevented by educating the owner about the side effects of a high-calcium diet during the last 15 days of pregnancy. A specific control program should be started in a flock if incidence is more than 10%, involving a concerted effort and money. Postparturient care should be undertaken for 48 hours. The parturient animal should be looked at and treatment given if needed. A high-phosphorous diet should be avoided, as it inhibits the renal enzyme that catalyzes the synthesis of vitamin D3 and also retards the absorption of calcium from the GIT. Maintaining a negative cation–anion balance leads to high intestinal calcium absorption, increases calcium resorption, and keeps the parathyroid gland active. The cation–anion balance should be negative or <10 meq/100 g of dry-matter feed. For this, ammonium chloride or ammonium sulfate 100 g each should be administered 21 days prior to parturition. In browsing or grain-fed goats, the addition of a calcium supplement (dicalcium phosphate, limestone, etc.) to the feed or to a salt or trace mineral–salt mixture usually meets calcium requirements. Care must be taken with feedstuffs containing a high level of oxalates.

Multiple-Choice Questions

1 The body condition score of goats in a flock should be maintained around what level to prevent metabolic diseases?
   A 2
   B 3
   C 4
   D 5

2 What biochemical alteration(s) are observed in pregnancy toxemia?
   A Hypoglycemia
   B Ketonemia
   C Both hypoglycemia and ketonemia
   D Both hyperglycemia and ketonemia

3 When is milk fever in goats mostly seen?
   A Preparturient
   B Postparturient
   C Equally pre- and postparturient
   D No correlation with parturition

4 Which of the following is false with regard to pregnancy toxemia?
   A Seen in late gestation
   B Occurs more in goats with multiple fetuses
   C Results in nervous signs, dystocia, and fetal mortality
   D Hyperglycemia is seen as the main biochemical change

5 Which of the following is false for hypomagnesemic tetany?
   A Goat milk contains magnesium at 14 mg/100 g of milk
   B High potassium decreases magnesium absorption
   C Magnesium plays a role in muscular conduction
   D Deficiency of magnesium results in discharge of acetylcholine

6 Which of the following is not a factor associated with milk fever?
   A Feeding a high-calcium diet during pregnancy
   B High milk yield
   C Oxalate in feed
   D High estrogen level after kidding

7 What is the range of total serum levels of calcium in cattle in mg/dl?
   A 2.2–6.6
   B 8.8–12.2
   C 10.4–14.2
   D 6.4–10.6

8 By what route should the first injection of calcium in milk fever be given?
   A Intravenous
   B Subcutaneous
   C Intradermal
   D Intraperitoneal

9 How can milk fever be prevented?
   A Maintaining a negative dietary cation–anion balance
   B Avoiding excess phosphorous in the diet
   C Careful feeding of feeds with oxalates
   D All of the above

10 How is pregnancy toxemia associated with parasitism classified?
   A Primary
   B Secondary
   C Starvation
   D Stress induced

11 Where is magnesium absorbed in ruminants?
   A Rumen
   B Small intestine
   C Abomasum
   D Large intestine

12 How is hyperesthesia in hypocalcemia initially seen?
   A Increased muscular tone
   B Muscle membrane instability
   C Decreased muscular tone
   D Increased vascularity

13 Which of the following is milk fever in goats not associated with?
   A Decreased gastrointestinal tract motility
   B Decreased stroke volume
   C Tetany and flaccid paralysis depending on magnesium concentration
   D Elevated body temperature

14 Which of the following is false with respect to the body condition score?
   A Indicates fat cover/fat reserve of body
   B Reflects nutritional status
   C Reflects animal welfare management
   D All of the above

15 Which of the following is false with respect to milk fever?
   A Ionized calcium level is more important than non-ionized calcium level
   B Fever is not evident in milk fever
   C Increased fetal calcium demand leads to preparturient hypocalcemia
   D Flaccid paralysis is evident in goats

References

Brozos, C., Mavrogianni, V.S., and Fthenakis, G.C. (2011). Treatment and control of peri-parturient metabolic diseases: pregnancy toxemia, hypocalcemia, hypomagnesemia. *Veterinary Clinics of North America: Food Animal Practice* 27 (1): 105–113. https://doi.org/10.1016/j.cvfa.2010.10.004.

Härter, C.J., Lima, L.D., Silva, H.G.O. et al. (2017). Energy and protein requirements for maintenance of dairy goats during pregnancy and their efficiencies of use. *Journal of Animal Science* 95: 4181–4193.

Hefnawy, E., Youssef, S., and Shousha, S. (2010). Some immunohormonal changes in experimentally pregnant toxemic goats. *Veterinary Medicine International* 2010: 768438. https://doi.org/10.4061/2010/768438.

Koyuncu, M. and Altınçekiç, S.O. (2013). Importance of body condition score in dairy goats. *Macedonian Journal of Animal Science* 3 (2): 167–173.

Martens, H. and Schweigel, M. (2001). Magnesium homeostasis and grass tetany. In: *Advances in Magnesium Research: Nutrition and Health* (ed. Y. Rayssiguier, A. Mazur, and J. Durlach), 475–481. London: John Libbey.

Moeini, M.M., Kachuee, R., and Jalilian, M.T. (2014). The effect of body condition score and body weight of Merghoz goats on production and reproductive performance. *Journal of Animal and Poultry Sciences* 3 (3): 86–94.

National Research Council (2007). *Nutrient Requirements of Small Ruminants: Sheep, Goats, Cervids, and New World Camelids*. Washington, DC: NRC.

Rook, J.S. (2000). Pregnancy toxemia of ewes, does, and beef cows. *Veterinary Clinics of North America: Food Animal Practice* 16: 293–317.

Further Reading

Fthenakis, G. (2022). Pregnancy toxemia in sheep and goats. *MSD Veterinary Manual*. Rahway, NJ: Merck. https://www.msdvetmanual.com/metabolic-disorders/hepatic-lipidosis/pregnancy-toxemia-in-sheep-and-goats

Gennari, C., Agnusdei, D., Nardi, P. et al. (1990). Estrogen preserves a normal intestinal responsiveness to 1,25-dihydroxyvitamin D3 in oophorectomized women. *Journal of Clinical Endocrinology & Metabolism* 71 (5): 1288–1293.

Dua, K. and Care, A.D. (1995). Impaired absorption of magnesium in the aetiology of grass tetany. *British Veterinary Journal* 151: 413–426.

Goff, J.P. (2009). Milk fever (parturient paresis) in cows, ewes, and doe goats. In: *Current Veterinary Therapy: Food Animal Practice*, 5e (ed. D.E. Anderson and D.M. Rings), 135–140. Philadelphia, PA: W.B. Saunders. doi: 10.1016/B978-141603591-6.10033-8.

Oetzel, G.R. and Goff, J.P. (2009). Milk fever (parturient paresis) in cows, ewes, and doe goats. In: *Current Veterinary Therapy: Food Animal Practice*, 5e (ed. D.E. Anderson and D.M. Rings), 130–134. Philadelphia, PA: W.B. Saunders https://doi.org/10.1016/B978-141603591-6.10033-8.

Radostits, O.M., Gay, C.C., and Hinchcliff, K.W. (2007). *Veterinary Medicine: A Textbook of the Diseases of Cattle, Horses, Sheep, Pigs, and Goats*, 10e. Philadelphia, PA: W.B. Saunders.

13

Poisoning in Goats

Kamlesh A. Sadariya, Shailesh K. Bhavsar, and Tamanna H. Solanki

Department of Veterinary Pharmacology and Toxicology, College of Veterinary Science and Animal Husbandry, Kamdhenu University, Anand, Gujarat, India

Goats are multipurpose animals that produce meat, milk, hide, fiber, and manure, and are also very versatile in nature as they can easily survive in different environmental conditions (Podder et al. 2020). The goat is regarded as the "poor man's cow" and the archeological evidence indicates an association of goats with humans in a symbiotic relationship for 10 000 years (Singh et al. 2020). Marginal and small farmers, landless rural and urban poor, and professional breeders leading a nomadic to semi-nomadic life are associated with goat-rearing in India and in several other countries (Sejian et al. 2021).

Poisoning in goats is seldom recorded and most poisoning accidents in food-producing animals occur in cattle, followed by sheep and goats. Poisoning appears to be an uncommon cause of illness in animals compared to other clinical problems such as infectious diseases, trauma, or neoplasia. One reason for this may be a lack of information on the most common toxicants affecting the veterinary species, so consequently there is little information available to guide and facilitate diagnosis, as reported toxicological incidence is very scarce for goats. It should be noted that most published cases of poisoning refer to special and/or unusual cases, since common causes of poisoning are rarely published, and reliable and complete toxico-epidemiological data are not easy to obtain for goats.

Similar to cattle and buffalo, small ruminant species like sheep and goats are likely to encounter many toxic agents. Sensitivity, clinical signs, and lesions can vary greatly between bovines and small ruminants (Schweitzer et al. 1984; Basaraba et al. 1999; Bozynski et al. 2009). A further difficulty with investigating causes of animal poisoning is that neither the veterinarian nor the animal owner is obliged to report the case nor to send samples for chemical analysis. Even when this does occur, the results are usually not published (even in annual reports) and there are only sporadic peer-reviewed papers dealing with regional incidences of animal poisoning. This limited reporting obscures the incidence of accidental or malicious poisoning, particularly when only a limited number of samples from the total number of animals involved, or only the baits used in poisoning attempts, are sent for analysis and the results recorded. Furthermore, only a few possible toxicants can be investigated in the designated laboratories, so that new chemicals are often not detected and, consequently, the real number of positive cases may be underestimated in goats and other farm animals (Guitart et al. 2010; Radke 2021).

Toxic plants and mycotoxins, heavy metals, and pesticides are most often suspected as toxic agents in the five countries that data has been obtained from: Belgium, France, Greece, Italy, and Spain. Limited attention is paid to small and large animal toxicology problems except when the economic loss is high (Guitart et al. 2010). The most common toxic agents are toxic plants, heavy metals, and pesticides, which are suspected of being involved in food-animal poisoning in Belgium, while pesticides are the most common class of toxicants in France, where insecticides and seed-coat products are involved, followed by drugs, plants, and nutritional disorders (e.g. urea poisoning, grain overload) (Royer and Buronfosse 1998).

Goats may be exposed to several toxicants, hence it is important to note what toxic agents species are susceptible to and how animals are affected in order to effectively diagnose and treat poisoning in goats. Common causes of poisoning in goats are depicted in Figure 13.1, while some toxicants causing poisoning in goats and their therapeutic management are outlined in Table 13.1.

The objective of this chapter is to provide a brief review of some of the more common toxicities in goats in India and across the world. It also summarizes several cases associated with toxicants for poisoning in goats and provides insight into situations practitioners may find themselves in for diagnosis and therapeutic management of common poisoning in goats.

Principles of Goat Disease and Prevention, First Edition. Edited by Tanmoy Rana.
© 2024 John Wiley & Sons, Inc. Published 2024 by John Wiley & Sons, Inc.

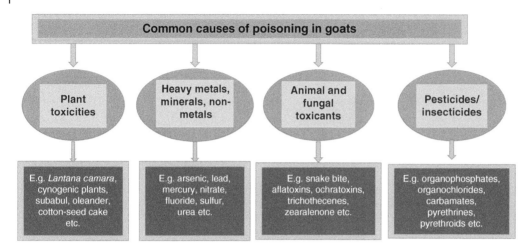

Common causes of poisoning in goats

Plant toxicities

E.g. *Lantana camara*, cynogenic plants, subabul, oleander, cotton-seed cake etc.

Heavy metals, minerals, non-metals

E.g. arsenic, lead, mercury, nitrate, fluoride, sulfur, urea etc.

Animal and fungal toxicants

E.g. snake bite, aflatoxins, ochratoxins, trichothecenes, zearalenone etc.

Pesticides/ insecticides

E.g. organophosphates, organochlorides, carbamates, pyrethrines, pyrethroids etc.

Figure 13.1 Common causes of poisoning in goats.

Table 13.1 Toxicants causing poisoning in goats and their therapeutic management.

Toxicants	Common toxic effect	Management of poisoning
Lantana camara poisoning	Hepatotoxicity, secondary photosensitization, and jaundice	Activated charcoal and supportive therapy along with provision of dark and cool place for animal, also take preventive measures
Cyanogenic glycosides/ cyanide poisoning	Cherry-colored blood, bitter almond-like smell from exhaled breath and ruminal contents	Sodium thiosulphate and sodium nitrite, also give supportive and symptomatic therapy
Subabul poisoning	Inappetence, complete loss of hair from all over the body, dryness and scaling of the skin	Mineral mixture, liver tonic, also take preventive measures
Urea poisoning	Ataxia, incoordination, muscle fasciculations, tremor, ptyalism, anuria, bloat, and convulsive seizures	Administration of cold water and diluted acetic acid (vinegar)
Nitrate/nitrite poisoning	Cyanotic mucous membranes and respiratory distress, chocolate brown-colored blood	Methylene blue, also give supportive and symptomatic therapy
Organophosphate poisoning	Salivation, tympany, tachypnea, polydipsia, urination, diarrhea, bradycardia, miosis, tremor, and convulsions	Atropine sulphate and symptomatic treatment

13.1 Toxic Plant Poisoning

Goats eat mostly woody and weedy plants and may be exposed to poisonous plants. Eating toxic plants can result in decreased productivity, animal deaths, and significant economic losses for producers. Knowledge of poisonous plants can help producers to identify and safely remove them from pastures before they cause harm to livestock. Animals can be poisoned by many different plant species, but an analytically confirmed diagnosis is not always easy and most cases are only suspected following necropsy and identification of leaves, stems, or pods in the rumen of an animal. Photographs of some of the toxic plants that cause poisoning in goats are provided in Figure 13.2.

Goats are very independent and curious creatures. As part of their curiosity, they explore their world by mouthing and tasting things, which has earned them the unfortunate reputation of eating everything and anything. Instead of grazing like sheep and cows, goats are browsers. This means that they tend to wander more and eat from plants that are at eye level. A few leaves from this, move on to another plant, and so on. Their ability to stand on their hind legs and their mobile upper lip allow them to reach tree leaves and other tasty greens that are not on the ground. Browsing is another defense against eating toxic plants, because if the goat does eat some, hopefully it is not too much. Here we discuss few of the plants that have the potential to produce toxicity in goats when they are eaten in excess quantity. These are the most common plant toxicities in goats.

(a)

(b)

(c)

(d)

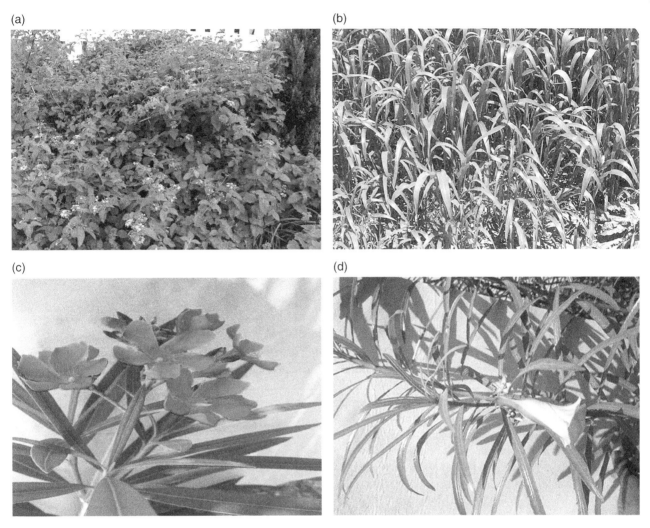

Figure 13.2 Common toxic plants causing poisoning in goats. (a) *Latana camara*; (b) *Sorghum vulgare*; (c) *Nerium indicum*; and (d) *Thevetia peruviana*.

13.1.1 *Lantana camara* Poisoning

Lantana camara is an exotic ornamental plant. Poisoning mainly occurs when stock unfamiliar with the plant are introduced to areas with *Lantana* weeds and toxicity occurs if the animal consumes 1% or more of its body weight, depending on the toxic content (Shafi et al. 2020). The leaves and immature berries of *Lantana* are more toxic to livestock (Haritha et al. 2019). Its toxicity is reported in cattle, buffalo, sheep, goats, camels, horses, dogs, guinea pigs, rabbits, ostriches, and rats (Sharma et al. 2007; Kumar et al. 2018; Ambica et al. 2020; Govindaiah et al. 2021).

L. camara causes toxicity in grazing animals due to the presence of active substances called lantadenes. It causes hepatotoxicity, photosensitization, and jaundice in grazing animals (Sharma et al. 2007). Other clinical signs are sluggishness, edematous ears and eyelids, cracks and fissures on the muzzle and other non-hairy parts, conjunctivitis, ulceration of the tip and under-surface of the tongue

(if unpigmented), and a pale conjunctival, vulvar, or vaginal mucous membrane. *L. camara* can cause secondary photosensitization due to the accumulation of phylloerythrin in the system because of compromised liver function. The animals die within two to four days in acute cases and dose-dependent mortality was reported in subacute poisoning (Parimoo et al. 2015).

Toxic effects can be managed by activated charcoal and supportive therapy, along with the provision of a dark and cool place, but this is not very effective in some severely affected or delayed diagnosis cases. A specific antidote for *Lantana* toxicity is still lacking. However, activated charcoal is an effective, quick, and economic chemical that adsorbs the toxins in the rumen and prevents further absorption of toxin in the body (Gupta et al. 2019; Haritha et al. 2019). Preventive measures are more effective than curative measures in *Lantana* toxicity. Prevention can be achieved by keeping the farm *Lantana* free (Gupta et al. 2019) and by providing ad libitum feed and water to animals before allowing them to graze during drought and scarcity periods (Ambica et al. 2020).

Deepa et al. (2017) reported clinical cases of acute *L. camara* poisoning in goats and their successful management. He reported that animals were fed with fresh *L. camara* plants unknowingly four days before showing symptoms like dullness, recumbency, jaundice, ruminal stasis, and photosensitization (showing discomfort and abnormal behavior when taken into sunlight). The mucous membrane and skin of the animals were icteric. They were treated with intravenous (IV) fluid mixed with B-complex vitamins and intramuscular injection of liver stimulants and prednisolone at 1 mg/kg body weight for six days. By the fifth day the animals had started taking food and became normal by two weeks.

Meena et al. (2022) reported *L. camara* poisoning associated with photosensitive dermatitis in Sirohi goats at the Livestock Research Station (LRS), Bojunda (Chittorgarh). Among 422 Sirohi goats in a herd, 19 (10 males, 9 females, aged 7–12 months) were presented with signs of anorexia, ruminal stasis, constipation followed by diarrhea, dehydration, icteric mucous membrane, and weakness in hind limbs, along with a history of grazing for the last four days on pastureland containing *Lantana* shrubs. The affected goats showed discomfort and abnormal behavior in sunlight. Clinical examination also revealed dermal signs including alopecia, erythema, edematous swelling, irritation of hairless areas, and sloughing of epidermis, especially ears, muzzles, neck, shoulder, and perianal, and perivulvar regions. For management of this toxicity, the affected goats were kept in sheds and dark and cool rooms to protect them from direct sunlight to avoid photosensitization, and were provided with adequate fresh water and good feed. The animals were not given green fodder during the course of the sickness. The management of toxic effects was achieved by oral administration of activated charcoal (universal antidote) at 5 g/kg body weight and a purgative.

13.1.2 Cyanogenic Glycoside/Cyanide Poisoning

Cyanide is one of the most potent and rapidly acting inorganic poisons and causes toxicity mainly in ruminants. Amygdalin, prunasin, linamarin, lotaustralin, dhurrin, taxiphyllin, vicianyn, proteacynve, and gynocardin have been detected as the most common glycosides in cyanogenic plants (Gracia and Shepherd 2004). The primary cause of cyanide poisoning in ruminants is the ingestion of plants containing cyanide-producing compounds called cyanogenic glycosides (Arnold et al. 2014).

Acute poisonings by plants containing cyanogenic glycosides are infrequently reported in goats. This is largely because of their browsing habits, which limit the amount of any one plant that is ingested. It is also likely that cases of acute death in goats are not evaluated and go undiagnosed. Cyanide is a highly lethal and rapidly acting toxin to which ruminants are more susceptible. The mechanism of cyanide toxicity is associated with inhibition of oxygen utilization by binding with ferric (trivalent) ion in cytochrome oxidase within mitochondria and resulting in histotoxic anoxia. Generally, signs quickly develop in acute cyanide intoxication, including hyperventilation, decreased blood pressure, hypoxemia-induced convulsions, coma, shock, respiratory failure, and death. Progression after the onset of convulsions is rapid and the animal has the characteristic bright cherry-red mucous membrane (Plumlee 2004). Many articles report that the blood, both arterial and venous, becomes cherry-red from accumulated oxyhemoglobin (Bingham et al. 2001). The rumen may be distended with gas; in some cases, the odor of "bitter almonds" may be detected after opening (Rhian 2012). Immediate diagnosis and treatments with sodium thiosulphate and sodium nitrite can be done together with supportive therapy for cases noticed early.

A clinical case of acute morbidity and mortality in a herd of goats after ingestion of *Heteromeles arbutifolia* is presented by Tegzes et al. (2003). A backyard herd of 60 goats was maintained long term on a diet consisting mostly of squash and cactus, and free access to a mineral block. After pruning what were believed to be olive trees, a neighbor donated the clippings that were subsequently fed to the goat herd. The clippings were later identified as *H. arbutifolia*. Within four hours of feeding, three animals died, and seven were moribund. The affected animals were tachycardic and had marked jugular pulses. Mucous membranes were pale pink. No treatment was instituted in the surviving affected goats. Field necropsies revealed multifocal hemorrhages in lungs and heart and congestion of the gastrointestinal tract.

13.1.3 Subabul Poisoning

Subabul (*Leucaena leucocephala*) is a tropical legume that is now widely distributed in India. In both sheep and goats, the palatability of *L. leucocephala* and inga dulce was ranked first and second, respectively (Gunasekaran et al. 2014). Mimosine, a non-protein free amino acid, is the main toxic principle of subabul. However, toxicity in ruminants depends on the amount and duration of subabul in the diet (Jones et al. 1976). Chronic or acute toxicosis can occur and removal of *L. leucocephala* from the diet is an effective way to treat the animals and hasten their recovery (Jones and Hegarty 1984). Fetal abortions, low fertility, and death were recorded after *Leucaena* feeding.

Effects of *Leucaena* feeding on reproductive performance, especially on the semen quality of goats, were found to reduce the concentration of spermatozoa (Zun Zun et al. 2017).

Many studies have reported natural occurrences of subabul toxicity in goats and its management under field conditions (Vijayakumar and Srinivasa 2018). Mimosine is also an iron chelator and affects metabolism of folate in mammalian cells (Oppenheim et al. 2000). Enzymes involved in blood clotting and fibrinolysis are inhibited by the serine protease inhibitor isolated from the seeds of *Leucaena* (Oliva et al. 2000). Because of high protein content and drought resistance, *L. leucocephala* can be used as an excellent fodder tree, especially during the summer season, but its use is limited due to the toxic principle mimosine. Hence proper measures should be followed to minimize the toxic effects of mimosine and retain protein levels at the optimum. The toxicity of subabul can be prevented by feeding it in the proportion of less than 40% in the diet, adding iodinated salt to subabul during feeding, mineral supplementation, and soaking the subabul in water and drying it off before feeding (Vijayakumar and Srinivasa 2018).

Hatzade et al. 2020 reported mimosine poisoning on the basis of history, clinical examination, and laboratory findings in a male goat. A 2-month-old non-descript male goat kid from the village of Shivani in the district of Akola was presented to the Teaching Veterinary Clinical Complex (TVCC) at the Post Graduate Institute of Veterinary and Animal Sciences, Akola, with the complaint of inappetence, complete loss of hair from all over the body, and dryness and scaling of the skin. History and clinical examination revealed continuous feeding of leaves of the subabul tree for a month, normal rectal temperature (100 °F), bradycardia on auscultation, pale mucous membranes, inappetence, weakness, lethargy, and alopecia all over the body. The case was diagnosed as mimosine poisoning on the basis of history, clinical examination, and laboratory findings. In this case the kid developed the clinical signs one month after feeding the subabul leaves, indicating chronic toxicity. Continuous feeding of subabul leaves for a period of one month manifested clinically as alopecia in this kid. Shivering and lethargy in this case may be due to subclinical deficiency of thyroid hormone and minerals. In this case the kid had diffuse alopecia, which indicated the toxic effect of mimosine. The case was treated with a mineral mixture consisting of vitamins A, D3, and E, iron, iodine, cobalt, manganese, copper, zinc, and sulfur and a liver tonic orally twice a day for a period of two weeks. The owner was advised to withdraw subabul tree leaves from the feed.

13.1.4 Oxalate Poisoning

When a ruminant consumes an oxalate-containing plant, the oxalate is metabolized in four possible ways. First, soluble oxalate may be degraded by rumen bacteria (Allison et al. 1977). Secondly, when calcium is taken with dietary feed that is high in soluble oxalate, oxalate ions in the rumen or intestine combine with calcium or magnesium to form insoluble oxalate crystals, which are then eliminated in the feces. This form of oxalate cannot be absorbed into the body. This leads to disturbances in calcium and phosphorus metabolism and causes excessive mobilization of bone mineral.

Ruminant animals are less affected, but prolonged grazing on some tropical grasses can result in severe hypocalcemia (Seawright et al. 1970). High levels of oxalate in pasture plants were considered as a major factor in urolith formation in grazing animals (McIntosh et al. 1974). In another study, high levels of oxalate in beet tops were related to the occurrence of hypocalcemia and hypomagnesemia in ewes (El-Khodery et al. 2008). Thirdly, when calcium is low in the diet, soluble oxalate remains soluble in the liquid portion of the intestine contents and is readily absorbed from the intestine into the bloodstream. If the oxalate ion concentration becomes very high in the blood being filtered by the kidney, it may combine with calcium or magnesium to form insoluble oxalate crystals that may block urine flow and cause kidney failure (Lincoln and Black 1980; Blaney et al. 1982). Fourthly, insoluble oxalate from ingested plants may pass through the digestive tract without any harmful effect on the body's metabolism (Ward et al. 1979).

In general, oxalate poisoning is a complex issue. Induction of acute oxalate intoxication depends on several factors, including the chemical form of oxalate, the age of the animal, the rate of consumption, the amount and quality of other feed consumed concurrently, the total amount of oxalate consumed, and adaptation to a diet containing oxalate (Burrows and Tyrl 1989). If large quantities of oxalate-rich plants are eaten, the rumen is overwhelmed and unable to metabolize the oxalate, and oxalate poisoning results. Based on published data, we consider that <2% soluble oxalate would be an appropriate level to avoid oxalate poisoning in ruminants, although the blood calcium level may decrease.

Wein Chang et al. (2004) and Rahman et al. (2011) reported that ruminants (cattle, goats, and sheep) fed on a high oxalate-containing grass had lower blood calcium levels when compared to animals fed on a low oxalate-containing grass. This data indicates that ruminant animals may efficiently utilize large amounts of oxalate without causing ill effects (although the blood calcium level is reduced) if proper management practices are followed.

A study with sheep and goats showed that administration of free oxalic acid led to changes in the rate of oxalic acid breakdown in the rumen, particularly in goats, thereby protecting the host animal from toxic symptoms (Duncan et al. 1997). It seems that ruminants, when adapted to oxalate-rich diets, are able to eat a wide array of plants without ingesting a harmful dose of oxalate.

Frutos et al. (1998) observed that goats could be adapted to oxalic acid by daily oral administration of 0.6 mM/kg live weight/day of free oxalic acid, which successfully generated an active oxalic acid–degrading rumen bacterial population, although the goats showed chronic mild hypocalcemia. Therefore, ruminants adapted to diets with high oxalate content can tolerate oxalate levels that may be toxic or lethal to unadopted ruminants.

13.1.5 Oleander Poisoning

Oleanders (*Nerium oleander*) are widely cultivated as ornamental plants, but all the parts of the plant are poisonous to humans, animals, and certain insects (Langford and Boor 1996; Soto-Blanco et al. 2006). This plant contains a mixture of very toxic cardiac glycosides, the cardenolides (Langford and Boor 1996). Cardenolides inhibit cellular membrane Na^+/K^+ ATPase, resulting in electrolytic disturbance that affects the electrical conductivity of the heart (Joubert 1989; Aslani et al. 2004). Toxic exposure of humans and different species of domestic animals to oleander cardenolides is common in regions where this plant grows (Aslani et al. 2004; Soto-Blanco et al. 2006). Classic symptoms of oleander intoxication are primarily heart and digestive disturbances and altered mental status (Langford and Boor 1996; Cheeke 1998; Knight and Walter 2001; Aslani et al. 2004).

Barbosa et al. (2008) evaluated the pathological effects of *N. oleander* on goats. They divided six healthy male goats, 6 months old, into two groups: test and control. The test group received 50 mg wet weight/kg/day of oleander leaves (red-flowered variety *N. oleander*) for six consecutive days. On the seventh day, the goats received an extra 110 mg/kg of oleander leaves, four times at one-hourly intervals. After the last dose, they received an additional 330 mg/kg dose of oleander leaves. The control group received water throughout the experimental period. As data for goats and sheep is lacking, dosing protocol in this study was based on a pharmacokinetic study in mice (Ni et al. 2002) and aimed to maintain high oleandrin levels in the brain for all days and high plasma levels on the last day. During the first six days, the only clinical sign was bradycardia one hour after dosing. On the seventh day, bradycardia was also present, followed by a moderate increase in heart rate. After the third administration of 110 mg/kg oleander leaves, clinical

signs such as distress, graded signs of apathy, colic, vocalizations, polyuria, moderate rumen distention, teeth grinding, and tachypnea were evident. Histological examination of kidneys in the goats indicated that there was no congestion or vascular disturbance. Necrosis was found in convoluted as well as in collecting tubules. Renal tubule necrosis is responsible for renal failure and is due to impairment of the K^+/Na^+-ATPase pump. The goats showed no significant liver alteration. It is widely known that oleander leaves are lethal to ruminants at a minimal dose of 50 mg/kg body weight (Knight and Walter 2001). The administration of such a dose did not produce any acute intoxication symptom in goats. Repeated daily doses failed to induce any chronic sign of poisoning. The additional 110 mg/kg doses (440 mg/kg total) did not lead to death in goats; interestingly, administration of a single dose of 110 mg/kg of oleander leaves to sheep caused death at between 4 and 12 hours (Aslani et al. 2004). Oleander poisoning in goats can induce kidney and heart failure in a manner similar to other species.

13.1.6 Gossypol Poisoning

Gossypol is the predominant pigment and probably the major toxic ingredient in the cotton plant (*Gossypium* spp.). Gossypol is found in cotton seed in both protein-bound and free forms; only the free form is toxic. Clinical signs of gossypol toxicosis may relate to effects on the cardiac, hepatic, renal, reproductive, or other systems. Prolonged exposure can cause acute heart failure resulting from cardiac necrosis. Also, a form of cardiac conduction failure similar to hyperkalemic heart failure can result in sudden death. Pulmonary effects, labored breathing, and chronic dyspnea are most likely secondary to cardiotoxicosis from congestive heart failure. Liver necrosis may be secondary to congestive heart failure. Hematological effects include anemia with reduced numbers of red blood cells (RBCs) and increased RBC fragility, decreased oxygen release from oxyhemoglobin, and reduced oxygen-carrying capacity of blood with lowered hemoglobin (Hb) and packed cell volume (PCV) values due to complexing of iron by gossypol.

Matondi et al. (2007) reported the effect of cotton-seed meal on goat erythrocyte membrane osmotic fragility. Goats given diets containing cotton-seed meal had higher erythrocyte fragility than those given the control diet that contained soybean meal. Erythrocyte fragility increased from week one to week six, which suggested a cumulative effect of free gossypol on erythrocyte fragility. Diets with high free gossypol content had correspondingly higher erythrocyte osmotic fragility. In this relatively short-term study, the only sign of gossypol toxicity observed was an increase in the erythrocyte osmotic fragility of RBCs. It was concluded that diets with less than 456 mg/kg of free gossypol can safely be used in complete diets of goats.

13.1.7 Water Hemlock Poisoning

Green et al. (2022) reported a case of water hemlock poisoning in Spanish goats. Water hemlock (*Cicuta douglasii*) is one of the most toxic plants to animals and little is known regarding the amount of the plant required to cause death in goats. The study was aimed at determining a lethal dose of water hemlock in a goat model. Plants were dosed to goats via oral gavage of freeze-dried ground plant material. Tubers are the most toxic part of the water hemlock plant. The results revealed that a dose of 0.25 g/kg body weight of dried water hemlock tubers can be lethal to goats, while a dose of 0.1 g/kg body weight is not toxic. A dose of 10 g/kg body weight of dried water hemlock above-ground parts can be toxic to goats. The results from this study suggest that one to two fresh tubers would be lethal to goats (Welch et al. 2020). Similarly, Green et al. (2022) evaluated diazepam as a drug treatment for water hemlock (*Cicuta* spp.) poisoning in Spanish goats. The results showed that diazepam provided nearly instant control of convulsions. Clinical signs of poisoning were completely controlled for the duration of the experiment in the goats that received a 10 mg/kg diazepam dose. These results suggest that diazepam is effective at managing the clinical signs of water hemlock poisoning in goats (Green et al. 2022).

13.2 Mycotoxin Poisoning

Mycotoxins are secondary metabolites of molds that have adverse effects on humans, animals, and crops that result in illnesses and economic losses. The worldwide contamination of foods and feeds with mycotoxins is a significant problem. Aflatoxins, ochratoxins, trichothecenes, zearalenone, fumonisins, tremorgenic toxins, and ergot alkaloids are the mycotoxins of greatest agroeconomic importance. Storing grains, feedstuffs, and forages at moisture levels beyond recommended ranges or in poor storage units may increase mold-related problems. Evaluation of the real exposure of small ruminants to mycotoxins is not always easy because the contaminants may not be distributed uniformly in feeds and they have an assorted diet composition (Whitaker et al. 2010). Cool, wet growing seasons may delay grain maturity, especially for corn, and result in mold and mycotoxin formation in the field. Fusarium toxins are more likely to occur in cool, wet conditions during growth, harvesting, and storage. Hot, humid conditions favor the development of aflatoxins. Delaying harvest to increase maturity and reduce moisture levels, or to avoid muddy

field conditions, may result in increased mold growth and mycotoxin formation. Mold-contaminated feed is also less palatable and may lower the intake of energy, dry matter, and critical nutrients in animals. This may considerably reduce milk production, growth, or weight gains, and depress resistance to metabolic and infectious diseases. The diseases caused by exposure to mycotoxins are known as mycotoxicosis. Reductions in production performance and increases in health problems from moldy feed are often moderate if mycotoxins are not present. For example, a 5–10% drop in performance may be typical with mold infestation, whereas mycotoxin contamination leads to greater losses in production, even when mold is not readily apparent.

Ruminants are generally more resistant to the adverse effects of mycotoxins than are monogastrics. This is because the rumen microbiota is capable of degrading mycotoxins (Adams et al. 1993). However, a number of mycotoxins resist rumen degradation, causing distinct clinical signs of intoxication in animals. Animals that consume feed contaminated with mycotoxins may suffer pathological changes in liver, kidneys, lungs, heart, and pancreas that have implications for their zootechnical performance (low weight gain and feed conversion), causing a great economic impact on livestock production. Another point of concern is the contamination of animal products once the mycotoxins and their metabolites are excreted in milk, meat, and eggs (Dorner et al. 1994; Rosmaninho et al. 2006). Moreover, goats may be exposed to a varying number of mycotoxins, originating from different feed materials. Such effects cause severe economic losses through clinically ambiguous changes in animal growth, feed intake reduction or feed refusal, alteration in nutrient absorption and metabolism, effects on the endocrine system, as well as suppression of the immune system.

13.3 Pesticide Poisoning

Most insecticides derived from plants (e.g. rotenone from *Derris* and pyrethrins from *Chrysanthemum* or *Pyrethrum*) have traditionally been considered safe for use on animals. Rotenone is present in a number of plants (*Derris*, *Lonchocarpus*, *Tephrosia*, and *Mundulea*). It is used worldwide because it has broad-spectrum insecticidal, acaricidal, pesticidal, and fish-killing properties. Rotenone's toxicity in animals is via inhibition of mitochondrial respiratory chain complex I, with cell death by apoptosis due to excess generation of free radicals. Following chronic exposure to rotenone, fatty acid synthesis is altered in the mitochondria, resulting in fatty changes in the liver and kidney. In poisoned animals, clinical signs may include pharyngitis, nausea, vomiting, gastric pain, clonic convulsions, seizures, muscle tremors, lethargy, incontinence, and respiratory stimulation followed by respiratory depression. The cardiovascular effects include tachycardia, hypotension, and impaired myocardial contractility. Toxicity is greater if the particles are smaller in size. Death occurs due to cardiorespiratory failure. Rotenone has the potential for reproductive toxicity and teratogenicity. Diagnosis of rotenone poisoning is based on detection of rotenone residue in blood, liver, urine, feces, and vomitus. There is no specific antidote for rotenone poisoning, so treatment is supportive.

Similarly, pyrethrins are insecticides obtained from the flowers of *Chrysanthemum cinerariaefolium*. Natural pyrethrins (pyrethrin I, pyrethrin II, jasmolin I, jasmolin II, cinerin I, and cinerin II) have been used as insecticides for decades. However, these compounds are very unstable in the body, so pyrethroids are preferred. Currently, the type II pyrethroid flumethrin is commonly used against ectoparasites (ticks, lice, and mites) in goats and other animals as a spray or as a 1% solution pour-on treatment. The toxicity of type II pyrethroids is greater than that of type I pyrethroids. Following oral ingestion, pyrethrins and pyrethroids are rapidly hydrolyzed in the gastrointestinal tract. Approximately 40–60% of an orally ingested dose is absorbed. As lipophilic compounds, pyrethroids distribute to tissues with a high lipid content such as fat and nervous tissue, in addition to liver, kidney, and milk. Clinical signs include salivation, vomiting, hyperexcitability, tremors, seizures, dyspnea, weakness, prostration, and death. Type II pyrethroids may also elicit signs such as choreoathetosis or salivation syndrome. Diagnosis of pyrethrin or pyrethroid poisoning is based on history of exposure, clinical signs, and determination of insecticide residue in body tissues and fluids. There is no specific antidote for pyrethrin or pyrethroid poisoning in animals. Generally, supportive treatment is required in poisoned goats.

Organophosphate insecticides are a major cause of animal poisoning. Organophosphates are derivatives of phosphoric or phosphonic acid. Currently, there are many organophosphate compounds in use, and they have replaced the banned organochlorine compounds. The chemistry of organophosphates is very complex. They vary greatly in toxicity, residue levels, and excretion in animals. Many organophosphates have been developed for plant and animal protection, and in general they offer a distinct advantage by producing few tissue and environmental residues. Some of the organophosphates developed initially as pesticides are also used as anthelmintics. Haloxon, naphthalophos, and crufomate are primarily used against parasitic infestations in ruminants. Organochlorine pesticides are synthetic pesticides widely used all over the world. They belong to the group of chlorinated hydrocarbon derivatives, which have vast application in chemical industries and in agriculture. These compounds are known for their high toxicity, slow degradation, and bioaccumulation. Even though many of the compounds that belong to organochlorine were banned in developed countries, the use of these agents has been rising (Jayaraj et al. 2016).

Giadinis et al. (2009) reported carbamate poisoning in a dairy goat herd. A total of 55 dairy goats in a herd exhibited signs of possible poisoning approximately one hour after the consumption of carnations from a nearby glasshouse. Clinical examination of the affected goats showed signs of salivation, tympany, tachypnea, polydipsia, urination, diarrhea, bradycardia, miosis, tremor, and convulsions. Treatment with atropine sulphate was initiated at a dose of 0.3 mg/kg body weight. The treatment was repeated for a few goats that relapsed, and was effective in all cases, with the exception of one goat kid that died.

13.4   Heavy Metal and Mineral Element Poisoning

Heavy metals are different from other toxic substances as they can be neither created nor destroyed. Anthropogenic activities are responsible for their redistribution into the environment and exposure to humans and animals. Heavy metal poisoning is one of the major non-infectious causes of adverse impacts on animal health and production. Biologically heavy metals are both beneficial and harmful. While a few heavy metals including copper, cobalt, iron, magnesium, manganese, selenium, and zinc are essential for vital physiological processes in trace amounts while excess amounts produce toxicities, others like lead, cadmium and mercury are better known for their toxicities. Toxic heavy metals refer to relatively dense metals/metalloids not actually beneficial to either humans or livestock, which in small amounts can lead to carcinogenicity, organ toxicity, and other deleterious health effects (Jaishankar et al. 2014). Examples like arsenic (As), cadmium (Cd), lead (Pb), and mercury (Hg) are among the top 10 toxic heavy metals of major public health concern according to the World Health Organization (Cheremisinoff 2006). The toxicity of toxic heavy metals has always been dependent on the dose, route of exposure, age, and nutritional statuses of the exposed animal. Acute heavy metal poisoning is associated with typical clinical symptoms culminating in the death of an individual animal or a group of animals with similar necropsy findings. Chronic toxicities are characterized by deterioration in general condition and loss of production. The presence of heavy metals above a critical level in edible animal products is a cause for public health concern. Early diagnosis, administration of a specific antidote, and management can effectively reduce the adverse impact of heavy metals on livestock health and production (Gupta et al. 2021).

Mineral elements are essential to animal health, survival, and production because they are part of physiological, structural, catalytic, and regulatory organism functions. Therefore, they should be present in the diet. However, they may be ingested in excessive doses due to errors in balancing mineral supplements and/or complete rations. An intake of plants with high mineral concentration may also result from the addition of fertilizers, herbicides, insecticides, or fungicides to pasture or cultivation where plants or grains will be used to feed animals, as well as decomposition of urban and industrial wastes, leaks and accidental spills of pollutants, leading to an accumulation of toxic mineral elements in the environment, poisoning the animals and potentially resulting in death. However, toxic doses, physiological changes during poisoning, symptoms, and mineral concentrations in the tissues of poisoned animals to confirm the diagnosis are not fully known. There are few research reports on the mineral element doses of cadmium, lead, copper, chromium, iodine, manganese, molybdenum, selenium, and zinc, and their concentration in the tissues of poisoned animals, or on their physiological effects, symptoms, diagnostic procedures, and treatment for poisoning, but they are considered toxic for animal intake (Reis et al. 2010).

Biswas et al. (2000) reported chronic toxicity of arsenic in goats. The results suggest that long-term exposure to inorganic arsenic at low levels in goats severe clinical signs of toxicity and toxico-pathological changes accompanied by mortality. The cytotoxic effect of arsenic is proportional to the quantitative accumulation of its residues in the organs. Since arsenic exerts cytotoxic changes on antibody-producing cells, efforts are needed to measure in depth both cell-mediated and humoral immune responses in animals exposed to chronic arsenic toxicity, as this element is rapidly becoming an unavoidable environmental pollutant.

Islam et al. (2011) reported effects of chronic arsenic toxicity on the hematology and histoarchitecture of the female reproductive system of the Black Bengal goat. There were significant differences in total erythrocyte count, Hb concentration, and total leukocyte count in goats chronically exposed to arsenic. Lymphocyte decreased with treatment by sodium arsenite, but neutrophil, eosinophil, and monocyte were increased. At the end of the study, the goats were euthanized. The ovary, uterine tube, uterus, cervix, and vagina were collected for gross and histopathological examinations. In the histopathological examination the ovarian follicles appeared to have degenerated and there was much stromal thickening around the follicle. A thickened myometrial layer and shortened mucosal folds in the uterine tube were observed. There was a reduction in the number and size of the endometrial glands. The mucosal cell lines appeared to have degenerated. Thin vaginal mucosa and proliferation of connective tissue, shortened cervical crypts, and thickened glandular epithelium of the cervix were also observed. It may be concluded that chronic arsenic exposure might have adverse effects on the female reproductive system.

Ortega-Morales et al. (2020) reported toxicity in goats exposed to arsenic in the region of Lagunera, northern Mexico. The Creole goats of the Lagunera that have been exposed to chronic arsenic toxicity did not show translocation of the metalloid to their milk, while the male goats did not show libido levels significantly different to the control group. However, the physiological parameters for goats exposed to drinking water with high concentrations of arsenic indicated weight loss, alterations in heart and respiratory rates, behavior changes, hair loss on their flanks, and keratosis on the nose and mouth.

13.5 Nitrite/Nitrate Poisoning

The occurrence of nitrate poisoning is difficult to predict because nitrate levels can change rapidly in plants and the toxicity of nitrate varies greatly among livestock due to prior exposure, age, health status, and diet. However, concern should certainly be raised when plant growth has been less than half of normal or nitrogen application more than twice that recommended. Nitrate is found in various plant species that are considered nitrate accumulators, including, but not limited to, corn, fireweed, lambs quarter, and pigweed (Wright and Davison 1964; Hall 2018). Usually nitrate is utilized by plants during photosynthesis. Excess nitrate accumulation occurs whenever the plant undergoes stress and photosynthesis is impaired. Common causes of nitrate accumulation include drought and increased fertilizer application.

Goats may be exposed to nitrate fertilizers through water supplementation or contaminated feeds (Sasu et al. 1970; Issi et al. 2009). Exposure of goats to nitrate fertilizers results in high mortality (Villar et al. 2003). Intoxication occurs when rumen microbes, metabolizing nitrate to nitrite for growth, become overwhelmed. Nitrite accumulates in the blood, oxidizes ferrous iron to the ferric form, and forms methemoglobin. Methemoglobin is unable to carry oxygen, and tissues undergo anoxia (Wright and Davison 1964). Onset of clinical signs is rapid and leads to death. Although often found dead, animals may be observed to exhibit signs associated with oxygen deprivation. Clinical signs include weakness, ataxia, tremors, and convulsions. Cyanotic mucous membranes and respiratory

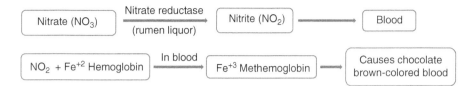

Figure 13.3 Mechanism of action of nitrate and nitrite poisoning in goats.

distress are characteristic of nitrate intoxication. Tissues and blood may have a chocolate brown-colored appearance due to methemoglobin formation (Casteel and Evans 2004). The mechanism of action of nitrate and nitrite poisoning in goats is illustrated in Figure 13.3.

In ruminants, postmortem ocular fluid is the optimal sample to evaluate for nitrate (Villar et al. 2003). Serum may be collected as an antemortem sample (Issi et al. 2009). Submission of suspect feed and water should be considered for evaluation. Forages possessing 10 000 ppm dry-matter nitrate are considered lethal and should be avoided entirely (Casteel and Evans 2004). Due to the acute nature of nitrate poisoning and rapid death, treatment may not be successful. Methylene blue 1% (20 mg/kg IV) and ascorbic acid (10 mg/kg IV) has been used successfully to treat goats following consumption of nitrate fertilizer (Issi et al. 2009).

13.6 Urea Poisoning

Urea-based fertilizers serve as a common source of exposure in goats through contaminated water or feed and consumption of urea-based fertilizers tends to lead to high mortality in goats (Villar et al. 2003). Urea is an economical source of non-protein nitrogen (NPN) in ruminants as it is incorporated into protein by ruminal microbes. Excess urea can occur in the ration through misformulation or high urea content within feedstuffs (Oruc et al. 2015). Surface water sources may also pose a threat following heavy rains and run-off from fields with recently applied fertilizer.

Urea intoxication in goats is due mostly to ruminal metabolism. Urease hydrolyzes urea to ammonia, and ammonia is protonated to ammonium. During this process, the pH of the rumen steadily becomes more alkaline and the production of ammonia is favored. Excess ammonia gets into the bloodstream, where the liver converts it to urea that is excreted in the urine. When urea is consumed in excess, the ensuing ammonia production overwhelms the liver. Ammonia is then able to cross the blood–brain barrier (Volmer 2004).

Acute death is common in urea intoxication, and clinical signs may not be observed. Onset of clinical signs observed in sheep may occur in as little as 15 minutes following

ingestion and include ataxia, incoordination, muscle fasciculations, tremoring, ptyalism, anuria, bloat, and convulsive seizures (Edjtehadi et al. 1978; Oruc et al. 2015). Characteristic gross and microscopic lesions are usually absent (Oruc et al. 2015). Ammonia analysis should be performed on postmortem ocular fluid and rumen content that is collected, sealed, and frozen immediately (Villar et al. 2003). Due to the volatile nature of ammonia, diagnostic value is lost as the postmortem sample collection interval increases. Animals that have been dead for more than 12 hours in a moderate climate have undergone too much autolysis to be diagnostically useful. This timeframe is dependent on the climate of the region. Suspect feed and water samples should also be submitted for urea analysis (Volmer 2004). Rumen pH can be measured in the field or through laboratory analysis. A rumen pH >8 is consistent with urea poisoning (Shaikat et al. 2012).

Due to the acute nature of poisoning, treatment may come too late to be effective. Treatment of urea poisoning centers around halting further formation of ammonia by inhibiting urease. Administration of cold water and acetic acid (vinegar) creates a suboptimal environment for urease to function (Shaikat et al. 2012). Due to the potential of limited resources for treatment and the acute nature of the intoxication, individuals should be triaged, as severity of signs and capacity to urinate may serve as prognostic indicators. Sheep that survived intoxication were observed to urinate frequently. Animas that retain the ability to urinate maintain a favorable prognosis.

13.7 Sulfur Poisoning

The maximum concentration of sulfur in concentrated rations for small ruminants is 0.3% and 0.5% in forage diets (National Research Council 2007). Water may contain high concentrations of sulfate. Elevated sulfur in the diet, accompanied by high-sulfate water, increases the potential for intoxication. It is likely that small ruminants would be affected at concentrations such as those given (Hamlen et al. 1993).

Clinical signs are similar to those observed with lead poisoning and water deprivation. The rumen may appear gray or black in color. Fluorescence of the laminar cortical region of the brain under ultraviolet light may be present, but is not definitive for sulfur-associated polioencephalomalacia. Absence of fluorescence also does not rule out the presence of laminar cortical necrosis. Diagnosis is often made through retrospective analysis of feed and water accompanied by clinical signs and lesions consistent with intoxication. Increased dietary thiamine can help reduce clinical signs associated with sulfur-induced polioencephalomalacia, but may not completely prevent microscopic lesions in the brain (Olkowski et al. 1992)

13.8 Fluorosis

A high fluoride level in drinking water causes different kinds of toxicosis in humans and animals (Choubisa 1999). One of these, dental fluorosis, characterized by enamel mottling, appears clinically at the maximum permissible level of fluoride, 1.5 ppm in drinking water (DenBesten and Li 2011). Its primary manifestations are mottling of teeth (dental fluorosis) and osteosclerosis of the skeleton (skeletal fluorosis). Besides these, non-skeletal fluorosis or toxic effects of fluoride in soft tissues – gastrointestinal discomfort, neurological disorders, impaired reproductive functions, and teratogenic effects – have also been reported in humans and animals. Calcium compounds (e.g. calcium gluconate), aluminum salts, or milk may be administered orally to bind excess fluoride in the gastrointestinal tract before absorption. Gastric aspiration and lavage are also effective. Adsorption therapy with activated charcoal is not helpful because fluoride does not bind to charcoal. As a preventive measure, change the feed and drinking water if it is high in fluoride.

Choubisa (1999) attempted to study chronic fluorosis intoxication in more than 2000 goats and sheep living in fluorosis-endemic areas of southern Rajasthan, India, but none of these animals or their lames was found to be affected with chronic fluorosis intoxication (Choubisa 2007). Later he traced a few isolated cases of fluorosis in animals from the same fluorosis-endemic areas, but its severity was found to be relatively less compared to bovines (cattle and buffalo) from these areas. It is evident that fluorosis toxicity occurs in any animal drinking fluoridated water, but its toxicity varies among species. In the reported study, three tribal villages, Fatehpura, Devala, and Dhunda of the Aspur Panchayat Samiti of the Dungarpur district of Rajasthan were selected as they have fluorosis concentrations in the range of 1.5–3.5 ppm in drinking water sources. Osteodental fluorosis was observed (Choubisa 2008) in native mature and immature goats and sheep who had been in these villages since birth. House-to-house surveys were undertaken in the early-morning and

late-evening hours when the animals were available, and in herds during the daytime. Findings on osteodental fluorosis were based on clinical signs only. However, the goats showed a relatively higher prevalence of these chronic fluorosis effects compared to sheep. In general, the prevalence and severity of osteodental fluorosis in these small ruminants were found to be less than in bovines.

13.9 Feed Additive/ Ionophore Toxicity

The ionophores monensin (Rumensin®, Elanco, Greenfield, IN, USA) and lasalocid (Bovatec®, Zoetis, Parsippany, NJ, USA) are common feed additives in caprine and ovine production, respectively, to improve feed efficiency and act as coccidostats. Ionophore intoxication can be easily misdiagnosed in small ruminant species as a result of its presentation. Intoxications, although not as common as in bovines, occur through feed misformulations, misuse, barn break-ins, and delivery errors. Feed misformulations may include excess being added to the ration through incorrect additive use, equipment failure, or antibiotic synergism (Hall 2004; National Research Council 2007).

Excessive ionophore consumption results in an increased influx of sodium into cells followed by an influx of calcium. The influx of ions creates a drastic change in pH, resulting in cellular damage. This, in addition to lipid peroxidation, results in membrane damage, allowing more calcium to enter. The excess calcium activates multiple enzymes that ultimately lead to muscle necrosis (Hall 2000).

The clinical signs exhibited by goats and sheep differ from those in cattle and may often be perceived as neurological in nature. Onset can occur within 24 hours. Sheep may go off their feed, exhibit lethargy, weakness, and stiff gait, and become recumbent. Surviving individuals may have decreased muscle mass in major muscle groups. Mortality may occur for an extended period of time following consumption (Nation et al. 1982).

Gross lesions may be difficult to discern on postmortem evaluation. Sheep afflicted with salinomycin exhibited pulmonary and skeletal muscle congestion and edema. Both hydrothorax and hydropericardium have been reported to be present. Microscopically, cardiac degeneration was also observed (Tafti et al. 2008). Ascites along with pulmonary and hepatic congestion may be observed. Skeletal muscle, not cardiac, is predominantly affected in small ruminant species. Generalized pallor or streaking may be evident in major muscle groups including the loins and those within the fore limbs and trunk region. Microscopically, myocyte degeneration and necrosis are observed. Fibrosis is evident in chronically affected individuals. In 1-month-old lambs, gastrointestinal hemorrhage is reported (Nation et al. 1982). Sections of skeletal muscle from the aforementioned groups, along with cardiac, lung, and liver, should be collected for microscopic evaluation (Nation et al. 1982; Tafti et al. 2008). Submission of suspect feed for ionophore analysis should be considered. Due to the delayed onset of signs and unlikeliness of feed remining or a retained sample, the submitted feed may not be representative of the feed consumed to inflict complications. No specific treatment is available for ionophore intoxication. Animals that survive intoxication should be handled with minimal stress, as mortality may persist in surviving individuals (Hall 2000).

13.10 Snake-Bite Envenomation in Goats

Snake-bite envenomation in humans and animals is an emergency that requires rapid examination and critical care for proper treatment. Snake envenomation is rare in goats and occurs during grazing in the field; it is more commonly observed in rural areas, especially area near to forests. The severity of the snake bite in animals depends on the type of snake, the age of the animal, the size of the animal, the number of bites, and the amount of venom injected. The clinical effects are more severe in small animals compared to large animals. In general, snake venom contains several toxins, including necrotizing, anticoagulant, and procoagulant fractions and neurotoxic, cardiotoxic, myotoxic, nephrotoxic, cytotoxic, hemolytic, and hemorrhagic fractions. Different snakes have varying combinations of these toxins in their venom. Snake envenomation is an emergency condition in animals and early clinical diagnosis and treatment should be initiated.

Venkatesakumar et al. (2020) reported a case of saw-scaled viper envenomation and its therapeutic management in a goat. A 3-year-old female non-descript goat was presented with a history of saw-scaled viper bite over the face, with the clinical signs of dullness, anorexia, epistaxis, and facial swelling. Clinical examination revealed pink and moist conjunctival mucous membrane, fang marks, and swelling over the right cheek and lower jaw. Elevated temperature, tachycardia, and tachypnea were observed. Hemato-biochemical evaluation of the goat revealed moderate anemia (decreased hemoglobin, packed cell volume, and RBCs) and thrombocytopenia. The 20-minute whole blood clotting test was prolonged. The goat was administered with two doses of 10 ml of polyvalent snake venom antiserum (contains snake venom antiserum against cobra, krait, Russell's viper, and saw-scaled viper) with normal saline IV. Strepto-penicillin and furosemide for three days and tetanus toxoid for one day were administered

intramuscularly. The goat was treated successfully with two doses of snake venom antiserum, strepto-penicillin, furosemide, and tetanus toxoid, and had an uneventful recovery.

Kumar et al. (2010) reported a snake-bite envenomation case in a goat. A Jamnapari goat aged about 2.5 years was presented with a history of sudden swelling in the tongue and periorbital region following a snake bite. Clinical examination revealed pale conjunctival mucous membrane, incoordination, frothy salivation, dullness, tympany with low pH, and swollen cyanotic tongue and periorbital region, with the presence of fang marks on the center of the tongue. The clinical parameters of body temperature, pulse, and respiratory rate were within the normal range. Administration of polyvalent snake venom antiserum, 5% dextrose, dexamethasone phosphate, normal saline, tetanus toxoid, and broad-spectrum antibiotic brought about an uneventful recovery in the goat.

Smith et al. (2015) reported cases of rattlesnake envenomation in three dairy goats. Usually cases of rattlesnake envenomation in dairy goats are lacking. These cases were presented to a veterinary referral hospital for envenomation of the Northern Pacific rattlesnake (*Crotalus oreganus*). Treatments and clinical characteristics reported in goats are similar to those for llamas, alpacas, and horses. Faster implementation of treatment with respect to the timing of the bite may lead to a more positive treatment response. These case descriptions provide basic information about rattlesnake envenomation that may be useful in managing cases of rattlesnake envenomation in dairy goats.

Prasanth et al. (2017) reported therapeutic management of cobra envenomation in a goat. A Malabari crossbred goat was presented with a history of cobra envenomation. The goat had fang marks on the lower mandible with considerable swelling around them. Subcutaneous administration of neostigmine was given to counteract the anticholinergic effect of cobra venom, followed by atropine sulfate to alleviate the side effects of neostigmine and bradyarrhythmia. Heart rate and SpO_2 level were monitored continuously. Antivenin was given via the IV route followed by another dose mixed with normal saline via constant-rate infusion over a period of one hour. IV injection of dexamethasone and amoxicillin-sulbactam was given. Tramadol was given intravenously to reduce pain and tetanus toxoid was administered intramuscularly. The animal made an uneventful recovery after three days.

13.11 Conclusion

There are numerous compounds and routes that small ruminants may access that can be detrimental to animal health and production. Many toxic compounds affect bovine, caprine, and ovine animals in similar ways. Due to variations among these species, the susceptibility, clinical presentation, and lesions associated with toxic agents may differ. Goats may be exposed to different toxicants or poisonous substances in a variety of ways. The poisonings in goats covered in this chapter are by no means all inclusive, as there are many other sporadic toxicities that may be encountered in goats that may not be reported or mentioned anywhere. Clinical presentation of individuals aids in deriving a list of differentials, and toxicants should always be considered. Recognition of sources, clinical signs, and lesions associated with toxicants in small ruminant species, particularly goats, can greatly help practitioners in differentiating toxicant and infectious etiologies. It is important to note what toxic agent species are susceptible to and how goats are affected to effectively diagnose and treat afflicted animals. The understanding that some intoxications in goats or small ruminants are presented differently than those in bovines is critical in proper sample collection and diagnosis.

Multiple-Choice Questions

1 Which is the toxic principle present in the *Lantana camara* plant?
   A Lantadenes
   B Dhurrin
   C Gossypol
   D Mimosine

2 *Lantana camara* can cause secondary photosensitization due to the accumulation of phylloerythrin in the system following compromise of which organ function?
   A Lung
   B Heart
   C Liver
   D Intestine

3 Which antidote is commonly used for cyanide poisoning in goats?
   A Sodium thiosulphate
   B Sodium nitrite
   C Both a and b
   D None of the above

4 A bitter almond-like smell is observed from the breath of the animal and during necropsy after opening the rumen due to poisoning by what?
   A Nitrate
   B Carbon monoxide
   C Cyanide
   D Phosphorous

5 What is the toxic principle present in subabul (*Leucaena leucocephala*)?
   A Mimosine
   B Dhurrin
   C Gossypol
   D Abrin

6 What can prolonged grazing by ruminants on some oxalate-rich tropical grasses result in?
   A Hypocalcemia
   B Hypercalcemia
   C Hyperphosphatemia
   D Anemia

7 In oxalate poisoning, oxalate is combined with which ions to form insoluble oxalate crystals that may block urine flow and cause kidney failure in animals?
   A Calcium and magnesium
   B Iron
   C Sodium
   D Potassium

8 What is the toxic principle that is present in oleander (*Nerium oleander*)?
   A Mimosine
   B Dhurrin
   C Cardenolides
   D Abrin

9 What is the mechanism of action of toxicity due to the oleander plant?
   A Inhibits cellular membrane Na^+/K^+ ATPase
   B Inhibits Ca^{++} channel
   C Inhibits angiotensin-converting enzyme
   D All of the above

10 Which plant contains the toxic constituent gossypol?
   A Subabul
   B Cotton-seed cake
   C Oleander
   D Groundnut cake

11 Which insecticide is commonly used against ectoparasites (ticks, lice, and mites) in goats?
  A Type I pyrethroid
  B Type II pyrethroid-flumethrin
  C Benzene hexachloride
  D Lindane

12 Pyrethrin insecticide is obtained from the flowers of which plant?
  A *Nerium oleander*
  B *Leucaena leucocephala*
  C *Chrysanthemum cinerariaefolium*
  D *Heteromeles arbutifolia*

13 A chocolate brown-colored appearance of blood is seen in poisoning due to which compound?
  A Oxalate
  B Cyanide
  C Nitrite
  D Fluoride

14 Which antidote is used for nitrite and nitrate poisoning in animals?
  A Methylene blue
  B Acetic acid
  C Sodium sulfate
  D Sodium nitrite

15 Which drug is used for the treatment of urea poisoning in animals?
  A Acetic acid
  B Sodium sulfate
  C Sodium nitrite
  D Methylene blue

16 What causes mottling of teeth and osteosclerosis of the skeleton in poisoning?
  A Nitrite
  B Urea
  C Fluoride
  D Cyanide

References

Adams, R. S., Kephart, K. B., Ishler, V. A., Hutchinson, L. J., & Roth, G. W. (1993). Mould and mycotoxin problems in livestock feeding. Extension Publication DAS 93–21. University Park, PA: Department of Dairy and Animal Science, Pennsylvania State University.

Allison, M.J., Littledike, E.T., and James, L.F. (1977). Changes in ruminal oxalate degradation rates associated with adaptation to oxalate ingestion. *Journal of Animal Science* 45 (5): 1173–1179.

Ambica, G., Reddy, G.A.K., Banotha, A.K., and Kumar, S.R. (2020). Therapeutic management of Lantana associated hepatic and renal toxicity in a bullock: a case report. *Journal of Entomology and Zoology Studies* 8 (2): 1502–1504.

Arnold, M., Gaskill, C., Smith, S.R., and Lacefield, G.D. (2014). Cyanide poisoning in ruminants. Report 168. Lexington, KY: Agriculture and Natural Resources Publications. https://uknowledge.uky.edu/anr_reports/168.

Aslani, M.R., Movassaghi, A.R., Mohri, M. et al. (2004). Clinical and pathological aspects of experimental oleander (*Nerium oleander*) toxicosis in sheep. *Veterinary Research Communications* 28 (7): 609–616.

Barbosa, R.R., Fontenele-Neto, J.D., and Soto-Blanco, B. (2008). Toxicity in goats caused by oleander (*Nerium oleander*). *Research in Veterinary Science* 85 (2): 279–281.

Basaraba, R., Oehme, F.W., Vorhies, M.W. et al. (1999). Toxicosis in cattle from concurrent feeding of monensin and dried distiller's grains contaminated with macrolide antibiotics. *Journal of Veterinary Diagnostic Investigation* 11: 79–86.

Bingham, E., Cohrssen, B., and Powell, C.H. (2001). *Patty's Toxicology*, 5e, vol. 9. New York: Wiley.

Biswas, U., Sarkar, S., Bhowmik, M.K. et al. (2000). Chronic toxicity of arsenic in goats: clinicobiochemical changes, pathomorphology and tissue residues. *Small Ruminant Research* 38 (3): 229–235.

Blaney, B.J., Gartner, R.J.W., and Head, T.A. (1982). The effects of oxalate in tropical grasses on calcium, phosphorus and magnesium availability to cattle. *Journal of Agricultural Science* 99 (3): 533–539.

Bozynski, C.C., Evans, T.J., Kim, D.Y. et al. (2009). Copper toxicosis with hemolysis and hemoglobinuric nephrosis in three adult Boer goats. *Journal of Veterinary Diagnostic Investigation* 21: 395–400.

Burrows, G.E. and Tyrl, R.J. (1989). Plants causing sudden death in livestock. *Veterinary Clinics of North America. Food Animal Practice* 5 (2): 263–289.

Casteel, S.W. and Evans, T.J. (2004). Nitrate. In: *Clinical Veterinary Toxicology*, 2e (ed. K.H. Plumlee), 127–130. St. Louis, MO: Mosby.

Cheeke, P.R. (1998). *Natural Toxicants in Feeds, Forages, and Poisonous Plants*, 2e. Prairie Village, KS: Interstate Publishers.

Cheremisinoff, N.P. (2006). *Agency for Toxic Substances and Disease Registry (ATSDR)*. Hoboken, NJ: Wiley.

Choubisa, S.L. (1999). Some observations on endemic fluorosis in domestic animals in Southern Rajasthan (India). *Veterinary Research Communications* 23 (7): 457–465.

Choubisa, S.L. (2007). Fluoridated ground water and its toxic effects on domesticated animals residing in rural tribal areas of Rajasthan (India). *International Journal of Environmental Studies* 64 (2): 151–159.

Choubisa, S.L. (2008). Dental fluorosis in domestic animals. *Current Science* 95: 1674–1675.

Deepa, C., Rajan, S.K., and Nikhila, M. (2017). Acute *Lantana camara* poisoning in goats-a case report. *Journal of Indian Veterinary Association, Kerala (JIVA)* 15 (2): 34–35.

DenBesten, P. and Li, W. (2011). Chronic fluoride toxicity: dental fluorosis. *Fluoride and the Oral Environment* 22: 81–96.

Dorner, J.W., Cole, R.J.C., Erlington, D.J. et al. (1994). Cyclopiazonic acid residues in milk and eggs. *Journal of Agricultural and Food Chemistry* 26: 1516–1518.

Duncan, A.J., Frutos, P., and Young, S.A. (1997). Rates of oxalic acid degradation in the rumen of sheep and goats in response to different levels of oxalic acid administration. *Animal Science* 65 (3): 451–455.

Edjtehadi, M., Szabuniewicz, M., and Emmanuel, B. (1978). Acute urea toxicity in sheep. *Canadian Journal of Comparative Medicine* 42 (1): 63.

El-Khodery, S., El-Boshy, M., Gaafar, K., and Elmashad, A. (2008). Hypocalcaemia in Ossimi sheep associated with feeding on beet tops (Beta vulgaris). *Turkish Journal of Veterinary and Animal Sciences* 32 (3): 199–205.

Frutos, P., Duncan, A.J., Kyriazakis, I., and Gordon, I.J. (1998). Learned aversion towards oxalic acid-containing foods by goats: does rumen adaptation to oxalic acid influence diet choice? *Journal of Chemical Ecology* 24 (2): 383–397.

Giadinis, N.D., Raikos, N., Loukopoulos, P. et al. (2009). Carbamate poisoning in a dairy goat herd: clinicopathological findings and therapeutic approach. *New Zealand Veterinary Journal* 57 (6): 392–394.

Govindaiah, K., Biradar, R., Gupta, V.M.D., and Munivenkatappa, B.S. (2021). Lantana toxicity in grazing cattle. *Indian Journal of Veterinary Sciences and Biotechnology* 17 (1): 85–88.

Gracia, R. and Shepherd, G. (2004). Cyanide poisoning and its treatment. *Pharmacotherapy* 24 (10): 1358–1365.

Green, B.T., Stonecipher, C.A., Welch, K.D. et al. (2022). Evaluation of diazepam as a drug treatment for water hemlock (Cicuta species) poisoning in Spanish goats. *Toxicon* 205: 79–83.

Guitart, R., Croubels, S., Caloni, F. et al. (2010). Animal poisoning in Europe. Part 1: farm livestock and poultry. *Veterinary Journal* 183 (3): 249–254.

Gunasekaran, S., Viswanathan, K., and Bandeswaran, C. (2014). Selectivity and palatability of tree fodders in sheep and goat fed by cafeteria method. *International Journal of Science, Environment and Technology* 3 (5): 1767–1771.

Gupta, R.K., Niyogi, D., Nayan, R. et al. (2019). Clinico-pathological study of *Lantana camara* toxicity in a sheep farm. *Journal of Pharmacognosy and Phytochemistry* 8 (4): 2219–2221.

Gupta, A.R., Bandyopadhyay, S., Sultana, F., and Swarup, D. (2021). Heavy metal poisoning and its impact on livestock health and production system. *Indian Journal of Animal Health* 60 (2): 01–23.

Hall, J.O. (2000). Ionophore use and toxicosis in cattle. *Veterinary Clinics of North America. Food Animal Practice* 16: 497–509.

Hall, J.O. (2004). Ionophores. In: *Clinical Veterinary Toxicology* (ed. K.H. Plumlee), 120–127. Maryland Heights, MO: Mosby.

Hall, J.O. (2018). Nitrate-and nitrite-accumulating plants. In: *Veterinary Toxicology* (ed. R.C. Gupta), 941–946. Cambridge, MA: Academic Press.

Hamlen, H., Clark, E., and Janzen, E. (1993). Polioencephalomalacia in cattle consuming water with elevated sodium sulfate levels: a herd investigation. *Canadian Veterinary Journal* 34 (3): 153.

Haritha, C.V., Khan, S., Manjusha, K.M., and Banu, A. (2019). Toxicological aspects of common plant poisoning in ruminants. *Indian Farmer* 6 (11): 812–822.

Hatzade, R.I., Salve, P.D., and Bhikane, A.U. (2020). Management of clinical case of subabul (*Leucaena leucocephala*) poisoning in a goat kid. *Pharma Innovation Journal* 9 (11): 98–100.

Hmohn, Z.Z.W., Kyaw, H., Phyu, S.H. et al. (2017). Effect of toxic levels of *Leucaena leucocephala* on semen quality of goats in Myanmar. *International Journal of VeterinarySciences and Animal Husbandry* 2 (6): 09–12.

Islam, M.T., Parvin, S., Pervin, M. et al. (2011). Effects of chronic arsenic toxicity on the haematology and histoarchitecture of female reproductive system of black bengal goat. *Bangladesh Journal of Veterinary Medicine* 9 (1): 59–66.

Issi, M., Gül, Y., Ilhan, S. et al. (2009). Acute nitrate poisoning in goats. *Kafkas Üniversitesi Veteriner Fakültesi Dergisi* 15 (5): 807–810.

Jaishankar, M., Tseten, T., Anbalagan, N. et al. (2014). Toxicity, mechanism and health effects of some heavy metals. *Interdisciplinary Toxicology* 7: 60–72.

Jayaraj, R., Megha, P., and Sreedev, P. (2016). Organochlorine pesticides, their toxic effects on living organisms and their fate in the environment. *Interdisciplinary Toxicology* 9 (3–4): 90–100.

Jones, R.J. and Hegarty, M.P. (1984). The effect of different proportions of *Leucaena leucocephala* in the diet of cattle on growth, feed intake, thyroid function and urinary excretion of 3-hydroxy-4 (1H)-pyridone. *Australian Journal of Agricultural Research* 35 (2): 317–325.

Jones, R.J., Blunt, C.G., and Holmes, J.H.G. (1976). Enlarged thyroid glands in cattle grazing Leucaena pastures [*Leucaena leucocephala* cv. Peru, tropical zone, Queensland, Western Australia, New Guinea]. *Tropical Grasslands* 10 (2): 113–116.

Joubert, J.P.J. (1989). Cardiac glycosides. In: *Toxicants of Plant Origin*, vol. II (ed. P.R. Cheeke), 61–96. Boca Raton, FL: CRC Press.

Knight, A.P. and Walter, R.G. (2001). *A Guide to Plant Poisoning of Animals in North America*. Jackson, WY: Teton NewMedia.

Kumar, M., Kumar, A., and Haque, S. (2010). Therapeutic management of snakebite envenomation in a goat. *VetScan* 5 (2): 1–2.

Kumar, R., Sharma, R., Patil, R.D. et al. (2018). Sub-chronic toxicopathological study of lantadenes of *Lantana camara* weed in guinea pigs. *BMC Veterinary Research* 14 (1): 1–13.

Langford, S.D. and Boor, P.J. (1996). Oleander toxicity: an examination of human and animal toxic exposures. *Toxicology* 109 (1): 1–13.

Lincoln, S.D. and Black, B. (1980). Halogeton poisoning in range cattle. *Journal of the American Veterinary Medical Association* 176 (8): 717–718.

Matondi, G.H.M., Masama, E., Mpofu, I.D.T., and Muronzi, F.F. (2007). Effect of feeding graded levels of cottonseed meal on goat erythrocyte membrane osmotic fragility. *Livestock Research for Rural Development* 19 (11): 169–172.

McIntosh, G.H., Pulsford, M.F., Spencer, W.G., and Rosser, H. (1974). A study of urolithiasis in grazing ruminants in South Australia. *Australian Veterinary Journal* 50 (8): 345–350.

Meena, V.K., Meena, S., and Choudhary, S.D. (2022). Lantana poisoning in Sirohi goats in Bojunda, Chittorgarh. *Haryana Veterinarian* 61 (SI): 128–130.

Nation, P.N., Crowe, S.P., and Harries, W.N. (1982). Clinical signs and pathology of accidental monensin poisoning in sheep. *Canadian Veterinary Journal* 23 (11): 323.

National Research Council (2007). *Nutrient requirements of small ruminants: sheep, goats, cervids, and new world camelids*. Washington, DC: NRC.

Ni, D., Madden, T.L., Johansen, M. et al. (2002). Murine pharmacokinetics and metabolism of oleandrin, a cytotoxic component of *Nerium oleander*. *Journal of Experimental Therapeutics and Oncology* 2 (5): 278–285.

Oliva, M. L. V., Souza-Pinto, J. C., Batista, I. F., Araujo, M. S., Silveira, V. F., Auerswald, E. A., Mentele, R., Eckerskorn, C., Sampaio, M.U. and Sampaio, C. A. (2000). Leucaena leucocephala serine proteinase inhibitor: primary structure and action on blood coagulation, kinin release and rat paw edema. *Biochimica et Biophysica Acta (BBA)-Protein Structure and Molecular Enzymology*, 1477(1–2), 64–74.

Olkowski, A.A., Gooneratne, S.R., Rousseaux, C.G., and Christensen, D.A. (1992). Role of thiamine status in sulphur induced polioencephalomalacia in sheep. *Research in Veterinary Science* 52 (1): 78–85.

Oppenheim, E.W., Nasrallah, I.M., Mastri, M.G., and Stover, P.J. (2000). Mimosine is a cell-specific antagonist of folate metabolism. *Journal of Biological Chemistry* 275 (25): 19268–19274.

Ortega-Morales, N.B., Cueto-Wong, J.A., Barrientos-Juárez, E. et al. (2020). Toxicity in goats exposed to arsenic in the region Lagunera, Northern Mexico. *Veterinary Sciences* 7 (2): 59.

Oruc, H.H., Celik, M., Sahinturk, P., and Gencoglu, H. (2015). Outbreak of Peracute urea toxicosis in sheep following the consumption of new packages of grain barley. *Uludağ Üniversitesi Veteriner Fakültesi Dergisi* 34 (1–2): 81–84.

Parimoo, H.A., Sharma, R., Patil, R.D., and Patial, V. (2015). Sub-acute toxicity of lantadenes isolated from *Lantana camara* leaves in Guinea pig animal model. *Comparative Clinical Pathology* 24 (6): 1541–1552.

Plumlee, K.H. (2004). Plants: cyanogenic glycoside. In: *Clinical Veterinary Toxicology* (ed. K.H. Plumlee), 391–392. St. Louis, MO: Mosby.

Podder, M., Dharma, S. and Jamatia, H. (2020). Housing management – an important key to success in goat rearing. *Pashudhan Praharee*, May 22. https://www.pashudhanpraharee.com/housing-management-an-important-key-to-success-in-goat-rearing.

Prasanth, C.R., Khan, S., and Ajithkumar, S. (2017). Therapeutic management of cobra envenomation in a goat. *Intas Polivet* 18 (1): 103–104.

Radke, S. (2021). Small ruminant toxicology and cases. *American Association of Bovine Practitioners Conference Proceedings*. https://bovine-ojs-tamu.tdl.org/AABP/article/view/8323.

Rahman, M.M., Nakagawa, T., Niimi, M. et al. (2011). Effects of feeding oxalate containing grass on intake and the concentrations of some minerals and parathyroid hormone in blood of sheep. *Asian-Australasian Journal of Animal Sciences* 24 (7): 940–945.

Reis, L.S.L.D.S., Pardo, P.E., Camargos, A.S., and Oba, E. (2010). Mineral element and heavy metal poisoning in animals. *Journal of Medicine and Medical Sciences* 1 (12): 560–579.

Rhian, B. (2012). Overview of cyanide poisoning. In: *MSD Veterinary Manual*. Rahway, NJ: Merck https://www.msdvetmanual.com/toxicology/cyanide-poisoning/cyanide-poisoning-in-animals.

Rosmaninho, J.F., Oliveira, C.A.F., Dos Reis, T.A., and Corrêa, B. (2006). Aflatoxina M1 e Ácido Ciclopiazônico em Leites de Consumo Comercializados no Município de São Paulo, SP, Brasil. *Brazilian Journal of Food Technology* 3: 55–59.

Royer, H. and Buronfosse, F. (1998). Epidemiologie descriptive des intoxications chez les ruminants (donnees ducnitv de lyon de janvier 1990 a aout 1998). *Le Point Vétérinaire* 29: 1205–1209.

Sasu, V., Hagiu, N., Tască, S. et al. (1970). Acute poisoning of sheep with ammonium nitrate fertilizer. *Revista de Zootehnie si Medicina Veterinaria* 20 (9): 62–67.

Schweitzer, D., Kimberling, C., Spraker, T. et al. (1984). Accidental monensin sodium intoxication of feedlot cattle. *Journal of the American Veterinary Medical Association* 184: 1273–1276.

Seawright, A.A., Groenendyk, S., and Silva, K.I.N.G. (1970). An outbreak of oxalate poisoning in cattle grazing Setaria sphacelata. *Australian Veterinary Journal* 46: 293–296.

Sejian, V., Silpa, M.V., Reshma Nair, M.R. et al. (2021). Heat stress and goat welfare: adaptation and production considerations. *Animals* 11 (4): 1–24.

Shafi, T.A., Siddiqui, M., Sakhre, M.P. et al. (2020). Successful treatment of *Lantana camara* poisoning in sheep. *EC Veterinary Science* 5 (2): 1–5.

Shaikat, A.H., Hasan, M.M., Hasan, S.A. et al. (2012). Non-protein nitrogen compound poisoning in cattle. *University Journal of Zoology, Rajshahi University* 31: 65–68.

Sharma, O.P., Sharma, S., Pattabhi, V. et al. (2007). A review of the hepatotoxic plant *Lantana camara*. *Critical Reviews in Toxicology* 37 (4): 313–352.

Singh, S., Kasrija, R., and Singh, P. (2020). A sight of present goat farming situation-a review. *International Journal of Current Microbiology* 9 (8): 1–9.

Smith, J., Kovalik, D., and Varga, A. (2015). Rattlesnake envenomation in three dairy goats. *Case Reports in Veterinary Medicine* 2015: 787534.

Soto-Blanco, B., Fontenele-Neto, J.D., Silva, D.M. et al. (2006). Acute cattle intoxication from *Nerium oleander* pods. *Tropical Animal Health and Production* 38 (6): 451–454.

Tafti, A.K., Nazifi, S., Rajaian, H. et al. (2008). Pathological changes associated with experimental salinomycin toxicosis in sheep. *Comparative Clinical Pathology* 17 (4): 255–258.

Tegzes, J.H., Puschner, B., and Melton, L.A. (2003). Cyanide toxicosis in goats after ingestion of California Holly (*Heteromeles arbutifolia*). *Journal of Veterinary Diagnostic Investigation* 15 (5): 478–480.

Venkatesakumar, E., Sivaraman, S., Vijayakumar, G. et al. (2020). Therapeutic management of saw scaled viper (*Echis carinatus*) snake envenomation in a goat. *Journal of Entomology and Zoology Studies* 8 (2): 1580–1582.

Vijayakumar, S. and Srinivasa, P. (2018). Clinical management of spontaneous *Leucaena leucocephala* (Subabul) poisoning in non descriptive goat. *International Journal of Current Microbiology and Applied Sciences* 7 (10): 1148–1151.

Villar, D., Schwartz, K.J., Carson, T.L. et al. (2003). Acute poisoning of cattle by fertilizer-contaminated water. *Veterinary and Human Toxicology* 45 (2): 88–90.

Volmer, P.A. (2004). Non protein nitrogen. In: *Clinical Veterinary Toxicology* (ed. K.H. Plumlee), 130–132. St. Louis, MO: Mosby.

Ward, G., Harbers, L.H., and Blaha, J.J. (1979). Calcium-containing crystals in alfalfa: their fate in cattle. *Journal of Dairy Science* 62 (5): 715–722.

Wein Chang, H., DeChi, W., ShenShyuan, Y., and YuKuei, C. (2004). Comparison of different oxalate contents of napiergrass fed to yellow cattle and goats. *Journal of Taiwan Livestock Research* 37: 313–322.

Welch, K.D., Stonecipher, C.A., Lee, S.T., and Cook, D. (2020). The acute toxicity of water hemlock (*Cicuta douglasii*) in a goat model. *Toxicon* 176: 55–58.

Whitaker, T., Slate, A., Doko, B. et al. (ed.) (2010). *Sampling Procedures to Detect Mycotoxins in Agricultural Commodities*. Dordrecht: Springer.

Wright, M.J. and Davison, K.L. (1964). Nitrate accumulation in crops and nitrate poisoning in animals. *Advances in Agronomy* 16: 197–247.

14

Genetic Diseases of Goats

Simant Kumar Nanda

Fisheries and ARD Department, Government of Odisha, Odisha, India

Goats were one of the earliest animals to be domesticated by humans. They are reared for milk and meat. In the Indian context, compared to large animal farming small ruminants are easier to rear, less capital intensive, and more remunerative. Moreover, sheep and goats are more adaptable to harsh climatic conditions than cows and buffalo. In many poor households small ruminants are often found to be the sole livelihood option, although small farmers also rear them to supplement household income. Small animal farming has become lucrative as the demand for meat has increased due to changes in food habits across society. Dairy breeds of goats, though fewer in number, are prized possessions in Rajasthan, Gujarat, Uttar Pradesh, Haryana, and the Punjab. Goat milk is preferred over cow/buffalo milk as baby food because it is easily digestible, but goat milk is not commercially marketed, although it may be available in limited quantities in certain regions. Dairy goat breeds like Barbari and Surti and dual-purpose breeds like Jamnapari and Beetal are primarily found in the Punjab, Haryana, Gujarat, and Uttar Pradesh. On the other hand, meat breeds like Black Bengal and Ganjam are reared in eastern India along with other local varieties, now recognized as breeds, and Mehsana, Sirohi, and Marwari in the northwest and Nellore in the south. There are nearly 200 breeds of domesticated goats worldwide, with India having the largest population in the world.

One of the major constraints among farmers is poor knowledge of farm practices, breeding, and nutrition, as well as of diseases that commonly affect flocks. These factors hamper productivity and consequently cause economic loss to beleaguered farmers. Diseases may be infectious or non-infectious. Infectious diseases may be due to bacterial, viral, or fungal agents and parasites, or may be non-infectious metabolic diseases. Some metabolic diseases have a genetic origin and could occur in all breeds. Together they reduce the vitality of animals, affecting the optimum level of growth and productivity and cause economic losses. Tracking and mapping different genetic diseases in sheep and goats and cataloging them is a difficult task, but scientists are at work to deliver this obligation in due course.

The modern concept of breeding has now begun to shift its focus to genetic diseases that have been overlooked in the past. Animals with hereditary abnormalities may prove more ruinous than those with diseases due to conventional causes because this unseen enemy may damage the quality of future generations. However, one common factor behind several diseases is the genetic factor. Genetic abnormalities have resulted in several congenital malformations, which will be discussed later in this chapter. One of the major constraints on successful goat-rearing at a farm level is the prevalence of non-descript animals or poor genetic quality in about 70% of animals, compounded by unorganized breeding programs. As a measure of comfort, genetic abnormalities in a carrier state are detectable with the aid of enzymes and surface protein markers and can be eliminated from goat populations, whereas common polygenic disorders including udder problems in does and gynecomastia in bucks are more difficult to eradicate because of the presence of the mutant genes responsible for them. This requires a change in breeder preference and selection regime. In making these changes, however, the beneficial traits will have to be balanced against the undesirable effects of the selected mutant genes (pleiotropy), which hold the key to the success or failure of domesticated goat breeding. Knowledge of the genetic bases of some livestock diseases has led to controlled breeding to eradicate them and has helped to create new avenues of learning for genetic engineering.

When we talk about this subject, we are precisely interested in knowing the importance and role of genetics in the art of plant and animal breeding. Genetics can be defined

Principles of Goat Disease and Prevention, First Edition. Edited by Tanmoy Rana.
© 2024 John Wiley & Sons, Inc. Published 2024 by John Wiley & Sons, Inc.

as a branch of biological science that deals with the scientific study of genes and heredity and how certain qualities are passed on from parents to offspring, whether in animals or plants or other living creatures including humans, as a result of changes in DNA sequence. It was commonly believed in the nineteenth century that an organism's traits were passed on to the offspring in a blend of characteristics "donated" by each parent, which in lay terminology is termed heredity. It was Gregor Mendel (1822–1884), the father of genetics, who gave this a more scientific explanation. Modern genetics has moved many steps farther and is no longer limited to the study of inheritance, but encompasses the study of the behavior and functions of genes. Applied genetics is a tool used to improve the quality of livestock and crop production. Cross-breeding and selective breeding are generally employed by breeders or farmers to derive the best from their stock. The process involves an intricate combination or assortment of characters in a compatible environment. Sophisticated research has led to a number of subfields like molecular genetics, epigenetics, and population genetics. Given this scenario, animal geneticists have a definitive role in planning for better breeds and production in all categories of animals, besides a good understanding of the subject to eliminate uneconomical and undesirable traits as far as possible.

14.1 Congenital Abnormalities

Congenital abnormalities that are inherited by progeny have become issues of great concern in sheep and goat breeding. The acquired traits may result in intrauterine fetal death, abortion, or stillbirth. These traits also affect their viability, performance, productivity, and value. A majority of the congenital defects in sheep and goats that have been studied so far tend to fall into the autosomal recessive category. The definitive etiology of congenital anomalies in small ruminants is unknown, but genetic, environmental (toxic, infectious, and nutritional), or inherited factors are suggested to be the probable causes. The domestic goat (*Capra hircus*) shares some of the congenital abnormalities generally seen in other domesticated ruminant animals (Hiraga and Dennis 1993). However, systematic studies of congenital anomalies in goats are relatively few and published literature consists almost entirely of case reports. The most frequently reported defects in goats are intersex, testicular hypoplasia, and unilateral cryptorchidism.

Environmental factors like food deficiency, infections (bacterial, viral, parasitic), drugs, poisonous plants, and chemicals have been known to interact with genes and alleles (Raoof et al. 2017) to cause abnormal development in growth or embryo formation during pregnancy. Interaction between genetic and environmental factors

may result in expression of some of the unexpressed diseases. The environmental factors listed have been reported to influence hormone production and receptors, and building proteins in addition to ion pathways in the body (Wagner et al. 2014), resulting in functional damage and also affecting the protein metabolism of the body.

Mutant genes are responsible for birth defects, metabolic errors, and reproductive problems in small ruminants due to undesirable traits. Sickness and birth imperfections in sheep and goats with heredity etiology may be categorized as (i) monogenic, (ii) polygenic, and (iii) chromosomal disorders. A mutation at a single locus that is transmitted from one generation to the next in a Mendelian ratio is referred as a monogenic disorder, whereas defects and diseases caused by mutant genes at several loci are considered polygenic in nature and may not have a detectable negative impact on an individual animal. The chromosomal diseases of genetic importance are characterized by the number or structure of the chromosomes that mostly cause reproductive problems in domesticated animals.

14.1.1 Congenital Abnormalities of Joints and the Skeleton

Goats (*C. hircus*) share some of the congenital abnormalities seen in other domesticated ruminants (Hiraga and Dennis 1993). The most frequent abnormalities reported in goats are intersex, testicular hypoplasia, and unilateral cryptorchidism.

14.1.2 Akabane Virus (*Bunyavirus*)

Akabane virus is associated with the epizootics of congenital deformities in cattle, sheep, and goats. It is a member of the Simbu serological subgroup of the Bunyaviridae family of arboviruses, which contains 25 viruses. It was isolated from *Aedes vexans* and *Culex tritaeniorhynchus* spp. of mosquitoes. Akabane virus demonstrates transplacental transmission that is limited to part of the gestation period and results in congenital malformations. All does inoculated with the virus completed their pregnancy in 140–148 days after mating ended with kyphosis, scoliosis, and brachygnathism. In such conditions there are marked changes in the skeletal musculature associated with loss of muscle mass. The carcass has depleted fat deposits, especially in the region of sternal and retroperitoneal brown fat. Brown adipose tissue or brown fat is one of two types of fat that humans and other mammals have. Its main function is to convert food into body heat. The midbrain, cerebellum, and medulla oblongata are found to be shrunken in size, whereas the spinal cord through the cervical region tapers off sharply from the thoracic region to the lumbar region. Studies, however, suggest that Akabane virus is in the list of teratogenic viruses and further studies are in progress to determine the mechanism by which it causes congenital deformities.

14.1.3 Hereditary Chondrodysplasia (Spider Lamb Syndrome)

Spider lamb syndrome is a lethal autosomal recessive genetic disorder that results in skeletal deformities in young sheep and goats. Suffolk and Hampshire breeds of sheep are primarily affected. Lambs may be normal at birth, but the deformities typically manifest by 4–6 weeks of age, including facial defects; kyphosis and scoliosis; overly long, bent, and/or splayed legs; a flat ribcage; and poor musculature (Figure 14.1). These defects were first observed in black-faced lambs in the 1970s. This disorder was subsequently ascribed to mutation in fibroblast growth factor receptor 3 gene (*FGFR3*). The animals that survive the perinatal period develop angular limb and facial deformities. Muscle atrophy is common. Marfan-like syndrome in humans is similar to hereditary chondrodysplasia in sheep. In Marfan-like syndrome in humans, physical features may include a long, narrow face; a curved spine or scoliosis; a breastbone (sternum) that may either stick out or be indented; joints that become dislocated; and flat feet.

14.1.4 Unilateral Carpal Flexion of Goats (Beta-mannosidosis)

Unilateral carpal flexion is due to an autosomal recessive gene, primarily seen in the Nubian breed, characterized by an inability to stand and flex the carpal joint and hyperextension of the pastern joint in the newborn. Sometimes

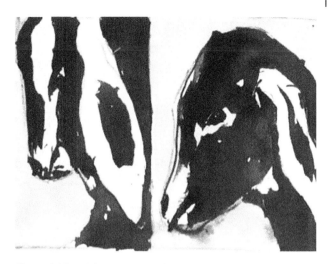

Figure 14.2 Unilateral carpal flexion of goats.

newborns are found to be deaf. Other symptoms include a domed skull, a small narrow muzzle, enophthalmos, and a depressed nasal bridge (Figure 14.2) (Smith and Sherman 2009). Clinically, beta-mannosidosis enzyme activity measured in plasma detects the carrier status in adults.

14.1.5 Caprine Arthritis Encephalitis Virus

Caprine arthritis encephalitis virus (CAEV) is antigenically related to Maedi-visna virus and genetically distinct from the *Lentivirus* of the Retroviridae family (Grego et al. 2002). There are chances of cross-species transfer of goat-adapted strains to sheep, where sheep and goats are reared in close contact. This virus causes arthritis, mastitis, encephalitis, and chronic pneumonia. It is found mostly in brain and lungs, but is also common in spleen, joints, lymph nodes, central nervous system (CNS), and mammary glands. Transmission mostly occurs by the oral route. Pregnant animals suspected of the disease may give birth to progeny with swollen knees and weak carpal joints. Arthrogryposis (crooked joints) is caused by Maedi-visna virus and CAEV. It is bilateral flexion rigidity of both carpi with outward rotation of the fore limbs. Femoral bending, scoliosis, hip subluxation, joint laxity, tibial/fibular agenesis, polydactyly, and inability to bear weight on hind limbs are some of the notable features (Figure 14.3).

14.1.6 Polydactyly (Supernumerary Digit)

Polydactyly may be found in the hind limbs. Extra digits are poorly developed, attached to a small stalk, and associated with mutations in a nonsense gene glioma-associated oncogne3 (*GLI-3*) with postaxial polydactyly.

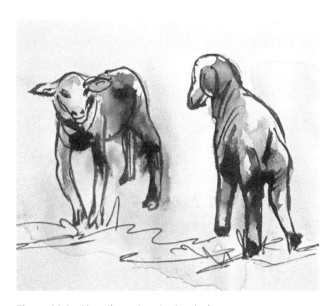

Figure 14.1 Hereditary chondrodysplasia.

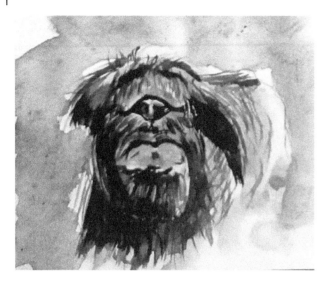

Figure 14.3   Caprine arthritis encephalitis virus.

14.2   Congenital Anomalies of the Head and Neck

14.2.1   Exencephaly (Defective Cranium with Brain Exposure)

Encephalocele denotes a condition where the brain is exposed due to a large opening in the skull. The brain together with the meninges may protrude through this opening. The condition is seen in many species and is believed to be inherited. Vitamin A deficiency and administration of albendazole during pregnancy have some relation to exencephaly. In kids the left ear is a hard limb-like shape and the right ear is relatively long. The kid has unilateral anophthalmia, a centrally located single eye with a bluish cloudy cornea (cyclopia – failure of division of orbits) and fissured lower eyelids. Nostrils and nasal cavity are absent.

14.2.2   Cyclopia

Cyclopia is a severe form of holoprosencephaly involving the craniofacial skeleton, and is characterized by the presence of a median orbita containing a single eyeball. The symptoms of cyclopia may include alopecia of the head, unequal ears, and dissimilar eyes or cornea. Generally, the kid is a stillbirth or else death of the animal occurs very early in its life (Rashed et al. 2014).

14.2.3   Entropion

Entropion is considered to have a complex genetic background involving a single significant single-nucleotide polymorphism (SNP). The SNP is located over the Bonferroni line in the region of chromosome 6. In this

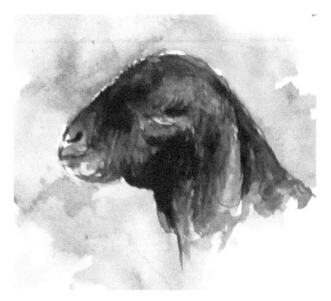

Figure 14.4   Entropion.

condition, the lower eyelid turns inward and traumatizes the conjunctiva and cornea. There is lachrymation, blepharospasm, and photophobia, leading to irritation of the eyeball and cornea (Figure 14.4). The inflammatory process thus damages the eye, causing loss of vision if untreated. Surgical intervention in the lower eyelid and cheek, by fixing a suture or a surgical staple to anchor the lid in an averted position, may correct the condition successfully.

14.2.4   Dermatosparaxis

Dermatosparaxis is also known as Ehlers–Danlos syndrome (EDS) and is classified as EDS type vii-c. It is caused by SNP in the *adamts2* gene, which is autosomal recessive (Zhou et al. 2012) and resembles the gene found in both humans and cattle (Colige et al. 1999). Heterozygous animals are phenotypically normal. The phenotypes in this disease are characterized by thin and hyperextensible skin, which is fragile, leading to hemorrhagic wounds and atrophic scars. It is otherwise described as cutis hyperelastica, hyperelastosis cutis, dermatosparaxis, dermal/collagen dysplasia, dermal/cutaneous asthenia, or EDS (Halper 2014). Such dermal defects prevent the affected animals from entering breeding systems, as they are either discarded or removed from their usual activities due to the presence of wounds or susceptibility to wound infections.

14.3   True Hermaphroditism

Freemartin or hermaphroditism in goats is not uncommon, especially in dairy goats. A true hermaphrodite only happens in mammals when an animal has the genes for being both female and male. This is typically the result of chimerism, or when two fertilized eggs or very young embryos of opposite sexes fuse together and develop into one offspring. Chimerism happens when two fraternal twins fuse; mosaicism happens when a single egg has a mutation after having split a few times, and that mutation is passed down to a larger percentage of the body's cells but not fully. Both principles are considered to be factors for hermaphroditism. A (pseudo-)hermaphrodite is usually genetically female, but has been masculinized. It displays either ovaries or testes but is infertile. The condition is prevalent in some goat breeds such as Alpine, Saanen, and Toggenburg. The low frequency of freemartins in goats is attributed to the infrequency of significant intraplacental vascular anastomoses. In freemartins, the development of the female reproductive system is inhibited by Müllerian-inhibiting substances (MIS).

14.4   Ovarian Dysgerminoma

Ovarian dysgerminoma is a neoplasm that originates from primordial germ cells of the ovary. Dysgerminoma is the female counterpart of seminoma in the testis, and occurs bilaterally in goats. The neoplastic cells are arranged as sheets or in a nest pattern. Mitotic figures and binucleated cells are present in the tumor. Hemorrhages, necrotic foci, and infiltrated lymphocytes are also observed. The male sex-specific genetic architecture may be either a ductus deferens-like structure embedded in the broad ligament with a thick muscular wall and a narrow star-shaped lumen. The tumor is composed of round to polygonal, finely granular to eosinophilic cytoplasm and distinct cell borders. In some cases, gonadal dysgenesis and hermaphroditism may be associated with dysgerminoma.

14.5   Complex Vertebral Malformation

The complex vertebral malformation (CVM) syndrome is a congenital lethal malformation, which in later stages develops into an aborted fetus or a perinatal malformed fetus. It is characterized by growth retardation and bilateral flexion of the carpal and metacarpophalangeal joints with rotation of the digits. Genomic analysis has identified a single base substitution of guanine to thymine at position 559 in the gene *slc35a3* to be the cause of CVM. The gene *slc35a3* codes for a nucleotide-sugar transporter, where the base mutation is reflected by an amino acid substitution at position 180; that is, valine to phenylalanine. This inhibits the function of the transporter and the defective transporter molecule leads to vertebral malformations. Defective calves possess this mutation in both alleles, which contributes to the autosomal recessive nature of the disorder.

14.6   Syndactylism ("Mule Foot")

Syndactylism is a congenital malformation of the distal parts of one or more limbs characterized by complete or partial fusion or no division of the functional digits (Figure 14.5). The inheritance of syndactylism in Holsteins has been determined as autosomal recessive. No studies have been found in goats for confirmation. Initial studies mapped the syndactyly locus to chromosome 15. Recent studies have demonstrated several mutations in the low-density lipoprotein receptor-related protein 4 gene (*lrp4*), impairing its function in distal limb development.

Figure 14.5   Syndactylism.

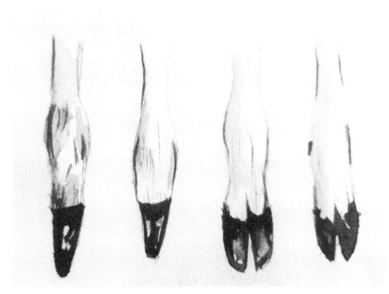

14.7   Acroteriasis

Acroteriasis is a lethal congenital malformation, morphologically characterized by severe facial dysplasia and tetrameric peromelia. Concurrent lesions are seen, such as hydrocephalus and palatoschisis. Affected individuals are mostly aborted or stillborn. The disorder is due to an inherited autosomal recessive gene.

14.8   Spinal Muscular Atrophy

Spinal muscular atrophy (SMA) is a neurodegenerative disease belonging to the group of lower motor neuron diseases. The age at disease initiation is difficult to determine and the speed of progression varies. The disorder is congenital in around 10% of cases. The clinical signs are dominated by progressive muscular weakness leading to recumbency and finally death. Muscular atrophy is especially conspicuous in the hind limbs.

14.9   Chromosomal Aberrations

These defects reduce the animals' fertility due to the development of gametes with unbalanced chromosome numbers, leading to non-viable embryos. The chromosomal aberrations, which are mostly identified in cultured blood lymphocytes, can be of one or two copies, designated as heterozygous and homozygous states, respectively.

14.9.1   Tandem Fusion Translocation

Tandem fusion translocation is characterized by the fusion of two chromosomes at the free end opposite the centromere, with simultaneous loss of one centromere.

- **Translocation**: This is a complicated translocation where chromosomal segments have been exchanged among chromosomes 1, 8, and 9.
- **Translocation 1/29**: This is a centromere fusion of chromosomes 1 and 29. This defect is the most common chromosomal translocation.

14.10   Classical Scrapie in Goats

Classical scrapie (caprine spongiform encephalopathy) is the prototype of transmissible spongiform encephalopathy (TSE). Prion diseases such as scrapie are neurodegenerative disorders with fatal consequences, caused by a conformational change of the cellular prion protein (PrPC) originating from the pathogenic form (PrPSc). Animals affected by it begin with behavioral changes that progress

to more obvious neurological signs such as ataxia pruritus, hyperesthesia, and cachexia. Clinical signs may vary between affected animals, but the most common behavioral alterations are restlessness, hyperexcitability to external stimuli, resistance to handling, and bruxism (Figure 14.6). In addition to these conditions, pruritus is a typical sign of classical scrapie. It can cause areas of alopecia by the animal continuously scratching or rubbing against hard objects (Figure 14.7). There is a clear influence of the PRNP genotype for codons 136, 154, and 171 in susceptibility to classical scrapie. On the other hand, studies have identified

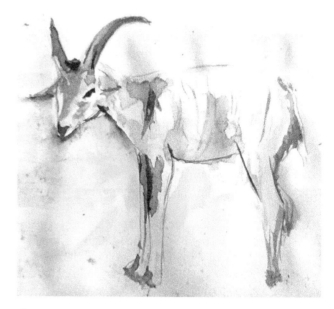

Figure 14.6   Classical scrapie.

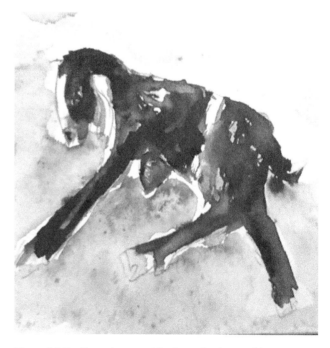

Figure 14.7   Alopecia caused by the animal scratching or rubbing against hard objects.

Table 14.1 Genotypes and phenotypes associated with scrapie in the goat.

PRNP genotype	Scrapie phenotype	References
VV21, LL23, GG49, SS49, HH143, HR143, RR154, PP168, PP240, SP240, and SS240	Variants found in scrapie-affected goats	Billinis et al. (2002)
R143 and H154	Moderately protective against scrapie	Billinis et al. (2002)
K222	Associated with healthy animals or scrapie resistance	Acutis et al. (2006), Vaccari et al. (2006)
Q168	Associated with scrapie susceptibility	Acutis et al. (2006)
M142	Associated with prolonged incubation period of scrapie and TSE in goats	Goldmann et al. (1996)

three polymorphic codons: 136 A (alanine)/V (valine), 154 R (arginine)/H (histidine) and 171 Q (glutamine)/R/H. Alanine, arginine, and arginine are at codons 136, 154, and 171, respectively, which are associated with protection against classical forms of scrapie (Table 14.1). The findings further described that the presence of methionine at codon 142 may represent a lower risk of the animal developing the disease.

14.11 Defects of Spermatozoa

Several defects of spermatozoa have been identified, but an inherited basis has only been established for the "Dag defect." This is characterized by spermatozoa with tails that are strongly coiled, extensively folded, or split into fibers. These abnormalities inhibit controlled motility. The fertility of affected sires reflects the level of abnormal spermatozoa. The sires often have severely reduced fertility, as the percentage of defective spermatozoa is mostly high. The tail abnormalities are not present in the spermatozoa as long as they are within the testicles, but develop during passage through the epididymidis. This has led to the hypothesis that the spermatozoa are normal but are damaged by an unfavorable biochemical environment within the tubules of the epididymidis.

14.12 Ectopic Heart (Ectopia Cordis Pectoralis)

The congenital condition ectopia cordis is characterized by complete or partial protrusion of the heart through a ventrally located defective wall of the thoraco-abdominal

region of the kid. In an ectopic heart condition a pulsating swelling is palpated, presternally, outside the chest.

Other defects include epitheliogenesis imperfecta with visceral eventration at the umbilicus. Umbilical hernias are soft, fluctuating, and painless reducible swellings of a lemon to water-melon size. The hernial rings range in diameter between one and three fingers.

14.13 Congenital Anomalies of the Pelvis and Perineum

- **Urethral dilatation with history of dysuria**: This is characterized by dilatation of the urethra extending to variable distances between the scrotum and free portion of the penis. The painless and fluctuating dilatations are of different sizes (small bean or duck-egg size), with urine dribbling from the tip of the penis by pressure on these diverticula. A double scrotum may also be found.
- **Ectopic testicles (cryptorchidism)**: This may be sub-cutaneous abdominal ectopic testicles, unilateral, or bilateral. Ectopic testicles can be surgically removed by the process of castration.
- **Scrotal hernia**: In this condition, the scrotum totally occupies the inguinal region and the testicles do not descend to the scrotal sack. The hernia contents may include portions of the omentum and intestine.
- **Rectal fistula into the tail**: Sometimes the kid has an anal opening into the tail. The tail is fatty, swollen, and doughy in consistency. Exploratory puncture yields a greenish, watery offensive fluid. Surgical reconstruction of the perianal part is done to repair the dorsal rectal wall and amputate the fatty tail.
- **Hypospadias**: A defect of the external genitalia, this is characterized by incomplete development of the prepuce with a ventral opening in the urethral fold. This condition was reported in a horned Saanen buck.

14.14 Metabolic Diseases Due to a Genetic Defect

The metabolism is a complex set of chemical reactions that the body uses to maintain life, including energy production. Special enzymes break down food or certain chemicals so that the body can utilize them in the right way for energy production or store them in some form or other; the metabolism also catalyzes substances that are no longer needed or makes those it lacks. When these chemical processes do not work properly due to a hormone or enzyme deficiency, metabolic disorders start manifesting. In most inherited metabolic disorders, a single enzyme is either not produced by the body at all or is produced in a form that does not work. The missing enzyme is like an absentee worker on the assembly line. Depending on that enzyme's job, its absence means toxic chemical build-up or absence of an essential product.

Generally, the presence or absence of an enzyme depends on the genetic materials and amino acids coded for the enzyme, which may come from either or both of the parents. The offspring who inherits two defective gene copies cannot produce enough effective enzymes and as a consequence develops a metabolic disorder. This type of genetic transmission is called autosomal recessive in inheritance. Genetic metabolic disorders can also be the result of mutation. However, these disorders are very rare in a population. Such diseases are often characterized by progressive brain and nerve deterioration. Depending on the specific disease, other organs of the body may be involved, such as heart, lungs, ears, nose, throat, and bones. Examples of metabolic disease conditions are cretinism, albinism, cystinuria (uroliths made from an amino acid called cysteine in the kidney, ureter, and bladder), phenylketonuria (PKU), some forms of gout, photosensitivity, and thyroid disease (Bacon and Garrod 1909).

14.14.1 Cretinism (Iodine Deficiency)

Iodine is an important mineral in the animal body and is incorporated in thyroid hormone, which is responsible for thermoregulation, metabolism, growth, reproduction, as well as production of different intermediate metabolites. Congenital iodine deficiency syndrome, also called cretinism, is a condition of severely stunted physical and neurological growth due to a congenital deficiency of thyroid hormone (congenital hypothyroidism), usually owing to maternal hypothyroidism (Bhardwaj 2018). Does or ewes grazing on iodine-deficient soil will have a deficiency of that mineral in their body, leading to deficiency in their offspring. If the ewes are allowed to graze on lucerne from the time of mating and receive a free-choice lick that includes iodine, the disease can be prevented. Investigations revealed that the condition was iodine responsive, and was probably caused by a goitrogen like thiocyanate. Goiter is the cardinal characteristic of clinical deficiency, whereas subclinical deficiency is difficult to diagnose.

14.14.2 Osteogenesis Imperfecta

Osteogenesis imperfecta is an inherited connective tissue disorder characterized by excessive bone fragility with a wide array of clinical signs and variations in severity. The majority of mutations are in either of the *COL1A1* or *COL1A2* genes, which code for type 1 collagen. Clinical findings can include spontaneous fractures, fragile iridescent teeth (dentinogenesis imperfecta), joint laxity, lung abnormalities, hypercalciuria, and occasional blue sclera. Osteogenesis imperfecta in cattle and small ruminants has

been documented in the Angus, Hereford, Charolais, Belgian Blue, and Holstein-Friesian cattle breeds and Romney sheep. Occurrence of this disease can also be attributed to the additive effects of three candidate genes, *ABCA13*, *QRFPR*, and *IFTIM5*, because all these genes are directly or indirectly involved in bone development (Zhang et al. 2020).

14.14.3 Photosensitization

Photosensitization is a clinical condition occurring in both humans and animals that causes significant injury to affected individuals. In livestock, outbreaks of photosensitization caused by ingestion of toxic plants such as *Lantana camara* are relatively common. The disease can also be congenital; however, congenital (type II) photosensitization is rare and is caused by abnormal heme synthesis resulting in the accumulation of photodynamic metabolites, including uroporphyrin, coproporphyrin, and protoporphyrin derivatives in the skin (Chen et al. 2019).

14.15   Breed-Specific Diseases

Some diseases are prevalent in some specific breeds that have genetic correlations. Examples are gangliosidosis (β-galactosidase deficiency) in Suffolk and Coopworth–Romney sheep; γ-glutamyl carboxylase deficiency in the Rambouillet breed; globoid cell leukodystrophy (Krabbe's disease or galactocerebroside β-galactosidase deficiency) in polled Dorset sheep; ceroid lipofuscinosis in South Hampshire, Swedish Landrace, and Rambouillet sheep; neuroaxonal dystrophy of the Suffolk breed; and primary cerebellar degeneration of Merino and Charolais sheep (Underwood et al. 2015).

14.15.1 Neoplastic Lesions

Some neoplastic lesions such as lymphoma of various organ systems are related to genetic factors due to their occurrence in some specific breeds of sheep and goats. The cancer metastasizes through the lymph system to major organs. Treatment in lymphoma is recommended only as a palliative measure, although enucleation may be successful if the disease is still localized.

14.15.2 G6-Sulfatase Deficiency Syndrome

G6-sulfatase deficiency is an inherited autosomal recessive metabolic defect that occurs in Nubian goats and related crosses. Goats affected by this enzyme deficiency exhibit delayed motor development, growth retardation, and early death. A mutation in the *G6-S* gene renders the enzyme incapable of degrading complex polysaccharides known as heparin-sulfate glycosaminoglycans (HS-GAGs), which then abnormally accumulate in the tissues such as CNS and viscera. As the disease is acquired in an autosomal passive style, the two sexes are similarly impacted and two duplicates of the blemished quality should necessarily be available as indications in the tissue. Breeders can evaluate the results by a device for determining mating matches and try not to create impacted kids. The test is suggested for Nubian goats and crosses of Nubian stock (Cavanagh et al. 1995).

14.15.3 Niemann-Pick Disease

Niemann-Pick disease is caused by mutations in specific genes related to metabolism of body fat (cholesterol and lipids). It is divided into four main types: type a, type b, type c1, and type c2. These are classified on the basis of genetic causes and according to clinical signs of the condition. In Niemann-Pick disease types a and b, mutations are caused by mutations in the sphingomyelin phosphodiesterase 1 (*smpd1*) gene and are passed from parents to offspring in a pattern called autosomal recessive inheritance. This means that both the mother and the father must pass on the defective form of the gene for the progeny to get affected.

SMPD1, also known as acid sphingomyelinase (ASM) enzyme, is accountable for the conversion of fats (lipid) referred to as sphingomyelin to ceramide. This enzyme is found in lysosomes, which are compartments within cells that break down and recycle different types of molecules. Mutations in *smpd1* result in a scarcity of ASM, a useful protein, which prevents motion of low-density lipoprotein cholesterol and different lipids. This leads to decreased rundown of sphingomyelin, inflicting build-up of fats in cells, which cause the cells to malfunction and die.

14.16 Other Genetic Disorders

14.16.1 Pendred Syndrome

Mutations in PDS (*slc26a4*) cause both Pendred syndrome and DFNB4, two autosomal recessive disorders that share hearing loss as a common feature. The hearing loss is because of temporal bone abnormalities along with isolated enlargement of the dilated vestibular aqueduct (DVA) to Mondini dysplasia, a complex malformation in which the normal cochlear spiral of 2½ turns is replaced by a hypoplastic coil of 1½ turns. In Pendred syndrome thyromegaly also develops, although affected animals usually remain euthyroid.

14.16.2 Myotonia Congenita (Congenital Myotonia)

Myotonia congenita is a heritable situation in goats where the animal develops tetanic muscle contraction when frightened or surprised. Occasionally the contraction is so intense that the goat collapses to the ground. Because of this phenomenon, affected animals are termed "fainting goats." Autosomal dominant myotonia congenita is a non-dystrophic skeletal muscle ailment characterized by muscle stiffness and inability of the muscle to loosen up after voluntary contraction.

14.16.3 Granulomatous Disease, Chronic, X-Linked

X-linked chronic granulomatous disease (CDGX) is a primary immunodeficiency condition characterized by onset of symptoms in the first months or years of life. The disorder results from impaired function of the phagocytic NADPH oxidase complex, which generates the microbiocidal respiratory burst. Laboratory studies using the dihydrorhodamine (DHR) assay show impaired phagocyte production of reactive oxygen species (ROS) in response to phorbol myristate acetate (PMA) stimulation. CDGX can be caused by mutation in several genes encoding structural or regulatory subunits of the phagocyte NADPH oxidase complex.

14.17 Identification of Genetic Traits and Known Causal Mutations

According to Online Mendelian Inheritance in Animals (www.omia.org), a compendium of inherited disorders, traits, and genes in animal species, sheep have 49 and goats have 17 genetic traits in which the causal mutation is known, whereas cattle have 268. Production phenotypes often follow a pattern of incomplete dominance where heterozygotes demonstrate an intermediate phenotype as compared to homozygotes. Most of the identified genetic disease phenotypes are produced in a simple autosomal recessive pattern. These diseases can be easily controlled with testing and selective breeding.

Genetic testing may play a pivotal role in the management of small ruminants. There are four classes of genetic testing currently available to producers and veterinarian geneticists. Parentage identification allows keeping of accurate pedigrees and therefore evaluation of offspring for desirable production traits. Genetic markers for specific production phenotypes can help producers to select animals with desired production traits. Many genetic diseases have been identified in sheep and goats. Genetic testing for known gene mutations associated with a disease phenotype can be used to control the prevalence of disease and for any resulting production losses. Lastly, testing has been developed for genetic mutations that have been identified that confer increased resistance to certain diseases.

14.17.1 Parentage Testing

Parentage testing is based on the principle of exclusion; that is, a DNA profile of an offspring is compared to that of its parents and if the profile does not match, the parent is excluded. If matches are made, each DNA marker is evaluated, leading to the conclusion that the parent is said to qualify. Parentage testing relies on genomic evaluation using SNPs or other important molecular markers to rule out individuals based on simple inheritance.

Understanding DNA structure is a key to understanding DNA-based parentage testing. DNA is made up of four bases, adenine (A), cystine (C), guanine (G), and thymine (T), put together in a linear structure to form chromosomes. Specific combinations of these bases form genes. Additionally, the animal genome contains sequences of bases that repeat in a tandem manner called microsatellite markers. The majority of parentage testing uses a specific type of microsatellite called short tandem repeat (STR), which has two bases repeating in tandem. Many STRs demonstrate length diversity within a population, allowing them to be used as markers for parentage.

14.17.2 Production Trait Genetic Testing

Some markers for a visible phenotype are also good indicators for a hidden malformation. The features found in animals with high-muscling phenotypes are similar regardless of genetic mutation. These animals demonstrate increase in muscularity, particularly of the loins and hindquarters, and leanness/low fat content. The GDF8 mutation is a point mutation, G to A transition, which creates a target site for microRNA highly expressed in skeletal muscles that block translation of myostatin. Polymorphism in the gene credited for the production of alpha-S1 casein in milk is an example. It results in variants associated with high and low production of casein. Animals carrying the high-casein variants also tend to have higher fat content in their milk and therefore these traits together are desirable for cheese producers, as they result in higher cheese yield.

14.17.3 Genetics of Disease Resistance in Small Ruminants

Disease resistance is used generically to cover resistance to infection – that is, a host's capacity to fight pathogens or a parasite life cycle – and additionally resistance to the aftereffects of infection, meaning how soon the animal can fully recover from illness. Sometimes tolerance is used to explain a host's capacity to face sequelae of infection. Resilience is associated with tolerance and describes an animal's capacity to hold its overall performance in the face of a disorder challenge. Genetic variations in the host animal versus nematode parasite resistance were determined in all fundamental manufacturing environments and against a number of parasite species, along with *Haemonchus contortus*, *Trichostrongylus colubriformis*, *Teladorsagia circumcinta*, and diverse *Nematodirus* spp. The Garole breed seems to confer more desirable resistance to nematodes than other breeds (Nimbkar et al. 2003) as a result of its genetic make-up. These authors additionally mentioned proof of more relative resistance of indigenous goats in opposition to parasitic infections in Thailand and the Philippines as compared to Anglo-Nubian–derived breeds and crosses. Further, Marshall et al. (2005) recorded numerous sizable quantitative trait loci for *H. contortus* in sheep from a Golden Ram flock inside which a primary gene for resistance was assumed to be segregating. The maximum continuously sizable location is that containing the interferon-γ locus on chromosome 3. In one study, Patterson and Patterson (1989) validated the breeding technique leading to higher resistance to foot rot in Merinos. In addition, Skerman and Moorhouse (1987) demonstrated the feasibility of using phenotypic observations in choosing sheep for foot rot resistance.

14.17.4 Future Prospects in Genetic Elimination of Diseases

Molecular markers are used to manipulate illnesses and to map quantitative trait loci that manipulate resistance to illnesses in farm animals. To accurately manipulate farm animals' diseases by using and exploiting genetic data, deeper know-how of genome versions is needed to improve alertness and to frame strategies for micro assay primarily and totally on genomics (DNA and mRNA), proteomics (protein), protein–protein interplay, and protein–DNA interplay and the position of small useful RNAs.

Epigenetic inheritance is the transmission of data from a one-mobileular or multicell organism to its descendants without that data being encoded inside the nucleotide series of the gene. Epigenetic mechanisms including DNA methylation, posttranslational changes of histone proteins, transforming of nucleosomes, and expression of small regulatory RNAs additionally make contributions to the law of gene expression, magnification of mobileular and tissue specificity, and warranty of inheritance of gene expression levels. All these could have an effect on disease resistance. Knowledge of the genetic bases of a few farm animals' illnesses has led to them being manipulated through breeding and is creating new avenues of manipulation through genetic engineering.

Exploitation of genetic data and engineering in controlling farm animals' diseases and the know-how of their molecular genetic foundations have afforded geneticists and breeders new platforms to tackle these illnesses effectively and cheaply.

It must be said that traditional strategies of manipulation inclusive of alternate control practices, culling, vaccinations, antibiotics, and different kinds of medicines have succeeded in manipulating many farm animals' diseases. However, they are facing more price-related and other problems, such as antibiotic resistance and residues in the environment, and hence are a chief reason for issues around environmental and human health.

With classical methods of breeding, disease traits with high heritability have been used successfully to reduce the incidence of some infectious diseases of farm animals. However, the heritability of most disease traits is very low and genetic control is not easily achievable through breeding.

Genetic recourse to manipulation is one course of action that could prove beneficial to animals, producers, and consumers. Genotyping of breeding animals for disease-inflicting mutations and removing them from the breeding herd may prove useful. Using this method, numerous such illnesses can be efficaciously managed or removed from the herd.

Diseases under multigenic control, which is complex, are not as easily determined and controlled as those under single-gene control. Also, the interaction of many host genes is further compounded by pathogenic and environmental factors.

14.18 Conclusion

Investigation into and studies of genetic diseases in sheep and goats indicate that there are around 30 genetic disorders that are monogenic in character. Most of the malformations in sheep and goats seem to be similar in nature. The common abnormalities in goats like intersexuality in dairy breeds, abortion in the Angora breed, and arthritis in Pygmy breeds may have resulted from breeders' preferences and selection errors. Sheep and goats have been given equal emphasis considering their role and value in the livelihood of farmers worldwide. Goat rearing relates to husbandry practices, breeding, diseases arising from genetic incompatibilities, and methods and technologies to detect and eradicate genetic etiology from sheep and goats. These may be achievable in due course.

While reviewing research papers on this complex subject, it was found that a number of research works have been carried out in sheep and goats in tandem and present an interesting and optimist vision of getting rid of genetic diseases in general. This will afford researchers and geneticists the opportunity to engage head-on with genetic diseases that could otherwise cripple generations of livestock including sheep and goats. Climate change and its effect on domestic animals and zoonotic diseases are of concern, which could influence animal-rearing systems and human health. This may completely change our outlook on animal farming and a new era is sure to emerge. The concept of a "One Health" approach may be just the beginning.

Multiple-Choice Questions

1   In which species are chromosomal defects of a structural nature (translocations) seen?
    A Cattle
    B Pig
    C Dog
    D Goat

2   In which species do transmissible spongiform encephalopathies (TSEs) occur?
    A Cattle
    B Goat
    C Pig
    D dog

3   How can genetic abnormalities for the carrier state be detected?
    A Enzymes
    B Surface protein markers
    C Both a and b
    D None of the above

4   What is it essential to do regarding congenital defects in order to determine their frequency and overall incidence?
    A Report
    B Document
    C Both a and b
    D None of the above

5   On what information are genetic tests becoming more and more reliant?
    A Quantity
    B Quality
    C Both a and b
    D None of the above

References

Acutis, P.L., Bossers, A., Priem, J. et al. (2006). Identification of prion protein gene polymorphisms in goats from Italian scrapie outbreaks. *Journal of General Virology* 87: 1029–1033.

Bacon, F. and Garrod, A.E. (1909). *Inborn Errors of Metabolism*. Oxford: Academic Press.

Bhardwaj, R.K. (2018). Iodine deficiency in goats. In: *Goat Science* (ed. S. Kukovics). London: IntechOpen, ch. 4.

Billinis, C., Panagiotidis, C.H., Psychas, V. et al. (2002). Prion protein gene polymorphisms in natural goat scrapie. *Journal of General Virology* 83: 713–721.

Cavanagh, K.T., Leipprandt, J.R., Jones, M.Z., and Friderici, K. (1995). Molecular defect of caprine N-acetylglucosamine-6-sulphatase deficiency. A single base substitution creates a stop codon in the 59-region of the coding sequence. *Journal of Inherited Metabolic Disease* 18 (1): 96.

Chen, Y., Quinn, J.C., Weston, L.A., and Loukopoulos, P. (2019). The aetiology, prevalence and morbidity of outbreaks of photosensitisation in livestock: a review. *PLoS One* 14 (2): e0211625.

Colige, A., Sieron, A.L., Li, S.W. et al. (1999). Human Ehlers-Danlos syndrome type VII C and bovine dermatosparaxis are caused by mutations in the procollagen I N-proteinase gene. *American Journal of Human Genetics* 65 (2): 308–317.

Goldmann, W., Martin, T., Foster, J. et al. (1996). Novel polymorphisms in the caprine PrP gene: a codon 142 mutation associated with scrapie incubation period. *Journal of General Virology* 77: 2885–2891.

Grego, E., Profiti, M., Giammarioli, M. et al. (2002). Genetic heterogeneity of small ruminant lentiviruses involves immunodominant epitope of capsid antigen and affects sensitivity of single-strain-based immunoassay. *Clinical and Vaccine Immunology* 9 (4): 828–832.

Halper, J. (2014). Connective tissue disorders in domestic animals. *Progress in Heritable Soft Connective Tissue Diseases* 802: 231–240.

Hiraga, T. and Dennis, S.M. (1993). Congenital duplication. *Veterinary Clinics of North America: Food Animal Practice* 9 (1): 145–161.

Marshall, K., van derWerf, J.H.J., Maddox, J.F. et al. (2005). A genome scan for quantitative trait loci for resistance to the gastrointestinal parasite *Haemonchus contortus* in sheep. *Proceedings of the Association for the Advancement of Animal Breeding and Genetics* 16: 115.

Nimbkar, C., Ghalasi, P.M., Swan, A.A. et al. (2003). Evaluation of growth rates and resistance to nematodes of Deccani and Bannur lambs and their crosses with Garole. *Animal Science* 76: 503–515.

Patterson, R.G. and Patterson, H.M. (1989). A practical approach to breeding for footrot resistant Merinos. *Journal of the New Zealand Mountain Lands Institute* 46: 64–75.

Raoof, S.O., Mhmud, K.I., Abdulkaream, A.A., and Mouhammed, K.Q. (2017). Estimation of the best linear unbiased prediction of rams depending on their progenys birth and weaning weight. *Iraqi Journal of Agricultural Sciences* 48 (6): 1405–1411.

Rashed, R., Al-kafafy, M., Abdellah, B. et al. (2014). Cyclopia of goat: micro and macroscopic, radiographic and computed tomographic studies. *Alexandria Journal for Veterinary Sciences* 42 (1): 1–10.

Skerman, T.M. and Moorhouse, S.R. (1987). Broomfield Corriedales: a strain of sheep selectively bred for resistance to footrot. *New Zealand Veterinary Journal* 35: 101–106.

Smith, M.C. and Sherman, D.M. (2009). *Goat Medicine*, 2e. Ames, IA: Wiley.

Underwood, W.J., Blauwiekel, R., Delano, M.L. et al. (2015). Biology and diseases of ruminants (sheep, goats, and cattle). In: *Laboratory Animal Medicine*, vol. 2015, 623–694.

Vaccari, G., Di Bari, M.A., Morelli, L. et al. (2006). Identification of an allelic variant of the goat PrP gene associated with resistance to scrapie. *Journal of General Virology* 87: 1395–1402.

Wagner, H., Eskens, U., Nesseler, A. et al. (2014). Pathologic anatomical changes in newborn goats caused by an intrauterine Schmalleaberg virus infection. *Berline and Münchener tierärztliche Wochenschrift* 2 (3–4): 115.

Zhang, X., Hirschfeld, M., Beck, J. et al. (2020). Osteogenesis imperfecta in a male Holstein calf associated with a possible oligogenic origin. *Veterinary Quarterly* 40 (1): 58–67.

Zhou, H., Hickford, J.G., and Fang, Q. (2012). A premature stop codon in the ADAMTS2 gene is likely to be responsible for dermatosparaxis in Dorper sheep. *Animal Genetics* 43 (4): 471–473.

15

Protozoan Diseases in Goats

Vikrant Sudan, Deepak Sumbria, and Rabjot Kour

Department of Veterinary Parasitology, College of Veterinary Science, Guru Angad Dev Veterinary and Animal Sciences University, Rampura Phul, Punjab, India

Goats are very sensitive to the effects of internal parasitism (such as anemia and low blood protein) (Table 15.1). Parasitism can cause decreased fertility, abortion, unthriftiness, increased susceptibility to other diseases, and death. Delay in puberty age due to parasitism is well documented. Besides this, parasitic diseases are known to cause decrease in fertility and reduced body weight gains in goats. The quality of hair is affected in parasitism, as rough hair is known to be associated with many parasites. Abortion in goats due to toxoplasmosis is a very well-known problem. Coccidiosis is also known to significantly alter health and production in goats. Moreover, quite a few of the goat parasitic infections are zoonotic in nature.

This chapter focuses on the haemoprotozoan diseases of goats. It will discuss each of them in turn and in detail, revolving around the causative agent, pathogenesis, clinical signs, diagnosis, and treatment, followed by general control strategies.

15.1 Babesiosis

Caprine babesiosis is caused by various species of genus *Babesia*. The parasite multiplies in red blood cells (RBCs) by asexual division, producing two, four, or more parasites. They are present in RBCs singly as round, ovoid, elongate, or amoeboid trophozoites (a growing stage in the life cycle of some sporozoan parasites), in pairs that are pyriform, or in tetrads that are cruciform. In general, *Babesia* are divided into two major groups: a *large form* with average length of more than 3 μm, and a *small form* at less than 2.5 μm. The large form makes an acute angle and the small form lies at an obtuse angle.

Common species in the goat are as follows:

- ***Babesia motasi***: This varies from 2.5 to 4×2 μm in size and mainly occurs singly or in pairs, forming an acute angle. Ticks such as *Dermacentra silvarum*, *Haemaphysalis punctate*, and *Rhipicephalus bursa* are responsible for its transmission.
- ***B. ovis***: This is smaller than *B. motasi* and ranges from 1 to 2.5 μm in size. It is found in the margins of RBCs and when present in a pair forms an obtuse angle. *R. bursa* is the main tick for its transmission.
- ***B. taylori***: This size ranges from 1.5 to 2 μm in length.

15.1.1 Life Cycle

In a vertebrate host – for instance, a goat – the *Babesia* organism occurs in RBCs and multiplies by binary fission, a budding process, or schizogony to form two, four, or more trophozoites. These are liberated from RBCs and invade other cells, and a large number of new young RBCs are parasitized. (A parasite liberated from an infected RBC is also known as a merozoite, a small amoeboid sporozoan trophozoite produced by schizogony that is capable of initiating a new sexual or asexual cycle of development.)

Babesia species are transmitted by ticks and the development of the parasite in a tick is either *transovarian* (occurring in one host tick) or *stage to stage* (occurring in two or three host ticks):

- **Transovarian**: After ingestion of an infected RBC by the tick, lysis of the RBC takes place and erythrocytic-form parasites are seen in the gut. They are generally irregular in shape with long rays and frequently are clumped together. Later on these differentiate into macro- and microgametes,

Table 15.1 Major parasites affecting goats.

Internal parasites

Roundworms – nematodes

Large stomach worm, barber pole worm, twisted worm – *Haemonchus*

Brown stomach worm – *Ostertagia*

Stomach/intestinal hairworm, small stomach worm – *Trichostrongylus*

Thread-necked worm – *Nematodirus*

Hookworm – *Bunostomum*

Nodular worm – *Oesophagostomum*

Large-mouthed bowel worm – *Chabertia*

Whipworm – *Trichuris*

Large lungworm – *Dictyocaulus filaria*

Cooperia

Strongyloides

Tapeworms (adult and larvae) – cestodes

Broad tapeworm – *Moniezia expansa*

Fringed tapeworm – *Thysanosoma actinioides*

Hydatid cysts – *Echinococcus granulosus*

Cysticercosis – *Taenia ovis*

Taenia hydatigena

Gid – *Taenia multiceps*

Flukes – trematodes

Liver fluke – *Fasciola hepatica, F. gigantica*

Amphistomes – *Paramphistomum, Cotylophoron, Fisherioderus*

Protozoa

Coccidia (coccidiosis) – *Eimeria*

Babesiosis – *Babesia* spp.

Theileriosis – *Theileria* spp.

Anaplasmosis – *Anaplasma marginale, Anaplasma centrale*

External parasites

Lice – *Damalinia*

Mites – *Chorioptes, Psoroptes, Sarcoptes, Demodex*

Flies – *Lucilia, Calliphora, Chrysomya*

Ked – *Melophagus ovinus*

Ticks – *Hyalomma* (mainly), *Dermacentor, Haemaphysalis*

Nasal bot – *Oestrus ovis*

which unite to form a zygote. The zygote undergoes further development and multiplication. Some forms also enter epithelial cells of the gut and transform into a spindle-shaped body. Inside the epithelial cell the parasite undergoes multiple fission processes and forms a "fission body." The mature fission body ruptures the epithelial cell and liberates club-shaped bodies or vermicules into the lumen of the gut. These vermicules enter the hemolymph and also reach the ovary, ova, and other tissues. The infective stages also reach the salivary gland of the tick and are able to infect the host during feeding of blood.

- **Stage to stage**: Multiplication of developmental forms is seen in phagocytes. Pseudocytes of the organism are formed after the nymph drops off and after 11–15 days club-shaped organisms are made. These are liberated from tick cells, migrate into the muscle sheath of the nymphal tick, and penetrate the muscle cell to make an ovoid form. Further development occurs after molting of the tick. On reaching the salivary gland, the parasite undergoes binary fission and forms the infective stages.

15.1.2 Pathogenesis

Activation of prekallikrein to kallikrein occurs 1–2 days before the parasite is seen in RBCs. Kallikrein increases vascular permeability and vasodilation, leading to circulatory stasis and shock. Kallikrein also triggers intravascular coagulation. The parasite mainly harms young RBCs, causes mechanical rupture of RBCs, and leads to anemia.

Another cause of excessive erythrocyte loss is due to absorption of the circulatory antigen–antibody complex on the surface of RBCs and its removal by phagocytosis.

15.1.3 Symptoms

Symptoms are fever (40–41 °C), followed by inappetence, increased respiratory rate, muscle tremors, anemia, jaundice, dry muzzle, salivation, cessation of rumination, fall in milk yield, and weight loss. In acute infection, a large number of RBCs are destroyed, which leads to hyperchromic normocytic anemia and hemoglobinuria. Initially there is diarrhea followed by constipation.

Postmortem examination shows emaciation, subcutaneous, and intramuscular edema, pale yellow discoloration of membranes, swelling and congestion of internal organs, enlargement of spleen and liver, and congestion of lymph nodes, kidney, and urinary bladder. There will be reddish, pink, or coffee-colored urine, and pale lungs with a reddish frothy fluid.

15.1.4 Diagnosis

Diagnosis is on the basis of clinical signs; blood smear examination; serological tests such as complement fixation, indirect fluorescent antibody, or enzyme-linked immunosorbent assay (ELISA); or molecular tests such as polymerase chain reaction (PCR).

15.1.5 Treatment

Diminazene (Berenil®, Merck, Rahway, NJ, USA) should be used at 3.5 mg/kg body weight intramuscularly (IM). Imidocarb should be used subcutaneously (SC) at 1.2 mg/kg.

Trypan blue (50–100 ml of 1–2% solution on normal saline).

Supportive treatment is desirable, which includes the use of anti-inflammatory drugs, corticosteroids, and fluid therapy. Blood transfusions may be life-saving in very anemic animals.

15.1.6 Control

Control is achieved by segregation and treatment of infected animals and control of ticks.

15.2 Theileriosis

Caprine theileriosis is caused by various members of the genus *Theileria*. Again, the parasite is seen in RBCs in a piroplasmic form or in lymphocytes in the macroshizont stage, known as Koch blue bodies. In RBCs they occur in round, oval, ring, and comma forms.

Common species are *T. hirci* and *T. ovis*:

- **T. hirci**: In RBCs the parasite is mainly oval in shape, but sometime a rod-shaped structure can be seen. Its size ranges from 0.6 to 2 μm. The parasites can be found in pairs or also in fours. In lymphocyte schizonts are seen and their size ranges from 4 to 8 μm. Transmission occurs by *R. bursa*.
- **T. ovis**: This looks like *T. hirci* and is transmitted by *R. bursa*, *Rhipicephalus evertsi*, *Dermacentor sylvarum*, etc.

15.2.1 Life Cycle

15.2.1.1 Development in the Goat

When an infected tick gets attached to a goat transmission does not occur immediately, because sporozoites develop in the salivary gland for 2–4 days. During blood feeding the sporozoite enters the blood circulation of the goat. The first visible stage occurs in a local lymph node 5–8 days after the infection. It is seen in lymphocyte and lymphoblast and an infected lymph node increases in size. For the next few days the parasites increase and multiply in the local lymph node, and elsewhere in lymphoid and reticuloendothelial tissue.

Macroschizonts (Koch blue bodies) are formed in lymphocyte (Figure 15.1). Microschizonts also appear in lymphocyte or in reticular cells or macrophage. The appearance of microschizonts coincides with the appearance of piroplasm in RBCs and on the basis of morphological similarities it is concluded that the piroplasm is derived from microschizonts. Two different forms are found in RBCs, the comma form and the ovoid form.

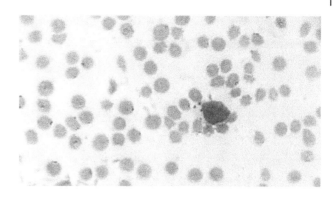

Figure 15.1 Koch blue bodies characteristic of theileriosis inside the lymphocyte of an infected goat.

15.2.1.2 Development in the Tick

After blood feeding, lysis of RBCs occur and merozoites come out and differentiate into the sexual stage. In the lumen, spindle-shaped microgamonts develop from ring forms, and break up to form many thread-like microgametes. The ring form also develop into the round form; that is, macrogametes. Macro- and microgametes fuse to form zygotes in epithelial cells.

Zygotes transform into club-shaped motile ookinetes. These ookinetes reach the salivary gland and combine into sporonts, from which sporogony occurs, with the production of infective particles.

15.2.2 Pathogenesis

The disease may occur in acute, subacute, or chronic forms. The acute form occurs in all breeds. The incubation period is 9–25 days, and there is high fever (40–41.5 °C), depression, lacrimation, nasal discharge, swelling of superficial lymph nodes, and anemia. A cerebral form of theileriosis is also noted.

Postmortem findings consist of enlarged spleen and liver, infarct on kidney, edematous lungs, swollen lymph nodes, pale mucus membranes, petechial hemorrhages, and ulcers (punched-out type) are seen in the abomasum and small intestine.

15.2.3 Diagnosis

Diagnosis is on the basis of symptoms and history; blood smear examination for RBC form and Koch blue bodies; serological tests such as immunofluorescence antibody (IFA), complement fixation (CF), ELISA; or molecular tests such as PCR.

15.2.4 Treatment

Treatment is with oxytetracycline or buparvaquone (Butalex®, Merck) at 2.5 mg/kg body weight. Supportive treatment is desirable, which includes the use of anti-inflammatory drugs, corticosteroids, and fluid therapy. Blood transfusions may be life-saving in very anemic animals.

15.2.5 Control

Control is via separation and treatment of infected animals and control of ticks.

15.3 Anaplasmosis in the Goat

Anaplasmosis is basically a disease of large and small ruminants in tropical and subtropical regions caused by rickettsia belonging to the genus *Anaplasma*. It affects cattle, sheep, goats, buffalo, and wild ruminants, and is mainly characterized by progressive anemia. *Anaplasma* is 0.2–0.5 μm in diameter with no cytoplasm. *Anaplasma ovis* are mainly transmitted to sheep and goats by *Rhipicephalus* spp. and *Dermacentor* spp.

15.3.1 Life Cycle

Anaplasma enters the RBC by invagination of the cytoplasmic membrane, leading to vacuole formation after which it multiplies by binary fission.

15.3.2 Transmission

Anaplasmosis is typically transmitted by ticks or biting flies. Iatrogenic transmission can also occur when instruments are reused without proper sanitation, including instruments used for dehorning, ear tagging, castrating, or vaccinating. In utero transmission has also been reported.

15.3.3 Clinical Signs

The acute phase of the disease is characterized by fever, progressive anemia, icterus, weight loss, milk yield decrease, and sometimes death. In addition, infection with *A. ovis* may predispose animals to other bacterial, viral, or parasitic infections that aggravate the condition of the animal and can lead to its death.

15.3.4 Pathogenesis

Parasitemia can be detected on days 3–8 post inoculation, with the parasitic load peak happening on days 12–36 post infection. Hematological changes include fall in packed cell volume (PCV), total erythrocyte count, and hemoglobin, and as the parasitemia drops there is gradual development of an autoimmune hemolytic anemia. Platelet count is also reduced.

15.3.5 Diagnosis

Anaplasmosis diagnosis is usually based on microscopic examination of Leishman or Giemsa-stained blood smears. Microscopic diagnosis may be difficult in carrier animals, thus various serological techniques have been used for the detection of *Anaplasma*-specific antibodies, including indirect IFA, ELISA, and CF. The competitive enzyme-linked immunosorbent assay (cELISA) is dependent on the use of a monoclonal antibody, ANAF16C1, which recognizes the conserved antigen MSP-5 of different *Anaplasma* species; it has high sensitivity and specificity values (Bhatia and Shah 2001).

15.3.6 Treatment

Treatment is with oxytetracycline at 10 mg/kg body weight. Other supportive therapy depends on the condition of the animal and may include phosphate supplementation, analgesics, antipyretics, and multivitamins.

15.4 Coccidiosis in the Goat

Coccidiosis is one of the major causes of morbidity and mortality in young goats. Older animals are immune to the infection. Seasonal prevalence of coccidiosis is determined by the availability of young goats for the development of the parasite. Freezing or low temperatures can either kill the oocysts or prevent them from sporulating. The species of coccidia that affect goats include *Eimeria arkhari*, *E. christenseni*, *E. faurei*, *E. gilruthi*, *E. hawkinsi*, *E. ninakohlyakimovae*, *E. pallida,* and *E. parva.*

15.4.1 Life Cycle

The sporulated oocysts are ingested by the host, which leads to liberation of sporozoites. Later on, first and second generations of schizogony occur with migration of schizonts to subepithelial tissues. Merozoites are formed and they initiate microgametocyte formation. Microgametes fertilize macrogametes with the formation of zygotes. Oocysts are shed from the cells and pass to the exterior to undergo sporogony.

15.4.2 Pathogenesis

Coccidiosis in goats is chiefly confined to animals of 4–6 months of age. It occurs due to overcrowding and poor hygiene conditions. The oocyst count reaches its peak after one month of infection (Figure 15.2).

Pathological changes are seen in the posterior part of the small intestine. The giant schizont and gametogenous stages lead to enlargement of the villi, where a polyp-like

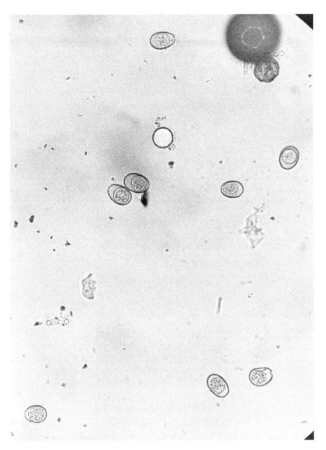

Figure 15.2 *Eimeria* oocysts in a fecal sample of a goat.

growth may be seen on the mucosa of the small intestine. In acute cases, the wall of the intestine is thickened, edematous, and hemorrhagic. Necrotic areas may also be seen on the mucosa. Intestinal mucosa is covered with petechial hemorrhages and the wall is thickened and inflamed.

15.4.3 Clinical Signs

Clinical signs consist of yellowish-green diarrhea, which is sometimes streaked with blood. The diarrhea may continue for two weeks accompanied by abdominal pain, anemia, weakness, and inappetence, and loss of weight may occur. Malabsorption may also occur due to coccidiosis.

15.4.4 Diagnosis

Diagnosis is based on the history of outbreaks and clinical signs, examination of feces, and postmortem findings.

15.4.5 Treatment

- Sulfonamides at 2 g/day for 6 days.
- Nitrofurazone at 7–10 mg/kg for 7 days.
- Amprolium at 100 mg/kg for 4–5 days.

15.4.6 Prevention and Control

Prevention and control consist of maintaining proper hygiene conditions. Regularly shifting food and water troughs, and covering them to prevent fecal contamination, can help reduce levels of infection.

15.5 Cryptosporidiosis

Cryptosporidiosis is one of the most common enteric protozoa found in young goats. The disease is particularly severe in young kids. It is associated with diarrhea and has immense zoonotic potential.

Cryptosporidium is a small, 4–8 μm parasite that undergoes development in parasitophorous vacuoles in the microvillar border of enteric epithelial cells, and is also seen in the gallbladder, respiratory, and renal epithelium, especially of immunocompromised hosts. Oocysts are thick walled, contain four sporozoites, are resistant to low and high temperatures (0–65 °C), and are colorless and transparent small oocysts. The first species, *Cryptosporidium muris*, was recognized by E.E. Tyzzer in 1907 in lab mice and now >20 species are reported in domestic and wild animals, birds, fish, reptiles, and humans.

15.5.1 Species

- *C. parvum* – humans, rhesus monkeys, calves, lambs, pigs, foals, cats, dogs, rabbits, guinea pigs, mice and rats, shellfish. The oocyst is 5–6 μm and has a prepatent period of 2–3 days.
- *C. andersoni* – cattle, rodents, etc.
- *C. baileyi* – chicken and other poultry.
- *C. meleagridis* – poultry, shellfish, humans.
- *C. muris* – mice, calves, cats, humans.
- *C. canis* – dogs, humans.
- *C. felis* – cats, humans.
- Other species occur in reptiles, snakes, and fish.

15.5.2 Life Cycle

The mode of infection is by ingestion of oocysts. The typical coccidiosis life cycle occurs in the brush border of infected epithelial cells. The sporozoites invade the microvillus brush border of enterocytes and two types of schizonts are produced. First-generation schizonts produce up to eight merozoites, which are recycled and produce either more first-type schizonts or a second generation of schizonts producing four merozoites that become gametocytes. Gametogomy occurs and oocysts are produced in 72 hours. The oocysts are minute, spherical, and colorless, lack a micropyle, and have a longitudinal suture at one pole.

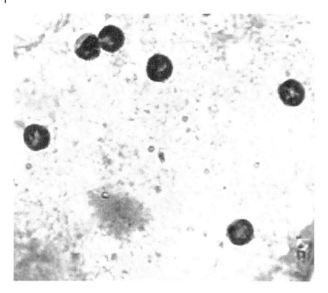

Figure 15.3 *Cryptosporidium* oocysts after modified Ziehl-Neelson staining.

15.5.3 Pathogenicity

Cryptosporidiosis is significant in kids (less than 3 weeks old) and lambs. It causes enterocolitis and is manifested by diarrhea of variable severity with clumps of mucous, and leads to depression, anorexia, and weight loss. In immunocompromised humans, symptoms of prolonged severe diarrhea and dehydration occur, persisting for 20–78 weeks. Death could occur in AIDS cases.

15.5.4 Diagnosis

The modified Ziehl-Neelson (MZN) staining method is the most common conventional method for the identification of oocysts in the feces (Figure 15.3).

15.5.5 Treatment

- Lasalocid sodium – 2 × 40 mg/kg body weight for three days for dairy cattle.
- Paromomycin – 100 mg/kg body weight/day orally for 11 days for kids.
- Nitazoxamide – 500 mg twice a day for three days for children.

15.6 Toxoplasmosis

Toxoplasma gondii was discovered by Nicolle and Manceaux in 1908. It is an obligate intracellular coccidian parasite of felines, which are the definitive hosts. It occurs as a facultative intracellular tissue cyst-forming parasite in a wide range of intermediate hosts, which include almost all warm-blooded animals, birds, and humans. *T. gondii* attacks all warm-blooded animals and infects every nucleated cell. It is not known to produce any toxin. The parasite is very common in goats and is associated with abortions.

T. gondii is transmitted in three ways:

- Congenital.
- Carnivorism.
- Fecal–oral route.

The resistant oocysts in cat feces aid in the dissemination of the parasite.

There are three infective stages of *T. gondii*:

- Tachyzoites in the pseudocysts.
- Bradyzoites in the tissue cysts.
- Sporozoites in the sporulated oocysts.

15.6.1 Life Cycle

There are two developmental cycles in the transmission of *T. gondii*.

15.6.1.1 Entero-epithelial Cycle

In felines, the definitive hosts, the entero-epithelial cycle leads to asexual reproduction by endodyogeny and endopolygeny and the formation of merozoites, gamonts, and oocysts in the intestinal epithelium when they ingest any one of the infective materials like pseudocysts, tissue cysts, or sporulated oocysts. A series of asexual generations from type A to E are produced in the intestines that multiply to form gametes and oocysts. Cats shed oocysts 3–5 days, 9–11 days, and 21–24 days after ingestion of tissue cysts, pseudocysts, and oocysts, respectively. Tissue cysts containing bradyzoites are most infective to felines.

15.6.1.2 Extra-intestinal Cycle

The extra-intestinal cycle occurs in non-felines, the intermediate hosts, when they ingest sporulated oocysts or infected meat or via the placenta.

15.6.2 Pathogenicity

Acute, subacute, or chronic disease occurs if the immune response is poor. Young, immunologically immature cats or older animals may be affected. Non-specific signs such as lethargy, inappetence, pyrexia, and weight loss are common. Severe dyspnea due to pneumonia may be seen, and ocular disease like anterior uveitis and chorioretinitis, as well as neurological signs including tremors, ataxia, and convulsions could occur.

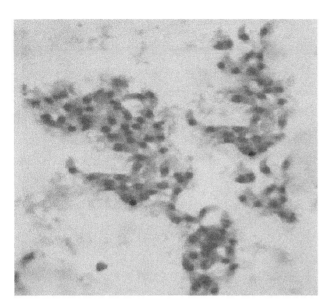

Figure 15.4 Purified tachyzoites from intraperitoneal lavage after staining with Giemsa stain.

15.6.3 Diagnosis

- Demonstration of organisms from biopsy material, lesions, organs, and on postmortem. Secretions, excretions, and body fluids can be used.
- Impression smears stained with Giemsa stain (Figure 15.4).
- Serological tests: indirect hemagglutination test (IHAT), CF, microscopic agglutination test (MAT), latex agglutination test (LAT), IFA, and ELISA.

15.6.4 Treatment

Treatment is with clindamycin. A vaccine, Toxovax® (Merck), is available.

15.7 Sarcocystosis

The genus *Sarcocystis* (Table 15.2) has an obligatory life cycle with the formation of asexual stages like tachyzoites and bradyzoites in the vascular endothelium of visceral organs and muscular and neural tissues of intermediate hosts like cattle, sheep, goats, pigs, horses, rabbits, chicken, and humans. The formation of sexual stages like gamonts and oocysts also occurs in the intestinal epithelial cells of definitive hosts like dogs and cats.

15.7.1 Life Cycle

Sarcocystis has an obligatory two-host life cycle. The definitive host gets infected by ingestion of infected muscles or organs containing sarcocysts. Sporulated oocysts or free sporocysts discharged in the feces of definitive hosts like dogs or cats infect the intermediate hosts orally by contamination of feed and water. They undergo schizogony to form first- and second-generation schizonts in the endothelial cells of the blood vessels of various visceral organs, leading to the formation of an actively multiplying type of merozoites called tachyzoites (Figure 15.5).

15.7.1.1 Pathogenesis

The early developmental phase is characterized by generalized lymphadenopathy, anorexia, fever, anemia, loss of weight and production, and abortion. Lesions occur in various organs – cysts in the myocardium, esophagus, tongue, and masseter muscles in chronic infections, and emaciation, submandibular edema, and exophthalmia are noticed. A powerful endotoxin called sarcocystin produced by the organisms acts on the central nervous system, cardiovascular system, and other organisms. A few species cause an increase in somatostatin levels and a decrease in somatomedin levels, and consequently reduce feed efficiency and growth.

15.7.2 Diagnosis

Clinical signs are not a true indicator of sarcocystosis. Liver enzyme levels and creatinine phosphokinase are elevated.

Tests for diagnosis include ELISA and acid pepsin digestion methods.

Table 15.2 Common species of *Sarcocystis* in the goat.

Intermediate host	*Sarcocystis* sp.	Location of cysts in the intermediate host	Size of cysts	Pathogenicity in the intermediate host	Definitive host
Goat	S. capracanis	All striated muscles	<1 mm	High	Canids
	S. hiricicanis	Central nervous system, Purkinje fibers	<2.5 mm	Intermediate	Dog
	S. moulei	All striated muscles	<12 mm	Non-pathogenic	Cat
	S. caprifelis	Esophageal muscles Diaphragmatic muscles	–	–	Cat

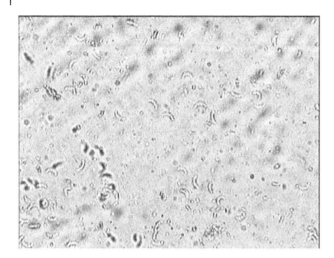

Figure 15.5 Metrozoites released after acid digestion of goat tissue (Percoll separation).

15.7.3 Treatment and Control

- Sulfadiazine – 20 mg kg orally once or twice a day for 12 weeks.
- Pyrimethamine – 1.0 mg/kg once a day for 120 days.

15.8 General Approaches to Minimizing Parasitic Infections on a Goat Farm

There are various strategies that should be strictly and stringently followed for the management and control of parasitic infections.

15.8.1 Integrated Parasite Management

Integrated parasite management (IPM) encourages a multi-disease control approach, integration with other disease control measures, and systematic application of a range of interventions, often in combination and synergistically (WHO 2004). The motive of IPM is to improve the efficacy, cost-effectiveness, ecological soundness, and sustainability of various methods of parasite control. IPM strategies have general similarities with integrated pest management systems that are commonly used in agriculture and deal with the adverse environmental and health effects of commonly used pesticides alongside the development of anthelmintic resistance. Such integrated approaches will surely help to preserve ecosystem integrity alongside encouraging the propagation of various natural enemies of pest species through biological control measures.

IPM favors the interrelated application of four approaches: (i) environmental management, which basically includes environmental manipulation for parasite control; (ii) biological control methods employing natural predators; (iii) chemical control methods consisting of the use of chemical compounds/drugs; and (iv) social and behavioral measures including public awareness.

15.8.1.1 Environmental Management

The environmental capability to maintain vectors can be reduced by long-term physical changes in temperature, often termed environmental modification (WHO 1982). The effectiveness of environmental management depends on how well the particular intervention is matched with the ecology of the particular disease-causing vector population. This also includes management practices like destruction of marshy areas for snail population control of trematode infections using molluscicides like copper sulphate and N-trityl morpholine.

15.8.1.2 Biological Control and Use of Natural Predators

Biological methods consist of the utilization of biological toxins and natural enemies to achieve effective vector management. An important advantage of biological control over chemical methods is the reduction in levels of ecosystem disturbance affecting other animal and plant species. Such methods have an advantage as they do not persist or accumulate in the environment or in body tissues, and are not toxic to vertebrates and other animal and plant fauna (WHO 1999). Targeted biological control using larvivorous fish (*Gambusa* for mosquito control) and copepods as well as the toxic products of bacterial agents have been successfully used to control vectors.

Research on the potential use of naturally occurring pathogens, parasitoids, and predators for the biological control of animal pests lags far behind that for plant pests. Among biological agents, entomopathogenic fungi played a uniquely important role in the history of microbial control of insects. Hemipterans and ants have been used to control ticks (Soulsby 2005). Certain plants like *Stylosanthes* are used for controlling ticks, while smoking with neem and eucalyptus has been traditionally been used to control flies and mosquitoes (Soulsby 2005). Tannin-rich plants are often used for control of gastrointestinal parasitism. Duck-rearing alongside a pond is recommended for snail control.

Traditional animal healthcare practices involve the use of medicinal plants to treat livestock diseases. Methanolic extracts of neem (*Azadirachtia indica*) leaves and bark, nochi (*Vitex negundo*) leaves, the vasharnbu (*Acorus calamus*) rhizome, and ptlngu (*Pongamia pinnata*) leaves possess acaricidal effects and are regularly used in goats.

15.8.1.3 Chemical Control

Chemical control methods are quick in response, and can be highly cost-effective if used efficiently. The insecticide

Table 15.3   Antiprotozoals for use in the goat.

Antiprotozoal	Use against
Buparvaquinone at 2.5 mg/kg body weight intramuscularly	Theileriosis
Imidocarb at 2–4 mg/kg body weight intravenously	Babesiosis
Tetracyclines	Rickettsial infections
Ivermectin	As an endectocide
Amprolium at 10 mg/kg body weight orally	Coccidiosis

Table 15.4   Acaricides for use in the goat.

Acaricide	Concentration and route of application
Coumaphos	1% dust, 0.34–0.46% spray, 10 mg/kg body weight as pour-on
Dichlorvos	8.9% as dog collar, 30–60 ml 1% solution as spray, 20% tag
Malathion	4–5% dust, 0.5–0.6% spray
Carbaryl	5% dust, 0.5% spray
Lindane	1% dust, 0.03% spray, 0.04–0.05% dip
Amitraz	250 ppm in water
Deltamethrin	1% solution as spray
Permethrin	0.25% dust, 0.05% spray, 10% tag
Ivermectin	0.2 mg/kg body weight as injection subcutaneously or liquid or paste or tablet

may be applied as a non-residual application (effective over a short timescale, killing only insects currently exposed) or as a residual (persistent) application (effective over a period of weeks or months). Insecticides remain an important tool (Table 15.3). A wide range of commercial acaricides is available on the market for topical application, some of which are outlined in Table 15.4.

Strategies for the use of chemical anthelmintics include the following:

- **Prophylactic treatments**: These treatments are done at regular intervals or drugs with a residual effect are used. A broad-spectrum anthelmintic like albendazole or a drug combination containing flukicide, anti-nematodal, and anti-cestodal preparations can be used for common dosing against trematodes, nematodes, and cestodes to prevent multiple drug resistance.
- **Curative treatment**: These treatments are based on clinical diagnosis. In this method there are reduced expenses on anthelmintics, the possibility of selection for resistance is significantly reduced if only some

animals are treated, and this will ensure the presence of a susceptible parasite population within the herd or flock. However, the disadvantage is that it requires regular monitoring, which increases labor input.

- **Measures against intermediate hosts**: Molluscicides like copper sulfate and N-trityl morpholine are used. Application in the spring is easy to apply and highly effective, killing off winter-infected snails and parent snails that would supply the nucleus of the year's breeding population.

15.8.1.4   Health Awareness and Behavior

Vector-borne diseases may be more serious when the affected animal or human host is malnourished, in ill health, or suffering from gastrointestinal diseases. In particular, improved awareness of hygiene and sanitation is important in reducing infectious diseases among susceptible goats. Awareness for early identification of diseases based on symptoms, the need to maintain attendance for drug delivery, and refraining from interfering with traps for vectors, as well as to some extent certain steps like indoor rearing of goats at night should be practiced in endemic areas.

15.8.2   Vaccines

A very few vaccines are available commercially on the market for parasite control. These include Rakshavac-T® (Indian Immunologicals, Hyderabad, India) for theileriosis, Anaplaz® (Fort Dodge Laboratories, Fort Dodge, IA, USA) for anaplasmosis, and Toxovac for toxoplasmosis.

15.8.3   Controlling Parasitic Infections of the Goat at a Grassroots Level

The following measures are recommended against free-living and parasitic stages of ticks and other vectors and for destruction of their microhabitats:

- Elimination of tick/fly shelters (cracks in the wall and perches, stagnant water sources) for larvae, nymphs, and adults.
- Pre-monsoon burning and/or rotation of pastures, or pasture spelling in the endemic area.
- Benefit from natural predators – birds, rodents, ants, shrews, spiders, especially fire ants, *Pheidole megacephala*, and *Hymenoptera* spp. wasps – that feed on engorged and free-living vectors and reduce their population.
- In indigenous and cross-bred animals, exposure to tick and fly infestations confers strong resistance.
- Periodic use of acaricides and insecticides (Tables 15.3 and 15.4) against the free-living stages of vectors.

- Destruction of breeding grounds of mosquitoes and flies such as stagnant water sources.
- Duck-rearing for snail control alongside use of chemicals like copper sulfate or N-trityl morpholone.
- Use of tannin-rich plants for control of gastrointestinal parasites as part of a herbal approach for control of parasitism.
- Regular deworming of infected animals throughout the year.

Multiple-Choice Questions

1 What is gall sickness associated with?
   A Anaplasmosis
   B Babesiosis
   C Trypanosomiosis
   D Theileriosis

2 Rakshavac-T is a cell culture vaccine against what?
   A Coccidiosis
   B Babesiosis
   C Trypanisomiosis
   D Theileriosis

3 A shuttle programme is associated with the treatment of what?
   A Coccidiosis
   B Babesiosis
   C Trypanisomiosis
   D Theileriosis

4 Which of the following anticoccidials is a thiamine analog?
   A Sulphonamide
   B Amprolium
   C Salinomycin
   D Monensin

5 What is coffee-coloured urine associated with?
   A Babesiosis
   B Theileriosis
   C Toxoplasmosis
   D Trypanosomiosis

6 What are intermittent fever, nervous signs, and petechial haemorrhages associated with?
   A Babesiosis
   B Theileriosis
   C Toxoplasmosis
   D Trypanosomiosis

7 Which of the following is a rapidly dividing stage?
   A Bradyzoites
   B Tachyzoites
   C Oocysts
   D All of the above

8 Which is the infective stage of *Toxoplasma gondii*?
   A Bradyzoites
   B Tachyzoites
   C Oocysts
   D All of the above

9 How many sporocysts and sporozoites, respectively, are there in *Cryptosporidium parvum*?
   A 2, 4
   B 4, 2
   C 0, 4
   D 0, 8

10 What is swelling of lymph nodes characteristic of?
   A Trypanosomosis
   B Theileriosis
   C Amoebiasis
   D Sarcocystosis

11 What are punched-out necrotic ulcers characteristic of?
   A Trypanosomosis
   B Theileriosis
   C Amoebiasis
   D Sarcocystosis

12 What is red-coloured urine characteristic of?
   A Trypanosomosis
   B Babesiosis
   C Amoebiasis
   D Sarcocystosis

13 What is neonatal diarrhoea in kids characteristic of?
   A Trypanosomosis
   B Cryptosporidiosis
   C Amoebiasis
   D Sarcocystosis

14 Buparvaquone is used in the treatment of what?
   A Trypanosomosis
   B Theileriosis
   C Amoebiasis
   D Sarcocystosis

15 Imidocarb is used in the treatment of what?
   A Trypanosomosis
   B Babesiosis
   C Amoebiasis
   D Sarcocystosis

16 Amprolium is used in the treatment of what?
   A Trypanosomosis
   B Coccidiosis
   C Amoebiasis
   D Sarcocystosis

17 Trypan blue is used in the treatment of what?
   A Trypanosomosis
   B Theileriosis
   C Amoebiasis
   D Babesiosis

18 Buparvaquone is used in the treatment of what?
   A Trypanosomosis
   B Theileriosis
   C Amoebiasis
   D Sarcocystosis

19 Parasitic infections are characterized by an increase in levels of what?
   A IgG
   B IgM
   C IgA
   D IgE

20 Rakshavac-T is prepared using what?
   A Attenuated schizonts
   B Attenuated sporozoites
   C Recombinant SPAG-1
   D Recombinant p67

21 What is the most important zoonotic species of *Cryptosporidium*?
   A *Cryptosporidium canis*
   B *Cryptosporidium felis*
   C *Cryptosporidium parvum*
   D *Cryptosporidium suis*

22 *Theileria annulata* infection in the salivary glands of tick can be visualized after what kind of staining?
   A Ponceau staining
   B Commassie brilliant blue staining
   C Acridine orange staining
   D Pyronin methyl green staining

23 Which of the following chemicals is used for cryopreservation of parasites?
   A Polyethylene glycol
   B Glycerol
   C Calcium chloride
   D Magnesium hydroxide

24 The MASP culture technique is used for the culture of what?
   A *Babesia* spp.
   B *Theileria* spp.
   C *Anaplasma* spp.
   D *Cowdria* spp.

25 What species does the smallest coccidian oocyst come from?
   A *Cryptosporidium* spp.
   B *Sarcocystis* spp.
   C *Toxoplasma gondii*
   D *Eimeria tenella*

References

Bhatia, B.B. and Shah, H.L. (2001). *Protozoa and Protozoan Diseases of Domestic Animals*. New Delhi: ICAR Publications.

Soulsby, E.J.L. (2005). *Helminths, Arthropods and Protozoa of Domesticated Animals*. London: Baillière Tindal.

WHO (1982). *Manual for Environmental Management for Mosquito Control, with Special Emphasis on Malaria Vectors*. Geneva: World Health Organization.

WHO (1999). *Bacillus thurinigiensis*. Environmental health criteria 217. Geneva: World Health Organization. https://apps.who.int/iris/bitstream/handle/10665/42242/WHO_EHC_217.pdf.

WHO (2004). *The World Health Report 2004: Changing History*. Geneva: World Health Organization.

16

Metabolic Diseases in Goats

Antônio C.L. Câmara[1] and Benito Soto-Blanco[2]

[1] *Large Animal Veterinary Teaching Hospital, Universidade de Brasilia, Brasilia, Brazil*
[2] *Department of Veterinary Clinics and Surgery, Veterinary School, Universidade Federal de Minas Gerais, Belo Horizonte, Brazil*

Small ruminants are typically purchased with little knowledge or instruction regarding appropriate care, such as age at castration, nutrition, and general husbandry practices. In general, metabolic diseases in goats are caused by an inability to meet their nutritional requirements. In does, late pregnancy and/or early lactation are the most frequent stages of toxemia, hypocalcemia, and hypomagnesemia. Bucks and male kids are more prone to obstructive urolithiasis due to early castration or inadequate feed management. The early stages of these diseases are characterized by reduced appetite, which leads to a further reduction in nutrient intake and increased morbidity. This chapter provides guidelines for the most common metabolic disorders (Figure 16.1) and their treatment and control in goats.

16.1 Polioencephalomalacia

Polioencephalomalacia (PEM), also known as cerebrocortical necrosis, is a neurological, metabolic disease with multiple etiologies and is typically related to thiamine (vitamin B1) deficiency or excessive sulfur intake (Figure 16.2). The disease may affect goats of all ages, but young goats appear to be particularly susceptible (Smith and Sherman 2009; Matthews 2016).

16.1.1 Etiology

PEM is a consequence of thiamine deficiency or excessive sulfur intake. In cattle, PEM is also related to excessive salt consumption associated or not with water deprivation, lead poisoning, bovine herpesvirus infection, and ingestion of cadaveric fragments containing thiaminase-rich clostridia (Sant'Ana and Barros 2010; Cebra et al. 2015).

Initially, PEM was only attributed to thiamine deficiency. Almost all the thiamine required by ruminants is produced by ruminal microbiota. The consumption of high-grain diets or carbohydrate-rich diets may result in ruminal acidosis. This reduction in the ruminal pH leads to a decrease in thiamine-producing bacteria and an expansion of thiaminase-producing bacteria (such as *Bacillus aneurinolyticus*, *Bacillus thiaminollyticus*, and *Clostridium sporogenes*) (Smith and Sherman 2009; Cebra et al. 2015; Constable et al. 2017). Another cause of thiamine deficiency is the consumption of thiaminase-containing plants, such as the ferns *Pteridium* spp., *Marsilea drummondii*, and *Cheilanthes sieberi*, but this is not common (Cebra et al. 2015) and has not been described in goats. Thiamine deficiency is believed to impair carbohydrate supply to the neurons in the brain due to reduced synthesis of the coenzyme thiamine pyrophosphate, a cofactor in the tricarboxylic acid cycle and pentose phosphate pathway (Smith and Sherman 2009).

Nowadays, most PEM cases are associated with excessive sulfur intake from food and water. In the rumen, ingested sulfur is normally reduced from sulfates to sulfides, which are used to synthesize sulfur-containing amino acids such as cysteine and methionine. Ruminal microorganisms may also use sulfate for energy production and release sulfide ions. In acidic ruminal fluid, sulfide ions become hydrogen sulfide (H_2S), which is extensively absorbed by the mucosa, transported through the bloodstream, and detoxified into sulfate in the liver. The concentration of sulfates can overwhelm the liver's ability to detoxify, and excess H_2S is released into the bloodstream and reaches the central nervous system. Neurons are very sensitive to H_2S, which suppresses oxidative phosphorylation by inhibiting cytochrome c oxidase (Gould 2000; Cebra et al. 2015; Constable et al. 2017).

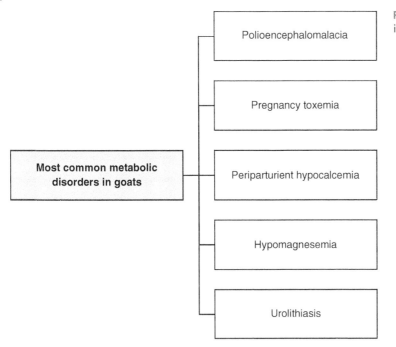

Figure 16.1   Most common metabolic disorders in goats.

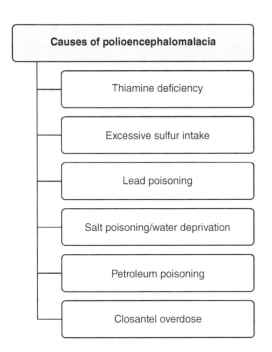

Figure 16.2   Main causes of polioencephalomalacia.

In goats, PEM also results from petroleum poisoning, probably due to sulfur toxicosis, but may also be caused by salt and lead poisoning (Batista et al. 2013; Câmara et al. 2018). One goat also developed PEM after an overdose of the anthelmintic closantel, which might have affected the neuronal metabolism (Sakhaee and Derakhshanfar 2010).

16.1.2   Clinical Signs

The initial clinical signs are variable and may include apathy, loss of appetite, separation from the flock, and diarrhea. The absence of rumen contractions was observed in goats with severe ruminal acidosis. During eructation, goats that present with sulfate poisoning may have a sulfite smell (similar to a rotten egg). Neurological signs develop progressively, including excitability, circling, or staggering gait, head pressing, ataxia, stargazing (staring upward at the sky with an upward lift of the head and neck), apparent blindness, and muscle trembling. Late signs include nystagmus, strabismus, lateral recumbency with opisthotonos, odontoprisis, muscle rigidity, and convulsions. Death occurs within 1–3 days of the first clinical signs (Lima et al. 2005; Smith and Sherman 2009; Sakhaee and Derakhshanfar 2010; Matthews 2016; Sivaraman et al. 2016; Constable et al. 2017; Câmara et al. 2018).

16.1.3   Ancillary Diagnostic Tests

Usually, no change is found in hematological analyses (Sivaraman et al. 2016; Sharma et al. 2021). Some goats present with hyperglycemia and consequent glucosuria (Matthews 2016). The only changes in cerebrospinal fluid (CSF) analysis in some animals are a slight increase in protein levels and mononuclear pleocytosis (Smith and Sherman 2009; Matthews 2016; Câmara et al. 2018). In cases of thiamine deficiency secondary to ruminal acidosis, rumen fluid analysis may reveal a reduced ruminal pH and microbial activity (Smith and Sherman 2009; Sivaraman et al. 2016).

Goats with PEM have reduced thiamine levels in the brain and liver. In live animals, thiamine levels can be estimated by the erythrocyte transketolase assay, which is determined using heparinized blood. However, determining blood thiamine levels is not helpful because they may remain unaffected. It is also possible to assess thiaminase activity in the feces or rumen content (Smith and Sherman 2009; Matthews 2016).

Sulfur poisoning can be confirmed by determining the H_2S concentration in the rumen gas cap. As the normal range of H_2S concentration is unknown for goats, it is necessary to determine these "normals" in unaffected goats from the flock to use as controls (Smith and Sherman 2009). However, anorexic animals may reduce the production and loss of ruminal H_2S by eructation or mucosal absorption (Cebra et al. 2015).

16.1.4 Pathology

At necropsy, the cerebrum, in severe cases, appears grayish-yellow or yellow. In cases of cerebral edema, the cerebral gyri are flattened, and the cerebellum may partially herniate through the foramen magnum. Examination under ultraviolet light reveals fluorescence on the cut surface of the affected areas of the cerebral cortex (Lima et al. 2005; Smith and Sherman 2009; Sant'Ana and Barros 2010; Matthews 2016; Câmara et al. 2018). The typical histological change is segmental laminar necrosis of the neurons from the cortical telencephalon, frequently accompanied by spongiosis (Sant'Ana and Barros 2010; Câmara et al. 2018).

16.1.5 Diagnosis

The diagnosis is based on the clinical signs of opisthotonos, nystagmus, blindness, strabismus, extensor rigidity, and response to thiamine treatment. A definitive diagnosis is obtained based on the PEM lesions observed on pathological examination. The differential diagnoses include pregnancy toxemia, enterotoxemia caused by *Clostridium perfringens* type D, caprine arthritis encephalitis, meningoencephalitis, tetanus, salt poisoning, and lead poisoning (Smith and Sherman 2009; Constable et al. 2017).

16.1.6 Treatment

Regardless of the cause of PEM, the intravenous (IV) administration of thiamine (usually thiamine hydrochloride) at 10 mg/kg in 5% dextrose-normal saline or other isotonic fluid is the specific therapy, repeated four times every six hours. Additional doses may be administered intramuscularly (IM) or subcutaneously (SC). Dexamethasone (1.0–2.0 mg/kg IM or SC) may be used to reduce brain edema and inflammation. Seizures can be controlled with anticonvulsants, such as diazepam (0.5–1.5 mg/kg) (Smith and Sherman 2009; Matthews 2016; Sivaraman et al. 2016).

Treatment response depends on the severity and extent of the brain lesions. Mildly affected goats show clinical improvement within 6–8 hours and recovery in up to 3 days, but moderately affected goats may recover within 9 days, and severe cases are not reversed by treatment (Smith and Sherman 2009; Matthews 2016; Sivaraman et al. 2016). Asymptomatic animals within the flock should receive supplementary thiamine as 50 mg/kg of feed for 2–3 weeks to prevent disease. It is important to ensure that the water and feed do not contain excessive amounts of sulfate (Constable et al. 2017).

16.2 Pregnancy Toxemia

Pregnancy toxemia, also known as gestational ketosis, is a highly lethal metabolic disease that affects goats in the third trimester of pregnancy. Affected goats develop a negative energy balance due to failing to meet the glucose requirements of the rapidly growing fetus(es). Its main effects are hypoglycemia, ketosis, metabolic acidosis, and nervous and digestive disturbances (Simões and Gutiérrez 2017; Sucupira et al. 2021).

16.2.1 Etiology

In the final third of pregnancy, the fetus(es) shows rapid growth and is responsible for consuming up to 40% of the glucose produced by the mother. However, the large volume occupied by the uterus with the fetus and placenta in the maternal abdomen reduces the volume occupied by the rumen, negatively affecting the total amount of feed consumed. When the energy supplied by the diet becomes lower than the body's demands, the body's glycogen reserves are used, mainly from the liver. Once that has been depleted, the body mobilizes amino acids from muscle proteins and fat from adipocytes for gluconeogenesis. Adipocytes release non-esterified fatty acids (NEFAs) that reach the liver via the bloodstream. NEFAs are oxidized in the mitochondria of hepatocytes for energy formation in a reaction that can generate ketone bodies if the supply of carbohydrates is insufficient. The ketone bodies formed are β-hydroxybutyrate (BHB), acetone, and acetoacetate, with BHB being the most important because it is the most stable. These compounds are used as energy sources by various tissues. When the ability of hepatocytes to oxidize NEFAs is exceeded, these compounds are converted into triglycerides and deposited in hepatocytes. Excess deposits eventually result in hepatic lipidosis and compromised liver function. Another factor seemingly involved in the etiology of pregnancy toxemia is the reduction in the ability of different tissues to use glucose. This reduction is associated with insulin resistance; however, the mechanism has not yet been fully elucidated (Simões and Gutiérrez 2017; Sucupira et al. 2021).

The main predisposing factors to pregnancy toxemia in goats are presented in Figure 16.3. This disease occurs in goats with two or more fetuses and occasionally in those with only one fetus. Pregnancy toxemia can occur in goats with a low or high body condition score (BCS). In goats with a BCS equal to or less than 2.0, the energy supply during pregnancy is insufficient, especially in the last third. In goats with BCS greater than 3.5, excess body fat in the final third of gestation impairs food consumption. Foods with low nutritional quality or unbalanced diets can favor the development of pregnancy toxemia, especially in late pregnancy, when food consumption decreases. Old animals or excessive wear of teeth can lead to failure in the consumption of food, predisposing to the disease. Concomitant diseases and stress in pregnant goats can trigger pregnancy toxemia by increasing the need for energy and reducing food consumption. The reduction in the movement of confined animals also seems to favor the occurrence of the disease. However, some females are more prone to developing the condition due to insulin resistance (Simões and Gutiérrez 2017; Sucupira et al. 2021).

16.2.2 Clinical Signs

The clinical signs show some variation according to body condition and the severity of the hypoglycemia and excess ketone bodies in the animal. Often, undernourished females present with a 10–20-day evolving condition, while those with good body condition and obesity present with a shorter (3–9-day) clinical evolution (Sucupira et al. 2021).

The disease usually starts with the goat isolating itself from the herd and losing its appetite, which contributes to the worsening of hypoglycemia and the production of ketone bodies. There is progressive impairment of consciousness, anorexia, apathy, difficulty in standing, and ataxia. Other possible signs include chewing movements, teeth grinding, swollen limbs, rumen atony, constipation, blindness, deafness, aimless wandering, and head pressing. There is an increase in heart and respiratory rates, and some goats show an increased body temperature; however, hypothermia may occur in a few animals. With the worsening of the disease, the goat presents with recumbency (initially sternal followed by lateral), flaccidity of the abdominal muscles, oliguria, deep depression, convulsions, coma, and death (Smith and Sherman 2009; Lima et al. 2016b; Harwood and Mueller 2018; Souza et al. 2020; Sucupira et al. 2021).

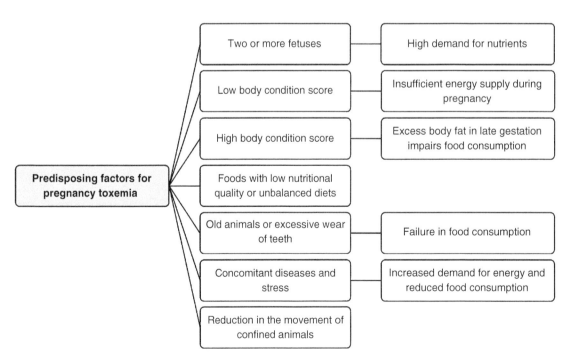

Figure 16.3 Main predisposing factors for pregnancy toxemia in goats.

Ketoacidosis can result in dystocic deliveries. Neonates are typically small and weak, with a high mortality rate. In cases of abortion, goats show gradual clinical improvement. If fetal death occurs without abortion, the doe may show an apparent improvement in clinical signs; however, fetal autolysis results in often fatal reproductive and systemic disorders (Smith and Sherman 2009; Harwood and Mueller 2018; Sucupira et al. 2021).

16.2.3 Ancillary Diagnostic Tests

Determining the serum of plasma BHB level is the best laboratory test to evaluate toxemia, as BHB is present in greater, more stable concentrations in the collected sample than are acetone and acetoacetate (Smith and Sherman 2009; Souto et al. 2013; Sucupira et al. 2021). BHB levels of up to 0.8 mmol/l are considered normal, while values of 0.8–1.6 mmol/l are associated with the subclinical form. Some clinical signs of toxemia can be seen when levels are >1.6 mmol/l, and the disease is evident when levels are >3.0 mmol/l. The semi-quantitative detection of ketone bodies in urine using urinalysis strips is also possible (Smith and Sherman 2009; Sucupira et al. 2021). In dead animals, it is possible to determine the levels of BHB in the vitreous humor and the CSF. In pregnancy, toxemia can present with levels >2.5 and >5.0 mmol/l, respectively (Sucupira et al. 2021).

Blood glucose is typically reduced in the initial phase of the disease; however, when the goat is in the prolonged recumbency phase, blood glucose may be normal or even elevated (Sucupira et al. 2021), which is associated with fetal death (Lima et al. 2012) and marked glucose intolerance (Lima et al. 2016a). Blood pH is reduced owing to progressive metabolic acidosis, which can lower urine pH (Sucupira et al. 2021). In the presence of kidney injury, goats have increased urea and creatinine levels (Souto et al. 2013). The activity of liver enzymes, such as aspartate aminotransferase (AST) and γ-glutamyl transferase (GGT), increases owing to hepatic lipidosis (Sucupira et al. 2021). Cortisol levels also increase (Smith and Sherman 2009; Souto et al. 2013; Souza et al. 2020), which may result in neutrophilia, lymphopenia, and eosinopenia on leucogram (Smith and Sherman 2009). Cardiac biomarkers, such as troponin I, creatine kinase, and creatine kinase-myocardial band (CK-MB), are increased in the serum of goats with pregnancy toxemia, indicating that some cardiac damage may occur (Tharwat et al. 2012; Souza et al. 2020).

16.2.4 Pathology

During necropsy, the carcass usually contains more than one fetus (Figure 16.4) and a large amount of abdominal fat. The liver is typically enlarged and pale pink or

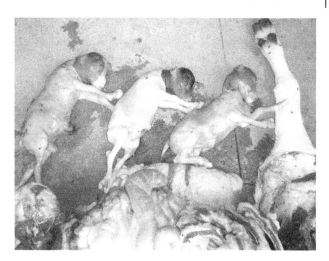

Figure 16.4 Three fetuses from a Boer doe that died from pregnancy toxemia.

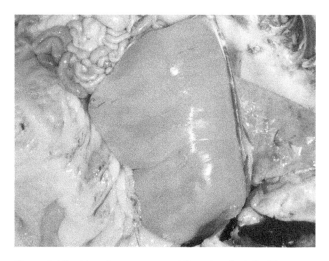

Figure 16.5 Liver from a pregnant Boer doe that died from pregnancy toxemia showing yellowish coloration due to fat infiltration.

yellowish due to fat infiltration (Figure 16.5) (Smith and Sherman 2009; Harwood and Mueller 2018; Sucupira et al. 2021). The adrenal glands are also often enlarged (Smith and Sherman 2009). Microscopically, the typical findings are hepatic lipidosis, marked fatty hepatocyte degeneration, and vacuolization of the renal tubular epithelial cells. Moreover, neurons in the cerebral cortex may exhibit ischemic degeneration and necrosis (Sucupira et al. 2021).

16.2.5 Diagnosis

The diagnosis is based on flock history, blood or urine BHB levels, clinical signs, and pathological findings. Increased BHB levels are the most important finding in diagnosing pregnancy toxemia. Differential diagnoses include periparturient hypocalcemia, polioencephaloma-lacia, rabies, listeriosis, brain abscess, acidosis, and hypomagnesemia (Harwood and Mueller 2018; Sucupira et al. 2021). It is important to emphasize that hypocalcemia may occur concomitantly with pregnancy-related toxemia.

16.2.6 Treatment

Treatment is not frequently administered owing to its high cost, and the mortality rates are high despite its effectiveness. To be effective, treatment should be initiated as soon as the clinical signs appear. Goats with hypoglycemia may receive IV glucose as an emergency therapy (Harwood and Mueller 2018; Sucupira et al. 2021), but with close monitoring during treatment because they may present with mild glucose intolerance (Lima et al. 2016a). For advanced cases of hyperglycemia, protamine zinc insulin (20–40 IU) can be used (Harwood and Mueller 2018), but its efficacy is questionable (Sucupira et al. 2021).

Treatment involves providing a source of energy for the goat and correcting other metabolic disorders. The main energy supply is propylene glycol (60 ml, orally two or three times a day), which is a precursor of glucose (Smith and Sherman 2009; Sucupira et al. 2021). Glycerin may be substituted for or associated with propylene glycol (Kalyesubula et al. 2019; Sucupira et al. 2021). Niacin (1 mg/day) seems to favor neurological recovery; in fact, some commercial propylene glycol-based products contain niacin in their composition (Smith and Sherman 2009).

As a reduction in serum calcium levels is present in many cases of pregnancy toxemia, administering 20% calcium borogluconate (1 ml/kg) is recommended (Sucupira et al. 2021). In sheep, recombinant bovine somatotropin (r-bST) can reduce maternal and fetal mortality by improving the cellular utilization of glucose and ketone bodies (Sucupira et al. 2021), but this treatment has not yet been tested in goats.

A cesarean section may be considered in late-gestation goats presenting with hypoglycemia; conversely, hyperglycemia may also result in fetal death, and surgical removal may be a lifesaving procedure (Lima et al. 2012; Sucupira et al. 2021).

16.2.7 Prevention

A nutritional plan should be adopted to prevent obesity during the last trimester of pregnancy. Does should have a BCS of at least 3 but no more than 4. Providing supplementary feed during the last few weeks of pregnancy may be necessary. Ultrasound may evaluate pregnant goats to identify twins that may be separated for special feeding and close monitoring (Smith and Sherman 2009; Harwood and Mueller 2018; Sucupira et al. 2021).

Overcrowding of animals in stalls must be avoided, as dominant animals make it difficult for others to feed properly. It is important to prevent physical stress, sudden changes in feed, and concurrent diseases in pregnant goats. When pregnancy toxemia occurs in the herd, the breeding conditions must be evaluated to avoid the occurrence of the disease in other goats (Smith and Sherman 2009; Harwood and Mueller 2018; Sucupira et al. 2021).

Pregnant goats should be monitored by measuring blood BHB levels or by semi-quantitative detection of ketone bodies in the urine. As assessing all the pregnant goats in the herd can be quite expensive, especially in large flocks, this monitoring can be performed through random sampling (10–15%). Goats in the last trimester of pregnancy that show increased BHB levels, reduced appetite, or abnormal behavior can be treated with propylene glycol (60 ml orally twice a day) (Smith and Sherman 2009; Harwood and Mueller 2018; Sucupira et al. 2021).

16.3 Periparturient Hypocalcemia

Hypocalcemia is a metabolic disorder characterized by reduced (*hypo*) blood calcium levels (*calcemia*), commonly known as parturient paresis, milk fever, and parturition sickness. This disease occurs in the periparturient period, mainly during the last weeks of pregnancy and the weeks following delivery. In contrast to cattle, the clinical condition is sporadic in goats; however, the subclinical form may be more common. Many cases are associated with hypomagnesemia (grass tetany) or pregnancy toxemia (Matthews 2016; Harwood and Mueller 2018).

16.3.1 Etiology

Blood calcium levels are controlled physiologically by the parathyroid hormone (PTH) and calcitonin, which modulate calcium mobilization from bones. Calcium mobilization is stimulated by the PTH, which increases blood calcium levels, while calcitonin inhibits it (Wilkens and Muscher-Banse 2020). Calcitriol (1,25-dihydroxycholecalciferol or 1,25-dihydroxyvitamin D3) improves calcium absorption in the gut (Herm et al. 2015; Wilkens and Muscher-Banse 2020) and may stimulate calcium mobilization from the bone depending on calcium blood levels (Wilkens and Muscher-Banse 2020). Goats show more effective control of calcium homeostasis than sheep because of higher calcitriol synthesis after dietary calcium restriction (Herm et al. 2015; Wilkens et al. 2012).

Fast-growing fetuses in late pregnancy and the onset of colostrum and milk production both increase calcium requirements. To compensate for this, the mineral is mobilized from the bones and absorbed more readily by the digestive system (Harwood and Mueller 2018). However, the increase in the rate of calcium absorption is slow. Parturition is usually responsible for mild hypocalcemia in goats (Smith and Sherman 2009). In dairy goats with high milk production, the imbalance between calcium demand and supply may be more accentuated, and serum levels may drop significantly, resulting in significant clinical consequences (Smith and Sherman 2009; Harwood and Mueller 2018). The highest frequency is observed in older goats from the fourth lactation (Smith and Sherman 2009), probably because of the reduced ability to absorb and mobilize calcium (Brozos et al. 2011).

Recent studies indicate that subclinical hypocalcemia presents with more intense fat mobilization and lipid peroxidation, causing metabolic and oxidative stress during the periparturient period while also retarding postpartum uterine involution (Bayoumi et al. 2021; Huang et al. 2021). Aged does (4–6 years), pregnant females with multiple fetuses, and dairy goats capable of heavy lactation are more prone to clinical hypocalcemia (Bayoumi et al. 2021).

16.3.2 Clinical Signs

Hypocalcemia in goats typically results in hyperesthesia and tetany, more so than the classic flaccid paralysis observed in dairy cattle (Bayoumi et al. 2021). Only periparturient goats are affected, and some cases may be complicated by hypomagnesemia or pregnancy toxemia. The initial signs include reduced appetite, lethargy, mild bloating, constipation, stumbling gait, and hypothermia. Many goats remain in sternal recumbency, with their heads turned to the flanks. Parturition may result in dystocia and a retained placenta due to weak uterine contractions. Other clinical signs include muscle tremors, lateral recumbency, mucous secretion in the nostrils, diminished pupillary light reflex, and a relaxed anal sphincter. Mild cases exhibit anorexia, lethargy, and reduced milk production (Smith and Sherman 2009; Matthews 2016; Harwood and Mueller 2018; Bayoumi et al. 2021). Severe cases may be found in a semi-comatose state.

16.3.3 Diagnosis

The presumptive diagnosis is based on herd history and clinical signs. The measurement of serum levels of calcium (normal range 8.9–11.7 mg/dl or 2.2–2.9 mmol/l) may be useful (Matthews 2016; Harwood and Mueller 2018); clinical signs are observed when these levels are lower than 6.0 mg/dl (Yamagishi et al. 1999). A quick response to treatment may confirm the diagnosis, but a temporary beneficial effect of calcium administration may occur in other diseases, such as enterotoxemia and mastitis (Matthews 2016; Harwood and Mueller 2018). Differential diagnoses include pregnancy toxemia, enterotoxemia, uterine rupture after dystocia, metritis, and rumen acidosis (Harwood and Mueller 2018).

16.3.4 Treatment

Therapy should be initiated as soon as possible. It consists of administering 20% calcium borogluconate solution (50–80 ml IV followed by 100 ml SC). Calcium may be administered intravenously only to hypocalcemic animals and in cases without concomitant pregnancy toxemia, as it can be lethal in cases without reduced calcium levels or damaged liver function. The heart must be monitored during calcium administration, stopping the administration if there is any sign of an arrhythmia. This administration results in a quick response in the affected goat, which stands up and walks within a few minutes (Matthews 2016; Harwood and Mueller 2018). While the doe is recovering, kids should be fed milk (Harwood and Mueller 2018).

16.3.5 Prevention

The critical period for hypocalcemia in goats is the last month of pregnancy and the first month of lactation. During this period, stress should be avoided because it may contribute to the initiation of hypocalcemia. Furthermore, the calcium content of the diet should be increased by using mineral supplements or calcium-rich ingredients. Attention to the oxalate content of the feed is recommended because it reduces calcium availability (Brozos et al. 2011).

16.4 Hypomagnesemia

Hypomagnesemia (*hypo*, reduced; *magnesemia*, blood magnesium levels) is a sporadic disease in goats (more common in beef cattle), known as grass tetany or lactation tetany for adult goats or milk tetany for kids fed a milk replacer.

16.4.1 Etiology

Hypomagnesemia mostly affects goats grazing fast-growing grasslands with low magnesium (Mg) concentrations, and the mobilization of magnesium from body stores is limited in goats; thus, any reduction in its absorption or increase in its demand by milk production may result in hypomagnesemia. Pastures fertilized with high amounts of potassium and nitrogen may also contribute to the disease because they reduce Mg absorption. Low concentrations of sodium in food also reduce availability (Foster et al. 2007; Martens and Schweigel 2000; Brozos et al. 2011; Simões and Gutiérrez 2017; Harwood and Mueller 2018). Moisture-rich forages that reduce the time of ruminal passage (Foster et al. 2007) and diets poor in fermentable carbohydrates (Martens and Schweigel 2000) impair Mg absorption. This deficiency may be partially counteracted in goats by reducing milk and urine production (Smith and Sherman 2009).

Low serum Mg affects neuromuscular transmission (Foster et al. 2007; Martens and Schweigel 2000; Brozos et al. 2011; Simões and Gutiérrez 2017), but the exact mechanism is unknown. The release of PTH after hypocalcemia, as well as the sensitivity of bone, intestines, and kidneys to PTH, is reduced with hypomagnesemia (Foster et al. 2007). Experimentally, in ewes insufficient body Mg might impair the immune system, impairing immune cell functions and the response to vaccination (Ahmed et al. 2020).

16.4.2 Clinical Signs

The first clinical signs are ataxia, stiffness, and hyperexcitability, which progress to tremors, tetanic spasms, recumbency, and paddling. Some goats exhibited concomitant hypocalcemia. Severe cases can be fatal within a few hours. Subclinical and chronic cases show reduced growth and milk yield (Foster et al. 2007; Matthews 2016; Harwood and Mueller 2018).

16.4.3 Diagnosis

Diagnosis is based on clinical signs and a quick response to treatment (Matthews 2016; Harwood and Mueller 2018). The serum Mg levels are typically lower than 1.1 mg/dl, from the normal range of 2.8–3.6 mg/dl (Smith and Sherman 2009; Simões and Gutiérrez 2017). Differential diagnoses include lead poisoning, pregnancy toxemia, lactational ketosis, and periparturient hypocalcemia (Harwood and Mueller 2018).

16.4.4 Treatment

The most efficient therapy is IV administration of 50 ml of 4–5% magnesium chloride with 20% calcium borogluconate, repeated by SC administration after 12–24 hours. Other formulations may be used depending on their availability. Affected goats responded quickly to treatment. Other goats from the flock should be preventively managed with magnesium oxide or calcinated magnesite (7 g/animal orally) (Brozos et al. 2011).

16.4.5 Prevention

Prevention is based on correcting the diet, providing good-quality fiber, and avoiding heavy fertilization of pastures with potassium and nitrogen. Dietary supplementation with Mg may be necessary for late pregnancy and lactation (Brozos et al. 2011; Matthews 2016). As many Mg supplements are not palatable, consumption must be checked (Brozos et al. 2011); therefore, mixing it with a palatable feed may be necessary.

16.5 Urolithiasis

Urolithiasis is defined as the formation of stones in the urinary tract. Obstructive urolithiasis is characterized by obstruction of the passage of urine by these stones. Obstructive urolithiasis is the most common urinary tract disease in small ruminants and is often the direct result of certain management practices (Stewart and Shipley 2021). As more goats and sheep are kept as pets, an increasing number develop urolithiasis. Unfortunately, these animals are typically purchased with little direction or instruction regarding appropriate care, such as age at castration, nutrition, and general husbandry practices (Scully 2021).

16.5.1 Etiology

Obstructive urolithiasis is primarily found in males due to their unique anatomy and is rarely seen in females (Scully 2021). This is especially common in castrated males and is even more common in males that are castrated at an early age. Urethral development depends on testosterone levels, and if the source of testosterone is removed before the urethra matures, the urethral diameter will not fully develop (Videla and Amstel 2016). Anatomically, the most common sites for uroliths to obstruct are the urethral process, distal sigmoid flexure, and ischial curvature (Guimarães et al. 2012; Riedi et al. 2018).

In addition to the anatomical factors that predispose small ruminants to urethral obstruction, numerous predisposing dietary factors can also contribute to urolith formation. For example, diets that are high in calcium (Ca), Mg, and/or phosphorus (P) result in an altered Ca : P ratio and can result in stone formation (Scully 2021). Non-dietary predisposing factors contributing to urolith development include increased urine concentration, urine stasis, increased urine pH, mineral excretion, desquamated epithelial cells, urinary tract infections, and urinary mucoproteins (Jones et al. 2012). In addition, limitation in the daily consumption or decreased renal elimination of water because of high environmental temperatures increases the concentration of urinary P and consequently favors the precipitation of phosphates. Another critical factor is the urinary pH, as phosphate precipitates when the pH is alkaline. Feeding with pelleted concentrates also favors the formation of uroliths because it increases the concentration of mucoproteins that form the organic matrix for depositing minerals. Less frequently, urolithiasis may occur in ruminants on pastures that contain excess oxalate, silica, or calcium. Vitamin A deficiency also increases epithelial desquamation, favoring stone formation (Lemos and Silveira 2008; Riet-Corrêa et al. 2008; Scully 2021).

Goats older than 1 year and breeds of African descent are at a greater risk of developing calcium carbonate uroliths than Anglo-Nubian, Nubian, and Toggenburg breeds. Nevertheless, other urolith types can affect very young small ruminants, putting every age category at risk (Nwaokorie et al. 2015).

16.5.2 Clinical Signs

Initially, clinical signs are non-specific and include reduced appetite or anorexia, isolation from the herd, intermittent recumbency with restlessness, apathy, congested ocular mucosa, dehydration, hyperthermia, tachycardia, tachypnea, hypomotility, or rumen atony. Subsequently, affected animals show signs of abdominal discomfort by adopting a micturition posture characterized by a broad base with the hind limbs stretched back (Riedi et al. 2018; Scully 2021). Owner and practitioner vigilance is necessary because such signs are commonly confused with constipation in the early stages (Scully 2021). Early intervention before complete obstruction requires careful examination and significantly improves prognosis (Riedi et al. 2018). Other signs of pain include bruxism, arching of the back, kicking of the abdomen, jerking, moaning, vocalization, touch sensitivity of the penile foreskin, and rapid movements with tail lifting (Guimarães et al. 2012; Riedi et al. 2018; Scully 2021; Videla and Amstel 2016). Repeated abdominal contractions for urination, spasmodic contraction of the penis, and visible movement of the preputial foreskin are often observed. Such efforts can result in passing a few drops of reddish urine (due to the presence of blood) and can predispose to rectal prolapse (Maciel et al. 2017; Scully 2021). Sometimes, the distended bladder can be palpated in the caudal abdomen (Videla and Amstel 2016). The absence of abdominal discomfort does not rule out obstructive urolithiasis, but may indicate an advanced stage of the disease (Riedi et al. 2018),

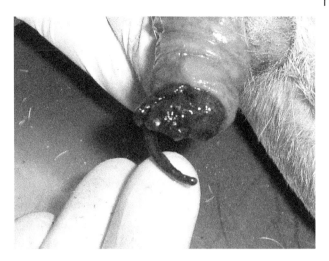

Figure 16.6 After penile exteriorization, observed necrosis of the urethral process and glans is observed due to obstruction by uroliths.

which can result in urethral or bladder rupture (Guimarães et al. 2012).

Physical examination should include exteriorization of the penis when possible. The following techniques can be used to exteriorize the penis in goats. The animal is restrained, with or without sedation, in a dog-sitting position, and 3 ml of 2% lidocaine solution is infused into the preputial orifice. This maneuver desensitizes the foreskin and the glans of the penis. The sigmoid flexure is pushed cranially, while the preputial skin is moved caudally, exposing the preputial mucosa with the glans, which is firmly held with the aid of gauze and pulled (Guimarães et al. 2012; Videla and Amstel 2016). The most common macroscopic findings are congestion, cyanosis, or necrosis of the urethral process and/or glans when this segment is the site of the obstruction (Figure 16.6) (Guimarães et al. 2012). If sedation is required to exteriorize the penis, diazepam (0.1–0.3 mg/kg IV) is recommended as an anxiolytic and for urethral relaxation. Other commonly used sedatives are acepromazine (0.05–0.1 mg/kg IV) or xylazine (0.05–0.1 mg/kg IV). However, both drugs can result in hypotension. Xylazine promotes diuresis, and its use is contraindicated until the obstruction is relieved (Videla and Van Amstel 2016).

16.5.3 Ancillary Diagnostic Tests

The most frequent hematological findings are leukocytosis with neutrophilia and hyperfibrinogenemia, which may occur in response to acute kidney infection, cystitis, and urethritis secondary to urolithiasis (Guimarães et al. 2012). Serum biochemistry reveals elevated urea and creatinine levels, especially in cases with postrenal azotemia

(Guimarães et al. 2012; Riedi et al. 2018). Other relevant biochemical changes include the increased activity of GGT and CK enzymes associated with hepatic lipolysis due to prolonged anorexia, and increased muscle activity due to frequent abdominal contractions, transport, cellulitis, and necrosis in cases of urethral rupture, respectively. Other biochemical alterations include hyperphosphatemia, hypermagnesemia, hypocalcemia, hypochloremia, hyponatremia, and imbalances in potassium and phosphorus (hyper- or hypo-) concentrations have also been reported (Maciel et al. 2017; Riedi et al. 2018).

Urinalysis is considered a vital laboratory test for the detection of nephropathies. However, in goats with anuria this test is possible only after an invasive urine sampling procedure (urethral process resection, cystocentesis, or laparotomy). The main physicochemical findings of urinalysis in patients with partial obstruction include a reddish color (hematuria), cloudy appearance, increased density, aciduria, proteinuria, and glycosuria (Guimarães et al. 2012). Sedimentoscopy reveals a high cell count, represented by an increase in the number of epithelial cells, erythrocytes, leukocytes, bacteria, mucus, and crystals (Maciel et al. 2017). Hematuria and the cloudy appearance of urine are due to hemorrhagic lesions caused by the presence of uroliths in the urinary tract mucosa, increasing cellularity in the urine (Lemos and Silveira 2008). Proteinuria and aciduria can be correlated with a diet with protein-rich grains or even associated with cases of concomitant glomerulonephritis, interstitial nephritis, pyelonephritis, or hydronephrosis (Riet-Correa et al. 2008; Guimarães et al. 2012).

Ancillary imaging tests, such as radiography, ultrasonography, and computed tomography, can help diagnose and confirm the presence of uroliths in the kidneys, ureter, bladder, and/or urethra. Transabdominal ultrasound, using a 3.5 or 5 MHz transducer, is a valuable tool for assessing urethral and bladder distention, assessing the kidneys, and identifying the presence of uroliths and free fluid in the abdomen, helping to define diagnosis and prognosis (Videla and Amstel 2016; Scully 2021). The bladder wall appears as a hyperechoic circle, and the white line enlarges when there is edema of the wall (Riedi et al. 2018). Ultrasound examination of the right kidney should be performed simultaneously, as continuous urinary pressure for 5–7 days can result in hydroureters and hydronephrosis, characterized by dilatation and fluid accumulation in the renal pelvis (Scully 2021).

Contrast radiography (retrograde urethrography, cyst urethrography, excretory urography, and normograde urethrocystography via tube cystotomy) is considered of great value for the diagnosis of obstructive urolithiasis in small ruminants. However, plain radiographs are sufficient for diagnosing radiopaque uroliths (e.g. calcium carbonate,

calcium oxalate, silicate). They are considered a less expensive means to better determine the surgical approach and prognosis (Kingsley et al. 2013; Riedi et al. 2018). Plain radiographs are used to locate and determine the number and size of uroliths in the urinary tract and assess the extent of urethral obstruction more accurately (Riedi et al. 2018).

16.5.4 Pathology

At necropsy, the urethral process and distal sigmoid flexure are the most common sites of obstruction by urolith(s) (Figure 16.7) (Scully 2021). Diffuse necrotic or hemorrhagic urethritis at the site of obstruction or along the entire length of the urethra after the obstruction, purulent and/or necrotizing urethritis, and urethral rupture are the most frequent findings in small ruminants (Guimarães et al. 2012; Riedi et al. 2018). Ureteritis and hydroureters are the most frequently reported pathologies (Lemos and Silveira 2008; Guimarães et al. 2012). Renal diseases include pyelonephritis, hydronephrosis, diffuse nephritis, renal abscesses, uroliths in the renal pelvis (Figure 16.8), hemorrhage, and renal rupture. Diffuse hemorrhagic cystitis, purulent cystitis, uroliths (Figure 16.9), necrotic foci, and vesical rupture have been reported in the bladder. Sand-like sediments are often observed instead of well-formed stones. Rupture of the

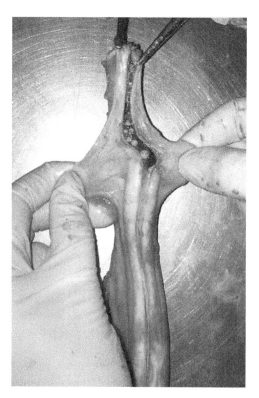

Figure 16.7 Urethral obstruction by uroliths at the sigmoid flexure. Note the necrotizing urethritis.

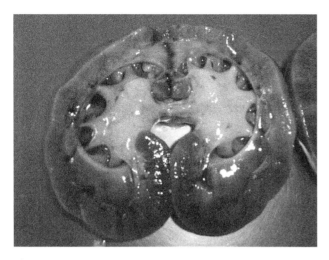

Figure 16.8 Kidney from a goat with urolithiasis showing hydronephrosis, diffuse nephritis, and uroliths in the renal pelvis.

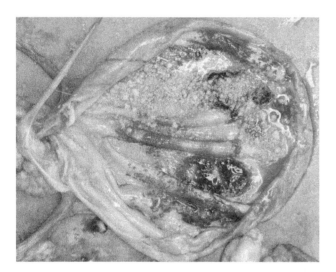

Figure 16.9 Urinary bladder presenting numerous uroliths and hemorrhagic cystitis with necrotic foci.

ventral wall of the bladder with hemorrhagic areas in the serosa and adherence to the pelvic cavity is observed. Additionally, if there is a rupture of the urethra, edema and cellulitis with an accumulation of urine are seen, which can then progress to subcutaneous necrosis (Guimarães et al. 2012).

16.5.5 Diagnosis

Presumptive diagnosis is based on clinical signs and epidemiological data, mainly those related to nutritional and management practices. Serum urea and creatinine levels can be used to assess the severity of the clinical condition and its evolution. The definitive diagnosis is obtained with the help of complementary imaging tests, surgical treatment, or necropsy, which allows visualization and confirmation of the obstructive process.

16.5.6 Treatment

Goats with obstructive urolithiasis should be treated promptly and be considered clinical and/or surgical emergencies, the primary goal being to restore urinary flow.

Percutaneous laparoscopic or laparotomy tube cystotomy have been reported to have the highest success rate for treating obstructive urolithiasis in small ruminants (Guimarães et al. 2012; Riedi et al. 2018). The main advantages include longer survival time and the return to reproductive function. However, there is a need for a longer hospital stay for follow-up, as clearance and recovery of urethral patency can occur within 2–3 weeks (Ewoldt et al. 2008). This may restrict their use to pet ruminants and breeders with high genetic value (Scully 2021).

If Ca uroliths (Ca carbonate or apatite) are suspected to be the primary cause of obstruction, better results can be obtained if another surgical approach is used, such as perineal urethrostomy (Ewoldt et al. 2008; Videla and Amstel 2016), bladder marsupialization, laser urethroscopy and lithotripsy (Videla and Amstel 2016), or vesicopreputial anastomosis (Cypher et al. 2017). Prepubic and perineal urethrostomy are considered emergency rescue procedures, as the incidence of stenosis can vary from 45% to 78% in up to eight months (Videla and Amstel 2016), and is recommended for beef goats, which will be referred to slaughter soon. Bladder marsupialization is an easy to perform technique; however, the risk of ascending urinary tract infections and skin irritation caused by urine leakage have been reported as important complications to be considered (Ewoldt et al. 2008, Videla and Amstel 2016). Recently, vesicopreputial anastomosis has been reported in goats as an alternative to redirect urine flow after failure to restore urination with other techniques, such as tube cystostomy and perineal urethrostomy, or as an alternative to bladder marsupialization, as skin lesions resulting from urine do not occur (Cypher et al. 2017). Other less routinely used techniques include penile amputation and prescrotal urethrotomy (Videla and Amstel 2016).

16.5.7 Prevention

The most important aspect of confined goats is disease prevention via a balanced diet. Feeds based on grains or bran must be supplemented with Ca such that the Ca : P ratio is at least 1.5 : 1. If the producer does not use balanced rations or does not consult a nutritionist for the formulation of the rations, the addition of 1–1.5% of calcium carbonate to grains or byproducts (bran) is a way to obtain an adequate Ca : P ratio. Attention should be paid to the mineral concentration in the feed, with recommended levels below 0.3% for Mg and 0.5% for P. Under no circumstances should mineral salt be offered to goats fed with grains and byproducts because, in addition to being unnecessary, it may predispose them to obstructive urolithiasis, fibrous osteodystrophy, and copper intoxication (Riet-Correa et al. 2008).

The addition of 2% ammonium chloride to the feed or at a dose of 200 mg/kg is recommended to acidify urine and prevent the precipitation of phosphates. Sodium chloride (NaCl) at 3–4% in the ration has also been used to avoid the formation of stones in confined animals, increasing water consumption and making it essential to maintain a permanent water supply (Riet-Correa et al. 2008). Additionally, to avoid urolithiasis in castrated ruminants, castration should be performed as late as possible, as testosterone promotes an increase in the diameter of the urethra during the sexual maturation phase (Videla and Amstel 2016).

Multiple-Choice Questions

1 What are the main causes of polioencephalomalacia in goats?
   A Thiamine deficiency and excessive sulfur intake
   B Copper poisoning and selenium deficiency
   C Fumonisin poisoning and biotin deficiency
   D Reduction in the movement of confined animals and excess body fat in late gestation

2 What is the specific therapy for polioencephalomalacia?
   A Amoxicillin (250 mg orally)
   B Ketamine (22 mg/kg intramuscularly)
   C Thiamine (10 mg/kg intravenously)
   D Fenbendazole (50 mg/kg orally)

3 Several factors are known to predispose goats to pregnancy toxemia. Which of these is *not* a predisposing factor?
   A Foods with low nutritional quality or unbalanced diets
   B Young goats (less than 5 years old)
   C Low body condition score
   D High body condition score

4 What does the best laboratory test to evaluate pregnancy toxemia seek to determine?
   A Plasma β-hydroxybutyrate (BHB) levels
   B Complete blood count
   C Plasma niacin levels
   D Presence of enterotoxins in urine

5 What is the typical clinical sign of periparturient hypocalcemia in goats?
   A Flaccid paralysis
   B Bilateral blindness
   C Teeth grinding, swollen limbs
   D Hyperesthesia and tetany

6 The specific therapy for periparturient hypocalcemia in goats consists of administering a solution of what substance?
   A Calcium hydroxyapatite
   B Calcium borogluconate
   C Magnesium chloride
   D Phosphorus pentasulfide

7 What are the clinical signs of hypomagnesemia?
   A Nystagmus, strabismus, lateral recumbency with opisthotonos, odontoprisis, muscle rigidity, and convulsions
   B Progressive impairment of consciousness, anorexia, apathy, difficulty in standing, and ataxia
   C Ataxia, stiffness, hyperexcitability, tetanic spasms, recumbency, and paddling
   D Excitability, staggering gait, head pressing, ataxia, apparent blindness, and muscle trembling

8 The prevention of hypomagnesemia includes avoiding heavy fertilization of pastures with what?
   A Sulfide and phosphorus
   B Phosphorus and potassium
   C Sulfide and nitrogen
   D Potassium and nitrogen

9 Diets with which dietary factors can contribute to urolith formation in goats?
   A Altered calcium : phosphorus ratio
   B Deficient in selenium
   C Deficient in magnesium
   D Rich in salt and carbohydrates

10 To prevent urolithiasis, confined male goats must be fed a balanced diet with what ratio?
   A Magnesium : phosphorus ratio of at least 2 : 1
   B Calcium : phosphorus ratio of at least 1.5 : 1
   C Phosphorus : magnesium ratio of at least 1.5 : 1
   D Phosphorus : calcium ratio of at least 2 : 1

References

Ahmed, M.H., Wilkens, M.R., Möller, B. et al. (2020). Blood leukocyte composition and function in periparturient ewes kept on different dietary magnesium supply. *BMC Veterinary Research* 16 (1): 484. https://doi.org/10.1186/s12917-020-02705-9.

Batista, J.S., Câmara, A.C.L., Almeida, R.D. et al. (2013). Poisoning by crude oil in sheep and goats. *Revue de Médecine Vétérinaire (Toulouse)* 164 (11): 517–520.

Bayoumi, Y.H., Behairy, A., Abdallah, A.A. et al. (2021). Peri-parturient hypocalcemia in goats: clinical, hematobiochemical profiles and ultrasonographic measurements of postpartum uterine involution. *Veterinary World* 14 (3): 558–568. https://doi.org/10.14202/vetworld.2021.558-568.

Brozos, C., Mavrogianni, V.S., and Fthenakis, G.C. (2011). Treatment and control of peri-parturient metabolic diseases: pregnancy toxemia, hypocalcemia, hypomagnesemia. *Veterinary Clinics of North America. Food Animal Practice* 27 (1): 105–113. https://doi.org/10.1016/j.cvfa.2010.10.004.

Câmara, A.C.L., Batista, J.S., and Soto-Blanco, B. (2018). Polioencephalomalacia in ruminants from the semi-arid region of Rio Grande do Norte, Brazil. *Semina Ciências Agrárias* 39 (1): 231–240. https://doi.org/10.5433/1679-0359.2018v39n1p231.

Cebra, C., Loneragan, G.H., and Gould, D.H. (2015). Polioencephalomalacia (cerebrocortical necrosis). In: *Large Animal Internal Medicine*, 5e (ed. B.P. Smith), 954–956. St. Louis, MO: Elsevier.

Constable, P.D., Hinchcliff, K.W., Done, S.H. et al. (2017). *Veterinary Medicine, a Textbook of the Diseases of Cattle, Sheep, Pigs and Goat*, 11e. St. Louis, MO: Elsevier.

Cypher, E.E., Van Amstel, S., Videla, R. et al. (2017). Vesicopreputial anastomosis for the treatment of obstructive urolithiasis in goats. *Veterinary Surgery* 46 (2): 281–288. https://doi.org/10.1111/vsu.12615.

Ewoldt, J.M., Jones, M.L., and Miesner, M.D. (2008). Surgery of obstructive urolithiasis in ruminants. *Veterinary Clinics of North America. Food Animal Practice* 24 (3): 455–465. https://doi.org/10.1016/j.cvfa.2008.06.003.

Foster, A., Livesey, C., and Edwards, G. (2007). Magnesium disorders in ruminants. *In Practice* 29 (9): 534–539. https://doi.org/10.1136/inpract.29.9.534.

Gould, D.H. (2000). Update on sulfur-related polioencephalomalacia. *Veterinary Clinics of North America. Food Animal Practice* 16 (3): 481–496. https://doi.org/10.1016/s0749-0720(15)30082-7.

Guimarães, J.A., Mendonça, C.L., Guaraná, E.L.S. et al. (2012). Estudo retrospectivo da urolitíase obstrutiva em ovinos: análise de 66 casos. *Pesquisa Veterinária Brasileira* 32 (9): 824–830. https://doi.org/10.1590/S0100-736X2012000900002.

Harwood, D. and Mueller, K. (2018). *Goat Medicine and Surgery*. Boca Raton, FL: CRC Press.

Herm, G., Muscher-Banse, A.S., Breves, G. et al. (2015). Renal mechanisms of calcium homeostasis in sheep and goats. *Journal of Animal Science* 93 (4): 1608–1621. https://doi.org/10.2527/jas.2014-8450.

Huang, Y., Wen, J., Kong, Y. et al. (2021). Oxidative status in dairy goats: periparturient variation and changes in subclinical hyperketonemia and hypocalcemia. *BMC Veterinary Research* 17: 238. https://doi.org/10.1186/s12917-021-02947-1.

Jones, M., Miesner, M.D., Baird, A. et al. (2012). Diseases of the urinary system. In: *Sheep and Goat Medicine* (ed. D.G. Pugh and A.N. Baird), 325–360. Maryland Heights, MO: Elsevier.

Kalyesubula, M., Rosov, A., Alon, T. et al. (2019). Intravenous infusions of glycerol versus propylene glycol for the regulation of negative energy balance in sheep: a randomized trial. *Animals* 9 (10): 731. https://doi.org/10.3390/ani9100731.

Kingsley, M.A., Semevolos, S., Parker, J.E. et al. (2013). Use of plain radiography in the diagnosis, surgical management, and postoperative treatment of obstructive urolithiasis in 25 goats and 2 sheep. *Veterinary Surgery* 42 (6): 663–668. https://doi.org/10.1111/j.1532-950x.2013.12021.x.

Lemos, R.A.A. and Silveira, A.C. (2008). Urolitíase e ruptura da bexiga. In: *Doenças de impacto econômico em bovinos de corte* (ed. R.A.A. Lemos and C.R.B. Leal), 337–346. Editora UFMS: Campo Grande, Brazil.

Lima, E.F., Riet-Correa, F., Tabosa, I.M. et al. (2005). Polioencefalomalacia em caprinos e ovinos na região semi-árida do Nordeste do Brasil. *Pesquisa Veterinária Brasileira* 25 (1): 9–14. https://doi.org/10.1590/S0100-736X2005000100003.

Lima, M.S., Pascoal, R.A., and Stilwell, G.T. (2012). Glycaemia as a sign of the viability of the foetuses in the last days of gestation in dairy goats with pregnancy toxaemia. *Irish Veterinary Journal* 65 (1): 1. https://doi.org/10.1186/2046-0481-65-1.

Lima, M.S., Cota, J.B., Vaz, Y.M. et al. (2016a). Glucose intolerance in dairy goats with pregnancy toxemia: lack of correlation between blood pH and beta hydroxybutyric acid values. *Canadian Veterinary Journal* 57 (6): 635–640.

Lima, M.S., Silveira, J.M., Carolino, N. et al. (2016b). Usefulness of clinical observations and blood chemistry values for predicting clinical outcomes in dairy goats with pregnancy toxaemia. *Irish Veterinary Journal* 69: 16. https://doi.org/10.1186/s13620-016-0075-4.

Maciel, T.A., Ramos, I.A., Silva, R.J. et al. (2017). Clinical and biochemical profile of obstructive urolithiasis in sheep. *Acta Scientiae Veterinariae* 45: 1515.

Martens, H. and Schweigel, M. (2000). Pathophysiology of grass tetany and other hypomagnesemias. Implications for clinical management. *Veterinary Clinics of North America. Food Animal Practice* 16 (2): 339–368. https://doi.org/10.1016/s0749-0720(15)30109-2.

Matthews, J. (2016). *Diseases of the Goat*, 4e. Oxford: Wiley.

Nwaokorie, E.E., Osborne, C.A., Lulich, J.P. et al. (2015). Risk factors for calcium carbonate urolithiasis in goats. *Journal of the American Veterinary Medical Association* 247 (3): 293–299. https://doi.org/10.2460/javma.247.3.293.

Riedi, A.K., Knubben-Schweizer, G., and Meylan, M. (2018). Clinical findings and diagnostic procedures in 270 small ruminants with obstructive urolithiasis. *Journal of Veterinary Internal Medicine* 32 (3): 1274–1282. https://doi.org/10.1111/jvim.15128.

Riet-Correa, F., Simões, S.D.V., and Vasconcelos, J.S. (2008). Urolitíase em ovinos e caprinos. *Pesquisa Veterinária Brasileira* 28 (6): 319–322. https://doi.org/10.1590/S0100-736X2008000600010.

Sakhaee, E. and Derakhshanfar, A. (2010). Polioencephalomalacia associated with closantel overdosage in a goat. *Journal of the South African Veterinary Association* 81 (2): 116–117.

Sant'Ana, F.J.F. and Barros, C.S.L. (2010). Polioencephalomalacia in ruminants in Brazil. *Brazilian Journal of Veterinary Pathology* 3 (1): 70–79.

Scully, C.M. (2021). Management of urologic conditions in small ruminants. *Veterinary Clinics of North America. Food Animal Practice* 37 (1): 93–104. https://doi.org/10.1016/j.cvfa.2020.10.003.

Sharma, N., Kumar, A., Singh, M.K. et al. (2021). Clinical management of polioencephalomalacia in goats – a retrospective study of 18 cases. *Veterinary Practitioner* 22 (2): 52–54.

Simões, J. and Gutiérrez, C. (2017). Nutritional and metabolic disorders in dairy goats. In: *Sustainable Goat Production in Adverse Environments*, vol. I (ed. J. Simões and C. Gutiérrez), 177–194. Cham: Springer.

Sivaraman, S., Vijayakumar, G., Venkatesakumar, E. et al. (2016). Clinical management of polioencephalomalacia in goats – a retrospective study of 18 cases. *Indian Veterinary Journal* 93 (5): 70–72.

Smith, M.C. and Sherman, D.M. (2009). *Goat Medicine*, 2e. Ames, IA: Wiley.

Souto, R.J.C., Afonso, J.A.B., Mendonça, C.L. et al. (2013). Achados bioquímicos, eletrolíticos e hormonais em cabras acometidas com toxemia da prenhez. *Pesquisa Veterinária Brasileira* 33 (10): 1174–1182. https://doi.org/10.1590/S0100-736X2013001000002.

Souza, L.M., Mendonça, C.L., Assis, R.N. et al. (2020). Changes in cardiac biomarkers in goats naturally affected by pregnancy toxemia. *Research in Veterinary Science* 130: 73–78. https://doi.org/10.1016/j.rvsc.2020.02.016.

Stewart, J.L. and Shipley, C.F. (2021). Management of reproductive diseases in male small ruminants. *Veterinary Clinics of North America. Food Animal Practice* 37 (1): 105–123. https://doi.org/10.1016/j.cvfa.2020.10.005.

Sucupira, M.C.A., Araujo, C.A.S.C., Souto, R.J.C. et al. (2021). Toxemia da prenhez em pequenos ruminantes. *Revista Brasileira de Buiatria* 2 (3): 65–83. https://doi.org/10.432 2/2763-955X.2021.012.

Tharwat, M., Al-Sobayil, F., and Al-Sobayil, K. (2012). The cardiac biomarkers troponin I and CK-MB in nonpregnant and pregnant goats, goats with normal birth, goats with prolonged birth, and goats with pregnancy toxemia. *Theriogenology* 78 (7): 1500–1507. https://doi.org/10.1016/j.theriogenology.2012.06.013.

Videla, R. and Van Amstel, S. (2016). Urolithiasis. *Veterinary Clinics of North America. Food Animal Practice* 32 (3): 687–700. https://doi.org/10.1016/j.cvfa.2016.05.010.

Wilkens, M.R. and Muscher-Banse, A.S. (2020). Review: Regulation of gastrointestinal and renal transport of calcium and phosphorus in ruminants. *Animal* 14 (S1): s29–s43. https://doi.org/10.1017/S1751731119003197.

Wilkens, M.R., Richter, J., Fraser, D.R. et al. (2012). In contrast to sheep, goats adapt to dietary calcium restriction by increasing intestinal absorption of calcium. *Comparative Biochemistry and Physiology. Part A, Molecular & Integrative Physiology* 163 (3–4): 396–406. https://doi.org/10.1016/j.cbpa.2012.06.011.

Yamagishi, N., Oishi, A., Sato, J. et al. (1999). Experimental hypocalcemia induced by hemodialysis in goats. *Journal of Veterinary Medical Science* 61 (12): 1271–1275. https://doi.org/10.1292/jvms.61.1271.

17

Nutritional Deficiency Diseases in Goats

Chinmoy Maji[1], Suman Biswas[2], and Jasleen Kaur[3]

[1] *North 24 Parganas Krishi Vigyan Kendra, West Bengal University of Animal & Fishery Sciences, Ashokenagar, West Bengal, India*
[2] *Department of Avian Sciences, Faculty of Veterinary & Animal Sciences, West Bengal University of Animal & Fishery Sciences, Mohanpur, West Bengal, India*
[3] *Department of Veterinary Microbiology, College of Veterinary Sciences, Lala Lajpat Rai University of Veterinary & Animal Sciences, Hisar, Haryana, India*

Goats and sheep are both small ruminants with worldwide distribution. The production system of these small ruminants also varies from backyards to highly commercialized to free range, intensive, or semi-intensive depending on various factors such as the place, agro-climatic condition, economic status of the owner, availability of feed, marketing channel, and so on. In terms of feeding pattern, sheep generally prefer grazing whereas goats are selective browsers or more precisely of the intermediate type (Spurlock and Ward 1991, pp. 461–469). Goats generally prefer to take the highly digestible portion of grasses at the height of their head, which gives natural protection to them against some helminths. Most ruminants prefer to collect their feed by grazing or browsing through different feeds or feed supplements like fishmeal, milk, and so on from animal origins; minerals, salts, or vitamins are also supplied to make up a balanced ration for these animals, with a common goal to improve production of meat, milk, or wool from an economic point of view. Though both small ruminants are very particular in taking feedstuffs, there is a common misunderstanding about goats that they eat anything. This lack of awareness, together with economic problems and non-availability of natural or compound feeds or rations leads to different deficiency symptoms in the goat. As most feedstuffs originate from plant or animal sources and contain very similar types of constituents, the main components may be classified grossly into six types: water, carbohydrate, protein, lipid, vitamins, and minerals. As most feedstuffs are complex in nature and these six compounds are often interconnected physiologically, so a particular deficiency of one feed component may be either too slight to observe or exhibit compound symptoms.

17.1 Deficiency of Water

Water is the most important element in the body's systems. Even a mere 10% deficit of water, which is generally expressed through the degree of dehydration, may be fatal. Water constitutes about two-thirds of the body, whereas carbohydrates, lipids, and protein mostly form the dry masses of feed, generally expressed through digestible crude protein (DCP), total digestible nutrient (TDN), and metabolizable energy (ME). Water constitutes about 65% of the body weight, in which extracellular water represents about 50% and the cellular fluid portion is 70%, though the water content of an animal's body varies with different ages and physiological conditions. Newborn and lactating animals exhibit a higher water percentage in their body than adult animals. It is also noteworthy to say that protoplasm-bound water is important, as it helps the animal to resist low temperatures and drought conditions, whereas extra- or intracellular free water acts as a solvent for different inorganic or organic compounds inside the body (Banerjee 1988, pp. 191–193). Goats generally obtain the required water from predominantly three sources: drinking water, water present in feed, and metabolic water. It has been found that if water is provided ad libitum, animals generally drink the required amount. For maintenance sheep and goats usually consume 3.5–15 l of water per day (Rankins and Pugh 2002, p. 20).

Water acts in cell rigidity and elasticity, as a solvent inside the body in electrolyte and buffer system regulation, as a lubricant to prevent friction and drying, for heat regulation through absorption, conduction, distribution, and heat loss, inside the body, and in the composition of different excretions and secretions.

A deficiency of water will affect the body's activities overall and is expressed through increased thirst, dryness in mucus-containing areas (like eyes, mouth cavity, tip of nose, etc.), weight loss, and altered skin tone. Until renal function is affected, the urine volume may be markedly reduced to conserve water. Hypovolemia and reduced effective circulatory volume due to water deficiency lead to increased pulse rate, decreased pulse pressure, rapid respiration rate, increased capillary refill time, increased packed cell volume (PCV), and total plasma protein concentration.

It is very interesting that the goat among all ruminants requires less water evaporation via perspiration to control the body temperature (Maloiy and Taylor 1971). It also has the ability to maintain a water reserve through reduced urine output and focal water losses. In summary, small ruminants should be given ad libitum quantities of fresh drinking water to ensure optimal production.

17.2 Deficiency of Energy

Energy deficiency is the most common limiting nutrient deficiency of the goat production system. A deficiency of energy is readily reflected through a marked drop in production and in the long run through lower body weight gain, reduced fertility, and metabolic disorders. Like water, the energy requirement also varies in different life stages of the goat. It also varies in pregnancy, lactation, and according to the level of activity and intended use of the animal for the desired production. The majority of energy in the goat comes from the breakdown of carbohydrates from feed sources, mainly roughage and feed supplements, whereas lipids are important as a major form of energy storage in the body. Energy is generally dependent on the digestible elements and thus most of the time it is expressed as TDN, which is the sum of DCP, digestible carbohydrate, and 2.25 × digestible crude fat (Smith and Sherman 1994). These deficits or requirements may also be expressed as energy units such as kcal of digestible energy (DE) or ME, though all these terms are interrelated (Table 17.1).

According to the requirements in the ration at different stages of life, net energy (NE) may be further classified for maintenance purposes (NE_M, i.e. 0.72*ME), lactation purposes (NE_L, i.e. 0.60*ME), and growth purposes (NE_G, i.e. 0.45*ME). NE_M is also proportion to the metabolic weight of the animal in kg: $NE_M = 65.3*W_{kg}^{0.75}$ (Vermorel 1978). Fat is an important supplement for energy, but total fat content should not exceed 8% of the diet.

Table 17.1 Interrelationship of gross energy (GE) and total digestible nutrients (TDN) with other energy units in a TDN system.

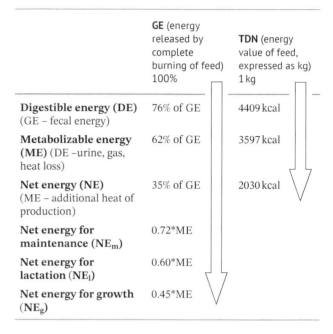

	GE (energy released by complete burning of feed) 100%	TDN (energy value of feed, expressed as kg) 1 kg
Digestible energy (DE) (GE – fecal energy)	76% of GE	4409 kcal
Metabolizable energy (ME) (DE –urine, gas, heat loss)	62% of GE	3597 kcal
Net energy (NE) (ME – additional heat of production)	35% of GE	2030 kcal
Net energy for maintenance (NE_m)	0.72*ME	
Net energy for lactation (NE_l)	0.60*ME	
Net energy for growth (NE_g)	0.45*ME	

An energy deficiency may arise from underfed or off-feed conditions, drought, starvation, environmental deviation from a thermoneutral zone (0–30 °C), excessive exercise, low quality of feed, poor digestibility of feed, more water-containing forages in the total ration, imbalanced rations for a doe with two or more kids, or any kind of stress.

Symptoms arising from a deficiency of energy vary according to the age of the animal, its physiological condition, availability of other nutrients, and environmental factors. In younger small ruminants, the symptoms are reflected within a short period through weak growth. An insufficient energy supply for a longer period in young animals result in retarded growth and delayed puberty.

In the case of an adult animal, a sudden deficiency of energy may lead to a marked drop in milk production. A prolonged energy deficiency result in a poor growth rate, lower body condition score, decreased immunity, decreased wool production, and deterioration of wool quality.

Pregnancy toxemia, a fatal metabolic disease in the goat in late pregnancy, occurs due to a low intake of an energy-rich diet and simultaneously caring for twins or triplets. It is characterized by hypoglycemia, ketonemia, and low liver glycogen content. Depression of consciousness, twitching of muscles, a stargazing posture, followed by paralysis and death are important clinical findings of pregnancy toxemia (Figure 17.1).

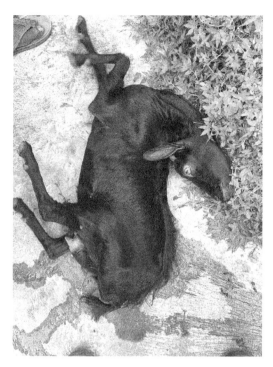

Figure 17.1 Pregnancy toxemia in a goat. *Source:* Courtesy of Dr. Satyaki Chakrabarti.

17.3   Deficiency of Protein

Protein is a major structural unit of animal tissue. It is needed throughout life for growth, repair of the body, and synthesis of various bio-products in the body's systems. It is essential in nerve function, immunity build-up, and metabolic regulation through hormones, enzymes, and oxygen transport (hemoglobin). Ruminants' protein requirement consists mainly of amino acids that come from two major sources: dietary protein and microbial protein. Most of the protein and non-protein nitrogen (NPN) in the diet are broken down to ammonia in the rumen, which is transformed to protein through rumen microbes. This microbial protein quality (amino and content) is surprisingly good. So, after the rumen development, it is not the quality but the quantity of dietary protein that is more important to the adult animal. NPN like urea incorporated into feed is a popular, inexpensive way to increase protein in the diet. Conditions like mixing of grain potentiate the fermentation of urea, whereas feedstuffs such as poor-quality roughage or urease-containing feed like raw soybean or wild mustard may inversely affect the fermentation process. Incorporation of urea in feed requires the utmost awareness to prevent urea toxicity in the goat. Sudden incorporation and improper mixing of ingredients sometimes have fatal consequences. It has been also observed that if crude protein exceeds 14% of dietary TDN, NPN is of no value (Rankins

and Pugh 2002, p. 22). Unlike carbohydrate and fat reserve, excess protein cannot be stored in the body's systems. Feeding of excess protein is undesirable because it results in increased feeding costs and a higher rate of disease (heat stress, evil-smelling feces, kidney dysfunction, etc.) (Banerjee 1988, p. 272).

Deficiency of protein is generally associated with deficiency of energy, and thus the term protein energy malnutrition is applied to ruminants, although it is less common in goats. In a young animal, reduced appetite, stunted growth, prolonged time for maturity, and muscle weakness may be observed in protein deficiency. In a mature animal, loss of weight, drop in production and reproduction performance, and edema associated with hypoproteinemia are observed. There is a marked alteration in the hemogram with chronic protein deficiency in a ruminant, in particular hemoglobin concentration, PCV, total protein, and total albumin content (Radostits et al. 2007, p. 1080). Protein requirement varies with age, physiological condition, and production performance. Body condition scoring in the goat may be used as a guideline to provide external supplements in case of protein deficiency in the goat.

17.4   Deficiency of Fiber

The fiber portion of a feed is very important due to its influence on digestibility. Fiber is actually cell wall material and consists mainly of hemicellulose, cellulose, lignin, and silica. Lignin and silica inversely affect digestibility. Goats can digest fiber like cellulose and hemicellulose and have the ability to convert these into volatile fatty acids by rumen fermentation. For healthy rumen functioning, the dietary fiber content should be greater than 50% and the minimum particle size of the fiber should be 1–2.5 cm (Rankins and Pugh 2002). So both the quality and quantity of the fiber content of feed are important for digestibility (Santini et al. 1991).

In a high-producing lactating goat, dietary fiber plays a pivotal role in milk fat digestion by maintaining the acetate–propionate ratio in the rumen, as acetate is a major precursor of fat in milk (Lu et al. 2005).

Thus a deficiency of fiber in the diet affects rumen function, influences salivation through mastication and milk-fat regulation, whereas the quality of fiber is influential in determining the degree of digestibility.

17.5   Deficiency of Minerals

The animal body contains of about 3% minerals, which remain mostly as ash. Out of about 30–40 minerals in the body, 23 elements have been proven to be essential in

Table 17.2 Essential minerals for the goat.

Major elements	Trace elements
Calcium (Ca)	Iron (Fe)
Phosphorus (P)	Iodine (I)
Magnesium (Mg)	Copper (Cu)
Potassium (K)	Manganese (Mn)
Sodium (Na)	Zinc (Zn)
Chlorine (Cl)	Cobalt (Co)
Sulfur (S)	Molybdenum (Mo)
	Selenium (Se)
	Chromium (Cr)
	Tin (Sn)
	Vanadium (V)
	Fluorine (F)
	Silicon (Si)
	Nickel (Ni)
	Arsenic (As)
	Lead (Pb)

Table 17.3 Interaction of minerals with other compounds.

Synergism interactions	Antagonism interactions
Ca–P, Na–Cl, Zn–Mo enhance the level of absorption within the gastrointestinal tract	P–Mg and Zn–Cu inhibit each other's absorption in the intestine
Ca and P combined form bone hydroxyapatite	K inhibits the absorption of Zn and Mn and not vice versa.
Fe and Cu combined form hemoglobin	Excess Mg and Cu form a complex with sulfate and reduce absorption of both
Mn and Zn combined form RNA	Excess Ca similarly forms Ca–P–Zn salt and affects absorption
Fe and Mo combined form xanthine and aldehyde oxide	Different minerals in the form of ions may compete with each other for the active center of the enzyme system (like Mg^{2+} and Mn^{2+} in the metallo-enzyme complex of alkaline phosphatase, cholinesterase, etc.)
Cu and Fe combined are part of cytochrome oxidase	ATPase is inhibited by Ca^{2+}
	Vitamin D affects the absorption of Mg and Ca
	Excess Mo reduces the biosynthesis of muscle protein

Note: See Table 17.2 for abbreviations.
Source: Adapted from Banerjee (1988).

the animal's body systems and six others may be essential. Out of all the essential minerals, calcium, phosphorus, sodium, chlorine, magnesium, potassium, and sulfur are considered macrominerals. The eight microminerals are cobalt, copper, molybdenum, iron, zinc, manganese, iodine, and selenium. The classification of major and minor or trace elements depends not on their relative importance, but on their concentration in the animal or the amount required in the feed (Table 17.2). A deficiency of these elements may result in metabolic disorders that can be rectified through timely supply of the deficient elements. Trace mineral deficiency develops slowly and sometimes become unnoticed and suppressed beneath other major deficiencies or disease conditions. Some of the mineral deficiencies may be traced through a liver biopsy.

There is a complex relationship between minerals and other substances. The interaction may be synergistic or antagonistic in nature (Table 17.3) and subsequently affects the availability and functioning of different biomolecules inside the body. Not all the minerals are important for goats, nor are the deficiency symptoms well studied in the case of goats. Some of the important mineral deficiencies in the goat production system are discussed here.

17.5.1 Copper

Copper (Cu) is a true "indicator" micromineral with an important role in goat nutrition (Haenlein and Anke 2011). It regulates different vital biochemical processes and is an

integral part of different body enzymes like ceruloplasmin, cytochrome C oxidase, superoxide dismutase, lysyl oxidase, galactosyl transferase ceramide, and dopamine β-hydroxylase. The physiological role of Cu in small ruminants is related to several functions, including cellular respiration, bone formation, connective tissue development, and being an essential catalytic co-factor of some metalloenzymes (Underwood and Suttle 2003). Cu requirements for goats have been reported to be between 8 and 10 mg/kg of dry matter (DM) intake, though a high regular intake leads to Cu toxicity (Anke and Seifert 2004). Sheep are more prone to Cu toxicity than goats, whereas goats are sensitive to Cu deficiency (Draksler et al. 2002).

In ruminants, Cu is absorbed partially in the forestomachs (dilatations and modifications of the esophagus) with the involvement of microflora, and in the stomach and the small intestine. The absorption and metabolism of Cu largely depend on molecular interaction with the presence of molybdenum (Mo) and sulfur (S) in the rumen. Thiomolybdates are produced in the rumen as a result of interaction between Mo and S, which depending on the ratios present can be distinguished as follows: monothiomolybdate (MoO_3S), dithiomolybdate (MoO_2S_2), trithiomolyibdate ($MoOS_3$), and tetrathiomolybdate (MoS_4) (Rocha and Bouda 2001). These thiomolybdates combine with free Cu molecules and form insoluble Cu complexes, which then result in the formation of Cu-Mo-S complexes. These complexes interfere with Cu consumption, which leads to secondary Cu deficiency. The amounts of dietary zinc (Zn) and iron (Fe) in goats also have a significant impact on copper absorption; if these levels are high, a competitive interaction will negatively impact copper absorption (Suttle 2010). Cu and Zn concentrations in the liver and ribs of experimental goats significantly decreased after the addition of a bentonite (clay) supplement (2 g/kg body weight) to a standard goat ration (Schwarz and Werner 1987). In cases of phosphorus (P) deficiency, the milk and heart muscle of goats contained more Cu than normal, and both had significantly higher Cu concentrations (Barhoum 1989).

Cu plays a multifactorial role in the body and its deficiency produces a variety of symptoms (Figure 17.2). In kids it produces two types of symptoms: congenital (swayback) and chronic/late (enzootic ataxia) (Banton et al. 1990). The congenital form develops within the growing fetus during the gestational period and the typical symptoms are noticed after birth. Swayback is characterized by prolonged recumbency, weakness, constant head shaking, and trembling. A histological examination of the brain reveals cavitation and the development of gelatinous maleic foci, as well as absence of or damage to the white matter in the cerebral hemisphere (Radwinsha and Zarczynsha 2014). Demyelination of the motor nerve in the white matter of the spinal cord is also noticed in kids. The late/chronic forms occur between 1 week to 6 months of age and are characterized by incoordination, ataxia, and paresis of the hind limbs (Radwinsha and Zarczynsha 2014). Reproductive disorders due to Cu deficiency are characterized by a low conception rate, abortion, a mummified fetus, and a hemorrhagic placenta with necrotic lesions (McDowell et al. 1997; Hidiroglou 1979). In addition, when does are exposed to long periods of Cu deficiency this produces nymphomaniac reproductive behavior, although in

the buck it does not affect reproductive performance (Hidiroglu 1979). The low conception rates are mostly associated with delayed or suppressed estrus or prolonged postpartum periods (Vázquez-Armijo et al. 2011).

17.5.2 Molybdenum

Mo is an important trace element in goat nutrition, but its role was not clear till 2000 (McDowell 2003). Because of its antagonistic interaction with Cu, excess Mo or its lack in particular soil or plants of various regions of the world has become a significant nutritional factor (Haenlein and Anke 2011).

Mo acts as a co-factor of different oxidase enzyme systems like xanthine oxidoreductase (Atmani et al. 2004). However, excess intake of Mo by goats from different sources like pasture, forage, industrial fallout, and aerial contamination affects health (it produces persistent scouring, emaciation, and depigmentation of hair) and overall performance (Radostits et al. 2007; Vázquez-Armijo et al. 2011). Among all animal species, goats are the most tolerant to Mo load in the body. The Mo requirement in the goat is about 100 μg/kg of DM intake (NRC et al. 2007). It is mostly deposited in liver and kidney, followed by lungs, hair, and brain (Anke and Risch 1989). Deficiency of Mo causes elevated production or expression of hormones such as estrogen, luteinizing hormone (LH), and follicular-stimulating hormone (FSH). This elevation has a significant negative impact on the reproductive efficiency and growth of the goats (Haenlein and Anke 2011).

17.5.3 Selenium

Selenium (Se) plays a key role in several functions of the animal body, mainly the formation of selenocysteine, which is the main component of about 30 selenoproteins, most of which are enzymes (Holben and Smith 1999). Glutathione peroxidase (GSH-Px), one of the major selenoproteins, destroys damaging peroxidases in the body tissue and contributes to cellular defense mechanisms by protecting the oxidation of fatty acids and hemoglobin, which is essential for the survival of animals. The daily requirement in goat rations is about 0.56 mg/kg DM intake (Szilagyi et al. 1986).

Deficiency of Se in small ruminants like goats leads to the development of "white muscle disease" or nutritional muscular dystrophy (NMD) (Figure 17.3). In NMD, skeletal muscles in a number of body parts, including the tongue, heart muscle, and diaphragm, experience hyaline degeneration (Beytut et al. 2002). NMD is also characterized by decreased concentration

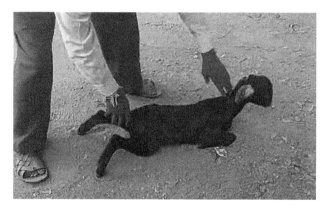

Figure 17.2 Copper deficiency in a kid showing posterior paralysis and inability to move.

(a)   (b)

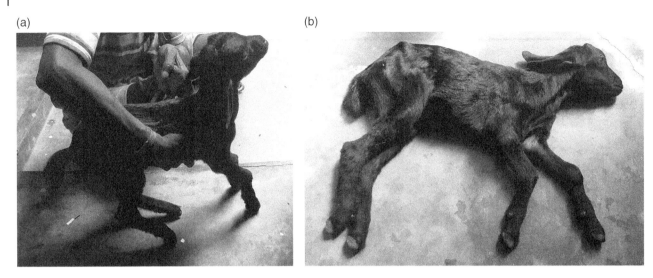

Figure 17.3 (a, b) Nutritional muscular dystrophy in a Bengal goat kid responsive to vitamin E and selenium treatment, showing inability to stand with elevated creatinine kinase and aspartate aminotransferase levels. *Source:* Courtesy of Dr. Soumen Samanta.

of GSH-Px with significant increase of creatinine kinase (CK), aldolase (ALD), lactate dehydrogenase (LDH), hydroxybutyrate dehydrogenase (HBDH), aspartate aminotransferase (AST), and alanine aminotransferase (ALT). In Se-deficient goats, an increase in AST activity was linked to liver damage, whereas an increase in CK activity was linked to the development of muscular dystrophy (Haenlein and Anke 2011). The disease is most often diagnosed in healthy kids younger than 6 months. The most typical signs include a hunched spine, widespread limbs in an improper posture, a stilted walk, and recumbency. The condition mostly affects the muscles in the thighs and crus. Changes in the muscles of the tongue hinder swallowing and cause milk to come out of the nostrils. In persistence of NMD, the goat may show dyspnea, a pulmonary murmur, and coughing, with improper cardiac function leads to mass animal deaths (up to 90% mortality) (Ghany-Hefnawy and Tortora-Perez 2009). Other less specific symptoms include debilitated kids, abortion, and retention of the placenta, which causes huge economic losses (Haenlein and Anke 2011).

17.5.4 Calcium and Phosphorus

Calcium (Ca) is the most abundant macromineral in the animal body, and 99% of it is found in bones as a complex form. Ca is a vital element for maintaining different bodily processes such as ossification of bone and cartilage, coagulation of blood, control of cardiac rhythm, cell membrane permeability, excitation of nerve and muscle, and activation and secretion of different growth hormones (GHs) and enzymes. The second most prevalent mineral in animals is phosphorus (P), and bones and teeth are where 80% of this mineral is found. In the ossification of bone, P works with Ca. It is also an essential component of nucleic acids and molecules rich in energy. Two parathyroid hormones, parathormone and calcitonin, as well as vitamin D3, play a major role in controlling the levels of Ca and P in animal bodies (Sobiech et al. 2010).

Goats frequently experience Ca and P deficiencies as a result of poor/inadequate nutrition, low vitamin D3 levels, complex interactions with other minerals like Zn and cadmium, or an incorrect Ca : P ratio (1.5 : 2.1) in the diet (Radostits et al. 2007; Radwinsha and Zarczynsha 2014). The recommended Ca and P requirements for goats are 3.3 and 4.0 g/kg DM intake, respectively (Anke and Seifert 2004). Lack of Ca and P leads to inappropriate bone mineralization, which is followed by decreased necrosis of cartilaginous cells and osteoblast penetration, resulting in loss of bone elasticity and deformation. This condition ultimately leads to osteomalacia or rickets in kids. The first signs of rickets include allotriophagy (pica) and stunted development. The condition may also be accompanied by a detectable thickening of circumferential rib segments and epiphyses, which results in the development of the rachitic rosary and is clinically presented by curvature of legs, impaired mobility, and lameness (Dittmer and Thomson 2011). The heart muscle and aorta in particular had significantly higher amounts of Zn, Fe, Cu, and manganese (Mn), indicating a shift in mineral content from the skeleton to many soft tissues in P-deficient goats (Haenlein and Anke 2011). In addition, P deficiency during gestation of the doe leads to the development of smaller and lighter kids, decreased conception rates with low milk production, and high kid mortality after parturition.

17.5.5 Magnesium

In mammals, magnesium (Mg) is the second most prevalent intracellular cation after potassium. In the animal body, Mg is principally found in bones and muscles. Mg is involved in many cellular metabolic pathways and is essential for almost all physiological processes. It is involved in the metabolism of proteins, nucleic acids, and carbohydrates by activating close to 30 enzymes (Radwinsha and Zarczynsha 2014). Mg regulates the development of ribosomal subunits, stabilizes DNA structure, and influences RNA transcription. Bivalent Mg ions are involved in the synthesis of ATP and stabilizing the cell membrane (Soetan et al. 2010). A dynamic relationship of Mg with Ca is necessary to maintain proportionate growth in kids. If Mg content remains high for a long period in the goat ration than Ca, it can stifle bone formation (Zimmermann et al. 2000). Mg enhances the absorption of potassium and defends heart muscle cells and neurons from free radicals and toxins.

Green succulent fodder contains a sufficient amount of Mg, but deficiency occurs due to prolonged low environmental temperatures, low food intake, chronic diarrhea, and long-standing disease conditions (Robson et al. 2004). Deficiency of Mg causes excitation of nerves and muscles. In long-term magnesium-deficient kids, this excitation leads to the development of hypomagnesemic tetany (Martens and Schweigel 2000). This affects mostly rapidly growing goats at the age of 1.5–4 months. The symptoms of tetany include anxiety, twitching of the ears, bulging eyes, jerking movements of the head, kicking at the abdomen, and a stiff and unsteady gait (Naik et al. 2010). These symptoms are followed by a contraction episode that lasts for 15–20 minutes. The heart and respiration rates visibly increase, the eyes bulge, and the head and neck are flung backward (opisthotonus) during this episode. Each episode leaves the animal weaker than before, with possible tremors and allotriophagic symptoms. One to two days later, contractions can recur, and death may occur.

17.5.6 Zinc

Zn is an essential component in animal nutrition because of its biological role in nearly 300 enzymes, protein synthesis, and other activities (Miao et al. 2013). Superoxide dismutase, alkaline phosphatase, carbonic anhydrase, LDH, RNA, and DNA polymerase all contain Zn as a structural component. It is crucial for the structural integrity of enzymes as well as the production of several hormones that are produced by the animal body, including GH, thyroid-stimulating hormone (TSH), glucagon, insulin, LH, adrenocorticotropic hormone, and FSH (Alves et al. 2012). Other functions include the synthesis of vitamin A, carbon dioxide (CO_2) transport, breakdown of collagen fibers, elimination of free radicals, maintenance of red blood cell membrane stability, fatty acid metabolism, carbohydrate metabolism, protein synthesis, and nucleic acid metabolism (Rubio et al. 2007).

Deficiency of Zn can be classified into two types: primary and secondary. Supplementation of Zn when insufficient can be done through milk and day-to-day rations when primary deficiency occurs, whereas secondary deficiency occurs when the goat is given feed containing sufficient Zn but its availability is suppressed by the presence of high number of Zn antagonists (Cu, Mg, phosphate, and divalent Fe compounds) and amino acids (Radwinska and Zarczynsha 2014). Under field conditions, interactions with Ca, cadmium (Cd), nickel (Ni), and phytic acid limit the bioavailability of Zn in goats and may cause secondary Zn deficiency (Haenlein and Anke 2011). A goat's daily Zn requirement is 90 mg/kg of DM intake (Haenlein and Anke 2011).

Some non-specific symptoms like reduced appetite, higher feed conversion ratio, and lower weight gains are observed in mild Zn deficiency of goats. Male kids with low Zn levels showed delayed testicular development as well as hypogonadism that resulted in oligospermia and a lack of testosterone (Bedwal and Bahuguna 1994). Lack of Zn results in testicular atrophy in bucks and this condition ultimately causes reduction of libido and sperm production (McDowell et al. 1997). However, spermatogenesis involves significant cell division, and to keep this process going sufficient Zn is needed for the metabolism of nucleic acids and proteins in cell replication (Hidiroglou and Knipfel 1984). Severe Zn deficiency in mature goats causes abnormalities of skin like scab formation on the low hairy part of the body (scrotum, udder, around the eyes, lips, vulva, and medial aspect of all four legs) with intense pruritus. This condition is popularly known as parakeratosis. Impaired protein synthesis and the activation of Zn-dependent enzymes, which are crucial for the metabolism of carbohydrates, lipids, and nucleic acids, are the most likely causes of parakeratosis (Al-Saad et al. 2010; Alves et al. 2012).

17.5.7 Cobalt

Co is an essential micromineral in ruminants and catalyzes different metabolic pathways (hydration, hydrogenation, and desulfurization). It also has a direct role in the formation of nucleic acids and stimulates the production of erythropoietin from the kidney. In the mammary gland, cobalt activates gluconolactonase and takes part in the pentose–phosphate pathway and glucose oxidation (Kennedy et al. 1994). About 50% of the Co supplied through goat rations is used in the formation of vitamin B12 (cobalamin). Structurally, cobalamin constitutes 4.5% Co and formation occurs in the rumen. Co is necessary for the healthy growth and functioning of the ruminal microbiota; however, goats are less susceptible to Co deficiency than are cattle or sheep (Sharman et al. 2008). When soil has less than 0.25 mg/kg of Co, it is more likely to yield pastures with insufficient Co levels. One of the key elements in reducing the Co content of soil is heavy liming (Radostits et al. 2007). This is known as primary Co deficiency. The presence of a high amount of fructans in the pasture leads to the development of hepatic insufficiency and limits the absorption of Co and vitamin B12 (Radostits et al. 2007). This is known as secondary Co deficiency. Overall data from many sources indicates that a concentration of 0.076 mg Co/kg of DM intake for goats appears to be appropriate (Dezfoulian and Aliarabi 2017).

Co deficiency symptoms are generally non-specific. A low level of cobalt in goat rations disrupts the symbiotic relationship of the ruminal microflora and causes the development of chronic indigestion and metabolic disorders. It is clinically evidenced by low body weight, emaciation, weakness, marked pallor of the visible mucous membrane (hyperchromic macrocytic anemia), and retardation of wool production (Digest 2007). Co deficiency reduces immunity in goats, especially their resistance to parasitic infections in the gastrointestinal system, and it decreases neutrophils' ability to kill pathogens (Schwarz et al. 2000). Long-term Co deficiency leads to the development of hepatic lipidosis in goats in conjunction with a low level of vitamin B12. It is mostly in seen Omani goats. The affected goat shows a complex syndrome of reduced body weight gains and a dry, scruffy hair coat, with a low erythrocytic count and consistent lesions in the liver (Radostits et al. 2007). Oral supplementation of Co in the form of cobalt sulfate (1 mg/day/animal) and parenteral administration of vitamin B12 (100–300 µg/animal) at weekly intervals are sufficient to treat the deficient goat.

17.5.8 Manganese

Mn actively contributes to the formation of the bone matrix and the production of chondroitin sulfate, which keeps connective tissue strong. In goat nutrition, it has been observed that redistribution of Mn among the various goat organs was based on a dietary phosphorus deficiency, especially in heart muscle and milk (Barhoum 1989). A deficiency of Mn relates to muscle weakness and congenital bone deformity, and is clinically manifested by a hopping gait. It is also related to infertility of the goat.

17.5.9 Bromine

Bromine (Br) as a bromide salt is mostly used in the treatment of epilepsy and sleeplessness. A deficiency of Br in animals is very rare due to its abundant presence in the biosphere, sea plants, and natural vegetation (Haenlein and Anke 2011). In experimentally produced Br-deficient goats, epithelial duct metaplasia is accompanied by mammary gland underdevelopment, and the clinical presentation includes high rates of abortion, decreased feed intake, and the birth of kids with low hemoglobin content (Zhavoronkov et al. 1996).

17.5.10 Cadmium

Cd is known as a dangerous heavy metal because of its carcinogenicity. Farm animals are not likely to exhibit symptoms of Cd deficiency because their typical feed intake of Cd is much higher than that of a deficiency ration. Its utility in goat nutrition remained unclear till 1986. Deficiency of Cd in kids causes mitochondrial degeneration of liver and kidney with a reduction of the contractile power of skeletal muscles (Anke et al. 1986). This ultrastructural modification leads to the development of fatal muscular weakness and low birth weight, which lead to high mortality in kids.

17.5.11 Nickel

Ni is a nutritionally essential micromineral for goats, but its importance was not established until 1970. It has been observed that goats with a Ni deficiency excrete more Ca and Fe in their feces but have a proportionate depletion of Zn in the body (Haenlein and Anke 2011). Deficiency of Ni produces a low hemoglobin content, which ultimately produces high mortality among kids and lactating goats (Anke et al. 1980). Goats with low Ni levels also had skin and hair abnormalities resembling parakeratosis.

17.5.12 Vanadium

No specific deficiency symptom had been observed and the nutritional requirement for vanadium (V) for animals was still unclear till 1980. It mostly acts as an analog of phosphorus and interferes with metabolism, cell proliferation, and angiogenesis in animals. Deficiency of V in kids causes deformation of the forefoot tarsal joint similar to P, Mn, or vitamin D deficiency. The blood profile of kids also shows high β-lipoprotein, triglyceride, and enzymes of the citrate cycle (Anke et al. 1986). Granulocystic hyperplasia of the endometrium is also observed in V-deficient goats (Mikhaleva 2000).

17.6 Deficiency of Vitamins

There is very scanty information about vitamin metabolism in the goat. Vitamins are organic components, required by animals in very small amounts compared to other nutritional components, and essential for normal growth and maintenance of animal life. These vitamins can be divided into two main categories according to their solubility pattern. The fat-soluble vitamins are vitamins A, D, E, and K, whereas vitamin B complex (B1–B12) and vitamin C are considered water-soluble vitamins. Among these vitamins, many have a tendency to be destroyed by oxidation, which may be accelerated by induction of heat, light, or minerals. Some biological compounds that produce vitamins after a certain biochemical alteration in the body are described as provitamins or vitamin precursors (like β -carotenoid is a precursor of vitamin A). Most of the vitamins are collected from plant sources as feed, from where some vitamins are synthesized in the animal body systems or ruminal microbial digestion system. Normally fat-soluble vitamins A, D, and E, and water-soluble vitamin B12 are well stored in the body in appreciable amounts (Tiwari et al. 2013, p. 164).

17.6.1 Deficiency of Vitamin A

Although all vitamins are necessary in goat nutrition, vitamin A is considered the most important from a practical point of view. Among different carotenoid and sterol precursors, β-carotenoid is the most important provitamin for vitamin A. Dark green leafy vegetables are a rich source of carotenoids in the case of the goat. Primary vitamin A deficiency arises mostly in young kids where the total ration lacks vitamin A or its precursor for a prolonged period. Secondary vitamin A deficiency appears when even after the required intake of vitamin A or its precursor, due to chronic diseases of the liver or intestine the absorption and transformation of vitamin A are hampered. Factors that may influence vitamin A utilization in the animal body include the following:

- The presence of a high temperature or light leading to oxidation of vitamin A supplement that has been stored for a long period. Pellet feed, which required high temperatures during processing, thus may be deficient in vitamin A.
- In summer or drought periods, the carotene content of leaves decreases due to thermal blocking.
- Hepatic insufficiency, biliary disorders, hypothyroidism rumen disorder, and intestinal mucosal health directly or indirectly affect the absorption and metabolism of vitamin A in the animal's body systems.
- Deficiency of antioxidants (including vitamin E, vitamin C, Se, phosphorus, and Zn) affects vitamin A absorption.
- The type of carotenoid in leafy vegetables or supplied feed directly regulates the conversion of carotene to vitamin A.
- Any disease condition mostly infectious or parasitic in origin interferes with the conversion of carotene.

In the case of the goat, the requirement for vitamin A per day is calculated by the National Research Council (NRC et al. 2007) on the basis of sheep and cattle requirements. Normally 5000 IU/kg DM of feed may be taken into account (Morand-Fehr 1991). According to the NRC's recommendation, a goat of 50 and 100 kg body weight requires 2000 IU and 3500 IU vitamin A/day, respectively. Additional supplementation is required in late pregnancy (1100 IU) and during the growth period (500 IU for weight gain of 100 g/day) or lactation period (3800 IU/l of milk production). While green leafy vegetables and colostrum are rich sources of vitamin A or its precursor, poor-quality old hay is deficient in vitamin A. Oral vitamin A in the form of palmitate is more desirable than injectable vitamin A, as the latter may be destroyed through rapid peroxidation at the injection site.

Vitamin A is essential for vision, maintenance of epithelial tissue, reproduction, proper skeletal development, and proper immune function. The physiological functions of vitamin A are as follows:

- **Vision**: This is the most evident and defined function of vitamin A. Retinol, which is the alcohol form of vitamin A, is utilized as the aldehyde retinal. This 11-cis-retinal combines with opsin protein to form rhodopsin (visual purple) in the retina of the eye, which is responsible for dim-light vision (Figure 17.3).
- **Bone development**: Vitamin A is essential for normal bone development through regulation of the activity of osteoclast of the epithelial cartilage. In deficiency of vitamin A, incoordination of shaping of bone is observed as osteoblast (depositing bone) functions become more functional than osteoclast (reabsorbing bone). As a result of disorganized bone growth, constriction at cranial openings affecting cranial nerves, herniation of brain increasing cerebrospinal fluid (CSF) pressure, and irritation of joints may occur.
- **Maintenance of epithelial tissue**: Epithelial secretory cells are protective linings of many systems of the body like respiratory, gastrointestinal, and urogenital systems as well as the eye. Vitamin A regulates the integrity of the lipoprotein membrane of these secretory epithelial cells. In deficiency of vitamin A, these secretory cells are replaced by stratified keratinizing epithelial cells. As a result of the changing character of the epithelium after keratinization, pathogens easily enter through the skin, respiratory organs, alimentary canal, urogenital surface, or eye. Subsequent inflammation or infection increases the severity of the disease, as deficiency of vitamin A may impair the regeneration of normal mucosal epithelium. Placental degeneration, corneal problems, and exophthalmia may develop due to mucosal changes because of hypovitaminosis A.
- **Reproductive efficiency**: The reproductive performance of both male and female goats is affected. In

adults, fertility is affected due to inadequate steroid hormone synthesis.

- **Immune mechanism**: Though unclear in the goat, vitamin A and β-carotene may be attributed to immunity against infection by both specific and non-specific defense mechanisms. This resistance may be associated with the role of vitamin A in the regulation of epithelial cell maintenance, corticosteroid production from the adrenal gland, and enhanced polymorphonuclear neutrophil function. Vitamin A deficiency affects antibody response to the T-cell-dependent antigenic process.

17.6.1.1 Deficiency Symptoms

- The liver can store vitamin A for months, though most conversion of β-carotene to vitamin A takes place in the upper part of the intestine, mainly the jejunum. Due to the hepatic storage supply, the adult goat does not exhibit clear clinical symptoms at vitamin A deficiency over a short period, while kids shows reduced growth (Figure 17.4), vision impairment, hair loss, diarrhea, and respiratory diseases.
- Visual problems due to xeropthalmia, corneal opacity, corneal ulcer, or serous mucoid discharge from the eye may develop.
- Bone deformity or increased CSF pressure may develop. Compression in the optic and auditory nerves may result in blindness and deafness.
- Keratinization may be observed of the eye, skin, respiratory system, reproductive system, or alimentary system, leading to corneal keratinization, pneumonia,

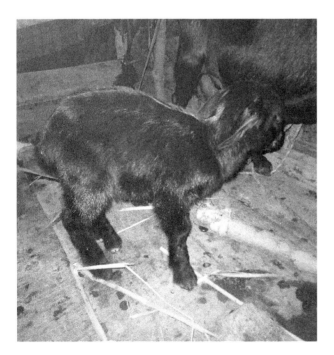

Figure 17.4 Deficiency of vitamin A in a kid showing skeletal weakness and inability to move. *Source:* Courtesy of Dr. Abhijit Barui.

degeneration of reproductive organs, or urinary calculi formation.

- Reproductive performance through spermatogenesis and oogenesis is hampered. Retained placenta, birth of abnormal offspring, and placental degeneration leading to abortion may occur in a deficient animal.
- Susceptibility to disease infection and inflammation increases with lower immunity.
- Congenital abnormalities like anophthalmos, microphthalmos, or congenital retinal changes may develop.

17.6.1.2 Treatment

Deficient animals may be treated with immediate vitamin A at a dose equivalent to 10–20 times the daily maintenance requirement (about 440 IU/kg body weight). Incorporation of vitamin A in the form of bolus powder in the ration is also prescribed and is readily fed to the goat.

17.7 Deficiency of Vitamin D

Vitamin D is not very common in feeds. Mostly vitamin D is biosynthesized inside the body through exposure of skin to sun rays. In the goat, except for young animals, the requirement is thus met naturally when the adult animal grazes in the sunlight. In the case of confined rearing and feeding practices, there may be a chance of vitamin D deficiency in kids. Winter hay contains very low amounts of vitamin D precursors.

Vitamin D2 (ergocalciferol) and D3 (cholecalciferol) are physiologically important for vitamin D activity and are referred to as provitamins. Ergocalciferol is formed from ergosterol, which is present in plants. Cholecalciferol is formed from 7-dehydrocholesterol, which is present in animal skin. This 7-dehydrocholesterol transformation to cholecalciferol in skin requires exposure to sunlight or ultraviolet (UV) rays to a limited extent. Excessive exposure to sunlight may lead to the generation of toxic compounds.

Vitamin D2 or vitamin D3 becomes biologically active after hydroxylation first at the liver (produces 25-OH D3) and secondly at the kidney (produces 1,25-dihydroxy cholecalciferol or calcitriol). Plasma Ca, P, and parathyroid hormone directly or indirectly control this activation pathway. Calcitriol or 1,25-dihydroxy cholecalciferol (1,25-DHCC) is the active form of vitamin D. Orally administered vitamin D is generally absorbed from the small intestine.

250–1000 IU vitamin D/day is required for goats (Kessler 1991a, 1991b). The functions of vitamin D are as follows:

- Calcitriol or 1,25-DHCC along with Ca and P is important for bone integrity.
- Vitamin D regulates the intestinal absorption of Ca and phosphate.

- Some researchers have pointed out that vitamin D has a significant role in cell proliferation and steroidogenesis in the goat (Yao et al. 2017).
- Vitamin D3 has a specific role in goat ovarian follicular development (Yao et al. 2020).
- Calcitriol is also involved in controlling the excretion of Ca and phosphate through the kidneys.

17.7.1 Deficiency Symptoms

- Deficiency of vitamin D in the goat is mainly observed through the imbalance of Ca and phosphorus in growing animals resulting in rickets. Joints are enlarged and legs become bowed in vitamin-deficient animals. The same may be observed in Ca deficiency in kids. Osteomalacia (demineralization of the bones) may be observed in adult goats exclusively kept indoors without vitamin D supplementation.
- Reduced productivity, reduced fertility, abnormal folliculogenesis, and poor body weight gain in young animals are important deficiency symptoms.

17.7.1.1 Treatment

Administration of vitamin D in deficient animals must be supplemented orally or parenterally with proper grazing in sunlight. Ca and P should be in the ration along with vitamin D.

17.7.2 Vitamin E Deficiency

Vitamin E is a lipid soluble organic alcohol that is also known as a "radical scavenger." Most of the time its importance is discussed alongside another antioxidant mineral, Se. Out of all isomers, alpha-tocopherol is the most biologically active. Generally deficiency of vitamin E and Se are observed when females consume poor-quality hay in Se-deficient areas. Sources of vitamin E may be of animal origin (eggs, milk, fish, etc.) or plant origin (soybean, alfalfa, cottonseed, leafy vegetables, etc.).

The 2007 NRC recommendation is 5.3 IU/kg body weight/day vitamin E for small ruminants (Rankins and Pugh 2002). Ruminants do not synthesize vitamin E. Exposure to oxidizing metals like Cu and Fe in feedstuffs decreases vitamin E availability (Frye et al. 1991). Corn- and sulfur-containing feeds also decreases vitamin E availability.

Vitamin E is a biological antioxidant acting in association with Se-containing glutathione peroxidase. It protects mammalian cells against oxidative damage by free radicals that are produced during cell metabolism. More particularly, it prevents oxidation of polyunsaturated fatty acids (PUFAs) of subcellular membranes and thus interrupts the chain reaction of lipid peroxidation that is detrimental to cellular health.

Vitamin E also plays an important role in maintaining the immune health of animals, inflammatory response, reproduction, and striated muscle function (Van Metre and Callan 2001).

17.7.2.1 Deficiency Symptoms

- The main deficiency of vitamin E in ruminants is expressed through the muscular degenerative changes of NMD. Two types of NMD are generally observed: skeletal muscle form and cardiac form. In the skeletal muscle form of NMD, lethargy, weakness, stiff or unsteady gait, firm and painful muscle, with paralytic symptoms and bilateral symmetrical involvement are seen. Muscle may have longitudinal white streaks or a parboiled appearance on postmortem. In the cardiac form weakness, tachypnea, tachycardia, pulmonary edema, and heart murmurs followed by death due to cardiac arrest may be observed.
- Deficiency of vitamin E in small ruminants has been shown to be associated with sterility, impaired fertility, reduced kidding, and impaired immunity. Vitamin E is also known as an anti-sterility factor.
- A single report of skin disease caused by deficiency of vitamin E has been reported so far. Periocular hair loss and diffuse, dandruff-like exfoliation of scales were important deficiency symptoms (Smith 1981).

17.7.2.2 Treatment

Vitamin E- and Se-containing medicine should be incorporated into feed in case of deficiency. Injectable vitamin E is available. In deficient animals, Smith and Sherman (1994) recommend that 25–50 IU vitamin E/kg in concentrate and 50–100 IU vitamin E/kg in concentrate should be given to adult goats and kids, respectively.

17.7.3 Vitamin K Deficiency

Generally healthy animals obtain their required vitamin K from rumen and the lower gut. Deficiency of vitamin K, which is important for blood clotting and vision, is generally not observed in small ruminants.

17.7.4 Deficiency of Water-Soluble Vitamins

Vitamin B complex and vitamin C are water-soluble vitamins. In most cases, goats do not require these vitamins as they are synthesized within the rumen by ruminal microorganisms. However, animals subjected to any clinical condition, a deficient diet, or drug interactions (like prolonged use of antimicrobials) may experience deficiency disorders. Perhaps for this reason, there are very rare investigation reports about deficiency of water-soluble vitamins in goats.

Notable water-soluble vitamin deficiencies cited in literature are listed in Table 17.4.

Table 17.4   Notable water-soluble vitamin deficiencies in the goat.

Water-soluble vitamin	Main function(s)	Deficiency symptom or function reported in the goat	References
Vitamin B$_1$ (thiamine)	Co-enzyme of pyruvate carboxylase, co-factor of transketolase	Polioencephalomalacia, goat polio, cerebrocortical necrosis, torticollis (Figure 17.5)	Dana et al. (2010), Nema et al. (2014), Simões et al. (2020)
Vitamin B3 (niacin)	Plays a central role in energy metabolism and oxidative phosphorylation Precursor of NAD$^+$/NADH and NADP$^+$/NADPH	Impaired regulation of β-hydroxyl butyrate and non-esterified fatty acid (NEFA) metabolism	Nelson et al. (2008), Saribay et al. (2020)
Vitamin B5 (pantothenic acid)	Acts as part of co- enzyme A (CoA) and acyl carrier protein (ACP)	Dermatitis, keratitis, adrenal hemorrhage, cortical fat deposition, depigmentation of hair in animals	Ball (2006), Ragaller et al. (2011), Novelli (1953)
Vitamin B6 (pyridoxine)	Co-enzyme for transaminase and deaminase, important for glucose production, hormone modulation, and neurotransmitter synthesis	Helps in improving sperm health	Daramola et al. (2015)
Vitamin B12 (cyanocobalamin)	Co-factor of methylmalonyl–CoA mutase and methionine synthase and thus regulates Krebs cycle, cell formation and function, and alteration of muscle protein	Although goats are more resistant to co-deficiency than sheep, hepatic lipidosis, white liver disease, muscle qualitative traits disbalance, and anemia may be observed	Johnson et al. (1999), Smith (2021)
Vitamin B7 (biotin)	Co-enzyme in the metabolism of fatty acids, isoleucine, and valine; vital for citric acid cycle, cell growth, metabolism of fat and amino acid	Dermatitis, diarrhea, poor growth rate	Pour (2017), Tahmasbi et al. (2007)
Vitamin C	Regulates oxidation reduction potential, acts as co-enzyme of oxidation of tyrosine and phenylalanine	Body weight loss, more prone to stress	Akinmoladun et al. (2020), Chakrabarti (2006)

(a)

(b)

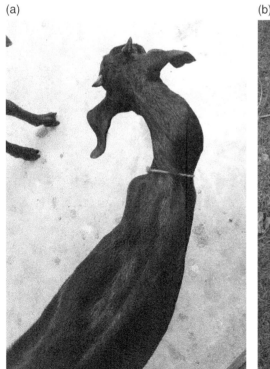
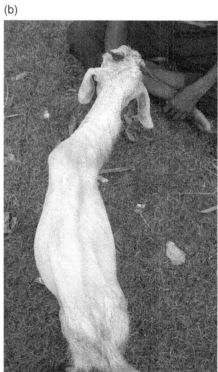

Figure 17.5   (a, b) Torticollis in goat due to thiamine deficiency. *Source:* Courtesy of Dr. Abhijit Barui.

Multiple-Choice Questions

1   Excessive dietary intake of calcium and copper causes deficiency of what?
    A Magnesium
    B Cobalt
    C Zinc
    D Iron

2   What is the most common parenteral form of iron?
    A Iron fumarate
    B Iron glutamate
    C Iron dextran
    D Iron dextrose

3   What deficiency is congenital chondrodystrophy in kids associated with?
    A Manganese deficiency
    B Magnesium deficiency
    C Calcium deficiency
    D Zinc deficiency

4   Hopping gait occurs in kids due to deficiency of what?
    A Vitamin E
    B Selenium
    C Vitamin E and selenium
    D Manganese

5   Spectacle disease most often occurs due to deficiency of what?
    A Zinc
    B Iron
    C Copper
    D Cobalt

6   What is the most common source of iron in case of iron deficiency in a grazing goat?
    A Ferrous sulfate solution
    B Ferric ammonium citrate
    C Molasses
    D Grass grown on fertile soil

7   What are peat scour, falling disease, and pine examples of?
    A Primary copper deficiency
    B Chronic copper deficiency
    C Tertiary copper deficiency
    D Secondary copper deficiency

8   Parakeratosis-like skin lesions are produced in deficiency of what?
    A Zinc
    B Cobalt

C Manganese
D Nickel

9   Granulocytic hyperplasia of the endometrium in goat occurs due to deficiency of what?
    A Vanadium
    B Calcium
    C Cadmium
    D Magnesium

10 What does the presence of a high amount of fructans in pasture lead to?
    A Copper deficiency
    B Chromium deficiency
    C Cobalt deficiency
    D Choline deficiency

11 Why does hepatic lipidosis in goats mainly occur?
    A Deficiency of cobalt and vitamin A
    B Deficiency of copper
    C Deficiency of cobalt and vitamin B12
    D Deficiency of selenium and vitamin E

12 Spermatogenesis in bucks is directly linked to which mineral?
    A Selenium
    B Zinc
    C Cobalt
    D Iron

13 Grass tetany in kids occurs due to deficiency of what?
    A Manganese
    B Magnesium
    C Molybdenum
    D Calcium

14 What should the ratio of calcium and phosphorus in goat rations be?
    A 2:1
    B 2.2:1.1
    C 3:1
    D 1.5:2.1

15 In nutritional muscular dystrophy, which muscles are commonly affected?
    A Smooth muscle
    B Cardiac muscle
    C Skeletal muscle
    D Abdominal muscle

16 What is absorption of copper directly related to?
  A Presence of zinc and iron in the rumen
  B Presence of molybdenum and sulfur in the rumen

C Presence of calcium and zinc in the rumen
D Presence of molybdenum and iron in the rumen

References

Akinmoladun, O.F., Fon, F.N., and Mpendulo, C.T. (2020). Stress indicators, carcass characteristics and meat quality of Xhosa goats subjected to different watering regimen and vitamin C supplementation. *Livestock Science* 238: 104083.

Al-Saad, K.M., Al-Sadi, H.I. and Abdul-Majeed, M.O. (2010). Clinical, hematological, biochemical and pathological studies on zinc deficiency (hypozincemia) in sheep. Veterinary Research (Pakistan) 3(2):14–20

Alves, C.X., Vale, S.H.L., Dantas, M.M.G. et al. (2012). Positive effects of zinc supplementation on growth, GH, IGF1, and IGFBP3 in eutrophic children. *Journal of Pediatric Endocrinology and Metabolism* 25 (9–10): 881–887.

Anke, M. and Risch, M.A. (1989). Importance of molybdenum in animal and man. In: *Proceedings 6th International Trace Element Symposium*, Jena, December 1989, 303–321. Jena: University of Jena.

Anke, M. and Seifert, M. (2004). Titanium. In: *Elements and their Compounds in the Environment* (ed. E. Merian, M. Anke, M. Ihnat, et al.), 1125–1140. Weinheim: Wiley.

Anke, M., Gruen, M., and Kronemann, H. (1980). The capacity of different organs to indicate the nickel level. In: *Proceedings 3rd Spurenelement Symposium*, Jena (7–11 July 1980), 237–244. Jena: University of Jena.

Anke, M., Groppel, B., Schmidt, A. et al. (1986). Cadmium deficiency in ruminants. In: *Proceedings 5th Spurenelement Symposium*, Jena (14–17 July 1986), 937–944. Jena: University of Jena.

Atmani, D., Benboubetra, M., and Harrison, R. (2004). Goats' milk xanthine oxidoreductase is grossly deficient in molybdenum. *Journal of Dairy Research* 71 (1): 7–13.

Ball, G.F.M. (2006). *Vitamins in Foods: Analysis, Bioavailability and Stability*. Boca Raton, FL: CRC Taylor & Francis.

Banerjee, G.C. (1988). *Feeds and Principles of Animal Nutrition*. Oxford: IBH Publishing.

Banton, M.I., Lozano-Alarcon, F., Nicholson, S.S. et al. (1990). Enzootic ataxia in Louisiana goat kids. *Journal of Veterinary Diagnostic Investigation* 2 (1): 70–73.

Barhoum, S. (1989). Der Einfluss des maessigen Phosphordefizites auf den Aschebestand und Mineralstoffstatus verschiedener Koerperteileder Ziege. In: *Proceedings 6th International Trace Element Symposium*, Leipzig, September 1989, 595–602. Jena: University of Jena.

Bedwal, R.S. and Bahuguna, A. (1994). Zinc, copper and selenium in reproduction. *Experientia* 50 (7): 626–640.

Beytut, E., Karatas, F., and Beytut, E. (2002). Lambs with white muscle disease and selenium content of soil and meadow hay in the region of Kars. *Turkey. Veterinary Journal* 163 (2): 214–217.

Chakrabarti, A. (2006). *Textbook of Clinical Veterinary Medicine*, 3e. New Delhi: Kalyani Publishers.

Dana, G.A., Peter, D.C., Peter, R.D. et al. (2010). Polioencephalomalacia: introduction (cerebrocortical necrosis). In: *Merck Veterinarian Manual* (ed. N.J. Whitehouse Station), 1174–1177. Merck.

Daramola, J.O., Adekunle, E.O., Oke, O.E. et al. (2015). Effects of pyridoxine supplementation or in combination with other antioxidants on motility, in vitro capacitation and acrosome reaction of goat buck spermatozoa during cryopreservation. *Small Ruminant Research* 131: 113–117.

Dezfoulian, A.H. and Aliarabi, H. (2017). A comparison between different concentrations and sources of cobalt in goat kid nutrition. *Animal* 11 (4): 600–607.

Digest, E.M. (2007). Hyperhomocysteinemia and cobalamin disorders. *Molecular Genetics and Metabolism* 90 (2): 113–121.

Dittmer, K.E. and Thompson, K.G. (2011). Vitamin D metabolism and rickets in domestic animals: a review. *Veterinary Pathology* 48 (2): 389–407.

Draksler, D., Núñez, M., Apella, M.C. et al. (2002). Copper deficiency in Creole goat kids. *Reproduction Nutrition Development* 42 (3): 243–249.

Frye, T.M., Williams, S.N., and Graham, T.W. (1991). Vitamin deficiencies in cattle. *Veterinary Clinics of North America: Food Animal Practice* 7 (1): 217–275.

Ghany-Hefnawy, A.E. and Tortora-Perez, J.R. (2009). The importance of selenium and the effects of its deficiency in animal health. *Small Ruminant Research* 89: 185–192.

Haenlein, G.F.W. and Anke, M. (2011). Mineral and trace element research in goats: a review. *Small Ruminant Research* 95 (1): 2–19.

Hidiroglou, M. (1979). Trace element deficiencies and fertility in ruminants: a review. *Journal of Dairy Science* 62 (8): 1195–1206.

Hidiroglou, M. and Knipfel, J.E. (1984). Zinc in mammalian sperm: a review. *Journal of dairy science* 67(6):1147–1156.

Holben, D.H. and Smith, A.M. (1999). The diverse role of selenium within selenoproteins: a review. *Journal of the American Dietetic Association* 99 (7): 836–843.

Johnson, E.H., Muirhead, D.E., Annamalai, K. et al. (1999). Hepatic lipidosis associated with cobalt deficiency in Omani goats. *Veterinary Research Communications* 23 (4): 215–221.

Kennedy, D.G., Kennedy, S., Blanchflower, W.J. et al. (1994). Cobalt-vitamin B12 deficiency causes accumulation of odd-numbered, branched-chain fatty acids in the tissues of sheep. *British Journal of Nutrition* 71 (1): 67–76.

Kessler, J. (1991a). Mineral nutrition of goats. *Goat. Nutrition* 46: 104–119.

Kessler, J. (1991b). Vitamin nutrition of goats. In: *Goat Nutrition* (ed. P. Morand-Fehr), 120–123. Pudoc: Wageningen.

Lu, C.D., Kawas, J.R., and Mahgoub, O.G. (2005). Fibre digestion and utilization in goats. *Small Ruminant Research* 60 (1–2): 45–52.

Maloiy, G.M.O. and Taylor, C.R. (1971). Water requirements of African goats and haired-sheep. *Journal of Agricultural Science* 77 (2): 203–208.

Martens, H. and Schweigel, M. (2000). Pathophysiology of grass tetany and other hypomagnesemias: implications for clinical management. *Veterinary Clinics of North America: Food Animal Practice* 16 (2): 339–368.

McDowell, L.R. (2003). *Minerals in Animal and Human Nutrition*. Amsterdam: Elsevier Science.

McDowell, L.R., Valle, G., Rojas, L.X. et al. (1997). Importancia de la suplementación mineral completaen la reproducción de vacas. In: *XXXIII Reuniónnacional de investigaciónpecuaria, XXIII Simposium de ganadería tropical: Interacciónnutrición-reproducciónenganadobovino*, 31–47. Veracruz, México.

Miao, X., Sun, W., Fu, Y. et al. (2013). Zinc homeostasis in the metabolic syndrome and diabetes. *Frontiers of Medicine* 7 (1): 31–52.

Mikhaleva, L.M. (2000). Tumourous and tumor-like lesions in goats with acquired and congenital experimental trace element deficiencies. *Mengen- und Spurenelemente* 20: 915–931.

Morand-Fehr, P. (ed.) (1991). *Goat Nutrition*. Wageningen: Pudoc.

Naik, S.G., Ananda, K.J., and Rani, B.K. (2010). Magnesium deficiency in young calves and its management. *Veterinary World* 3 (4): 192–193.

National Research Council, Division on Earth and Life Studies, Board on Agriculture and Natural Resources et al (2007). *Nutrient Requirements of Small Ruminants: Sheep, Goats, Cervids, and New World Camelids*. Washington, DC: National Academies Press.

Nelson, D.L., Lehninger, A.L., and Cox, M.M. (2008). *Lehninger Principles of Biochemistry*. London: Macmillan.

Nema, A., Nema, V., Kumar, D. et al. (2014). Polioencephalomalacia in goats: a case study. *Veterinary Clinical Science* 2 (3): 48–51.

Novelli, G.D. (1953). Metabolic functions of pantothenic acid. *Physiological Reviews* 33 (4): 525–543.

Pour, H.A. (2017). Vitamin H and their role in ruminant: a review. *Cancer Biology* 7 (4): 53–56.

Radostits, O.M., Gay, C.C., Hinchcliff, K.W. et al. (2007). *Veterinary Medicine: A Textbook of the Diseases of Cattle, Horses, Sheep, Pigs and Goats*, 10e. St. Louis, MO: Elsevier Saunders.

Radwinska, J. and Zarczynska, K. (2014). Effects of mineral deficiency on the health of young ruminants. *Journal of Elementology* 19 (3): 915–928.

Ragaller, V., Lebzien, P., Südekum, K.H. et al. (2011). Pantothenic acid in ruminant nutrition: a review. *Journal of Animal Physiology and Animal Nutrition* 95 (1): 6–16.

Rankins, D.L. Jr. and Pugh, D.G. (2002). Feeding and nutrition. In: *Sheep and Goat Medicine* (ed. D.G. Pugh), 20–22. Philadelphia, PA: W.B. Saunders.

Robson, A.B., Sykes, A.R., McKinnon, A.E. et al. (2004). A model of magnesium metabolism in young sheep: transactions between plasma, cerebrospinal fluid and bone. *British Journal of Nutrition* 91 (1): 73–79.

Rocha, G.F.Q. and Bouda, J. (2001). Fisiopatología de las deficiencias de cobreenrumiantes y sudiagnóstico. *Veterinaria México* 32 (4): 289–296.

Rubio, C., González Weller, D., Martín-Izquierdo, R.E. et al. (2007). El zinc: oligoelementoesencial. *Nutrición Hospitalaria* 22 (1): 101–107.

Santini, F.J., Lu, C.D., Potchoiba, M.J. et al. (1991). Effects of acid detergent fiber intake on early postpartum milk production and chewing activities in dairy goats fed alfalfa hay. *Small Ruminant Research* 6 (1–2): 63–71.

Saribay, M.K., Köse, A.M., Özsoy, B. et al. (2020). The effects of supplemental niacin and methionine on serum glucose, βhydroxybutyric acid, and non-esterified fatty acid levels during late gestation and early postpartum period in Damascus dairy goat. *Turkish Journal of Veterinary & Animal Sciences* 44 (2): 266–272.

Schwarz, T. and Werner, E. (1987). Die WirkunglaengerfristigerBentonitapplikationen auf den StoffwechselausgewaehlterSpurenelementebeiderZwergzi ege. In: *Proceedings 7th Arbeitstagung Mengen- und Spurenelemente*, Leipzig, December 21–22, 99–106. Leipzig: University of Leipzig.

Schwarz, F.J., Kirchgessner, M., and Stangl, G.I. (2000). Cobalt requirement of beef cattle—feed intake and growth at different levels of cobalt supply. *Journal of Animal Physiology and Animal Nutrition* 83 (3): 121–131.

Sharman, E.D., Wagner, J.J., Larson, C.K. et al. (2008). The effects of trace mineral source on performance and health of newly received steers and the impact of cobalt concentration on performance and lipid metabolism during the finishing phase. *Professional Animal Scientist* 24 (5): 430–438.

Simões, P.B.A., Bexiga, R., Lamas, L.P. et al. (2020). Pregnancy toxaemia in small ruminants. In: *Advances in Animal Health, Medicine and Production* (ed. A.F. Duarte and L.L. da Costa), 541–556. Cham: Springer.

Smith, M.C. (1981). Caprine dermatologic problems: a review. *Journal of the American Veterinary Medical Association* 178: 724–729.

Smith, G.W. (2021). Nutritional myopathies in ruminants and pigs. In: *MSD Veterinary Manual*. Rahway, NJ: Merck https://www.msdvetmanual.com/musculoskeletal-system/myopathies-in-ruminants-and-pigs/genetic-myopathies-in-ruminants-and-pigs.

Smith, M.C. and Sherman, D.M. (1994). Nutrition and metabolic diseases. In: *Goat Medicine* (ed. M.C. Smith and D.M. Sherman), 528–560. Hoboken, NJ: Wiley.

Sobiech, P., Rypula, K., Wojewoda-Kotwica, B. et al. (2010). Usefulness of calcium-magnesium products in parturient paresis in HF cows. *Journal of Elementology* 15 (4): 693–704.

Soetan, K.O., Olaiya, C.O., Oyewole, O.E. (2010). The importance of mineral elements for humans, domestic animals and plants: A review. *African journal of food science* 4(5): 200–222.

Spurlock, S.L. and Ward, M.V. (1991). Parenteral nutrition in equine patients: principles and theory. *Compendium on Continuing Education for the Practising Veterinarian* 13: 461–467.

Suttle, N.F. (2010) Mineral Nutrition of Livestock. Wallingford UK: CABI.

Szilagyi, M., Anke, M., Szentmihalyi, S. et al. (1986). Serum enzyme status of goats with selenium deficiency. In: *Proceedings Macro and Trace Element Seminar*, December, 194–201. Leipzig: University of Leipzig-Jena.

Tahmasbi, M., Galbraith, H., and Scaife, J. (2007). The effect of biotin deficiency in the pre-ruminant and immediately post-ruminant Angora and Cashmere kids. *Journal of Animal and Veterinary Advances* 6 (4): 539–548.

Tiwari, S.P., Sahu, T., and Agnihotri, M.K. (2013). *Mineral and Vitamin Nutrition of Livestock*. New Delhi: SSPH.

Underwood, E.J. and Suttle, N.F. (2003). *The Mineral Nutrition of Livestock*. Wallingford: CABI Publishing.

Van Metre, D.C. and Callan, R.J. (2001). Selenium and vitamin E. *Veterinary Clinics of North America: Food Animal Practice* 17 (2): 373–402.

Vázquez-Armijo, J.F., Rojo, R., López, D. et al. (2011). Trace elements in sheep and goats reproduction: a review. *Tropical and Subtropical Agroecosystems* 14 (1): 1–13.

Vermorel, M. (1978). Feed evaluation for ruminants. II. The new energy systems proposed in France. *Livestock Production Science* 5 (4): 347–365.

Yao, X., Zhang, G., Guo, Y. et al. (2017). Vitamin D receptor expression and potential role of vitamin D on cell proliferation and steroidogenesis in goat ovarian granulosa cells. *Theriogenology* 102: 162–173.

Yao, X., Wang, Z., El-Samahy, M.A. et al. (2020). Roles of vitamin D and its receptor in the proliferation and apoptosis of luteinised granulosa cells in the goat. *Reproduction, Fertility and Development* 32 (3): 335–348.

Zhavoronkov, A., Kaktursky, L., Anke, M. et al. (1996). Pathology of experimental hypobromosis and hypolithiosis in goats. In: *Proceedings 16th Arbeitstagung Mengen- und Spurenelemente*, Jena, December 6–7, 670–678. Jena: University of Jena.

Zimmermann, P., Weiss, U., Classen, H.G. et al. (2000). The impact of diets with different magnesium contents on magnesium and calcium in serum and tissues of the rat. *Life Sciences* 67 (8): 949–958.

18

Diagnostic Techniques in Goats

Mohammad I. Yatoo[1], Oveas R. Parray[2], Rather I. Ul Haq[2], and Mohsina Mushtaq[1]

[1] *Division of Veterinary Clinical Complex, Faculty of Veterinary Sciences and Animal Husbandry Shuhama, Sher E Kashmir University of Agricultural Sciences and Technology of Kashmir, Srinagar, Jammu and Kashmir, India*
[2] *Division of Veterinary Medicine, Faculty of Veterinary Sciences and Animal Husbandry Shuhama, Sher E Kashmir University of Agricultural Sciences and Technology of Kashmir, Srinagar, Jammu and Kashmir, India*

18.1 Diagnosis of Infectious Diseases

Definitive diagnosis of any disease is not possible by using a single test alone, therefore one should go for a cluster of tests for accurate diagnosis (Radostits et al. 2009, p. 2). Disease diagnosis should be done via thorough examination of the animal for typical clinical signs, physical examination, case history, response to treatment, culture and isolation of the organism, serological tests, molecular tests, and necropsy of the dead animals.

18.1.1 Case History

The case history should include recording of age, weight, number of animals affected, number of deaths, nutrition, change in feed, reproductive management, vaccination, and treatment history.

18.1.2 Clinical Signs

There are a number of diseases that can be diagnosed by the typical clinical signs, including contagious caprine pleuropneumonia, peste des petits ruminants (PPR), listeriosis, mastitis, anthrax, brucellosis, acidosis, bloat, ovine progressive pneumonia, ecthyma/sore mouth (Figure 18.1), goat pox (Figure 18.2), tetanus, polioencephalomalacia, and scrapie (Table 18.1).

18.1.3 Physical Examination

Physical examination includes recording of vital signs:

- Temperature: normal range goats, 100.5–103.5 °F (38–40 °C), kids 102–104 °F (39–40 °C).

- Heart rate in beats per minute: normal range goats 70–90, kids 90–150.
- Respiration rate in breaths per minute: normal range goats 15–30, kids 20–40.
- Rumen motility: normal range goats 2/min.
- Color of mucous membrane: pink = normal, pale white = anemia, pale = hypovolemic shock.
- FAMACHA score (1–5): normal 1–2.
- Body condition score (1–5).
- Examination of goat for pus, swelling, pain, abscess, or any other lesion (Jackson and Cockcroft 2002, p. 281; Pugh and Baird 2012, p. 18).

18.1.4 Culture and Isolation of Organism

Culture and isolation of the pathogenic organism remains the gold standard test for most infectious diseases (Pugh and Baird 2012, pp. 87–92; Radostits et al. 2009, p. 2). Samples from diseased animals including nasal swabs, skin scrapings, milk, urine, pus, and other discharges should be taken for inoculation in broth at 37 °C, followed by culture on specific agar using the streaking or spread-plate technique, and subsequently observed for their characteristic colonies:

- Medusa head colonies on nutrient agar are indicative of *Bascillus anthracis*.
- Metallic green sheen on eosin methylene blue (EMB) agar is specific for *Escherichia coli*.
- Fried egg colonies on pleuropneumonia-like organisms (PPLO) agar are typical of *Mycoplasma capricolum* subsp. *capripneumoniae* (Figure 18.3).
- *Staphylococcus aureus* produces small colonies surrounded by yellow zones on mannitol salt agar.

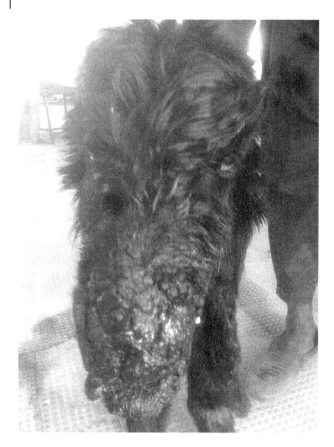

Figure 18.1 Contagious ecthyma in a goat.

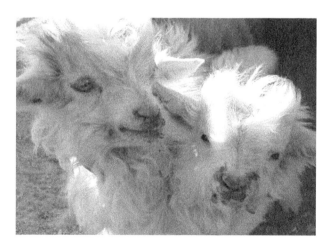

Figure 18.2 Goat pox in Pashmina goats.

18.1.5 Staining

Staining procedures are used to diagnose bacterial, protozoal, and fungal diseases (Clark 1972, p. 10). The commonly used staining procedures are described here.

18.1.5.1 Gram Staining

Gram staining is used to distinguish between Gram-positive and Gram-negative bacteria based on the structure of their cell walls. Gram-positive bacteria lack an outer lipid membrane and have a thick peptidoglycan layer, thus they retain the crystal violet and appear purple under a light microscope, while Gram-negative bacteria have a thin peptidoglycan layer and outer lipid membrane, do not retain crystal violet, and appear reddish in color.

The smear is flooded with crystal violet and left for one minute, then rinsed with water. Gram's iodine is poured and left for one minute and again the slide is rinsed with water. Decolorizer 95% ethyl alcohol or acetone is added to the slide and left for 5–10 seconds until the alcohol runs almost clear and the slide is again rinsed with water. Then the slide is flooded with safranin and left for 45 seconds and again rinsed, dried, and observed under oil immersion.

18.1.5.2 Ziehl–Neelsen Staining

This stain is used for the identification of mycobacteria that are acid fast and are not decolorized after staining red by carbol fuchsin. The procedure is as follows:

- Heat-fix the smear and allow it to cool.
- Put carbol fuchsin over the slide and heat for five minutes.
- Wash the slide with distilled water.
- Cover the slide with 25% sulfuric acid and leave for five minutes.
- Cover the slide with methylene blue counter stain for ten seconds.
- Wash the slide, air dry, and examine under oil immersion.
- Tubercle bacilli appear bright red on a blue background.

18.1.6 Blood Smear Examination

Blood smear examination is valuable for determination of differential leukocyte counts, hemolysis, and detection of various infectious protozoa including *Babesia*, *Theileria*, *Anaplasma*, *Ehrlichia* and so on. Various stains like Giemsa's stain, Wright's stain, and Leishman's stain are used. Thick and thin smears should be prepared from capillaries in the ear or tail tip in live animals.

18.1.6.1 Giemsa Staining

There are two methods for staining with Giemsa stain: fast (10% Giemsa stain) and slow (3% Giemsa stain). The procedure is as follows:

- Methanol fix the air-dried smear.
- Pour the stain over the slide.
- Leave for 10 minutes for fast staining and 45 minutes for slow staining.
- Pour off the remaining stain, rinse with clean water, and allow the slide to dry.
- Observe under oil immersion.

Table 18.1 Common infectious diseases of the goat.

Bacterial	Viral	Hemoprotozoal	Fungal	Endoparasites	Ectoparasites
Anthrax	Peste des petits ruminants (PPR –ovine rinderpest)	Anaplasmosis	Candidiasis	**Flatworms**	**Ticks**
Enterotoxemia	Variola caprina (goat pox)	Ehrlichiosis	Cryptococcosis	Liver flukes (*Dicrocoelium dendriticum, Fasciola hepatica, Fasciola gigantica, Fascioloides magna*)	*Amblyomma*
Blackleg	Caprine arthritis encephalitis (CAE)	Babesiosis	Facial eczema	Stomach flukes (*Schistosoma bovis*)	*Boophilus*
Braxy	Foot and mouth disease	Theileriosis	Fungal placentitis		*Dermacentor*
Infectious necrotic hepatitis	Orf, also known as contagious ecthyma	Cryptosporidiosis	Sporotrichosis	**Tapeworms**	*Hemaphysalis*
Tetanus	Contagious pustular dermatitis	Coccidiosis	Zygomycosis	*Echinococcus granulosus*	*Hyalomma*
Gas gangrene	Infectious labial dermatitis	Giardiosis		*Moniezia*	*Ixodes*
Caseous lymphadenitis	Thistle disease	Neosporosis		*Taenia ovis, Taenia hydatigena*	*Rhipicephalus*
Listeriosis	Sore mouth or scabby mouth	Sarcocystosis			Mites (mange)
Tuberculosis	Akabane virus infection	Toxoplasmosis		**Roundworms**	*Chorioptes bovis*
Pasteurellosis/mannheimiosis	Bluetongue disease	Trypanosomiasis		*Haemonchus contortus*	*Demodex ovis, Demodex caprae*
Brucellosis	Border disease (hairy shaker disease)			*Chabertia ovina*	*Psorobia ovis*
Foot rot	Cache Valley virus infection			*Dictyocaulus filarial*	*Psoroptes ovis*
Contagious caprine pleuropneumonia	Enzootic nasal adenocarcinoma			*Elaeophora schneideri*	*Sarcoptes scabiei* var. *caprae, Sarcoptes scabiei* var. *ovis*
Colibacillosis	Dermatophilosis, also known as cutaneous streptothricosis			*Cooperia*	
Salmonellosis	Nairobi sheep disease			*Muellerius capillaris*	**Lice**
Chlamydiosis, also known as enzootic abortion of ewes (EAE)	Ovine orthonairovirus (NSDV) infection			*Nematodirus*	Chewing lice
Dermatophilosis, also known as cutaneous streptothricosis	Ovine encephalomyelitis (louping ill)			*Neostrongylus linearis*	*Damalinia caprae, Damalinia crassipes, Damalinia limbata, Damalinia ovis*
Rainscald, rain rot, lumpy wool, or strawberry foot rot	Ovine progressive pneumonia (OPP)			*Oesophagostomum*	Sucking lice *Linognathus africanus, Linognathus ovillus, Linognathus pedalis, Linognathus stenopsis*
Enzootic posthitis and vulvitis, also known as sheath rot, pizzle rot, or enzootic balanoposthitis	Ovine pulmonary adenocarcinoma			*Protostrongylus refescens*	
Leptospirosis	Rift Valley fever			*Teladorsagia circumcincta*	**Flies and Mosquitoes**
Listeriosis	Schmallenberg virus infection			*Trichostrongylus*	*Aedes Anopheles Culex*
Mastitis	Ulcerative dermatosis			*Trichuris ovis*	Myiasis
Mycoplasmosis	Variola ovina (sheep pox)				Fly strike
Paratuberculosis (Johne's disease)	Wesselsbron virus infection				*Chrysomya*
Q fever					*Lucilia*
Tularemia ulcerative balanoposthitis and vulvitis, also known as necrotic balanoposthitis/vulvitis, pizzle disease, knobrot, or peestersiekte					*Oestrus ovis* (sheep bot fly)
Vibriosis					Sheep ked (*Melophagus ovinus*)

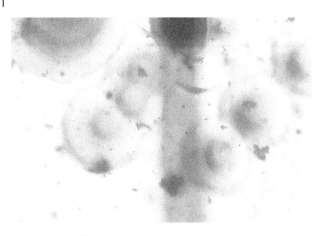

Figure 18.3   *Mycoplasma* colony.

18.1.6.2   Leishman's Stain

Leishman's stain is used to identify leukocytes, malaria, and trypanosomes. The procedure is as follows:

- Add Leishman's stain to the dried smear and allow it to act for one minute.
- Add twice the volume of distilled water to the slide.
- Allow the stain to act for 10–12 minutes.
- Wash the slide with distilled water, air dry, and examine.
- The stain contains methanol, therefore there is no need to fix the slide.

18.1.6.3   Wright's Stain

Wright's stain is used for staining blood cells for differential leukocyte counts. The procedure is as follows:

- Pour 1 ml stain over the smear and leave for one to three minutes.
- Add 2 ml distilled water and keep for six minutes.
- Rinse the smear, dry, and examine.

18.1.7   Serological Tests

Serological tests are used to detect antigen or antibodies against a particular disease. Common serological tests include enzyme-linked immunosorbent assay (ELISA), slide agglutination test/latex agglutination test, complement fixation test (CFT), and *Brucella* agglutination test.

18.1.7.1   Enzyme-Linked Immunosorbent Assay

Capture antibody specific to the target protein is attached to the microplate. Standards and samples are then added. Washing to remove unbound substances is done. Detection antibody is then added that binds with the immobilized target protein. Excess antibody is then washed away and horseradish peroxidase (HRP) conjugate is added. Substrate is added for indirect detection of bound protein. Figure 18.4 demonstrates an ELISA test.

18.1.7.2   Slide Agglutination Test

This test is used for detection of an unknown antigen or antibody in a sample. The antigen/antibody and serum are mixed in a definite proportion and formation of a clump indicates a positive slide agglutination test result (Figure 18.5). A latex agglutination test has a similar principle but is more specific than a slide agglutination test.

18.1.7.3   Complement Fixation Test

CFT is used for the detection of a specific antigen or antibody. It consists of the following two steps:

- A known antigen and test serum are mixed with the inactivated complement. If serum contains the specific antibody, complement will be activated by the antibody antigen complex and will be not available to react at the second stage.
- Unutilized complement is detected by adding the indicator system and observing lysis of red blood cells (RBCs).

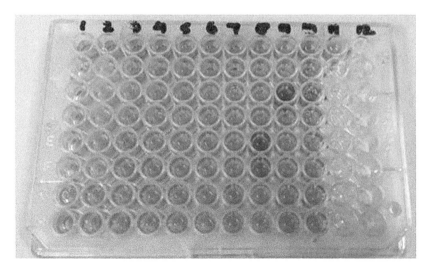

Figure 18.4   Enzyme-linked immunosorbent assay (ELISA).

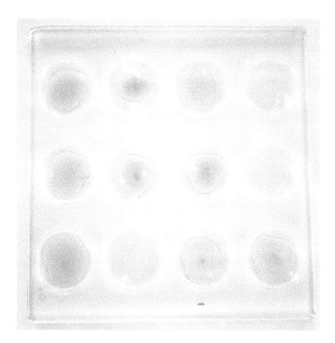

Figure 18.5 Agglutination test.

18.1.7.4 *Brucella* Agglutination Tests

In this test a suspension of *Brucella melitensis* smooth cells stained with Rose Bengal dye (pink color) are used to detect *Brucella* agglutinins. Briefly, the stained bacterial suspension agglutinates when mixed with samples containing specific immunoglobulin (Ig)G or IgM antibodies present in the patient sample.

18.1.8 Paratuberculosis Testing

Johne's testing is done by fecal smears, fecal and tissue culture, intradermal/skin testing, DNA probes using feces or tissues, serology, necropsy, and histology.

A skin test is carried out by intradermal inoculation of 0.1 ml of antigen (avian PPD tuberculin or johnin) into a clipped or shaven site, usually on the side of the middle third of the neck. The skin thickness is measured with calipers before and 72 hours after inoculation. Increases in skin thickness of over 2 mm should be regarded as indicating the presence of delayed-type hypersensitivity (DTH).

18.1.9 Molecular Tests

Molecular diagnostic tests are highly specific and aid in confirmation of disease. Commonly these include polymerase chain reaction (PCR), restriction fragment length polymorphism (RFLP), basic local alignment search tool (BLAST), polyacrylamide gel electrophoresis (PAGE), and gene sequencing.

PCR is used for amplification of sequences of DNA using primers that are complementary to the template. PCR cycle steps include denaturation of template DNA for separation of two strands by heating to 95 °C, primer annealing at a temperature of around 55 °C, elongation, and extension. This step requires a temperature of 72 °C for optimum polymerization using deoxynucleoside triphosphates (dNTPs), magnesium, and taq polymerase.

RFLP is used to identify unique patterns of DNA fragments (variable number of tandem repeats) in order to differentiate between organisms. DNA is extracted from the cells and subjected to digestion using restriction enzymes to cut it. PAGE or electrophoresis of DNA fragments is done and bands are seen using a GelDoc apparatus. Gene sequencing is done to determine the order of bases in DNA for identifying unique DNA fingerprints or patterns.

BLAST is a tool used to detect regions of similarity between biological sequences.

18.1.10 Necropsy

Necropsy can be an important tool for diagnosing a significant number of diseases. Many diseases produce characteristic pathognomonic lesions that can help in diagnosis. Specific findings may confirm the disease and cause of death of the animal. Common findings associated with certain diseases are mentioned here.

- **Johne's disease**:
  - Thickening of small intestines (ileum).
  - Enlarged ileocecal lymph nodes.
  - Nodules in liver.
- **Coccidiosis**:
  - Thickening of intestines (colon).
  - Presence of irregular raised nodules in intestinal mucosa.
- **Hemorhagic enteritis**:
  - Intestinal contents with blood.
  - Dark red mucosa.
- **Contagious ecthyma**: Vesicles and ulcers on muzzle and in oral cavity, teats and lesions in rumen.
- **Caseous lymphadenitis**: Enlarged cervical lymph nodes with white pasty material.
- **Copper toxicity (for differential diagnosis)**:
  - Icterus.
  - Thin blood.
  - Orange-yellow liver.
  - Gun-metal gray kidneys.
- **Pregnancy toxemia (for differential diagnosis)**:
  - Fatty liver that floats in formalin.
  - Twins or triplets.
  - Excess body fat.

18.1.11 California Mastitis Test

The California mastitis test (CMT) is a widely used and rapid animal-side test that detects both change in somatic cell count and pH. It involves a reagent that is sodium lauryl sulphate and bromocresol purple dissolved in distilled water.

An equal amount of milk and CMT reagent are added to CMT paddle wells. The paddle is rotated gently clockwise and anticlockwise. The stringing or gel formation indicates a positive test for mastitis and the result is graded as 0 (no mastitis), + (slight), ++ (moderate mastitis), and +++ (severe or acute mastitis). Figure 18.6 demonstrates CMT of a milk sample.

18.1.12 Somatic Cell Counting

Somatic cell counting (SCC) is most accurate in goats when performed through a dye procedure, as automated SCC methods performed for cattle are not valid in goats. The procedure is as follows:

- Take a clean slide marked with a $1\,cm^2$ area.
- Take 10 μl of milk and spread evenly on the slide.
- Air dry and fix the slide.
- Pour Newmann Lampert stain on it and keep there for two minutes.
- Drain the stain, air dry, and observe under oil immersion.

18.1.13 Culture and Isolation

Culture and isolation enable identification of an organism by observing characteristic colony features, therefore enabling prescription of specific antibiotic against the pathogen. It is usually done by initial culturing in nutrient broth followed by isolation in specific media. Briefly,

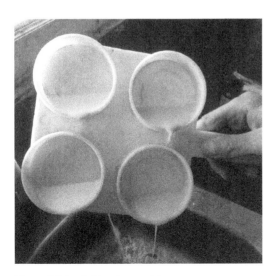

Figure 18.6 California mastitis test.

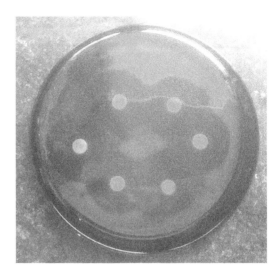

Figure 18.7 Antibiotic sensitivity test.

the milk sample collected aseptically in a sterile vial or tube is cultured in nutrient broth and incubated for overnight culture. The growth is checked and biochemical tests are carried out. Simultaneously subculturing is done in specific media like MacConkey agar (for Gram-negative bacteria), EMB agar (*Escherichia coli*), salt-mannitol agar, tryptic soy broth (TSB) and brain heart infusion (BHI) (*Staphylococcus aureus*), PPLO media, and so on. Besides elucidating the sensitivity of isolated microbes, an antibiotic sensitivity test can also help in deciding on mastitis therapy (Figure 18.7).

Some convenient mastitis-detecting and field-applicable diagnostics like the Draminski mastitis detector can also help in the diagnosis of mastitis. This is based on the electrical resistance of milk and indirectly gives an indication of subclinical mastitis. In subclinical mastitis there is a change in electrolytes, thus that is explored for diagnosis. Draminski mastitis detector cups are marked as per teats of the udder and filled to more than half, the switch is pressed, and readings are taken. Readings less than 250 indicate subclinical mastitis.

18.2 Diagnosis of Parasitic Diseases

Parasitic diseases are highly prevalent in small ruminants and are mostly associated with gastrointestinal disorders, weakness, itching, alopecia, anemia, and weight loss in affected animals, thus resulting in huge economic losses. Early and proper diagnosis may help to select the specific drug therapy and save the life of the animal, plus it may reduce the risk of drug resistance (Craig 2018, p. 185). Common diagnostic tests include fecal examination (consistency, egg, parasite), blood smear examination, culture, and necropsy findings.

There are main two types of parasites in goats: internal and external. Internal parasites include stomach worms (*Haemonchus contortus*, commonly called the barber pole worm), liver flukes (*Dicrocoelium*, *Fasciola hepatica*), intestinal coccidia (*Eimeria*), and lung worms (*Dictyocaulus* spp. or *Muellerius capillaris*) (Keeton and Navarre 2018, p. 201; Zajac 2006, p. 529). External parasites include ticks, mites, and lice. The diagnosis of parasitic infestation can be based on clinical signs or fecal or skin sample examination.

18.2.1 Clinical Signs and Symptoms

Common signs and symptoms of parasitism include:

- Diarrhea.
- Weight loss.
- Rough hair coat.
- Anemia and weakness.
- Fever.
- Bottle jaw.
- Inappetence/anorexia.
- Itching, scab or crust formation (ectoparasites).

18.2.2 Fecal Examination

This involves direct examination, sedimentation, and flotation (Urquhart et al. 1996, p. 276).

18.2.2.1 Direct Examination

Fecal samples are collected directly or in plastic bags and then smeared on a glass slide. They are examined under a microscope and on the bases of egg shape and size the parasites are identified. *H. contortus* eggs are oval and medium sized; *Ascaris* eggs are oval to round in shape; eggs of *Fasciola* are ellipsoidal in shape and are operculated; *Trichuris* eggs are barrel shaped and have a pair of polar

plugs on both sides. Figure 18.8 demonstrates the shape of few parasitic eggs in a fecal sample.

18.2.2.2 Sedimentation Technique

This technique is used for the identification of fluke eggs. Take a few grams of fecal matter and mix it with the desired amount of tap water, then filter the mixture by using porous material or filter paper in a 50 ml centrifuge tube. Centrifuge the mixture and allow the mixture to stand for 10 minutes. Discard the supernatant and resuspend the sediment in water again. Centrifuge again until you get clear sample. Then make a slide, put a cover slip on it, and examine under a microscope.

18.2.2.3 Flotation Technique

The flotation technique is the most important and common for the detection of parasites. It is based on the specific gravity between the solution and a parasitic egg. All parasites cannot be identified by this method. A desired amount of fecal sample is taken, titrated, and saturate solution added to it. The sample is strained and poured into a tube. After that a cover slip is placed over the top of tube in such a way that the cover slip touches the solution. Then the cover slip is examined under a microscope.

18.2.2.4 Eggs per Gram

The fecal egg count also helps in determining the severity of infection, although it does not give the total infection of the flock. It is important that samples are evaluated by a quantitative method like modified McMaster method, one of the best methods for quantitative analysis of fecal matter. It measures the number of eggs per gram (epg) of feces. If epg is <500 the infection is low. If epg lies between 500 and 1000 it indicates moderate infection. If epg is >1000 it indicates severe infection.

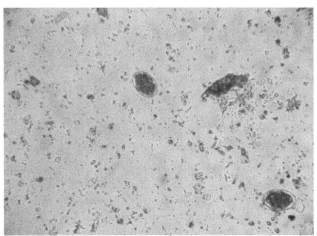
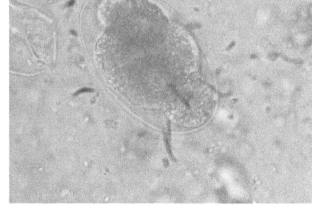

Figure 18.8 Parasitic eggs in a fecal sample.

The consistency of fecal matter (pellet, liquid diarrhea, hard, semi-solid) also reveals the parasitic load, but in some parasitic infections diarrhea is absent (acute haemonchosis).

18.2.3 Fluorescent Peanut Agglutination Technique

Different parasites are responsible for gastrointestinal tract infection. In order to identify which type of parasite is responsible, the peanut agglutination technique is used. For instance, it is used to stain and identify *Haemonchus* eggs. Briefly, parasitic eggs are purified by routine sugar centrifugation methods and lectin conjugated to fluorescein isothiocyanate. Binding to *Haemonchus* eggs can be visualized under ultraviolet illumination.

18.2.4 Culturing

This method involves culturing of eggs of different species and then polymerase chain reaction (PCR) is used to detect the parasitic DNA.

18.2.5 Baermann Technique

The Baermann technique is used for the identification of lung larval worms. In this method a desired amount of feces are taken and wrapped in a porous cloth and suspended in warm water overnight. The temperature of the water activates larva migration out of the feces through the porous cloth. These larvae are concentrated and collected in a collecting vessel, then aspirated and placed on a microscope slide for identification.

18.2.6 Skin Scraping

Skin scraping is used for the identification of ectoparasites. Deep skin scrapings are taken with the help of a scalpel. The scalpel blade is dipped into mineral oil or glycerin before collection.

The cellophane tape technique is more accurate than skin scraping for identification of parasites. Skin biopsy is also sometimes used for diagnosis of ectoparasites.

18.2.7 Trichogram Method

In addition to skin scraping, another method of finding parasites is the trichogram or hair plucking method. This is used for the identification of deep parasites. In this method a small drop of mineral oil is placed on a slide and then a tuft of hair is placed on the slide, a cover slip is put on, and it is examined under a microscope.

18.2.8 Postmortem Examination

Postmortem examination is a very important tool for the diagnosis of parasitic disease when an animal dies due to a parasitic load. For instance, *Haemonchus* are large, *Trichostrongylus* are small, and *Ascaris* form bunches or coils when in large numbers.

18.3 Diagnosis of Metabolic and Production Diseases

Animals often undergo a negative energy balance during the transition period (three weeks before to three weeks after parturition), which results in numerous metabolic/production diseases. Common diseases encountered in goats due to metabolic imbalances include pregnancy toxemia, fatty liver disease, periparturient hypocalcemia, hypomagnesemia, lactic acidosis, alkalosis, low milk-fat syndrome, and urolithiasis. This section highlights the diagnostic aspects of these diseases in detail.

Metabolic diseases, now known as production diseases, result from an imbalance between the rates of input of dietary nutrients and the output of production. Like any other living animal, goats must be supplied with a feed containing essential nutrients for maintenance and activity of the body, as well as to fulfill growth, pregnancy, and lactation needs. These essential nutrients include water, energy (carbohydrate), amino acids (protein), minerals, and vitamins. To support bodily functions, all essential nutrients are required within optimum limits on a daily basis.

Some metabolic diseases commonly encountered in goats include the following (Saun 2022, pp. 1–12):

- Pregnancy toxemia/ketosis/acetonemia/twin kid disease/pregnancy disease/pregnancy ketosis.
- Fatty liver disease/lactational ketosis.
- Periparturient hypocalcemia (milk fever).
- Hypomagnesemia (grass tetany/lactation tetany/milk tetany).
- Lactic acidosis (grain overload).
- Alkalosis.
- Low milk-fat syndrome.
- Urolithiasis/urinary calculi/water belly.
- Other mineral deficiencies (macro and micro).
- Vitamin deficiencies.

The general diagnostic approach for all diseases includes history taking, clinical signs, physical examination, and response to treatment (Smith and Sherman 2011, pp. 9–13). Specific diagnostic tests are outlined in the following.

18.3.1 Pregnancy Toxemia

18.3.1.1 Blood Glucose Level

Blood glucose level below 25 mg/dl is a good diagnostic indicator. The procedure for estimation of blood glucose using the enzymatic (glucose oxidase and peroxidase or GOD-POD) kit method is as follows:

- Mark three test tubes as blank, standard and sample.
- Add 1000 µl of working reagent to all three test tubes, followed by the addition of 10 µl standard and 10 µl sample in the standard and sample test tubes respectively.
- Mix and incubate at 20–30 °C for 20 minutes or 37 °C for 10 minutes.
- Read the absorbance at 546 nm wavelength against the reagent blank.

Calculation:

$$G = 100 \times \frac{\text{Absorbance of sample}}{\text{Absorbance of standard}} (\text{mg} / \text{dl})$$

18.3.1.2 Blood Ketone Level

Plasma or serum β-hydroxybutyrate (BHBA) level in SI units is used for analysis of ketonemia, as BHBA is the predominant circulating ketone body. Serum BHBA concentrations in excess of 3000 µmol/l indicate ketosis.

18.3.1.3 Urine and Milk Ketone Levels

BHBA test strips and nitroprusside powders can be used to detect the presence of BHBA in milk and urine.

Rothera's test or the Ross test for detection of ketone bodies in urine/milk is conducted as follows:

- Saturate 1 ml urine/milk with ammonium sulfate.
- Add 1–2 mg sodium nitroprusside and mix well.
- Stratify 1 ml strong ammonia solution.
- Read the reaction after five minutes.

A positive test is indicated by the presence of permanganate, a purple color.

Ketosis dipsticks can also be used to identify ketone bodies in the urine or plasma.

18.3.1.4 Plasma Cortisol Level

Concentrations above 10 ng/ml indicate pregnancy toxemia.

18.3.1.5 Necropsy Findings

- Severe fatty degeneration of liver.
- Concentrations of BHBA in the aqueous humor or the cerebrospinal fluid (CSF) >2500 or 500 µmol/l,

respectively, are suggestive of pregnancy toxemia in sheep and goats.

18.3.2 Hypocalcemia

18.3.2.1 Blood Biochemical Analysis

Serum calcium concentrations >4–5 mg/dl in sheep and goats are fairly diagnostic of hypocalcemia. The procedure for blood calcium estimation using the Arsenazo III kit method is as follows:

- Three test tubes are marked blank, standard, and sample.
- 1000 µl of Arsenazo reagent is added to all three test tubes, followed by 20 µl of standard and 20 µl of sample in the standard and sample test tubes, respectively.
- Mix and incubate for two minutes at 20–30 °C.
- Read the absorbance against the reagent blank at 650 nm wavelength.

Calculation:

$$C = 8 \times \frac{\text{Absorbance of sample}}{\text{Absorbance of standard}} (\text{mg} / \text{dl})$$

18.3.2.2 Sulkowitch Test

This is for detecting calcium in urine:

- In test tube A (control), take 5 ml urine and add 5 ml distilled water to it.
- In test tube B (test), mix 5 ml urine and 5 ml Sulkowitch reagent.
- Read the test for turbidity as follows:
  - No precipitate: calcium <5 mg%.
  - Mild precipitate: 5–10 mg%.
  - Cloudy: 10–15 mg%.
  - Milky white: 15–20 mg%.
  - Heavy chalky: 20 mg% and above.

18.3.3 Hypomagnesemia

18.3.3.1 Blood Biochemical Analysis

Serum magnesium levels <1.5 mg/dl are indicative of this disease and levels >1 mg/dl are considered diagnostic.

18.3.3.2 Postmortem Tests

Magnesium concentrations in CSF (for 12 hours after death), urine (for 24 hours after death), or anterior eye chamber fluid (for 48 hours after death) are also useful postmortem tests.

18.3.4 Urolithiasis

Necropsy findings include severe hemorrhage and inflammation of the bladder wall, urine in the abdomen with bladder or urethral rupture, and calculi or struvite crystal sediment in the bladder and urethra.

18.3.5 Fatty Liver Disease

18.3.5.1 Serum Biochemistry
Elevated levels of liver-specific enzymes consisting of γ-glutamyl transferase (GGT), aspartate aminotransferase (AST), and sorbitol dehydrogenase (SDH) along with increased serum bilirubin concentrations are highly suggestive of liver damage.

18.3.5.2 Ultrasonography of Liver
Diffuse nature and echogenicity are roughly proportional to the volume of fat vacuoles and the amount of triglyceride in the liver.

18.3.5.3 Necropsy Findings
Grossly enlarged liver, pale yellow, friable, and greasy along with infiltration of fat in the liver cells. Histopathological changes include presence of fatty cysts (lipogranulomas), enlarged hepatocytes, compressed hepatic sinusoids, decreased volume of rough endoplasmic reticulum, and evidence of mitochondrial damage.

18.3.6 Lactic Acidosis

18.3.6.1 Rumen pH Estimation
In lactic acidosis the pH of rumen fluid of the affected animal falls <5.

The procedure for rumen pH estimation is as follows:

- Rumen fluid is collected by left flank puncture using a 16 G or 18 G needle.
- A drop of the rumen fluid is put on the pH meter strip and allowed to dry for a minute.
- The color is matched with the pH strip and the rumen pH recorded.

18.3.6.2 Microscopic Examination of Protozoa
The procedure is as follows:

- Place a drop of rumen fluid on a clean glass slide.
- Put on a cover slip and examine under low-power microscope.
- Count the number of live protozoa and assess their motility.
  - No. of protozoa >30 indicates healthy rumen, 10–30 indicates mild ruminal dysfunction, 1–10 indicates moderate ruminal dysfunction, and 0 indicates severe ruminal dysfunction.
  - Protozoal motility: swirls/vigorous indicates healthy rumen, moderate indicates straw feeding, slow/ wagging/sluggish indicates ruminal disorder, and no motility indicates severe ruminal disorder.

18.3.7 Low Milk-Fat Syndrome

The fat % in milk from the affected doe is determined using a Lactoscan. Milk fat is often reduced to <50% of normal.

18.3.8 Alkalosis

Alkalosis can be diagnosed by determining rumen pH as discussed earlier. A pH >7 can be diagnostic of alkalosis when correlated with history and clinical signs.

18.3.9 Mineral Deficiency

Estimation of serum mineral concentration by atomic absorption spectrophotometer, spectroscopy, or spectrophotometer and correlating these to history and clinical manifestations can help in diagnosing mineral deficiency diseases. The samples of choice for diagnosis are blood (serum, plasma), hair, and tissue (bone, liver).

18.3.10 Urolithiasis

Urolithiasis is mostly diagnosed on clinical examination or ultrasonography.

18.4 Diagnostic Tests Relevant to Cerebrospinal Fluid Alterations and Organ Functions

For diagnosis of alterations in CSF in goats in infectious or non-infectious diseases, the following tests can be done.

18.4.1 Cytological Examination

18.4.1.1 Total Leukocyte Count
The diluting fluid consists of:

- Glacial acetic acid 10 ml.
- Distilled water 90 ml.
- Crystal violet 0.1 g.

  Filter the diluting fluid before use.
  The procedure is as follows:

- Fill the total leukocyte count (TLC) pipette up to mark 1 with diluting fluid.
- Suck CSF up to mark 11.
- Discard the first two drops and charge the Neubauer chamber.

- Count the cells in the ruled areas on both the sides of chamber.
- Multiply the counted cells by 0.6 to get the total number of cells/cmm.

  The interpretation is:

- Normal count: ≤15 cells/cmm.
- High count (pleocytosis): meningitis, encephalitis, myelitis.
- Extremely high count: pyogenic meningitis.

18.4.1.2   Differential Leukocyte Count

The technique for the differential leukocyte count (DLC) is as follows:

- Centrifuge the fluid and discard the supernatant.
- Prepare the smear from sediment.
- Stain it with Giemsa/Leishman's stain.
- Examine under a microscope and count 100 cells.

  The interpretation is:

- Presence of neutrophils: brain abscess, suppurative encephalitis, meningitis.
- Increase in number of lymphocytes: viral, fungal, or chronic infections.

18.4.2   Chemical Examination of Proteins

18.4.2.1   Pandy's Method

The reagent is carbolic acid 10 g + distilled water 100 ml.
  The technique is as follows:

- Take 1 ml reagent in a test tube.
- Add a few drops of CSF and mix properly.

  The interpretation is:

- Slight turbidity: normal.
  1) Marked turbidity: brain abscess.

18.4.2.2   None-Apelt Test

The procedure is as follows:

- Take 1 ml saturated ammonium sulfate in a test tube.
- Overlay 1 ml CSF.
- Allow it to stand for few minutes.
- A grayish-white ring at the junction indicates the presence of globulin.

18.5   Liver, Kidney, and Pancreatic Function Tests

These tests give indications about the normal and abnormal functions of organs like the liver, kidney, and pancreas. They are based on estimation of biochemicals, enzymes, hormones, or metabolites related to these organs. They can help in diagnosis of disease and hence act as diagnostic biomarkers.

For liver function, bilirubin, AST (serum glutamic oxaloacetic transaminase, SGOT), alanine aminotransferase (ALT or serum glutamate pyruvate transaminase, SGPT), GGT, and alkaline phosphatase (ALP) are some of the diagnostic biomarkers, whereas blood urea nitrogen (BUN), creatinine, and urine characteristics can act as renal diagnostic markers. Exocrine pancreatic function is detected by trypsin, amylase, or lipase activity, whereas endocrine action is evaluated by insulin, glucagon, and somatostatin estimation. Inulin, sodium sulfanilate, and phenolphthalein (PSP) are used for renal function tests, whereas bromsulphthalein (BSP) is used for hepatic function tests (Underwood 2015, p. 628).

18.5.1   Enzymes for Detection of Tissue or Organ Function

Enzymes play an important role in the functioning of an organ or tissue (Underwood 2015, p. 628). Estimating their concentration can help detect normal or abnormal function. They serve as diagnostic biomarkers for vital organs or diseases. AST (formerly SGOT, not specific), ALT (formerly SGPT, more relevant), GGT, ALP, sorbitol dehydrogenase (SDH), and glutamate dehydrogenase (GDH) are diagnostic enzymes for the liver. Muscle injury also results in a rise in enzymes. Creatine kinase, ALP, and AST are indicative of muscle-related problems. For diagnosis of bone-related afflictions, ALP has diagnostic significance. Arginase is related to udder (mastitis) and liver disease. ALP also has relevance for renal function. Functions of the pancreas can be diagnosed by levels of amylase, lipase, and trypsin. Serum lactic acid and lactate dehydrogenase (LDH) can be diagnostic for liver, skeletal muscle, heart muscle, and erythrocyte afflictions.

For diagnosing abnormalities of urinary system functions, urinalysis (examination of urine) forms an important part of clinical diagnosis. It involves macroscopic and microscopic examination. Macroscopic examination involves physical and chemical examination. Physical examination is based on color, transparency, odor, foam, and specific gravity. Chemical examination involves pH, protein, glucose, ketone bodies, hematuria, hemoglobinuria, bile pigments, or calcium.

For diagnosing rumen functions, other relevant tests are cellulose digestion time (CDT) and sedimentation activity time (SAT).

In CDT a thread of cotton with known diameter is suspended with a button or glass or metal bead in about 50 ml strained centrifuged rumen fluid and kept at 37 °C.

A 16% glucose solution at 0.3 ml per 10 ml rumen fluid may be added. It should be observed at one-hour intervals. The normal time for digestion of the thread is 48–54 hours. This may be prolonged in ruminal disorders or inactive rumen fluid.

In SAT about 50 ml rumen fluid is collected and strained through double-fold muslin cloth. The strained fluid is kept in a glass cylinder or small beaker at room temperature or at 37 °C in an incubator. It should be observed from time to time. The time required for flotation of particulate material is to be noted. The normal time for flotation ranges between four and eight minutes. Setting of the particulate materials rapidly and prolongation of time required for flotation indicate abnormality of rumen function (indigestion).

For protozoal activity, a drop of fresh ruminal fluid is taken on a clear glass slide, a cover slip is placed over it, and it is examined under a low-power microscope (100× magnification). The motility is graded arbitrarily as +, ++, +++, depending on motility. Moderate (++) to vigorous (+++) indicates normal protozoal activity. The ratio of live to dead protozoa should be noted for clinical purposes.

Multiple-Choice Questions

1 What are Medusa-head colonies characteristic of?
   A *Bascillus antracis*
   B *E. coli*
   C *Brucella*
   D None of the above

2 What are fried-egg colonies characteristic of?
   A *Mycobacterium*
   B *Rickettsia*
   C *Mycoplasma*
   D None of the above

3 Lipopolysaccharide is present in the cell wall of what type of bacteria?
   A Gram +ve
   B Gram –ve
   C Both
   D None

4 On Gram staining how do Gram +ve bacteria appear?
   A Purple
   B Red
   C Blue
   D Gray

5 What is Ziehl-Neelson staining used for?
   A Anthrax
   B *Mycoplasma*
   C *Mycobacterium*
   D None of the above

6 Which of the following stains does not require fixing?
   A Gram stain
   B Giemsa stain
   C Leishman's stain
   D None of the above

7 What condition are gunmetal gray kidneys seen in?
   A Arsenic poisoning
   B Lead poisoning
   C Copper toxicity
   D None of the above

8 What concentration of dextrose is recommended for pregnancy toxemia treatment?
   A 50%
   B 30%
   C 20%
   D None of the above

9 What plasma cortisol level indicates pregnancy toxemia?
   A 5 ng/ml
   B 10 ng/ml
   C 20 ng/ml
   D All of the above

10 What does the Sulkowitch test detect in urine?
   A Magnesium
   B Protein
   C Calcium
   D Glucose

11 What is the serum magnesium level below which hypomagnesemia is indicated?
   A 4 mg/dl
   B 3 mg/dl
   C 2.5 mg/dl
   D 1.5 mg/dl

12 What is the normal pH of rumen?
   A 4
   B 5
   C 6
   D 7

13 Feeding what with the diet can stabilize propionate : acetate levels?
   A Monensin
   B Tylosin
   C Amprolium
   D None of the above

14 Calcium below what level can result in hypocalcemia?
   A 8 mg/dl
   B 10 mg/dl
   C 12 mg/dl
   D None of the above

15 What can be used to treat postparturient hemoglobinuria?
   A Sodium acid phosphate
   B Dicalcium phosphate

   C Both of the above
   D None of the above

16 What are two forms of pregnancy toxemia?
   A Nervous form and gastric form
   B Wasting form and taxemic form
   C Nervous form and wasting form
   D None of the above

17 What is Rothera's test used for?
   A Pregnancy toxemia
   B Milk fever
   C Acidosis
   D Alkalosis

References

Clark, G. (ed.) (1972). *Staining Procedures*. Baltimore, MD: Williams and Wilkins.

Craig, T.M. (2018). Gastrointestinal nematodes, diagnoses and control. *Veterinary Clinics of North America: Food Animal Practice* 34 (1): 185–199.

Jackson, P.C.G. and Cockcroft, P.D. (2002). *Clinical Examination of Farm Animals*. Oxford: Wiley.

Keeton, S.T.N. and Navarre, C.B. (2018). Coccidiosis in large and small ruminants. *Veterinary Clinics of North America: Food Animal Practice* 34 (1): 201–208.

Pugh, D.G. and Baird, A.N. (2012). *Sheep and Goat Medicine*. St. Louis, MO: Elsevier.

Radostits, O.M., Gay, C.C., Hinchcliff, K.W., and Constable, P.D. (2009). *Veterinary Medicine: A Textbook of the Diseases of Cattle, Sheep, Goat, Pigs and Horses*. St. Louis, MO: Elsevier Saunders.

Saun, R.V. (2022). Common nutritional and metabolic diseases of goats. State College, PA: Pennsylvania State University. http://goatdocs.ansci.cornell.edu/Resources/GoatArticles/GoatFeeding/GoatNutritionalDiseases1.pdf.

Smith, M.C. and Sherman, D.M. (2011). *Goat Medicine*. Hoboken, NJ: Wiley.

Underwood, W.J. (2015). Biology and diseases of ruminants (sheep, goats, and cattle). *Laboratory Animal Medicine* 2015: 623–694.

Urquhart, G.M., Armour, J., Duncan, J.L. et al. (1996). *Veterinary Parasitology*. Oxford: Blackwell Science.

Zajac, A.M. (2006). Gastrointestinal nematodes of small ruminants life cycle anti helminthics, and diagnoses. *Veterinary Clinics of North America: Food Animal Practice* 22: 529–541.

19

Management of Pain from Surgery and Lameness in Goats

Joe S. Smith and Pierre-Yves Mulon

Department of Large Animal Clinical Sciences, University of Tennessee, Knoxville, TN, USA

19.1 Pathophysiology of Pain

Pain is conducted through the body via a complex pathway of neurotransmission. Nociception is the neural processes of deciphering and processing noxious stimuli, and as such comprises the initial stages of pain management, ending with a signal arriving at the central nervous system. Various sensory receptors (nociceptors) function with the peripheral nervous system in these initial stages (Coetzee 2013). The pain pathway begins with transduction of painful signals into electrical impulses at the initial site of injury; from this step the electrical signal is transmitted through nerves to the spinothalamic tracts (Muir and Woolf 2001). Modulation of the painful stimuli then occurs in the dorsal horn of the spinal cord (Muir and Woolf 2001). This impulse is projected into the brain, where perception of the pain occurs (Gottschalk and Smith 2001). Figure 19.1 displays this pain pathway. After injury, changes may occur in the central nervous system where hypersensitivity to pain occurs, known as nociceptive windup or "wind-up" (Coetzee 2013; Gottschalk and Smith 2001; Kissin 2000). These wind-up effects can result in increased sensitivity to pain, mainly allodynia (where a previously non-painful trigger now causes pain) and hyperalgesia (where a previously painful stimulus now results in more pain than it initially would have) (Ochroch et al. 2003).

One way in which this wind-up can be mitigated is in the management of surgical pain. There are typically two phases to surgical pain: pain from the incision, and then pain from prolonged inflammation that arises from the ensuing tissue damage (Ochroch et al. 2003). Effective preoperative pain management therefore can lead to decreased wind-up and improve animal welfare in goats undergoing surgery. There are multiple drug combinations (multimodal analgesia) that can be utilized in this respect. Figure 19.1 lists various analgesic drugs effective in various parts of the pathway.

19.2 Arthritis

One concern of older goats, or goats with an orthopedic condition, is arthritis or osteoarthritis (OA). Across all species, including humans and goats, hundreds of billions of dollars are spent annually in the management, treatment, and prevention of arthritis; despite this significant investment, the pathogenesis of the disease is not completely understood (McCoy 2015). Arthritis can manifest as a degenerative joint disease from multiple conditions, such as natural wear and tear over time, or be related to an orthopedic condition, or have an inflammatory or infectious nature. The differentiation between orthopedic conditions and inflammatory conditions is essential for the management of arthritis in caprine patients. OA is traditionally defined as "an inherently noninflammatory disorder of movable joints characterized by deterioration of articular cartilage and by the formation of new bone at the joint surfaces and margins" (Renberg 2005). Joint pain is unique as hyaline cartilage has no innervation: the pain is solely transmitted by the peripheral tissues containing a rich proportion of free nerve endings, which are either thermal, mechanical, or chemical afferent receptors. Known pain-inducing intraarticular mediators are substance P and bradykinin, alongside with pro-inflammatory mediators such as interleukin 1 and prostaglandin E2.

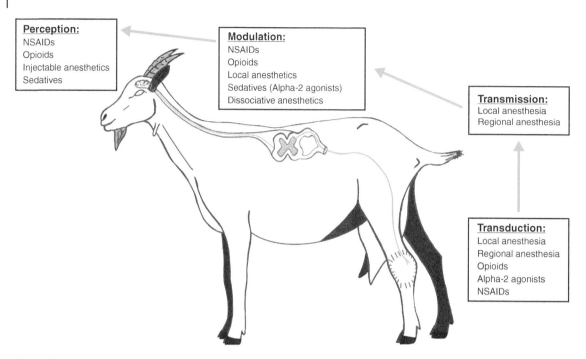

Figure 19.1 An example of the pathway of nociception in the goat, and a listing of different analgesic agents based on activity of anatomical location. Initially the painful stimulus leads to transduction at the site of injury or trauma. Once transduction has occurred, it is followed by transmission to the spinal cord, where modulation may occur. At this point the impulse is transmitted to the brain where perception of the stimuli occurs. NSAIDs, non-steroidal anti-inflammatory drugs. *Source:* Adapted from Coetzee (2013).

Arthritis of inflammatory origin is different to OA, as it is characterized by an influx of inflammatory cells (Renberg 2005). Inflammation within the joint leads to an increased volume of synovial fluid, secondary to a fluid egress from an increase in vascular permeability of the synovial membrane. The resultant joint distension stretches the synovial membrane and peripheral tissue, stimulating the mechanoreceptors and lowering the threshold of pain during locomotion and motion of the joint. Sepsis into the joint is directly responsible for a severe presence of cytokines responsible for the recruitment of polynuclear cells. Figure 19.2 displays bony and soft tissue changes associated with arthritis in goats.

19.3 Recognition of Pain

Recognition of pain can be challenging in ruminant species such as goats. As prey species, goats do not always show discomfort, especially in the early stages of a painful stimulus. Producers should be observant for slight changes in behavior and habits, such as deviations from normal ambulation, appetite, defecation, and urination. Multiple resources are available for pain recognition strategies in livestock species, such as the Guidelines for Recognition and Assessment of Animal Pain, published online by the Royal School of Veterinary Studies in Edinburgh (https://www.vet.ed.ac.uk/animalpain).

19.4 Analgesics Available

19.4.1 Non-steroidal Anti-inflammatory Drugs

Non-steroidal anti-inflammatory drugs (NSAIDs) provide analgesia in an indirect manner by decreasing the inflammatory responses to injured tissues (Table 19.1). This damage to the tissue results in the production of inflammatory mediators such as prostaglandins, which act on primary afferent neurons to lead to pain. NSAIDs function by blocking the cyclooxygenase (COX) pathway to prevent the formation of prostaglandins and other pro-inflammatory signals (Thurmon et al. 1996; Plummer and Schleining 2013). In this manner, the analgesic potency of NSAIDs can be increased by utilization before surgery or potentially painful management procedures to avoid or diminish wind-up.

The NSAID class has several benefits when compared to other analgesic drug classes such as opioids and α_2 adrenergic agonists. Primarily, the NSAID class does not result in sedation of the patient, a side effect of the other two classes of drugs (Smith et al. 2021b). Secondly, the NSAID class provides a longer duration of analgesia and a slower elimination half-life, partially due to the ability to sequester in inflamed tissues. NSAIDs are generally considered most effective against pain of low to moderate intensity and originating from the somatic or integumentary systems

(a)

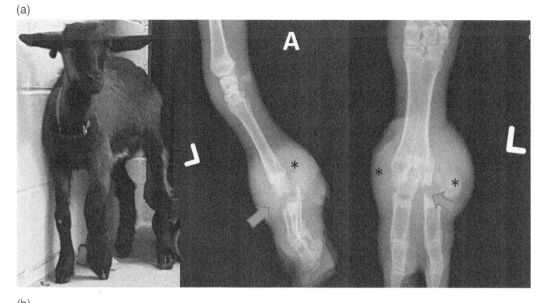

(b)

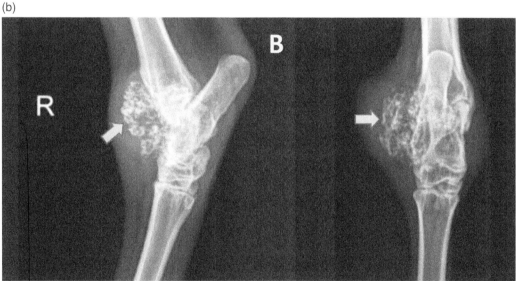

Figure 19.2 Various presentations of arthritis in goats. (a) Septic arthritis presenting in the left carpus of a goat kid. Note the profound soft tissue swelling of the pancarpal region (*) as well as the bony destruction (blue arrow). (b) Right tarsal view of an adult goat with arthritis from caprine arthritis and encephalitis (CAE) virus, a small ruminant lentivirus. Notice all of the mineral opacity proliferation in the soft tissue of the pantarsal region (green arrow).

(Plummer and Schleining 2013). Adverse effects of NSAIDs include gastrointestinal (abomasal) ulceration and nephropathy (especially in goats that are hypovolemic, shocky, or dehydrated).

NSAIDs may be helpful in the management of chronic painful conditions; however, the clinician should consider adverse effects in developing therapeutic plans and should monitor for complications when long-term therapy is necessary (Smith et al. 2021b). Caution should be considered in cases where goats present with azotemia or severe dehydration, and in these cases fluid therapy to restore perfusion and glomerular filtration should be considered

before the initiation of NSAID therapy due to the potential risk of causing renal injury. For cases where clinicians suspect abomasal (gastric) ulceration from NSAID administration, consideration should be given to administration of coating agents, potentially sucralfate (for juvenile patients that are not ruminating yet), altering feeding strategies, and administration of gastroprotectants (Hund and Wittek 2018). Among gastroprotectant therapies, the proton pump inhibitor (PPI) class of drugs is considered the most effective in veterinary use. In mature, ruminating goats pantoprazole and esomeprazole have been studied for this purpose (Smith et al. 2020a; Smith et al. 2021a, Fladung et al. 2022).

Table 19.1 Analgesic dose table for goats.

Drug	Reference	Analgesic drug class	Dose	Route	Frequency	Comments
Opioids						
Morphine		Opioid: μ agonist				
	George (2003), Gordon et al. (2022)		0.05–0.1 mg/kg	IV or SC	q 4–6 hr	
	Gordon et al. (2022)		0.25 mg/kg	SC	q 2–3 hr	
	Gordon et al. (2022)		0.4 mg/kg	IM	q 3–4 hr	
	Hendrickson et al. (1996)		0.1 mg/kg	EP		
				PO		Not recommended PO
Fentanyl	Carroll et al. (1999)	Opioid: μ agonist; κ antagonist		TD		Not supported by EBM
	Carroll et al. (1999)			IV	Not recommended due to rapid clearance	
Butorphanol	Carroll et al. (2001)	Opioid: μ antagonist to partial agonist; κ agonist	0.1 mg/kg	IV	4–6 hr	Altered behavior in less painful animals
	Carroll et al. (2001)		0.1 mg/kg	IM	4–6 hr	Altered behavior in less painful animals
Tramadol	De Sousa et al. (2007)	Opioid: weak μ agonist; inhibitor of serotonin reuptake	2–4 mg/kg	IV	q 6 hr	
	De Souza et al. (2007)		2 mg/kg	PO		Not recommended
Naloxone						
NSAIDs						
Phenylbutazone		Non-selective COX inhibitor		IV, SC, PO		Not recommended
Meloxicam	Shukla et al. (2007)	Slightly/moderately selective COX-2 inhibitor	0.5 mg/kg	IV	q 8 hr	
	Ingvast-Larsson et al. (2010)		0.5 mg/kg	PO	q 24 hr	
	Ingvast-Larsson et al. (2010)		0.5 mg/kg	IM	q 24 hr	
Flunixin meglumine	Smith et al. (2020b), Reppert et al. (2019)	Non-selective COX inhibitor	1.1 mg/kg; 2.2 mg/kg	IV	q 12 hr (1.1 mg/kg)	
	Konigsson et al. (2003)		2.2 mg/kg	PO	Once	Note: for an oral granule formulation
	Smith et al. (2020b)		1.1 mg/kg	SC	q 12 hr	
	Reppert et al. (2019)		3.3 mg/kg	TD	Once	Low bioavailability
Firocoxib	Stuart et al. (2019)	Highly selective COX-2 inhibitor	0.5 mg/kg	IV. PO	Once	High volume of distribution could lead to residue risk; currently no clinical studies
Grapriprant	Halleran et al. (2021)	Prostaglandin E2 P4 receptor inhibitor	2–4 mg/kg	PO	Once	Based on achieving levels that are comparatively therapeutic in other species.

Table 19.1 (Continued)

Drug	Reference	Analgesic drug class	Dose	Route	Frequency	Comments
Local anesthetics						
Lidocaine	Ivany and Muir (2004)[a]	Local anesthetic: sodium channel blocker	1 ml/50kg	EP		
	Van Metre (2010)[a]		1 m/15kg	EP		
	Hellyer et al. (2007)		1–2 mg/kg	SC		
	Doherty et al. (2007)		2.5 mg/kg	IV	Loading dose	Administer slowly
	Doherty et al. (2007)		0.1 mg/kg/min	IV	CRI following loading dose	

COX, cyclooxygenase; CRI, continuous-rate infusion; EP, epidural; IM, intramuscular; IV, intravenous; NSAID, non-steroidal anti-inflammatory drug; PO, oral; q, every; SC, subcutaneous; TD, transdermal.
[a] Indicates published doses that are based on clinical experience.

19.4.1.1 Flunixin Meglumine

Flunixin is available in an injectable formulation, transdermal formulation, and oral granule form that have been evaluated for use in goats (Konigsson et al. 2003; Smith et al. 2020a; Graves et al. 2020). While commonly administered by intravenous (IV) injection, recent research has demonstrated that subcutaneous (SC) administration achieved similar concentrations to IV, and does not appear to lead to myositis as seen in other large animal species (Smith et al. 2020b). The transdermal formulation was not very bioavailable in goats, and was not adequate by itself to mitigate the pain from castration (Graves et al. 2020; Reppert et al. 2019). Flunixin is clinically used for short-term analgesia for pain from soft tissue origins, and use for longer than three days may require monitoring for adverse effects.

19.4.1.2 Meloxicam

Meloxicam is available as an injection as well as an oral tablet (human generic) (Karademir et al. 2016). Both are commonly used in goats, with the human generic tablet having the advantage of being very cost-effective. With respect to adverse effects, meloxicam is thought to be safer than flunixin for long-term usage, as well as more effective for musculoskeletal pain. Long-term usage should focus on identifying the lowest effective dose and/or the longest duration between administrations that still achieves therapeutic efficacy in order to minimize adverse effects.

19.4.1.3 Other Non-steroidal Anti-inflammatory Drugs

Diclofenac, aspirin, phenylbutazone, and acetaminophen are sometimes considered for usage in goats. Practitioners should make evidence-based decisions regarding their use and consider prior to use the potential for residues that could be harmful to human health (phenylbutazone) or wildlife health (diclofenac) (Smith et al. 2021b; Plaza et al. 2022). While aspirin has been considered the prototype NSAID, it is currently lacking evidence to support its use for analgesia in goats (Plummer and Schleining 2013).

19.4.2 Opioids

This class of drugs, which acts on opioid receptors in the central nervous system, is quite broad. Classification of opioids is based on their action as agonist, agonist–antagonist, or antagonist of one of several opioid receptors that have been identified (Smith et al. 2021b), with common opioid receptors including mu (μ), delta (δ), and kappa (κ) (Smith et al. 2021b). Activity by receptor varies, an example being mu receptor action typically resulting in analgesia and sedation, whereas kappa receptor activation can lead to central analgesia (Smith et al. 2021b). Similar to the α_2 adrenergic agonists, stimulation of the opioid receptors results in stimulation of the G-coupled protein pathways and the ultimate hyperpolarization of postsynaptic neurons (Smith et al. 2021b). The opioid class of drugs is generally believed to provide potent visceral analgesia.

When considering the potential for adverse effects, the opioid class of drugs has the potential to induce some degree of sedation, respiratory depression, decreased gastrointestinal motility, and decreased appetite. Opioids have been reported to induce a hyperexcitable state that will mask their sedative properties (Galatos 2011). Opioids have potent analgesic activity, with some degree of variation in potency noticeable between the different specific opioid class members.

19.4.2.1 Morphine

Morphine is considered the prototype of the opioid agonist. It is generally administered as an injectable product by either IV, intramuscular (IM), or epidural routes in goats, with oral administration not recommended (Smith et al. 2021b). It has a relatively short plasma half-life and hence must be readministered frequently, with durations varying by route. In most locations it is a scheduled drug due to the potential for human abuse and can require additional licensing and record keeping. In comparison to some of the other opioids it can be less expensive; however, its analgesic potency is also less than many of the other opioids that are currently available.

19.4.2.2 Butorphanol

Butorphanol is a synthetic opioid that, in comparison to morphine, is three to five times more potent in its analgesic effects and has both agonist and antagonist properties (Galatos 2011). Butorphanol also has a less negative respiratory effect in comparison to morphine, but costs considerably more at the present time. In recent years, increased use of a combination of butorphanol, xylazine, and ketamine for restraint in goats has demonstrated potent analgesic effects for short procedures. Butorphanol is typically a regulated narcotic, and can require additional licensure and regulatory paperwork.

19.4.2.3 Fentanyl

Fentanyl is a potent opioid analgesic (approximately 100 times as potent as morphine) that is available as an injectable solution as well as a transdermal patch. Limitations of the use of fentanyl include expense, as well as the potential diversion for human abuse. The injectable formulation is rarely used in small ruminants or camelids; however, the transdermal patch formulation can provide for moderately long and extremely potent analgesia. The patch can be applied to a clipped area of the skin in a portion of the body where the animal is not likely to consume the patch, and where the patch will be unlikely to come into contact with a heat source such as a heating pad or heat lamp. The patch can provide stable plasma concentrations for two to three days (Smith et al. 2021c). Figure 19.3 demonstrates application of a fentanyl transdermal patch in a 2-year-old goat as part of a pain management plan after it was attacked by a dog.

19.4.2.4 Other Opioids

Hydromorphone, buprenorphine, tramadol, and nalbuphine are among other opioids discussed for use in goats. Currently, these drugs can be cost-prohibitive and clinicians should utilize evidenced-based approaches prior to employing them.

19.4.3 α₂ Adrenergic Agonists

The α₂ adrenergic agonists are routinely used in goats for both their sedative and analgesic properties, and xylazine, detomidine, and medetomidine are examples of this class of drug (Smith et al. 2021b). The analgesic potency of these compounds is generally considered to be similar to that of the less potent opioids (such as morphine), given that they utilize the same effector mechanisms and are located on many of the same neurons of the brain as the mu opioid receptor (Thurmon et al. 1996). On binding to the α₂ adrenergic receptor in neurons of the brain, the drug induces signaling of the membrane-associated G-coupled proteins that results in activation of potassium channels in the postsynaptic neuron (Plummer and Schleining 2013). This process allows an influx of potassium into the cell, resulting in hyperpolarization making the receptors unresponsive to stimulation (Thurmon et al. 1996).

Ruminants such as goats are generally more sensitive to α₂ adrenergic agonists than other species like horses, pigs, and small animals. For this reason, appropriate dosing is of importance when administering. On should consider when using large animal preparations of xylazine (i.e. 100 mg/ml xylazine) that these formulations may not be appropriate for use in animals with a small body mass. Utilizing the 20 mg/ml xylazine formulation, this can be diluted even further with sterile water as needed to a 1–2 mg/ml concentration (Plummer and Schleining 2013). Similar dilution of other α₂ adrenergic agonists may be necessary to avoid administration of too high dosages. These drugs are rapidly eliminated from the plasma and, as such, have quick elimination half-lives. For this reason, use of these drugs in an IM or epidural manner may prolong the period of analgesia over that of IV dosing, albeit it will be slower in onset than IV (Smith et al. 2021b; Kastner 2006).

With regard to xylazine, there is limited data on the duration of analgesia, but what data is available suggests that IM dosing of xylazine provides roughly 60 minutes of analgesia, with the onset of action and the magnitude of effect being dose dependent (Smith et al. 2021b; Grant et al. 1996). Xylazine does cause cardiovascular depression, with a dose-dependent decrease in heart rate and cardiac output (Kastner 2006). In pregnant does the drug will result in decreased heart rates of the fetuses. Xylazine has also been associated with decreased lung compliance, tachypnea, pulmonary edema, and hypoxia (Kastner 2006), although pulmonary edema is a more commonly observed adverse effect in sheep rather than goats. A transient hyperglycemia is often observed following use of xylazine in goats. This hyperglycemia will result in increased urine output and this class of drugs does have a propensity to induce a short-term diuresis. While this side effect can have a

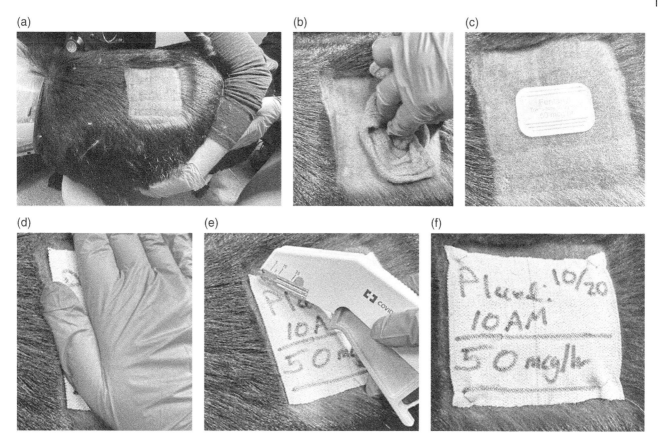

Figure 19.3 Placement of a fentanyl transdermal patch (FTP) on a 2-year-old Nigerian Dwarf doe as part of a treatment plan after being attacked by a dog. (a) An area is clipped over the thorax. Care should be taken to select an area that will not be exposed to excessive heat (from a heating lamp, vent, or other source). (b) The clipped area is lightly blotted with a damp cloth to remove residual hair and debris, but care is taken not to scrub excessively, as this may remove oils from the skin that can alter absorption. (c) The FTP is applied to the center of the clipped region. (d) An elastic bandage is applied over the FTP, and pressure is used for 30–60 seconds to insure good contact between the patch and the skin. A non-adherent dressing can be placed inside the elastic bandage to avoid contact with the FTP if desired. (e) The elastic bandage is secured with skin staples. (f) Patch after application. Note that the time and date of application, as well as the dosage, are listed on the elastic bandage for easy reference.

minimal impact on the patient, it should be considered if the drug is being used to provide analgesia for a goat that is experiencing a suspected or confirmed urethral obstruction, as this diuresis may increase urethral pressure.

The analgesic effects and adverse side effects of detomidine and medetomidine are similar to those described for xylazine (Kastner 2006). Due to the short duration of potent analgesia, these drugs are most useful for acute pain and surgical pain in goats. For some cases of chronic severe pain, a loading dose followed by continuous-rate infusions (CRI) of these drugs is employed; however, this analgesia is typically accompanied by sedation in a dose-dependent fashion. With these dose-dependent characteristics in mind, high-dose analgesia typically results in accompanying significant sedation. The use of the epidural route in administering these drugs may lessen the sedation compared to other routes, but clinicians should be aware of potential systemic adverse effects from epidural administration.

A benefit of the use of α_2 adrenergic agonists is that the effects of this class (including the adverse effects) can be reversed rapidly with the use of α_2 adrenergic antagonists such as yohimbine and tolazoline. It is critical to realize that when the α_2 adrenergic antagonists are utilized the analgesic properties of the α_2 adrenergic agonists are also reversed, potentially leaving the goat painful if alternate means of analgesia are not simultaneously instituted. Considering this, multimodal analgesia protocols are encouraged when feasible and appropriate, as if the α_2 adrenergic agonists are reversed then residual analgesia from other agents can be expected.

19.4.4 Ketamine

While ketamine has profound dissociative effects, commonly used for anesthesia, it also has a potent analgesic effect at doses lower than required for anesthesia. There is evidence to support that the analgesia is more effective for somatic pain than for visceral pain (Lin 1996). Ketamine has a short plasma half-life, so to mitigate this CRIs and epidural use can be employed in combination with other analgesics to provide long-term analgesia. It should be noted that unlike opioids, ketamine does not depress the respiratory system and actually stimulates the cardiovascular system. It is a regulated drug in most locations.

19.4.5 Gabapentin

Gabapentin is a γ-aminobutyric acid (GABA) analog that was initially developed to treat epilepsy in humans. It is also effective as an analgesic for chronic or neuropathic pain and is used for this function in human medicine. The drug binds to calcium voltage-gated channels and inhibits neuroexcitation. Initial studies done in beef calves have demonstrated synergism with NSAIDs (meloxicam) in relieving pain associated with an induced lameness model (Coetzee et al. 2011). The authors have used the drug several times for treating chronic lameness in sheep, goats, and llamas with apparent success; however, no formal clinical trials have been done at this time.

Table 19.1 includes doses, routes, and frequencies for various classes of analgesic drugs routinely used in goats.

19.5 Non-pharmacological Therapies

Several non-pharmacological therapies exist for the management of pain in goats. Most notably, acupuncture (AP) and electroacupuncture (EAP) are becoming more popular for the management of pain in large animal species. While AP and EAP are not exhaustively studied in goats, these techniques have been comparatively studied and demonstrated to increase endogenous opioid production (Ali et al. 2019), as well as to increase regional microcirculation and facilitate healing of nerve injuries (Smith et al. 2021c). Figure 19.4 demonstrates the application of electroacupuncture as part of a multimodal pain management approach for a goat recovering from a metatarsal fracture.

19.6 Regulatory Concerns

Veterinarians should be aware of the local, regional, and national regulations regarding the use of analgesic drugs in goats, which can be considered food animal species. As such, regulatory limitations could exist regarding the use of certain drugs in animals that could potentially enter the food chain. Additionally, few drugs are approved for goats, as well as for the management of pain in livestock, so use

of these drugs in these species may constitute "extra-label" drug usage, and have additional regulatory responsibilities, such as zero tolerance for residues at slaughter (Smith et al. 2021b). Clinicians should be cognizant of these regulations and use existing resources to provide withdrawal recommendations as appropriate. For example, Canadian veterinarians can solicit withdrawal advice from the Canadian Global Food Animal Residue Avoidance Databank (CgFARAD; https://cgfarad.usask.ca) for extra-label use in food animal species. Veterinarians should also be aware of local laws/regulations regarding the storage, transport, use, and disposition of controlled substances, as several of the drugs mentioned in this chapter (opioids for example) have additional paperwork requirements due to the potential for diversion and human drug abuse.

19.7 Strategies for Analgesia in Goats

19.7.1 Preoperative Analgesia

Prior to surgery, clinicians should consider a multimodal approach to analgesia. Preemptive administration of an NSAID such as flunixin meglumine or meloxicam helps reduce nociceptive wind-up (Smith et al. 2021b). Anesthesia of the surgical site by local or loco-regional blocks should be associated with NSAID administration prior to husbandry procedures. Preoperative drugs such as the α_2 agonists, ketamine, and opioids can also be utilized to minimize the overall painful stimulus of the planned procedure.

19.7.2 Epidural

Access to the epidural space is by either the lumbosacral space (for "high" or cranial epidural) or via the sacrococcygeal or first coccygeal space (for "low" or caudal epidural). For administration via the cranial approach, the site should be identified by localization of a palpable depression on the dorsal midline between the wings of the ilium and caudal to the dorsal process of the sixth lumbar vertebra (Smith et al. 2021b). Clipping the hair and an aseptic preparation are recommended. A 1.5 in., 20–18-gauge needle is typically adequate to access the space at this location. Advanced in a perpendicular manner, the space is reached when a "pop" is felt, and the practitioner should be aware that some animals will react when the space is reached. A drop of the drug to be given can be then placed in the hub of the needle, and if the epidural space has been reached the negative pressure should lead to aspiration into the space (Smith et al. 2021b). When the drug is administered into the epidural space, no resistance should be encountered and the injection should be given over approximately

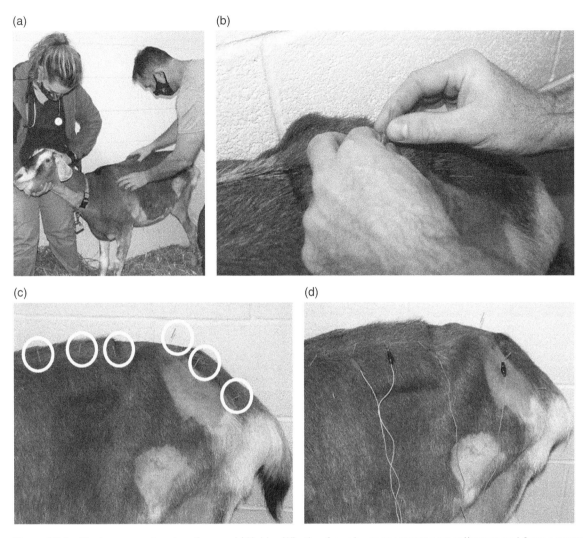

Figure 19.4 Electroacupuncture in a 3-year-old Nubian Whether for pain management post splint removal from a metatarsal fracture. (a) Examination by palpation for "trigger points" and other focal areas of sensitivity. (b) An 0.3 × 30 mm silicone-coated needle (Seirin Inc.) is being placed at Bai hui (a point at the dorsal midline of the lumbosacral spine). (c) Additional needles are placed along the left bladder line. (d) Electrical current being applied with an Ito ES-130 three-channel electrical stimulation unit (Ito Co. Ltd).

one to two minutes to prevent rapid cranial migration of the drug. The goat's head should be secured and preferably elevated for this procedure.

The site for a caudal epidural can be located by moving the tail dorsal and ventral in a "pumping" fashion and feeling for the most cranial space between the coccygeal or sacrococcygeal processes while doing so. Clipping the hair and aseptic preparation are again recommended for this procedure. The needle is placed into the most cranial identified space, and inserted at a 45° angle to the spinal cord. Similar to the lumbosacral technique, the administration of a drop of the drug to check for negative pressure is useful in identifying the epidural space.

For repeated administration of drugs into the epidural space an epidural catheter can be considered. These devices offer advantages in that the drug can be very easily administered, they can be in place for several days, and they are simple to remove. It should be noted that these catheters are designed for short-term administration, and prolonged placement can lead to inflammation. The catheter site itself should be kept as clean as possible, and consideration should be given to covering it with a protective film and securing the catheter to the skin. The ideal patient for an epidural catheter is one that is relatively easily handled and confined to a small space for several days while the catheter is in place. An epidural catheter applied to a non-tractable patient could lead to damage to the catheter and risk to the patient.

There are several steps in the placement of an epidural catheter, as described by Smith et al. (2021b). First, the patient should be sedated or anesthetized to facilitate optimal location of landmarks and catheter insertion.

This involves sternal placement with the pelvic limbs securely positioned. The site should be clipped and sterile-prepped and the use of a sterile drape should be considered. A Tuohy needle should be passed into the epidural space, and feeling a "pop" will indicate that the needle has passed through the ligamentum flavum. This is not a hanging drop technique, and the catheter is then fed through the Tuohy needle. After the catheter is advanced to its appropriate destination, the needle is removed over the catheter, and the catheter is secured to the skin. Keeping the catheter and its cap sterile is essential, so a bandage or adhesive film should be considered. If kept sterile these epidural catheters can be employed for several days. Figure 19.5 demonstrates the position of an epidural catheter in a doe that suffered trauma after being hit by a car.

19.7.3 Regional Local Anesthesia

Local anesthesia can be considered to improve postoperative comfort. Care should be taken not to exceed a total dose of 5–7 mg/kg of lidocaine in goats, as this could lead to toxicity (Cattle and Lin 2022). Clinicians can even consider not exceeding 4 mg/kg total dosing (Edmondson 2016). Diluting the commercially available 2% lidocaine solution to 1% is a very effective way to achieve enough volume injection for sufficient diffusion around the nerves without reaching toxicity in smaller patients. In addition to cornual blocks for disbudding and local blocks for flank laparotomy procedures, several more recent techniques such as a Bier block or soaker catheter can also be considered (Van Metre, 2010).

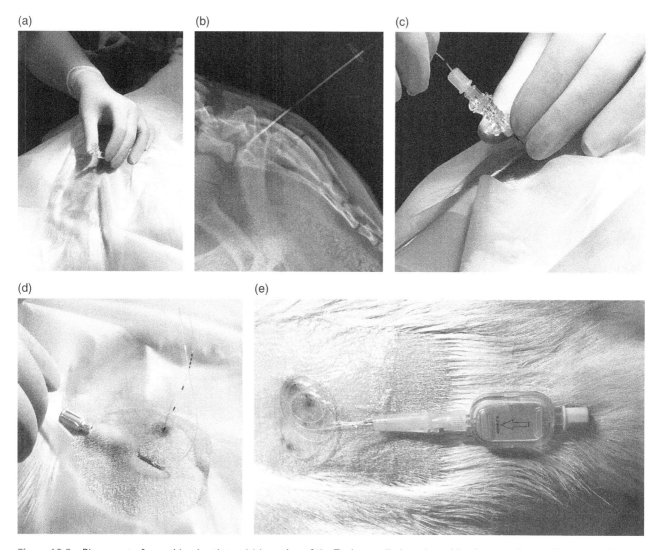

Figure 19.5 Placement of an epidural catheter. (a) Insertion of the Tuohy needle into the epidural space after sterile preparation and draping. (b) Radiographic image of the Tuohy needle placement. (c) Feeding of the epidural catheter through the Tuohy needle. (d) Securing the epidural catheter under the skin after removal of the Tuohy needle. (e) Securing the final assembly of the catheter with sterile adhesive film. Note: missing from E is further securing of the catheter with tape and suture.

The Bier block technique is a form of distal limb regional anesthesia that can be used as an aid to surgical procedures, or potentially as a diagnostic method. For this technique a tourniquet (rubber surgical tubing or similar) is placed proximal to the region of the limb that is being manipulated. Often this location is the cephalic or recurrent tarsal vein with the tourniquet placed above the tarsus or elbow. After clipping and aseptic prep, a small butterfly catheter (19 gauge or smaller) can be introduced into the vein and an approximate 1 ml 2% lidocaine/5 kg body weight dosage can be administered for local anesthesia of the distal limb. After administration the authors remove the catheter and typically apply a pressure bandage to the site where the catheter was introduced for the duration of the procedure. The tourniquet can typically be placed for 30 minutes, and this technique has been reported with no adverse effects relative to the limb perfusion being observed (Babalola and Oke 1983).

19.7.4 Topical Agents

Topical analgesics have been recently explored and utilized in ruminant patients. The transdermal formulation of flunixin meglumine has been used for the improvement of welfare in cattle (Kleinhenz et al. 2018). This formulation has been useful as the ease of administration (pouring over the topline) is convenient compared to injection or oral administration. Unfortunately, due to the low bioavailability of this product in the goat, it is not currently recommended for use in caprine patients (Reppert et al. 2019). Other topical formulations of analgesics, such as buprenorphine (Freise et al. 2022) and ketoprofen (Mills et al. 2022), have been developed for veterinary species, and in the future these may be adjunctive therapies for analgesia in goats.

19.8 Management of Osteoarthritis

Arthritis and osteoarthritis can be challenging to manage clinically because of the remodeling of the joint structure as well as the potential for wind-up from the chronic painful stimuli. Drugs chosen for analgesia of arthritis should be selected for ease of administration, low potential for adverse effects, and comparative evidence for their use. The authors have routinely used meloxicam for the treatment of osteoarthritis in goats. An example of an initial plan would be 1 mg/kg orally every 24 hours for 5–7 days, and then instructing the client or producer either to decrease the dose to the lowest that is still effective, or to increase the time between administrations to the longest that is still effective. This allows the animal to benefit while

reducing overall exposure to the drug, which will reduce the potential for adverse effects. Gabapentin can also be used for cases where an NSAID alone is not satisfactory. Anecdotal reports suggest that doses of 5–15 mg/kg orally every 8–12 hours can be used in combination with an NSAID. Practitioners should be aware of the potential for sedation from gabapentin, and the fact that it may be controlled in some locations. Polysulfated glycosaminoglycans have been associated with an inhibition of the pro-inflammatory cytokines present in the synovial fluids in other species, and its use may participate synergistically with the other drugs of the analgesic protocol.

Since osteoarthritis is a chronic, degenerative condition, focus should also be on management of the patient and the environment. Weight reduction for overconditioned animals is key in reducing mechanical stress on damaged joints. Environmental changes, such as application of rubber mats or softer surfaces, reduction of stocking density, as well as easily accessible water and food sources should also be considered in the management of osteoarthritic animals.

19.9 Future Directions

With the multifaceted role that goats perform in society, multiple future directions exist for approaches to mitigation of pain in the species. Several new classes of drugs warrant further investigation in goats, examples being prostaglandin receptor antagonists and soluble epoxide hydrolase inhibitors (Tucker et al. 2021). Grapriprant is a new drug in the canine market that functions by binding to and inhibiting the actions of the prostaglandin receptor. Benefits of this drug include NSAID-like actions without the adverse effects of NSAIDs. While this drug has not been investigated in adult goats at the time of publication, preliminary work in alpacas shows poor oral bioavailability with other mature ruminating species, suggesting that development of injectable formulations would be a priority for caprine use. Grapriprant has been demonstrated to achieve comparative therapeutic plasma levels when administered orally in pre-ruminating kid goats (Halleran et al. 2021). Soluble epoxide hydrolase inhibitors function by reducing the breakdown of epoxyeicosatrienoic acids into harmful and inflammatory dihydroxyeicosatrienoic acids (Tucker et al. 2021). The benefit of these compounds is prevention of chondrocyte apoptosis, protection of the cartilage matrix, and, when combined with an NSAID, optimized pain control (Tucker et al. 2021). As such, these drugs present potentially powerful options for the management of pain and osteoarthritis in goats.

Recognition of pain is another area where future research endeavors should focus. Pain can be assessed by visual scoring (example: grimace scale), measurement of biomarkers associated with pain (examples: prostaglandin, substance P), mechanical nociceptive threshold, as well as behavior. While multiple grimace scale systems have been developed for sheep (Hager et al. 2017), these systems are currently lacking for goats. A stall-side or point-of-care biomarker assay would allow for clinicians to monitor pain in a more comprehensive manner, but currently these assays are laboratory and time intensive. Future research in "user-friendly" systems for detection of pain in goats would greatly benefit practitioner and patient alike.

19.10 Conclusion

Multiple options exist for practitioners regarding the management of pain in goats. NSAIDs, opioids, and other drugs can be used in sole or multimodal therapies, depending on the circumstances. Clinicians should consider preemptive and regional analgesia to decrease nociceptive wind-up prior to painful stimuli through practices such as preoperative administration of an NSAID as well as regional practices such as epidural drug administration and soaker catheters. Pain management is a rapidly evolving field, and diligence is required for new developments that would benefit analgesia in caprine patients.

Multiple-Choice Questions

1 Which of the following steps of pain transmission is not affected by local anesthetics?
   A Transduction
   B Transmission
   C Modulation
   D Perception

2 Which of the following is/are concerns regarding the use of a transdermal fentanyl patch in a goat?
   A An external heat source altering absorption
   B The animal potentially consuming the patch
   C Human abuse of the patch
   D All of the above

3 Which of the following is not an identified benefit of acupuncture or electroacupuncture therapy?
   A Prostaglandin inhibition
   B Increases in regional microcirculation
   C Accelerated nerve injury healing
   D Increases in endogenous opioid production

4 What is the phenomenon of increased pain sensitivity that is observed after a painful stimulus?
   A Wash-out
   B Nociceptive wind-up
   C Drug withdrawal
   D Wind-down

5 What is the approximate absolute bioavailability of transdermal flunixin in meat goats (i.e. compared to intravenous administration)?
   A 100%
   B 75%
   C 50%
   D 25%

6 Which of the following analgesic drugs would not be expected to cause sedation in a patient?
   A Xylazine
   B Flunixin meglumine
   C Butorphanol
   D Ketamine

7 Which of the following is considered a toxic dose of lidocaine for goats?
   A 3 mg/kg
   B 2 mg/kg
   C 8 mg/kg
   D 1 mg/kg

8 How many mg of lidocaine are in 1 ml of 2% lidocaine solution?
   A 0.2 mg
   B 2 mg
   C 20 mg
   D 200 mg

9 Which of the following could be employed for management of a goat with chronic osteoarthritis?
   A Body weight reduction
   B NSAID administration
   C Padded floor surfaces
   D All of the above

10 Which of the following is considered a potential adverse effect from the NSAID drug class in goats?
   A Seizures
   B Decreased renal perfusion (decreased glomerular filtration rate)
   C Respiratory depression
   D Tachycardia

11 Which of the following could be used to treat suspected abomasal ulceration from NSAID administration in an adult goat?

A A proton pump inhibitor (e.g. pantoprazole)

B Lidocaine

C Grapriprant

D Morphine

12 Which of the following drugs do not influence the perception component of the physiology of pain?

A Sedatives

B Local anesthetics

C Opioids

D NSAIDs

13 Which of the following is not a component of pain from osteoarthritis?

A Nerve endings in the hyaline cartilage

B Thermal afferent receptors

C Chemical afferent receptors

D Mechanical afferent receptor

14 Which of the following routes would not be an effective way to deliver flunixin meglumine in a goat?

A Intravenous

B Subcutaneous

C Transdermal

D Oral

15 Which of the following NSAIDs is associated with residues that are harmful to scavenging wildlife?

A Diclofenac

B Meloxicam

C Flunixin meglumine

D Aspirin

16 Which of the following is/are receptor(s) that interact with opioids?

A Mu (μ)

B Delta(δ)

C Kappa (κ)

D All of the above

17 Which of the following receptors does morphine interact with?

A Mu

B Delta

C Kappa

D Omega

18 Which of the following opioids has the greatest potency?

A Morphine

B Butorphanol

C Fentanyl

D All have equal potency

19 Which of the following could be used to reverse an α_2 adrenergic agonist?

A Yohimbine

B Xylazine

C Detomidine

D Romifidine

20 Which of the following drugs has been demonstrated in livestock to have synergism for pain management when administered with gabapentin?

A Butorphanol

B Fentanyl

C Meloxicam

D Xylazine

21 Which of the following adverse effects could potentially occur with the use of opioids in goats?

A Respiratory depression

B Decreased gastrointestinal mobility

C Hyperexcitation

D All of the above

22 Which of the following drugs functions by direct action on the prostaglandin receptor?

A Meloxicam

B Grapriprant

C Flunixin meglumine

D Ketamine

23 Which of the following could be utilized to reverse an opioid?

A Yohimbine

B Tolazoline

C Naloxone

D Ketamine

24 Which of the following is not a mediator associated with pain from osteoarthritis?

A Substance P

B Bradykinin

C Interleukin-1

D Gastrin

25 Which stage of the pain pathway are opioids not thought to be effective in?

A Transduction

B Transmission

C Modulation

D Perception

References

Ali, U., Apryani, E., Ahsan, M.Z. et al. (2019). Acupuncture/electroacupuncture as an alternative in current opioid crisis. *Chinese Journal of Integrative Medicine* 26 (9): 643–647.

Babalola, G.O. and Oke, B.O. (1983). Intravenous regional analgesia for surgery of the limbs in goats. *Veterinary Quarterly* 5 (4): 186–189.

Carroll, G.L., Hooper, R.N., Boothe, D.M. et al. (1999). Pharmacokinetics of fentanyl after intravenous and transdermal administration in goats. *American Journal of Veterinary Research* 60 (8): 986–991.

Carroll, G.K., Boothe, D.M., Hartsfeld, S.M. et al. (2001). Pharmacokinetics and selected behavioral responses to butorphanol and its metabolites in goats following intravenous and intramuscular administration. *Veterinary Anaesthesia and Analgesia* 28: 188–195.

Cattle, S.R. and Lin, H. (2022). *Farm Animal Anesthesia: Cattle, Small Ruminants, Camelids and Pigs*. Chichester: Wiley Blackwell.

Coetzee, J.F. (2013). A review of analgesic compounds used in food animals in the United States. *Veterinary Clinics of North America: Food Animal Practice* 29 (1): 11–28.

Coetzee, J.F., Mosher, R.A., Kohake, L.E. et al. (2011). Pharmacokinetics of oral gabapentin alone or co-administered with meloxicam in ruminant beef calves. *Veterinary Journal* 190 (1): 98–102.

Doherty, T.J., Kattesh, H.G., Adcock, R.J. et al. (2007). Effects of a concentrated lidocaine solution on the acute phase stress response to dehorning in dairy calves. *Journal of Dairy Science* 90 (9): 4232–4239.

Edmondson, M.A. (2016). Local, regional, and spinal anesthesia in ruminants. *Veterinary Clinics of North America: Food Animal Practice* 32 (3): 535–552.

Fladung, R., Smith, J.S., Hines, M.T. et al. (2022). Pharmacokinetics of esomeprazole in goats (Capra aegagrus hircus) after intravenous and subcutaneous administration. *Front. Vet. Sci.* 9: 968973. https://doi.org/10.3389/fvets.2022.96897.

Freise, K.J., Reinemeyer, C., Warren, K. et al. (2022). Single-dose pharmacokinetics and bioavailability of a novel extended duration transdermal buprenorphine solution in cats. *Journal of Veterinary Pharmacology and Therapeutics* 45 (Suppl 1): S31–s9.

Galatos, A.D. (2011). Anesthesia and analgesia in sheep and goats. *Veterinary Clinics of North America: Food Animal Practice* 27 (1): 47–59.

George, L.W. (2003). Pain control in food animals. In: *Recent Advances in Anaesthetic Management of Large Domestic Animals* (ed. E.P. Steffey). Ithaca, NY: International Veterinary Information Service https://www.ivis.org/library/recent-advances-anesthetic-management-of-large-domestic-animals/pain-control-food-animals.

Gordon, E., Dirikolu, L., Liu, C.C. et al. (2022). Pharmacokinetic profiles of three dose rates of morphine sulfate following single intravenous, intramuscular, and subcutaneous administration in the goat. *Journal of Veterinary Pharmacology and Therapeutics* 45 (1): 107–116.

Gottschalk, A. and Smith, D.S. (2001). New concepts in acute pain therapy: preemptive analgesia. *American Family Physician* 63 (10): 1979–1984.

Grant, C., Upton, R.N., and Kuchel, T.R. (1996). Efficacy of intra-muscular analgesics for acute pain in sheep. *Australian Veterinary Journal* 73 (4): 129–132.

Graves, M.T., Schneider, L., Cox, S. et al. (2020). Evaluation of the pharmacokinetics and efficacy of transdermal flunixin for pain mitigation following castration in goats. *Translational Animal Science* 4 (4): txaa198.

Hager, C., Biernot, S., Buettner, M. et al. (2017). The Sheep Grimace Scale as an indicator of post-operative distress and pain in laboratory sheep. *PloS One* 12 (4): e0175839.

Halleran, J., Magnin, G., Mzyk, D. et al. (2021). Pharmacokinetics of grapiprant in goat kids at two different dosing regimens. *Small Ruminant Research* 205: 106531.

Hellyer, P.W., Robertson, S.A., and Fails, A.D. (2007). Pain and its management. In: *Lumb & Jones Veterinary Anesthesia and Analgesia*, 4e (ed. J.C. Thurmon, W.J. Tranquilli, and K.A. Grimm), 31–57. Ames, IA: Blackwell.

Hendrickson, D.A., Kruse-Elliott, K.T., and Broadstone, R.V. (1996). A comparison of epidural saline, morphine, and bupivacaine for pain relief after abdominal surgery in goats. *Veterinary Surgery* 25: 83–87.

Hund, A. and Wittek, T. (2018). Abomasal and third compartment ulcers in ruminants and South American camelids. *Veterinary Clinics of North America: Food Animal Practice* 34 (1): 35–54.

Ingvast-Larsson, C., Högberg, M., Mengistu, U. et al. (2010). Pharmacokinetics of meloxicam in adult goats and its analgesic effect in disbudded kids. *Journal of Veterinary Pharmacology and Therapeutics* 34: 64–69.

Ivany, J.M. and Muir, W.W. (2004). Farm animal anesthesia. In: *Farm Animal Surgery. St* (ed. S.L. Fubini and N.G. Ducharme). Louis, MO: W.B. Saunders, ch. 5.

Karademir, U., Erdogan, H., Boyacioglu, M. et al. (2016). Pharmacokinetics of meloxicam in adult goats: a comparative study of subcutaneous, oral and intravenous administration. *New Zealand Veterinary Journal* 64 (3): 165–168.

Kastner, S.B. (2006). A2-agonists in sheep: a review. *Veterinary Anaesthesia and Analgesia* 33 (2): 79–96.

Kissin, I. (2000). Preemptive analgesia. *Anesthesiology* 93 (4): 1138–1143.

Kleinhenz, M., Van Engen, N., Smith, J. et al. (2018). The impact of transdermal flunixin meglumine on biomarkers of pain in calves when administered at the time of surgical castration without local anesthesia. *Livestock Science* 212: 1–6.

Konigsson, K., Torneke, K., Engeland, I.V. et al. (2003). Pharmacokinetics and pharmacodynamic effects of flunixin after intravenous, intramuscular and oral administration to dairy goats. *Acta Veterinaria Scandinavica* 44 (3–4): 153–159.

Lin, H.C. (1996). Dissociative anesthetics. In: *Lumb and Jone's Veterinary Anesthesia*, 3e (ed. J. Thurmon, W. Tranquilli, and G.J. Benson). Philadelphia, PA: Williams and Wilkins.

McCoy, A.M. (2015). Animal models of osteoarthritis: comparisons and key considerations. *Veterinary Pathology* 52 (5): 803–818.

Mills, P.C., Owens, J.G., Reinbold, J.B. et al. (2022). A novel transdermal ketoprofen formulation for analgesia in cattle. *Journal of Veterinary Pharmacology and Therapeutics* 45 (6): 530–542.

Muir, W.W. 3rd and Woolf, C.J. (2001). Mechanisms of pain and their therapeutic implications. *Journal of the American Veterinary Medical Association* 219 (10): 1346–1356.

Ochroch, E.A., Mardini, I.A., and Gottschalk, A. (2003). What is the role of NSAIDs in pre-emptive analgesia? *Drugs* 63 (24): 2709–2723.

Plaza, P.I., Wiemeyer, G.M., and Lambertucci, S.A. (2022). Veterinary pharmaceuticals as a threat to endangered taxa: mitigation action for vulture conservation. *Science of the Total Environment* 817: 152884.

Plummer, P.J. and Schleining, J.A. (2013). Assessment and management of pain in small ruminants and camelids. *Veterinary Clinics of North America: Food Animal Practice* 29 (1): 185–208.

Renberg, W.C. (2005). Pathophysiology and management of arthritis. *Veterinary Clinics of North America: Small Animal Practice.* 35 (5): 1073–1091.

Reppert, E.J., Kleinhenz, M.D., Montgomery, S.R. et al. (2019). Pharmacokinetics and pharmacodynamics of intravenous and transdermal flunixin meglumine in meat goats. *Journal of Veterinary Pharmacology and Therapeutics* 42 (3): 309–317.

Shukla, M., Singh, G., Sindhura, B.G. et al. (2007). Comparative plasma pharmacokinetics of meloxicam in sheep and goats following intravenous administration. *Comparative Biochemistry and Physiology, Part C* 145: 528–532.

Small Ruminant Tips (2010). 128th Annual Meeting of the Iowa Veterinary Medical Association. September 16–17, Pages 69–173, Ames, IA.

Smith, J.S., Kosusnik, A.R., and Mochel, J.P. (2020a). A retrospective clinical investigation of the safety and adverse effects of pantoprazole in hospitalized ruminants. *Frontiers in Veterinary Science* 7: 97.

Smith, J.S., Marmulak, T.L., Angelos, J.A. et al. (2020b). Pharmacokinetic Parameters and Estimated Milk Withdrawal Intervals for Domestic Goats (Capra Aegagrus Hircus) After Administration of Single and Multiple Intravenous and Subcutaneous Doses of Flunixin Meglumine. *Front. Vet. Sci.* 7: 213. https://doi.org/10.3389/fvets.2020.00213.

Smith, J.S., Mochel, J.P., Soto-Gonzalez, W.M. et al. (2021a). Pharmacokinetics of Pantoprazole and Pantoprazole Sulfone in Goats After Intravenous Administration: A Preliminary Report. *Front. Vet. Sci.* 8: 744813. https://doi.org/10.3389/fvets.2021.744813.

Smith, J.S., Schleining, J., and Plummer, P. (2021b). Pain management in small ruminants and camelids: analgesic agents. *Veterinary Clinics of North America: Food Animal Practice* 37 (1): 1–16.

Smith, J.S., Schleining, J., and Plummer, P. (2021c). Pain management in small ruminants and camelids: applications and strategies. *Veterinary Clinics: Food Animal Practice* 37 (1): 17–31.

de Sousa, A.B., Santos, A.C.D., Schramm, S.G. et al. (2007). Pharmacokinetics of tramadol and o-desmethyltramadol in goats after intravenous and oral administration. *Journal of Veterinary Pharmacology and Therapeutics* 31: 45–51.

Stuart, A.K., KuKanich, B., Caixeta, L.S. et al. (2019). Pharmacokinetics and bioavailability of oral firocoxib in adult, mixed-breed goats. *Journal of Veterinary Pharmacology and Therapeutics* 42 (6): 640–646.

Thurmon, J., Tranquilli, W., and Benson, G.J. (1996). Preanesthetics and anesthetic adjuncts. In: *Lumb and Jones' Veterinary Anesthesia*, 3e (ed. J. Thurmon, W. Tranquilli, and G.J. Benson), 183–209. Philadelphia, PA: Williams and Wilkins.

Tucker, L., Trumble, T.N., Groschen, D. et al. (2021). Targeting soluble epoxide hydrolase and cyclooxygenases enhance joint pain control, stimulate collagen synthesis, and protect chondrocytes from cytokine-induced apoptosis. *Frontiers in Veterinary Science* 8: 685824.

Van Meter, M. E. M., McKee, K. Y., & Kohlwes, R. J. (2010). Efficacy and Safety of Tunneled Pleural Catheters in Adults with Malignant Pleural Effusions: A Systematic Review. Journal of General Internal Medicine, 26(1), 70–76. https://doi.org/10.1007/s11606-010-1472-0

20

Antimicrobial Resistance in Goat Production Practices

Bhupamani Das[1], Kruti Debnath Mandal[2], Abhinav Suthar[3], and Chinmoy Maji[4]

[1] Department of Clinics, College of Veterinary Sciences & Animal Husbandry, Sardarkrushinagar, Kamdhenu University, Gandhinagar, Gujarat, India
[2] Teaching Veterinary Clinical Complex, Faculty of Veterinary and Animal Sciences, Institute of Agricultural Science, Benaras Hindu University, Mirzapur, Uttar Pradesh, India
[3] Department of Medicine, College of Veterinary Sciences & Animal Husbandry, Sardarkrushinagar, Kamdhenu University, Gandhinagar, Gujarat, India
[4] North 24 Parganas Krishi Vigyan Kendra, West Bengal University of Animal & Fishery Sciences, Ashokenagar, West Bengal, India

The domestic goat (*Capra hircus*) has been raised by livestock owners for milk, meat, and skin purposes. More than 300 breeds of goat have been identified and domesticated worldwide. The unique ability of the goat to thrive on any type of food resources makes it the most economical dairy animal. Goat-keepers enjoy decent profits with minimum input costs. Most goat-keepers in developing countries have a poor economic status. Therefore, for developing countries like India, the goat is considered as the poor man's cow. Apart from that, the good fecundity rate, easy breeding management, and comparatively short gestation period are the attractive side of goat farming. Peste des petits ruminants, contagious ecthyma, coccidiosis, and haemonchosis are the major diseases of goats responsible for high morbidity and mortality. Due to poor economic status, scarcity of veterinary services and lack of proper diagnostic facilities lead to indiscriminate use of various antimicrobials in goats. After poultry farming, reports of antimicrobial resistance (AMR) frequently come from goat farms. All over the world, other than milk consumption, goat meat is widely preferred by most of consumers. The development of AMR in the goat population creates a serious threat to public health.

AMR is recognized as an emerging issue in the practice of veterinary medicine, especially in developing countries like India. More than two million illnesses and deaths are registered annually. An antimicrobial agent encompasses a broad range of natural or synthetic products that either kill or prevent the growth of microorganisms. AMR, also known as a superbug, is defined as the capacity of an organism to resist the growth inhibitory or killing capacity of drugs beyond the normal susceptibility of the specific microbe species (Acar and Röstel 2001; Mathur and Singh 2005; McDonnell and Russell 1999).

20.1 Causes of Antimicrobial Resistance

Microbes such as bacteria, virus, fungi, and parasites are living organisms that evolve over time. Therefore, they adapt to a new environment quickly and efficiently by a constant process of reproduction, thriving, spread, and change, so that they can survive in any harsh conditions. However, if something stops their ability to grow, such as the use of antimicrobials, they immediately enable changes in their living system that ensure their survival. To better appreciate the causes of AMR, we need to understand the various sequential steps involved for a drug to get to a patient and its eventual use, which include production, distribution, prescription, dispensing, and finally consumption of the drug by the patient or its use in animal production (Adefarakan et al. 2014; Quick and Bremer 1997). Consequently, any imprudent practice along this flow may result in the emergence of resistance.

There are several biological means for this to happen (Figure 20.1).

20.1.1 Indiscriminate Use of Drugs

Overuse of antimicrobials in livestock health and production beyond therapeutic needs has been highlighted in recent years. It is considered one of the most common causes for acceleration of AMR in small ruminants (Haulisah et al. 2021).

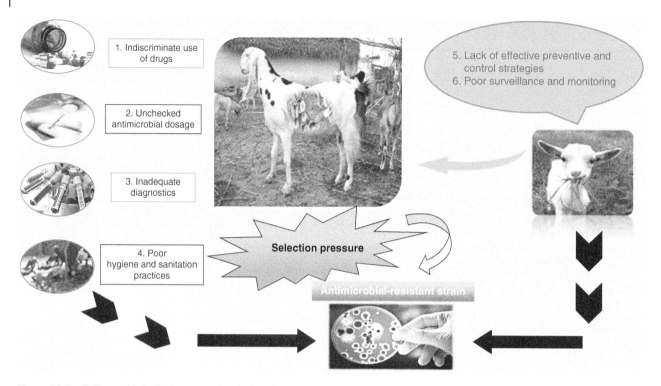

Figure 20.1 Different biological causes of antimicrobial resistance in the goat. NoSystem images/Getty Images; Alexander Raths/ Adobe Stock.

20.1.2 Unchecked Antimicrobial Dosage

Antimicrobials – including antibiotics, antivirals, antifungals, and antiparasitics – are medicines used to prevent and treat various infections in animals. Antibiotic dosing must aim to address not only the bacteria isolated, but also the most resistant subpopulation in the colony, to prevent the advent of further resistant infections because of the inadvertent selection pressure of current dosing regimens (Roberts et al. 2008).

20.1.3 Inadequate Diagnostics

The timely diagnosis and availability of routine antimicrobial sensitivity testing (AMST) to provide information on resistance trends, including emerging resistance, is very necessary in veterinary clinical practice. However, AMST is not possible to perform in rural laboratories or in field conditions due to a lack of necessary facilities (Ayukekbong et al. 2017). There is also a need for the development of effective policies against AMR. Therefore, use of antimicrobial agents without proper testing is believed to contribute to the resistance problem.

20.1.4 Veterinary Practitioners

Veterinarians or clinicians play an essential role in the treatment and prevention of diseases, but may jeopardize this if their practices are not evidence based. For example,

the practices of prescribing antimicrobials vary among clinicians in most countries. In some cases antimicrobial prescriptions are inappropriate (i.e. inappropriate drug, inappropriate doses, or use of an antimicrobial without any indications). Due to the high animal–doctor ratio in most developing countries, veterinary doctors are overwhelmed and there is often inadequate time for meaningful education, and also miscommunication occurs with the animal owner or keeper on drug dosage and administration guidelines. In that case, treatment consists of administering broad-spectrum antimicrobials without a proper diagnosis, which in the long term may result in resistance in treated animals. In a cross-sectional study, it was shown that in 52% and 48% of cases, respectively, the antimicrobial and the dosage was inappropriate (Odoi et al. 2021).

20.1.5 Poor Hygiene and Sanitation Practices

Usually, AMR arises when there is overuse of antimicrobials or non-completion of treatment duration. However, in recent research published in the journal *Scientific Reports*, scientists found that poor hygiene and sanitation could also be reasons for the increasing AMR (Ramay et al. 2020). Environmental conditions such as overcrowding and poor sanitation contribute to the circulation of resistant microbes and contagious diseases from one animal to another. Transmission of resistant pathogens is facilitated by contaminated water or food, vectors, or close contact (Ayukekbong et al. 2017).

20.1.6 Lack of Effective Preventive and Control Strategies

AMR is an increasingly serious phenomenon, where diseases causing microorganisms develop the capacity to resist the efforts of medicines hitherto used to successfully treat them. This includes antibiotic resistance, which is one of the most common forms of AMR. It is important to note that the growing incidence of AMR is a matter of global health concern. Lack of effective preventive strategies like availability of vaccines for only a few diseases, a paucity of effective antimicrobials to control drug-resistant pathogens, and a shortage of new quality-assured antimicrobials have resulted in worsened outcomes for infectious diseases and also jeopardize modern clinical procedures such as chemotherapy and invasive surgery (Table 20.1) (WHO 2021).

20.1.7 Poor Surveillance and Monitoring

The accuracy of AMR burden estimates depends on the quality and availability of input data (Hay et al. 2018). The present global surveillance system remains disconnected and underdeveloped and there is an urgent need to strengthen surveillance and monitoring. Only 70 countries have enrolled in the World Health Organization's (WHO) Global AMR Surveillance System (GLASS). There have been fewer than 50 reported AMR rates in recent years, where the data pertaining to small ruminants, especially goats, is negligible (WHO 2018). The current data is self-reported, heterogeneous, and based on a few isolates from a handful of surveillance sites.

20.2 Types of Antimicrobial Resistance

AMR can be broadly classified into natural resistance and acquired resistance.

20.2.1 Natural Resistance

Natural resistance can be intrinsic resistance, the innate ability of a microbe to resist the action of certain antimicrobial agents as a consequence of structural or functional characteristics, or induced resistance, where genes are naturally occurring in the microbe but are only expressed after exposure to an antimicrobial agent. In this type of resistance, microorganisms do not possess

Table 20.1 Resistant antimicrobials along with infectious pathogens in the goat.

Antimicrobials	Infectious pathogen	Reference
Ampicillin, amoxycillin-clavulanic acid, tetracycline, chroramphenicol, ceftrixone	*Escherichia coli*	Njoroge et al. (2013)
Tetracycline, erythromycin	*Salmonella* spp.	Igbinosa (2015)
Penicillin, clindamycin, oxacillin	*Pasteurella multocida*	Tahamtan et al. (2014)
Azole	*Candida* spp., *Cryptococcus gattii*, *Malassezia pachydermatis*, *Aspergillus fumigatus*	Álvarez-Pérez et al. (2021)
Ivermectin	*Oestertagia* spp.	Badger and McKenna (1990)
Ivermectin	*Haemonchus contortus*	Hall et al. (1981)
Ivermectin	*Teladorsagia circumcincta*	Eysker et al. (2006)
Ivermectin, levamisole	*Vernonia amygdalina*	Adediran and Uwalaka (2015)
Ivermectin, eprinomectin, albendazole sulfoxide, albendazole	Nematode	Arece-García et al. (2017)
Diminazene aceturate, isometamidium chloride	*Trypanosoma vivax*	Boma et al. (2022)

the target site for drugs, so the drugs do not affect them, or they have naturally low permeability to those agents because of the chemical nature of the drugs and the microbial membrane structure, especially for those that require entry into the microbial cell in order to effect their action. For instance, *Staphylococcus aureus* is naturally resistant to polymyxin; *Candida* spp. are naturally resistant to fluconazole.

20.2.2 Acquired Resistance

Acquired resistance occurs when a particular microorganism obtains the ability to resist the activity of an antimicrobial agent to which it was previously susceptible. Methicillin-resistant *S. aureus* (MRSA) and vancomycin-resistant *S. aureus* (VRSA) are two examples of the link between antimicrobial dosage and resistant development.

AMR can be further classified into side resistance, cross-resistance, and multiple resistance.

20.2.3 Side Resistance

If a microbe population becomes resistant to an active ingredient, it is obvious that it becomes tolerant to other active ingredients that have the same mode of action.

20.2.4 Cross-Resistance

Cross-resistance occurs when the microbe strain has the ability to survive therapeutic doses of chemically unrelated drugs with different modes of action.

20.2.5 Multiple Resistance or Multiple Drug Resistance

Multiple resistance is a type of simultaneous AMR shown by a species of microorganism to at least two or more antimicrobial drugs with different modes of action. It develops when any drug is taken for longer than necessary or when it is not needed. It is important to note that multidrug-resistant microbes are resistant to almost all antimicrobials, which makes them even more difficult to treat, therefore they can cause severe illness or even death in small ruminants (Nipane et al. 2008). Several sheep and goat farms have been closed because of multiple drug resistance in Australia, South Africa, and New Zealand (Kaplan 2004; Geary 2005; Abbott et al. 2012).

20.3 Mechanism of Antimicrobial Resistance

Understanding the mechanism of resistance of microbes (Figure 20.2) can help researchers better predict how quickly resistance will emerge, as well as provide tools for studying the biology of the microbe and therapeutic target.

20.3.1 Natural Resistance

Natural resistance of microbes to an antimicrobial agent typically includes the following elements.

20.3.1.1 Permeability Barrier

One of the most important natural resistance mechanisms is reduced susceptibility due to the chemical structure and composition of the outer cell layers of vegetative bacteria and bacterial endospores. This natural resistance is a chromosomal-controlled characteristic of the bacterial cell. The ability to withstand an antimicrobial attack, due to this natural resistance, varies between species and sometimes also between various strains of the same species. These strains can become tolerant to antimicrobials and resist higher antimicrobial concentrations than are needed for killing most of the bacteria of the same species. The most susceptible Gram-positive bacteria have no extra layers outside their peptidoglycan layer, which makes them the most sensitive of the bacteria. Gram-negative bacteria have the presence of a lipid bilayer and a lipopolysaccharide (LPS) layer outside the outer membrane, making them

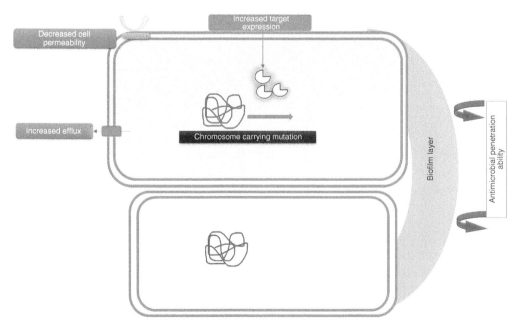

Figure 20.2 Mechanism of natural resistance in antimicrobial resistance.

less susceptible to antimicrobial attack. They can also regulate permeability through the synthesis of porins, the proteins that are involved in the uptake of antibiotics (Poole 2002).

For example, the most resistant mycobacteria have a complex cell wall outside their peptidoglycan polysaccharide layer – a waxy layer and a lipid layer – making them the least susceptible of the vegetative bacteria (Anderson and O'Toole 2008). Again, the bacterial endospores of *Bacillales* and *Clostridiales* spp. are far more resistant to antimicrobials than are all vegetative bacteria. Their spore wall is composed of layers that differ from the vegetative cell, which protects them against biocide action (Leggett et al. 2012). Microorganisms other than bacteria and bacterial endospores – fungi and enveloped viruses – are more susceptible to biocides than are Gram-positive bacteria, the enveloped viruses being the most susceptible. Fungi-like bacteria can develop antibiotic resistance where germs like bacteria and fungi develop the ability to defeat the drugs designed to kill them. Antifungal resistance is intrinsically genetically coded, seen in fungal species that are inherently non-susceptible to certain antifungals (Ben-Ami and Kontoyiannis 2021). For example, the drug fluconazole does not work against infections caused by the fungus *Aspergillus*, a type of mold. Some studies have indicated that antibiotics that include antifungal agents may also contribute to antifungal resistance in *Candida*.

20.3.1.2 Biofilm Formation
Another important form of natural resistance in bacteria is the formation of biofilms. Bacteria naturally prefer to live together in close contact with each other. Biofilms are highly organized communities of bacteria cohabiting in extracellular polymeric substance (EPS) slime, consisting of polysaccharides, protein, lipids, phospholipids, nucleic acids, and humid substances (Jahn and Nielsen 1998; Sutherland 2001; Tsuneda et al., 2003). The EPS protects the biofilm community against threats from outside, such as biocides and topical antibiotics. The position of the bacteria in a biofilm reflects their susceptibility to biocides, the most susceptible strains living underneath and the least susceptible strains on the top.

20.3.2 Acquired Resistance
Acquired resistance is mediated through vertical gene transfer and horizontal gene transfer.

20.3.2.1 Vertical Gene Transfer
Vertical gene transfer by mutation is a spontaneous change in the DNA sequence within the gene that may lead to a change in the trait that it codes for. Any change

in a single base pair may lead to a corresponding change in one or more of the amino acids for which it codes, which can then change the enzyme or cell structure that consequently changes the affinity or effective activity of the targeted antimicrobials. In the prokaryotic genome, mutation occurs due to base changes caused by exogenous agents, DNA polymerase error, deletions, insertions, and duplications. For prokaryotes, there is a constant rate of spontaneous mutation of about 0.0033 mutations per DNA replication that is relatively uniform for a diverse spectrum of organisms. The mutation rate for individual genes varies significantly among and within genes. Here, the group of susceptible microbes develop mutation in genes that subsequently results in survival in the presence of an antimicrobial agent (Courvalin 1996; McManus 1997; Tenover 2006). Generally, mutation occurs through one of the following mechanisms (Figure 20.3):

- **Modification of antimicrobial target**: Modification of target sites of antimicrobial agents is a common mechanism of acquired resistance. It results from spontaneous mutation of a gene in the chromosome and selection in the presence of an antimicrobial agent (Lambert 2005).
- **Decrease in drug uptake**: Drug uptake into any cell is a continuous process of passive influx of drug into cytoplasm coupled to trapping or through active transport in the porin channel. Reduced uptake of the drug signals a reduction or alteration in the porin channel or efflux pumps.
- **Modification of metabolic enzymes**: In enzymatic modification, an acetyl, adenyl, or phosphate group is added to a specific site of antimicrobial agent in order to modify it chemically and inactivate the antimicrobial agent, making it unable to bind to the target site.

20.3.2.2 Horizontal Gene Transfer
Horizontal gene transfer is another process by which resistance can be established. It is the movement of genetic information between organisms, a process that includes the spread of a resistant gene among microbes, fueling pathogen evolution (Burmeister 2015). Gene transfer results in genetic variation in bacteria and is a large problem when it comes to the spread of drug-resistant genes. The mechanism of horizontal gene transfer was earlier thought to be important for prokaryotic evolution, but is now becoming a common and widespread phenomenon for eukaryotes as well. The process is quite complex, mainly because acquired DNA must pass through both the outer cell membrane and the nuclear membrane to reach the eukaryote genome.

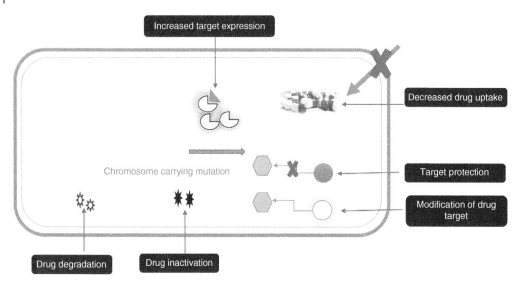

Figure 20.3 Mechanism of vertical gene transfer in antimicrobial resistance.

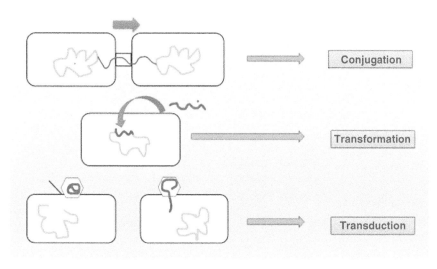

Figure 20.4 Mechanism of horizontal gene transfer in antimicrobial resistance.

There are three well-understood mechanisms of horizontal gene transfer (Figure 20.4), and these are discussed here.

20.3.2.2.1 Conjugation Bacterial conjugation is a process that involves the transfer of DNA via a plasmid from a donor cell to a recombinant recipient cell during cell-to-cell contact. This is thought to be the main mechanism of horizontal gene transfer. This process is encoded by plasmids or transposons (Cafini et al. 2017). It involves a donor bacterium that contains a conjugative plasmid that is self-transmissible, in that it possesses all the necessary

genes for that plasmid to transmit itself to another bacterium by conjugation and a recipient cell that does not. Conjugation genes known as *tra* genes enable the bacterium to form a mating pair with another organism, while *ori*T (origin of transfer) sequences determine where on the plasmid DNA transfer is initiated by serving as the replication start site, where DNA replication enzymes will nick the DNA to initiate DNA replication and transfer. In addition, mobilizable plasmids that lack the *tra* genes for self-transmissibility but possess the *ori*T sequences for initiation of DNA transfer may also be transferred by conjugation if the bacterium containing them also possesses a conjugative plasmid. The *tra* genes of the conjugative plasmid enable a mating pair to form, while the *ori*T sequences of the mobilizable plasmid enable the DNA to move through the conjugative bridge.

Transposons or jumping genes are small pieces of DNA that encode enzymes that enable the transposon to move from one DNA location to another, either on the same molecule of DNA or on a different molecule. Transposons may be found as part of a bacterium chromosome or in plasmids and are usually between 1 and 12 genes long. Each contains a number of genes, such as those coding for antibiotic resistance or other traits, flanked at both ends by insertion sequences coding for an enzyme called transposase that catalyzes the cutting and resealing of DNA during transposition. Many conjugative plasmids and conjugative transposons possess rather promiscuous transfer systems that enable them to transfer DNA not only to like species, but also to unrelated species. The ability of bacteria to adapt to new environments as part of bacterial evolution most frequently results from the acquisition of large DNA sequences from another bacterium by conjugation.

20.3.2.2.2 Transformation Microbes like bacteria can take up pieces of DNA directly from the environment around the cell. This process is relatively common in bacteria, but less so in eukaryotes. A few bacteria such as *Neisseria gonorrhoeae*, *Neisseria meningitidis*, *Hemophilus influenzae, Legionella pneomophila*, *Streptococcus pneumoniae*, and *Helicobacter pylori* tend to be naturally competent and transformable. Competent bacteria are able to bind much more DNA than non-competent bacteria. Some of these genera also undergo autolysis that then provides DNA for homogenous recombination.

In addition, some competent bacteria kill non-competent cells to release DNA for transformation. During transformation, DNA fragments (usually about 10 genes long) are released from a dead degraded bacterium and bind to DNA-binding proteins on the surface of a competent living recipient bacterium. Depending on the bacterium, either both strands of the DNA penetrate the recipient, or a nuclease degrades one strand of the fragment and the remaining DNA strands enter the recipient. This DNA fragment from the donor is then exchanged for a piece of the recipient's DNA by means of RecA proteins and other molecules and this involves breakage and reunion of the paired DNA segments (Winter et al. 2021).

20.3.2.2.3 Transduction Transduction is the process in which bacterial DNA is moved from one bacterium to another by a virus. During the replication of lytic

bacteriophages and temperate bacteriophages, occasionally the phage capsid accidently assembles around a small fragment of bacterial DNA (De la Cruz and Davies 2000). When this bacteriophage, called a transducing particle, infects another bacterium, it injects the fragment of donor bacterial DNA it is carrying into the recipient, where it can subsequently be exchanged for a piece of the recipient DNA by homologous recombination. Transduction can be of generalized and specialized types. Generalized transduction occurs in a variety of bacteria, including *Staphylococcus*, *Escherichia*, *Salmonella*, and *Pseudomonas*. Plasmids, such as the penicillinase plasmid of *S. aureus*, may also be carried from one bacterium to another by this process. Specialized transduction may occur occasionally during the lysogenic life cycle of a temperate bacteriophage. During spontaneous induction, a small piece of bacterial DNA may sometimes be exchanged for a piece of the bacteriophage genome, which remains in the bacterial nucleoid. This piece of bacterial DNA replicates as part of the bacteriophage genome and is put into each phage capsid. The bacteriophages are released, adsorb to recipient bacteria, and inject the donor bacterium DNA/phage DNA complex into the recipient, where it inserts into the bacterial chromosome (Talavera-González et al. 2021).

The whole process of horizontal gene transfer by conjugation, transformation, and transduction is summarized in Figure 20.4.

20.4 Barriers to Effective Surveillance of Antimicrobial Resistance

- Limited staff capacity as well as trained clinical and laboratory personnel, especially microbiologists and health professionals, affects the adequacy of data management (Jayatilleke 2020).
- Poor communication between laboratory stuff and clinical teams leads to delays in reporting results (Ombelet et al. 2018).
- Lack of consumables, diagnostics, and reagents again affects laboratory results (Ombelet et al. 2018).
- There is a shortage of external funding from government and national and international agencies to strengthen laboratory capacity and surveillance (Gandra et al. 2020).
- Quality assurance regarding selection, sampling, and transport of specimens is questionable (Ombelet et al. 2018).
- A weak laboratory infrastructure also greatly influences the quality and reliability of pathogen detection and AMST (Opintan et al. 2015; Dar et al. 2016).

Table 20.2 Antimicrobial resistance reported from different geographical locations (2012–2022).

Year of publication	Year of study	Geographical location	Name of bacteria	Isolate number	Antibiotic resistance	Author
2012	–	Ghana	*Escherichia coli*	27/51	Tetracycline 100% Cefuroxime >90% Chloramphenicol >90% Gentamicin 80% Cotriaxole 65% Amikacin 60% Ampicillin <10% Cefotaxime 0%	Donkor et al. (2012)
2012	–	Iran	*Staphylococcus aureus*	11/44	blaZ gene-6/11 (54%) (blaZ gene-Beta lactamase producing genes responsible for penicillin resistance) blaZ + tetM – 1/11 (9%) (tetM, responsible for tetracycline resistance)	Askari et al. (2012)
2013	–	Kenya	*E. coli*	54/400	Tetracycline 15% Amoxicillin clavulanate 17% Chloramphenicol 4% Sulphamethoxazole-trimethoprim 2% Ampicillin 27% Ceftriaxone 2%	Maina et al. (2013)
2013	–	DG Khan and Lahore districts of Pakistan	*E. coli* *S. aureus* *Streptococcus* spp. *Bacillus* spp. *Corynebacterium* spp. *Pseudomonas* spp.	16/400 90/400 14/400 10/400 6/400 10/400	**For *E. coli*** Streptomycin 87% Tetracycline 50% Norfloxacin/ciprofloxacin 75% Ceftezole/penicillin 62.5% Amoxicillin/enrofloxacin/trimethoprim-sulfamethoxazole 37.5% Gentamicin 25% **For *S. aureus*** Ciprofloxacin 75% Streptomycin/tetracycline/norfloxacin 62.5% Ceftezole 50% Penicillin/enrofloxacin/trimethoprim-sulfamethoxazole 37.5% Amoxycillin 25% Gentamicin 12.5% **For *Streptococcus* spp.** Streptomycin/tetracycline/ciprofloxacin 71.42% Penicillin/norfloxacin 57.14% Ceftezole 42.85% Amoxycillin/enrofloxacin/gentamicin/trimethoprim- sulfamethoxazole 28.57%	Najeeb et al. (2013)

Year		Location	Organism	Isolates	Antibiotic resistance	Reference
2014	–	Grenada and Carriacou island	Corynebacterium jejuni	8/252	Tetracycline 42.9% Metronidazole 28.5%	Stone et al. (2014)
2014	–	Nigeria	E. coli	70/166	Tetracycline 91.43% Cotrimoxazole 94.29% Nitrofurantoin 95.71% Gentamicin 84.28% Ciprofloxacin 15.7% Ofloxacin 1%	Adefarakan et al. (2014)
2015	2005–2007	England and Wales	E. coli	13 isolates	Tetracycline 76.9% Trimethoprim-sulfamethoxazole 69.2% Sulfonamide 76.9% Streptomycin 61.5%	Cheney et al. (2015)
2015	2014	Grenada	E. coli	140 isolates	Streptomycin 19% Tetracycline 7% Nalidixic acid 4% Trimethoprim-sulfamethoxazole 2%	Amadi et al. (2015)
2016	2015	Tanzania	E. coli	2736 isolates	Ampicillin 21.5% Amoxicillin 11.1% Streptomycin 4.7% Sulfamethoxazole 5.7% Tetracycline 7.6% Trimethoprim 4.6%	Mwanyika et al. (2016)
2016	–	Central Java and Riau	S. aureus	24 isolates	Oxacillin 58.33% Tetracycline 16.67 Gentamicin 25% Ampicillin 41.67% Erythromycin 20.83%	Widianingrum et al. (2016)
2016	–	Switzerland	S. aureus	12/34	Tetracycline 35%	Merz et al. (2016)
2016	2015	Tanzania	Salmonella spp.	120 isolates	Ampicillin 2.9% Amoxicillin 0.82% Streptomycin 3.7% Sulfamethoxazole 2.9% Trimethoprim 1.2%	Mwyankiya et al. (2016)
2017	–	Kumaris, Ghana	Campylobacter spp.	32/134	Erythromycin 100% Ampicillin 88% Tetracycline 76% Chloramphenicol 64% Trimethoprim-sulfamethoxazole 60%	Karikari et al. (2017)

(Continued)

Table 20.2 (Continued)

Year of publication	Year of study	Geographical location	Name of bacteria	Isolate number	Antibiotic resistance	Author
2018	–	Pakistan	S. aureus	143/384	**For coagulase-positive _S. aureus_** Ampicillin 60% Amoxicillin 50% Cefotaxime 40% Sulfamethoxazole-trimethoprim 20% Gentamicin 30% Enrofloxacin 20% Chloramphenicol 20% **For coagulase-negative _S. aureus_** Ampicillin 40% Amoxicillin 30% Cefotaxime 20% Gentamicin 20% Ciprofloxacin 10%	Aqib et al. (2018)
2018	2015–2017	China	Corynebacterium pseudotuberculosis	40/102	Nitrofurantoin 100% Furazolidone 100% Streptomycin 100%	Li et al. (2018)
2018	2015	Saudi Arabia	S. aureus		MDR 4.7% MRSA 2%	El-Deeb et al. (2018)
2018	–	Iran	S. aureus		_ermC_ 50% _tetK_ 100% _tetM_ 18% _blaZ_ 100%	Rahmdel et al. (2018)
2018	2015–2016	Jordan	S. aureus	38 isolates	Penicillin 90% Ampicillin 76% Clindamycin 66% Gentamicin 26% Tetracycline 32% Rifampicin 29% Erythromycin 21% Cefotaxime 21% Doxycycline 13% Amoxicillin-clavulanate 21%	Obaidat et al. (2018)

Year		Location	Organism			Reference
2019	–	Eastern Nepal	*E. coli*		**For *E. coli*** Amoxicillin 100% Tetracycline 93% Nalidixic acid 25% **For *Salmonella* spp.** Amoxicillin 100% Tetracycline 24% Chloramphenicol 11% **For *Shigella*** Amoxicillin 100% Chloramphenicol 80% Tetracycline 60% Nalidixic acid 20% **For *Vibrio* spp.** Amoxicillin 100% Tetracycline 40%	Bantawa et al. (2019)
2019	2015–2016	Iran	*Acinetobacter baumannii*	9/162	Streptomycin 7% Gentamicin 8% Amikacin 10% Tobramycin 4% Ciprofloxacin 7% Levofloxacin 3% Chloramphenicol 3% Trimethoprim 14% Cotrimoxazole 11%	Askari et al. (2019)
2019	2017	Virginia University, USA	*E. coli*	408 isolates	Tetracycline 51% Streptomycin 30% Ampicillin 19% Amoxicillin-clavulanate 5%	Ndegwa et al. (2019)

(Continued)

Table 20.2 (Continued)

Year of publication	Year of study	Geographical location	Name of bacteria	Isolate number	Antibiotic resistance	Author
2019	2018	Malaysia	*S. aureus, S. agalactiae, E. coli*	145 milk samples	**For *S. aureus*** Penicillin 93.55% Tetracycline 93.55% Gentamicin 31% Norfloxacin 31% **For *S. agalactiae*** Vancomycin 100% Tetracycline 100% Clindamycin 100% Penicillin 66.67% **For *E. coli*** Gentamicin 100% Chloramphenicol 100% Norfloxacin 100%	Ariffin et al. (2019)
2020	–	Saudi Arabia	*E. coli*	77 (diarrhoea samples)	Kanamycin 20.7% Gentamicin 9.4% Amikacin 1.2% Cefuroxime 2.5% Ceftrazidime 2.5% Norfloxacin 11.3% Nalidixic acid 17.6% Ciprofloxacin 22.6%	Shabana and Al-Enazi (2020)
2020	–	Malaysia	*S. aureus*	198/664	Penicillin 26% Tetracycline 6% Amoxycillin 4% MRSA Penicillin 60% Tetracycline 100%	Chai et al. (2020)
2021	–	Qena, Egypt	*Enterococcus fecalis* *E. faecium* *E. casseli* *E. hirae*	11/34 4/38	**For *Enterococcus fecalis*** Penicillin 64.9% Oxacillin 89.22% Vancomycin 75.7% **For *E. faecium*** Erythromycin 64% Tetracycline 18.9% Linezolide 70.3% Nitrofurantoin 43.2%	El-Zamkan and Mohamed (2021)

MDR, multidrug resistance; MRSA, methicillin-resistant *Staphylococcus aureus*.

20.5 Present Status of Antimicrobial Resistance in Goat Production Practices

There is scant literature available regarding antibiotic resistance among goats in different parts of the world, as goats are regarded as minor livestock for meat production. However, in the previous decade people realized the importance of transmission of antibiotic-resistant genes through the meat and milk of livestock. Most work on it is carried out in Iran, Ethiopia, Ghana, Kenya, Grenada, India, and European countries. The recent published data (2012–2022) on the antibiotic resistance pattern shown by different bacterial isolates collected from goats of different areas is detailed in Table 20.2.

20.6 Conclusion

The indiscriminate use of antibiotics without proper knowledge regarding proper dosing and withdrawal periods by different types of livestock owners, farm managers, and drug practitioners is contributing to developing more and more antibiotic resistance. We need to undertake more research on antibiotic resistance patterns developed in different geographic areas of the world to ascertain the current antibiotic resistance status. We need to educate livestock owners about effects of antibiotic resistance and stop the incremental use of antibiotics in goats.

Multiple-Choice Questions

1   What is the most common cause of acceleration of antimicrobial resistance in small ruminants?
    A   Indiscriminate use of drugs
    B   Unchecked antimicrobial dosage
    C   Inadequate diagnostics
    D   Poor hygiene and sanitation practices

2   What must antibiotic dosing be aimed at?
    A   Only the bacteria isolated
    B   The most resistant subpopulation in the colony
    C   Preventing the advent of further resistant infections
    D   All of the above

3   What are the characteristics of natural antimicrobial resistance?
    A   There can be intrinsic resistance
    B   There can be induced resistance
    C   It does not possess the target site for drugs
    D   All of the above

4   Which of the following feature in acquired antimicrobial resistance?
    A   Microbes obtain the ability to resist the activity of an antimicrobial agent
    B   It does not possess the target site for drugs
    C   Both a and b
    D   None of the above

5   What is an example of acquired resistance?
    A   Methicillin-resistant *Staphylococcus aureus* (MRSA)
    B   Vancomycin-resistant *Staphylococcus aureus* (VRSA)
    C   Polymyxin-resistant *Staphylococcus aureus*
    D   Both a and b

6   If a microbe population becomes resistant to an active ingredient, what is it called?
    A   Side resistance
    B   Acquired resistance
    C   Innate resistance
    D   Cross-resistance

7   What are the features of antimicrobial cross-resistance?
    A   Microbes have the ability to survive therapeutic doses of chemically unrelated drugs with different modes of action
    B   Microbes obtain the ability to resist the activity of an antimicrobial agent
    C   Microbes do not possess the target site for drugs
    D   All of the above

8   When does multiple resistance or multiple drug resistance occur?
    A   Any drug is taken for longer than necessary or when it is not needed
    B   Microbes obtain the ability to resist the activity of an antimicrobial agent
    C   Microbes do not possess the target site for drugs
    D   None of the above

9   What are the mechanisms required for natural resistance?
    A   Permeability barrier
    B   Biofilm formation
    C   Both of the above
    D   None of the above

10   What are the characteristics of Gram-positive bacteria?
   A   No extra layers outside their peptidoglycan layer
   B   Increased susceptibility of bacteria to antimicrobial attack
   C   Presence of lipid bilayer and lipopolysaccharide layer
   D   Both a and b

11   What are the characteristics of Gram-negative bacteria?
   A   Presence of lipid bilayer and lipopolysaccharide layer outside the outer membrane
   B   Reduced susceptibility of bacteria to antimicrobial attack
   C   Increased susceptibility of bacteria to antimicrobial attack
   D   Both a and b

12   What are the characteristics of biofilm formation?
   A   Important form of natural resistance in bacteria
   B   Highly organized communities of bacteria cohabiting in extracellular polymeric substance (EPS) slime
   C   EPS protects the biofilm community against threats from outside, such as biocides and topical antibiotics
   D   All of the above

13   What is acquired resistance mediated through?
   A   Vertical gene transfer
   B   Horizontal gene transfer

   C   Both of the above
   D   Neither of the above

14   What is the common mechanism of acquired resistance?
   A   Modification of antimicrobial target
   B   Decrease in drug uptake
   C   Modification of metabolic enzymes
   D   None of the above

15   How is enzymatic modification of an antimicrobial agent achieved?
   A   Addition of acetyl, adenyl, or phosphate groups
   B   Inactivation of the antimicrobial agent
   C   Inability to bind to the target site
   D   All of the above

16   Which of the following are described correctly?
   A   *tra*Genes enable the bacterium to form a mating pair with another organism
   B   *ori*T (origin of transfer) sequences of the mobilizable plasmid enable the DNA to move through the conjugative bridge
   C   Transposons or jumping genes are small pieces of DNA that encode enzymes that enable the transposon to move from one DNA location to another, either on the same molecule of DNA or on a different molecule.
   D   All of the above

References

Abbott, K.A., Taylor, M.A., and Stubbings, L.A. (2012). *SCOPS–Sustainable Worm Control Strategies for Sheep: A Technical Manual for Veterinary Surgeons and Advisers*, 4e. Madison, MS: Context Publishing.

Acar, J. and Röstel, B. (2001). Antimicrobial resistance: an overview. *Revue Scientifique et Technique* 20 (3): 797–810.

Adediran, O.A. and Uwalaka, E.C. (2015). Effectiveness evaluation of levamisole, albendazole, ivermectin, and *Vernonia amygdalina* in West African Dwarf Goats. *Journal of Parasitology Research* 706824. https://doi.org/10.1155/2015/706824.

Adefarakan, T.A., Oluduro, A.O., David, O.M. et al. (2014). Prevalence of antibiotic resistance and molecular characterization of *Escherichia coli* from faeces of apparently healthy rams and goats in Ile-Ife, southwest, Nigeria. *IFE Journal of Science* 16 (3): 447–460.

Álvarez-Pérez, S., García, M.E., Anega, B. et al. (2021). Antifungal resistance in animal medicine: current state

and future challenges. In: *Fungal Diseases in Animals* (ed. A. Gupta and N. Pratap Singh). Cham: Springer.

Amadi, V., Watson, N., Onyegbule, O. et al. (2015). Antimicrobial resistance profiles of Escherichia coli recovered from feces of healthy free-range chickens in Grenada, West Indies. *International Journal of Current Microbiology and Applied Sciences* 4 (6): 168–175.

Anderson, G.G. and O'Toole, G.A. (2008). Innate and induced resistance mechanisms of bacterial biofilms. *Current Topics in Microbiology Immunology* 322: 85–105.

Aqib, A., Nighat, S., Ahmed, R. et al. (2018). Drug susceptibility profile of Staphylococcus aureus isolated from mastitis milk of goats and risk factors associated with goat mastitis in Pakistan. *Pakistan Journal of Zoology* 51(1). https://doi.org/10.17582/journal.pjz/2019.51.1.307.315.

Arece-García, J., López-Leyva, Y., González-Garduño, R. et al. (2017). Effect of selective anthelmintic treatments on health and production parameters in Pelibuey ewes during lactation. *Tropical Animal Health and Production* 48 (2): 283–287.

Ariffin, S.M.Z., Hasmadi, N., Syawari, N.M. et al. (2019). Prevalence and antibiotic susceptibility pattern of Staphylococcus aureus, Streptococcus agalactiae and Escherichia coli in dairy goats with clinical and subclinical mastitis. *Journal of Animal Health and Production* 7 (1): 32–37.

Askari, E., Soleymani, F., Arianpoor, A. et al. (2012). Epidemiology of mecA-methicillin resistant Staphylococcus aureus (MRSA) in Iran: a systematic review and meta-analysis. *Iranian Journal of Basic Medical Science* 15 (5): 1010–1019.

Askari, N., Momtaz, H., and Tajbakhsh, E. (2019). *Acinetobacter baumannii* in sheep, goat, and camel raw meat: virulence and antibiotic resistance pattern. *AIMS Microbiology* 5 (3): 272–284.

Ayukekbong, J.A., Ntemgwa, M., and Atabe, A.N. (2017). The threat of antimicrobial resistance in developing countries: causes and control strategies. *Antimicrobial Resistance and Infection Control* 6: 47.

Badger, S.B. and McKenna, P.B. (1990). Resistance to ivermectin in a field strain of Ostertagia spp. in goats. *New Zealand Veterinary Journal* 38 (2): 72–74.

Bantawa, K., Sah, S.N., Subba Limbu, D. et al. (2019). Antibiotic resistance patterns of Staphylococcus aureus, Escherichia coli, Salmonella, Shigella and Vibrio isolated from chicken, pork, buffalo and goat meat in eastern Nepal. *BMC Research Notes* 12 (1): 766.

Ben-Ami, R. and Kontoyiannis, D.P. (2021). Resistance to antifungal drugs. *Infectious Disease Clinics of North America* 35 (2): 279–311. https://doi.org/10.1016/j.idc.2021.03.003.

Boma, S., Vitouley, S.H., Somda, M.B. et al. (2022). In vivo analysis of trypanocidal drug resistance in Sahelian goats infected by Trypanosoma vivax strains collected in northern Togo. *Veterinary Parasitology* 306: 109723.

Burmeister, A.R. (2015). Horizontal gene transfer. *Evolution, Medicine, and Public Health* 29 (1): 193–194. https://doi.org/10.1093/emph/eov018.

Cafini, F., Romero, V.M., and Morikawa, K. (2017). Mechanisms of horizontal gene transfer. In: *The Rise of Virulence and Antibiotic Resistance in Staphylococcus aureus* (ed. S. Enany and L.E. Crotty), 61–79. London: IntechOpen https://doi.org/10.5772/65967.

Chai, M.H., Faiq, T.A.M., Ariffin, S.M.Z. et al. (2020). Prevalence of methicillin resistant *Staphylococcus aureus* in raw goat milks from selected farms in Terengganu. *Malaysia. Tropical Animal Science Journal* 43 (1): 64–69.

Cheney, T.E., Smith, R.P., Hutchinson, J.P. et al. (2015). Cross-sectional survey of antibiotic resistance in Escherichia coli isolated from diseased farm livestock in England and Wales. *Epidemiology and Infection* 143 (12): 2653–2659.

Courvalin, P. (1996). The Garrod lecture: evasion of antibiotic action by bacteria. *Journal of Antimicrobial Chemotherapy* 37: 855–869.

Dar, O.A., Hasan, R., Schlundt, J. et al. (2016). Exploring the evidence base for national and regional policy interventions to combat resistance. *Lancet* 387 (10015): 285–295. https://doi.org/10.1016/S0140-6736(15)00520-6.

De la Cruz, F. and Davies, J. (2000). Horizontal gene transfer and the origin of species: lessons from bacteria. *Trends in Microbiology* 8: 128–133.

Donkor, E.S., Newman, M.J., and Yeboah-Manu, D. (2012). Epidemiological aspects of non-human antibiotic usage and resistance: implications for the control of antibiotic resistance in Ghana. *Tropical Medicine & International Health* 17: 462–468.

El-Deeb, W., Fayez, M., Elmoslemany, A. et al. (2018). Methicillin resistant Staphylococcus aureus among goat farms in Eastern province, Saudi Arabia: prevalence and risk factors. *Prevention in Veterinary Medicine*, vol. 156, 84–90.

El-Zamkan, M.A. and Mohamed, H.M.A. (2021). Antimicrobial resistance, virulence genes and biofilm formation in Enterococcus species isolated from milk of sheep and goat with subclinical mastitis. *PLoS One* 16 (11): e0259584.

Eysker, M., van Graafeiland, A.E., and Ploeger, H.W. (2006). Ivermectineresistentie bij teladorsagia circumcincta bij geiten in Nederland [Resistance of Teladorsagia circumcincta in goats to ivermectin in the Netherlands]. *Tijdschrift voor diergeneeskunde* 131 (10): 358–361.

Gandra, S., Alvarez-Uria, G., Turner, P. et al. (2020). Antimicrobial resistance surveillance in low- and middle-income countries: progress and challenges in eight south Asian and southeast Asian countries. *Clinical Microbiology Review* 33 (3): e00048–e00019.

Geary, T.G. (2005). Ivermectin 20 years on: maturation of a wonder drug. *Trends in Parasitology* 21 (11): 530–532.

Hall, C.A., Ritchie, L., and McDonell, P.A. (1981). Investigations for anthelmintic resistance in gastrointestinal nematodes from goats. *Research in Veterinary Science* 31: 116–119.

Haulisah, N.A., Hassan, L., Bejo, S.K. et al. (2021). High levels of antibiotic resistance in isolates from diseased livestock. *Frontiers in Veterinary Science* 8: 652351. https://doi.org/10.3389/fvets.2021.652351.

Hay, S.I., Rao, P.C., Dolecek, C. et al. (2018). Measuring and mapping the global burden of antimicrobial resistance. *BMC Medicine* 416 (1): 78. https://doi.org/10.1186/s12916-018-1073-z.

Igbinosa, I.H. (2015). Prevalence and detection of antibiotic-resistant determinant in Salmonella isolated from food-producing animals. *Tropical Animal Health and Production* 47 (1): 37–43.

Jahn, A. and Nielsen, P.H. (1998). Cellbiomass and exopolymer composition in sewer biofilms. *Water Science and Technology* 37 (1): 17–24.

Jayatilleke, K. (2020). Challenges in implementing surveillance tools of high-income countries (HICs) in low middle income countries (LMICs). *Current Treatment Options in Infectious Diseases* 12 (3): 191–201. https://doi.org/10.1007/s40506-020-00229-2.

Kaplan, R.M. (2004). Drug resistance in nematodes of veterinary importance: a status report. *Trends in Parasitology* 20 (10): 477–481.

Karikari, A.B., Obiri-Danso, K., Frimpong, E.H. et al. (2017). Antibiotic resistance of *Campylobacter* recovered from faeces and carcasses of healthy livestock. *Biomedical Research International* 2017: 4091856.

Lambert, P.A. (2005). Bacterial resistance to antibiotics: modified target sites. *Advanced Drug Delivery Review* 57 (10): 1471–1485.

Leggett, M.J., McDonnell, G., Denyer, S.P. et al. (2012). Bacterial spore structures and their protective role in biocide resistance. *Journal of Applied Microbiology* 113: 485–498.

Li, H., Yang, H., Zhou, Z. et al. (2018). Isolation, antibiotic resistance, virulence traits and phylogenetic analysis of Corynebacterium pseudotuberculosis from goats in southwestern China. *Small Ruminant Research* 168: 69–75.

Maina, D., Makau, P., Nyerere, A. et al. (2013). Antimicrobial resistance patterns in extended-spectrum β-lactamase producing Escherichia coli and Klebsiella pneumoniae isolates in a private tertiary hospital. *Kenya. Microbiology Discovery* 1 (5): 1–4.

Mathur, S. and Singh, R. (2005). Antibiotic resistance in food lactic acid bacteria—a review. *International Journal of Food Microbiology* 105: 281–295.

McDonnell, G. and Russell, A.D. (1999). Antiseptics and disinfectants: activity, action and resistance. *Clinical Microbiology Reviews* 12: 147–179.

McManus, M.C. (1997). Mechanisms of bacterial resistance to antimicrobial agents. *American Journal of Health-System Pharmacy* 54: 1420–1433.

Merz, A., Stephan, R., and Johler, S. (2016). Staphylococcus aureus isolates from goat and sheep milk seem to be closely related and differ from isolates detected from bovine milk. *Frontiers in Microbiology* 7: 319.

Mwanyika, G., Call, D.R., Rugumisa, B. et al. (2016). Load and prevalence of antimicrobial-resistant Escherichia coli from fresh goat meat in Arusha. *Tanzania. Journal of Food Protection* 79 (9): 1635–1641.

Najeeb, M.F., Anjum, A.A., Ahmad, M.U.D. et al. (2013). *Journal of Animal & Plant Sciences* 23 (6): 1541–1544.

Ndegwa, E., Almehmadi, H., Kim, C. et al. (2019). Longitudinal shedding patterns and characterization of antibiotic resistant *E. coli* in pastured goats using a cohort study. *Antibiotics* 8 (3): 136.

Nipane, S.F., Mishra, B., and Panchbuddhe, A.N. (2008). Anthelmintic resistance—clinician's present concern. *Veterinary World* 1 (9): 281.

Njoroge, S., Muigai, A.W.T., Njiruh, P.N. et al. (2013). Molecular characterisation and antimicrobial resistance patterns of *Escherichia coli* isolates from goats slaughtered in parts of Kenya. *East African Medical Journal* 90 (3): 72–83.

Obaidat, M.M., Salman, A.E., Davis, M.A. et al. (2018). Major diseases, extensive misuse, and high antimicrobial resistance of Escherichia coli in large- and small-scale dairy cattle farms in Jordan. *Journal of Dairy Science* 101 (3): 2324–2334.

Odoi, A., Samuels, R., Carter, C. et al. (2021). Antibiotic prescription practices and opinions regarding antimicrobial resistance among veterinarians in Kentucky, USA. *Plos One* 16 (40): e0249653.

Ombelet, S., Ronat, J.B., Walsh, T. et al. (2018). Clinical bacteriology in low-resource settings: today's solutions. *Lancet Infectious Diseases* 18 (8): e248–e258. https://doi.org/10.1016/S1473-3099(18)30093-8.

Opintan, J.A., Newman, M.J., Arhin, R.E. et al. (2015). Laboratory-based nationwide surveillance of antimicrobial resistance in Ghana. *Infection and Drug Resistance* 8: 379–389.

Poole, K. (2002). Mechanisms of bacterial biocide and antibiotic resistance. *Journal of Applied Microbiology* 92: 55S–64S.

Quick, J. and Bremer, K. (1997). Quality control of essential drugs. *Lancet* 350: 1106.

Rahmdel, S., Hosseinzadeh, S., Shekarforoush, S.S. et al. (2018). Safety hazards in bacteriocinogenic *Staphylococcus* strains isolated from goat and sheep milk. *Microbial Pathogenesis* 116: 100–108.

Ramay, B.M., Caudell, M.A., Cordón-Rosales, C. et al. (2020). Antibiotic use and hygiene interact to influence the distribution of antimicrobial-resistant bacteria in low-income communities in Guatemala. *Scientific Reports* 10 (1): 1–10.

Roberts, J.A., Kruger, P., Paterson, D.L. et al. (2008). Antibiotic resistance – What's dosing got to do with it? *Critical Care Medicine* 36 (8): 2433–2440.

Shabana, I.I. and Al-Enazi, A.T. (2020). Investigation of plasmid-mediated resistance in *E. coli* isolated from healthy and diarrheic sheep and goats. *Saudi Journal of Biological. Science* 27 (3): 788–796.

Stone, D.M., Chander, Y., Bekele, A.Z. et al. (2014). Genotypes, antibiotic resistance, and ST-8 genetic clone in Campylobacter isolates from sheep and goats in Grenada. *Veterinary Medicine International* 2014: 212864.

Sutherland, I. (2001). Biofilm exopolysaccharides: a strong and sticky framework. *Microbiology* 147: 3–9.

Tahamtan, Y., Hayati, M., and Namavari, M.M. (2014). Isolation and Identification of Pasteurella multocida by PCR from sheep and goats in Fars province. *Iran. Archives of Razi Institute* 69 (1): 89–93.

Talavera-González, J.M., Talavera-Rojas, M., Soriano-Vargas, E. et al. (2021). In vitro transduction of antimicrobial resistance genes into *Escherichia coli* isolates from backyard poultry in Mexico. *Canadian Journal of Microbiology* 67 (5): 415–425. https://doi.org/10.1139/cjm-2020-0280.

Tenover, F.C. (2006). Mechanisms of antimicrobial resistance in bacteria. *American Journal of Medicine* 119: 3–10.

Tsuneda, S., Aikawa, H., Hayashi, H. et al. (2003). Extracellular polymeric substances responsible for bacterial adhesion onto solid surface. *FEMS Microbiology Letters* 223: 287–292.

Widianingrum, D.C., Windria, S., and Salasia, S.I.O. (2016). Antibiotic resistance and methicillin resistant *Staphylococcus aureus* isolated from bovine, crossbred Etawa goat and human. *Asian Journal of Animal Veterinary Advances* 11: 122–129.

Winter, M., Buckling, A., Harms, K. et al. (2021). Antimicrobial resistance acquisition via natural transformation: context is everything. *Current Opinion in Microbiology* 64: 133–138. https://doi.org/10.1016/j.mib.2021.09.009.

World Health Organization (2018). *Global Antimicrobial Resistance Surveillance System (GLASS) Report: Early Implementation 2017–2018*. Geneva: WHO.

World Health Organization (2021). Antimicrobial resistance. Geneva: WHO. https://www.who.int/health-topics/antimicrobial-resistance.

21

Prevention and Control Strategy in Combating Diseases of Goats

Amita Tiwari[1], Shivangi Udainiya[1] and Tanmoy Rana[2]

[1] *Department of Veterinary Medicine, College of Veterinary Science & Animal Husbandry, Nanaji Deshmukh Veterinary Science University, Jabalpur, Madhya Pradesh, India*
[2] *Department of Veterinary Clinical Complex, West Bengal University of Animal & Fishery Sciences, Kolkata, West Bengal, India*

Goats contribute substantially to the Indian economy in terms of production of meat, wool, hide, milk, and so on. In terms of goat population and milk production, India occupies first position in the world. Not only that, but goat rearing also ensures self-employment and acts as a cushion during natural calamities like drought and famine. It therefore serves as an important means of livelihood and nutritional security for small marginal farmers and landless rural households (Figure 21.1). The main constraints hindering the productivity of the livestock sector in most countries are diseases, poor nutrition, breeding policies, and management.

There are various kinds of diseases that affect the health of the goat and important steps needs to be taken to prevent and control these diseases. Prevention is the basic principle for controlling any disease. The introduction of diseases onto farms is a major concern of every goat-keeper. The goat-farm owner or individual goat-raisers in small rural areas are cautious about the control and management of goats to prevent any unusual occurrence of diseases. The farm or individual shelter should be disease free. Diseases can enter the property from many sources (Figure 21.2). The introduction of new animals to the farm is one of the importance sources for introduction of any disease. Breeding services; goat shows; entry of visitors; infectious materials like clothing, shoes, skin, and hair; unclean conditions in pens and pastures; and poor health management practices are also sources for the introduction of disease. Goats new to the farm/shelter should be quarantined for a minimum of four weeks, during which time they should be dewormed and observed closely.

Quarantine of new animals brought from outside the property is an essential step to protect goats from bacteria, viruses, and other organisms that new animals might be carrying (Figures 21.3–21.5). This chapter discusses the prevention and control of goats from any incidence of disease. There are various measures to be undertaken for the prevention and control of diseases of goats.

21.1 Control of Infectious Diseases

Most diseases in goats are self-limiting and do not require any specific treatment or preventive measures, but a few of them have severe effects on goat health and production. Some infectious diseases are of economic importance and also hence require special attention (Figure 21.6). There are various means by which these diseases can be prevented. Most can be prevented by proper sanitation, a controlled diet, suitable housing, and also by vaccinating animals against these diseases at the right time and age.

21.1.1 Biosecurity Measures

Biosecurity mainly focuses on preventing the spread of infectious agents from an infected animal to susceptible animals. A biosecurity plan must take into account all modes of transmission, including direct animal contact within a herd, contact with wild animals or other domesticated species, airborne transmission, contaminated feed or water, and visitors or vehicles that come onto the farm. The most common and important method of disease control in an individual herd is to avoid introduction of disease agents. Most diseases of a contagious nature are introduced into operations when new animals are added. Disease agents can be introduced when breeding animals are added to an operation; when animals mingle at a fair, show, or sale; or when animals come into contact with wildlife.

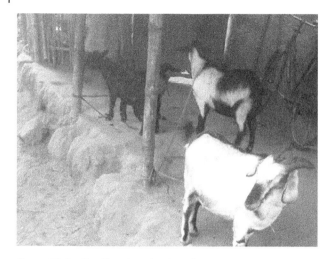

Figure 21.1 Small-scale animal rearing.

If a closed herd or flock is not feasible, then use an animal quarantine program. A useful isolation program consists of a facility that prevents mingling of animals for at least 30 days, including separate water supplies.

The issues an effective biosecurity program must address can be complicated because of all the potential routes of disease transmission. An effective disease control program must address traffic control, sanitation, food safety, personal hygiene, good management practices (GMP), generally accepted (GA) hygiene, quality assurance and herd health, bioterrorism, and isolation or quarantine. Although the issues that a biosecurity program must address are diverse and complicated, the management practices that are part of an effective program are usually simple and easy to incorporate into a normal production system.

Figure 21.2 An organized animal farm.

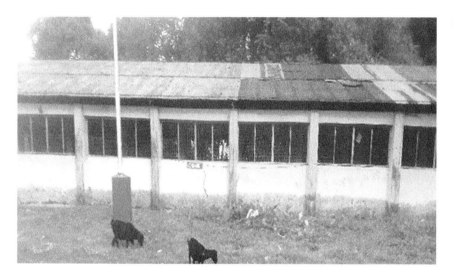

(a)

(b)

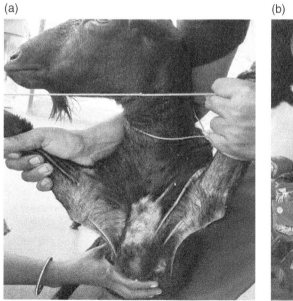
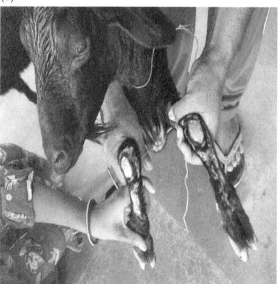

Figure 21.3 (a, b) Various manifestations of disease.

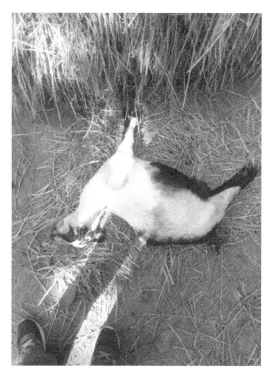

Figure 21.4 A goat that died due to disease.

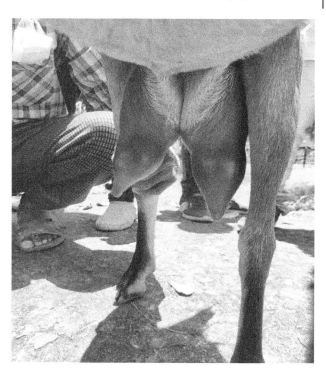

Figure 21.5 A swollen udder.

Figure 21.6 Preventive strategy to control disease before the entrance of new animals.

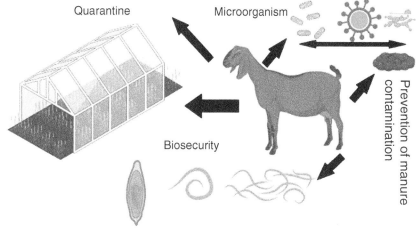

The following are some measures and practices that should be adopted by producers to ensure safety and herd health (Figure 21.7):

- Prevention is better than cure – prevent problems occurring rather than correcting them.
- Implement individual and premises animal identification programs.
- Good record-keeping helps in better and effective management practices.

- The health history of the herds should be maintained when new animals are purchased.
- Attempt to prevent manure contamination by never stepping into feed bunks.
- Quarantine and isolate new and sick animals.
- Routinely clean and disinfect feeding equipment, which can be done with chlorine, iodine, or quaternary ammonia products.
- Routinely clean and disinfect equipment used to medicate animals, especially equipment used on multiple animals.

Good herd health

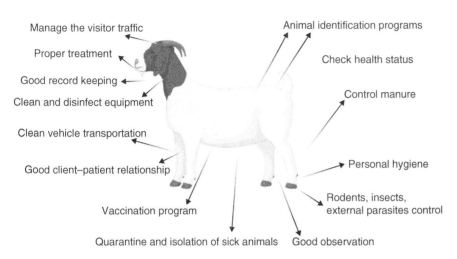

Manage the visitor traffic

Proper treatment

Good record keeping

Clean and disinfect equipment

Clean vehicle transportation

Good client–patient relationship

Vaccination program

Quarantine and isolation of sick animals

Good observation

Animal identification programs

Check health status

Control manure

Personal hygiene

Rodents, insects,
external parasites control

Figure 21.7 Maintenance of good herd management.

- Provide a clean area for restraint, treatment, and isolation of sick animals.
- Consult with a veterinarian or animal health personnel when goats are ill or die unexpectedly.
- It is very important to monitor and manage visitor traffic.
- Know the health status of animals brought into the herd.
- Transport animals in clean vehicles.
- Properly dispose of carcasses of dead animals.
- Have a control program for other animals that could spread disease (rodents, insects, external parasites, etc.).
- Control manure and dispose of it frequently.
- Maintain good personal hygiene.
- Be observant.
- Maintain a good relationship with a veterinarian.
- Have a sound vaccination program.

21.1.2 Vaccination

When we rear a number of animals in one place and have insufficient pasture facilities, an intensive system of rearing leads to the spread of many diseases. This causes reduced production potential and more mortality, which in turn results in economic losses to farmers. Hence identification of diseases in goat and their prevention are very important (Table 21.1).

Vaccination is important in animals for several reasons:

- Veterinary vaccines have had, and continue to have, a major role in protecting animal health and public health, reducing animal suffering, enabling efficient production of food animals to feed the burgeoning human population, and greatly reducing the need for antibiotics to treat food and companion animals.

- Vaccinating animals helps in stimulating an immune response without causing the disease itself. This creates early exposure to disease-causing organisms, where the animals' immune system is able to recall the infectious agent against which the animal is vaccinated.
- Vaccination helps provide sustainable and economic stability for farmers and the communities they serve.
- When animals are not well cared for it leads to reduced resistance to diseases and leads to the development of clinical diseases.
- Vaccines are efficient in preventing the transmission and spread of contagious animal diseases (zoonotic diseases) from animals to people and from animal to animal.
- Vaccination is a cost-effective method used in preventing animal diseases; vaccines are generally safe, efficient, and are associated with few severe side effects.
- Vaccination is good for long-term prevention because diseases and illnesses that may cost more than the vaccines are avoided.

Certain measures need to be taken before, during, and after the vaccination of animals:

- Deworming should be done at least one week before vaccination so that parasites do not interfere in the immune response.
- The cold chain of the vaccine should be maintained.
- Only sterilized and disposable syringes and needles should be used for vaccination and disposed of properly after use.
- The vaccine should be given at a proper dose and route, as mentioned on the vial of the product.
- Avoid vaccinating sick and stressed animals.
- Any kind of antibiotic or immunosuppressant drug should not be given to the animal post vaccination.

Table 21.1 Bacterial and viral diseases.

Disease	Symptoms	Prevention	Vaccine	Dose and route
Bacterial diseases				
Anthrax	Sudden fever and death Dark-colored bloody discharge from natural orifices such as nose, anus, and vagina	Vaccination once a year in affected areas Disposal of carcass by either burying or burning Do not open the carcass as the germs spread through air	Anthrax live spore vaccine	0.5 ml IM
Hemorrhagic septicemia	Fever Dysentery Swelling of lower mandible and death Higher occurrence in rainy season	Vaccinate once a year before onset of the rainy season	H·S oil adjuvant vaccine	2 ml IM or SC
Brucellosis	Abortion during late pregnancy Infertility Scrotal swelling in male Joint swelling	Disposal of dead fetus and placenta Use gloves while handling infected items as it affect human beings	*Brucella abortus* Strain-19 live vaccine	
Enterotoxemia	Sudden death in young growing kids Mucous diarrhea may also be seen during death	Vaccinate once a year before the onset of the monsoon Do not feed on young grass	Enterotoxemia vaccine	3–5 ml SC
Pneumonia	Fever Respiratory distress Mucous discharge from nostril Reduced feed intake Weight gain Cough	Clean water, well-ventilated house		
Foot rot	Wound in foot region	Keep animals in a dry clean house		
Mastitis	Swelling of udder Change in milk	Clean shed, wash udder with disinfectant solution		
Viral diseases				
Peste des petits ruminants (PPR)	Fever Ocular and nasal mucous discharge Mouth lesion Respiratory distress	Yearly vaccinationSeparation of infected from healthy animals	Live attenuated PPR vaccine	1 ml SC
Foot and mouth disease (FMD)	Fever Wound lesion in foot and mouth Excess salivary secretion Difficulty in walking	First vaccination at 3rd month and then once at 4–6-month interval	FMD inactivated polyvalent vaccine	1 ml IM
Goat pox	Fever Ocular and nasal mucous discharge Respiratory distress Pox lesions on non-hairy parts such as lips, thigh, udder, etc.	Yearly vaccination (optional)	Sheep and goat pox vaccine	0.3 g triturated vaccine mixed with 30 ml glycerine for 100 animals SC or IM route

IM, intramuscular; SC, subcutaneous.

21.2 Control of Endoparasites/ Internal Parasites

Goats are considered to be very sensitive to the effects of endoparasites, which are responsible for various ill effects in goats such as increased susceptibility to disease, anemia, hypoproteinemia, decreased fertility, abortion, unthriftiness, and death (Figure 21.8 and Table 21.2). The effect of parasitism is determined by the interactions between the type of parasites present in a geographic area, the parasite life cycles, the environment including weather patterns and type of farm management, and the host factors.

Goats are usually affected by all three types of worms: nematodes, cestodes, and trematodes.

21.2.1 Nematodes

There are a large number of species of nematodes that live at different levels of the gastrointestinal tract. Most infections are mixed, but three species stand out in their pathogenicity: *Haemonchus*, *Ostertagia*, and *Trichostrongylus*.

- ***Haemonchus contortus***: This is also known as the barber pole worm and is one of the most common worms in goats. This parasite is economically important, one of the most serious parasite pathogens, and fourth-stage larvae and adults are aggressive blood feeders and live in the abomasum. Severely afflicted goats develop anemia, bottle jaw, weakness, reluctance to move, exercise intolerance, and weight loss.
- ***Ostertagia circumcincta***: The larvae of this parasite live in the gastric glands of the stomach and are responsible for causing inflammation and leakage of protein into the intestinal tract, resulting in low protein, bottle jaw, and diarrhea.
- ***Trichostongylus* spp.**: Larvae live in either the abomasum or the small intestine and cause problems similar to *Ostertagia*. Severely afflicted goats develop loss of condition and appetite, poor growth, dull attitude, diarrhea, bottle jaw, pot-bellied appearance, and death. Treatment

includes supportive care (fluids, good nutrition) and deworming with anthelminthics.

21.2.2 Cestodes

Goats are also subject to cestode or tapeworm infestation.

- ***Moniezia* spp.**: This is the most common cestode and usually does not cause clinical disease except with heavy infections. Eggs passed in proglottid segments in feces are taken up by mites living on pasture. An intermediate stage develops in the mite over four months, which matures to the adult tapeworm in the host after the mites are consumed during grazing. Rarely, it causes ill thrift and weight loss in kids during their first summer on pasture. Very severe infections can cause intestinal obstruction predisposing to enterotoxemia and, potentially, intestinal rupture. Treatment is fenbendazole at 15 mg/kg orally; albendazole 10 mg/kg; oxfendazole (10 mg/kg); or oral niclosamide 50 mg/kg.

21.2.3 Trematodes

- ***Fasciola hepatica***: This is known as the common liver fluke. It needs the right snail host, and the right combination of temperature and moisture. Goat saffected with liver fluke infestation show poor appetite, lethargy, and weight loss; acute cases die suddenly. Treatment mainly includes triclabendazole (not in first three months of pregnancy) at 15 mg/kg orally.
- ***Fascioloides magna***: Known as the large American liver fluke, the parasite's natural hosts are deer and elk and it is found in the Adirondacks. Goats become infected in late summer when grazing swampy areas also inhabited by wild ruminants, and develop clinical signs (usually sudden death) in January or February. One fluke can kill a goat. Control by fencing off marshy pastures or prophylactic treatment with albendazole one month after the first killing frost.

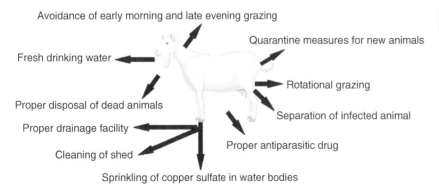

Figure 21.8 Control measures for endoparasites on the farm.

Table 21.2 Endoparasites affecting the goat.

Endoparasite	Symptoms	Anthelmentic drug	Dose	Route	Remarks	Prevention
Nematodes	Fever, anemia, edema in lower jaw, reduced growth	Piperazine	110–200 mg/kg	Oral	First dose to be given within 5–6 days of birth Repeat at 45-day intervals	Deworming at regular intervals
		Tetramisole	15 mg/kg BW	Oral		
		Morantel Citrate	10 mg/kg BW	Oral		
		Levamisole	7.5 mg/kg BW	Oral once		
Trematodes	Emaciation, anemia, edema in lower jaw	Oxyclozanide	10–15 mg/kg BW	Oral once	Deworming at 4–6-month intervals	Control of snails, avoid grazing in early morning and late evening, deworming of animals periodically
		Fenbendazole	5–7.5 mg/kg BW	Oral		
		Albendazole	5–10 mg/kg BW			
		Tricalbebdazole	10–12 mg/kg BW	Oral		
		Rafoxanide	7.5 mg/kg BW	Oral		
Cestodes	Reduced growth, fever, kid mortality	Dichlorophen	0.5 mg/kg BW	Oral	Deworming at 4–6-month intervals	Deworming at regular intervals
		Albendazole	5–10 mg/kg BW	Oral once		
		Fenbendazole	5–7.5 mg/kg BW	Oral once		

BW, body weight.

- ***Dicrocoelium dendriticum***: This is the small liver fluke, whose life cycle includes snails and ants. Clinical signs such as chronic weight loss and depression are rare, but livers may be condemned at slaughter. Treatment is with albendazole (not in the first three months of pregnancy) at 15 mg/kg orally.

21.2.4 Lungworms

Goats are also subject to lungworm infestation from three main types of lungworm: *Dictyocaulus filaria*, *Protostrongylus*, and *Parelaphostrongylus tenuis*:

- ***Dictyocaulus filaria***: This lungworm has a direct life cycle and is the most pathogenic; adults live in the bronchi. Adults produce eggs within one month. Clinical signs include increased respiratory rate, difficult breathing, and coughing. Ivermectin, levamisole, and fenbendazole will kill larval stages and adults.
- ***Protostrongylus***: This lives in the bronchi and usually does not cause clinical disease except in kids. Levamisole is not effective. Two doses of fenbendazole at 15 mg/kg or of ivermectin will kill the larval stages.
- ***Parelaphostrongylus tenuis***: The meningeal worm in goats causes severe neurological disease due to aberrant migration of the parasite through the spinal cord. The life cycle is indirect, with terrestrial snails as intermediate hosts. Keeping goats off fields frequented by deer will limit infections. Ivermectin is generally used to treat lungworm infestation (Stehman and Smith 2004, pp. 1–9).

21.2.5 Deworming Schedule for Goats

- Deworming of kids should be done at the age of 1 month and then once a month up to 6 months of age.
- Dewormer should be given according to the weight of the animal.
- In adult goats, deworming should be done at an interval of 2–3 months.
- Deworming should be done with the advice of a veterinary doctor.
- Dewormers should be changed at regular intervals. Excess or low dosage and the repeating of a deworming drug may lead to the development of drug resistance. This may reduce the effect of the dewormer.
- It is better to give a combination of dewormers for multiple worms than one for a specific worm.

21.2.6 Common Measures for Control of Endoparasites

- Proper drainage and sprinkling of copper sulfate near water bodies will help to control fluke infection
- Avoid early-morning and late-evening grazing.
- Keep the shed clean and provide clean, good-quality drinking water.
- Separate infected animals from healthy ones.
- Provide proper quarantine measures when purchasing new animals.
- Ensure proper disposal of dead animals.
- Practice rotational grazing to control infection.

21.3 Control of Ectoparasites/ External Parasites

Ectoparasites must be treated carefully because they not only affect growth, they also affect skin quality, which leads to economic loss to producers (Figure 21.9). Common external goat parasites include ticks, lice, and mites. Some parasites feed on blood, causing blood-loss anemia, especially in young animals. The result is unthrifty, poor-performing sheep and goats. A regular program of treatment and prevention of external parasites should be an important part of a flock health program. An effective external parasite control program must include increased comfort for animals, improved performance, and higher quality of products (Table 21.3).

21.3.1 Ticks

Ticks may be divided into two major groups: soft ticks (Argasidae) and hard ticks (Ixodidae). Hard ticks can further be divided into three (one-host, two-host, and three-host ticks) depending on the number of hosts involved in their life cycle. Their effects are various, including reduced growth, milk, and meat production; damaged hides and

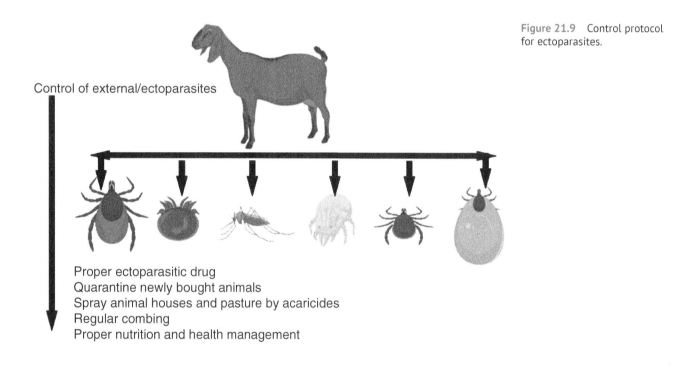

Figure 21.9 Control protocol for ectoparasites.

Control of external/ectoparasites

Proper ectoparasitic drug
Quarantine newly bought animals
Spray animal houses and pasture by acaricides
Regular combing
Proper nutrition and health management

Table 21.3 Common pesticides used for control of ectoparasites in animals.

Pesticides	Uses	Doses
Cypermethrin 10% w/v	Ticks, lice, flies, mites, midges, and keds	Dilute 1–2 ml in 1 l water and apply on whole body as spray or bath Repeat after 15 days to kill newly emerged larva and adults from egg For animal houses: dilution rate is 20 ml/l water
Deltamethrin 12.5 mg/ml	Ticks, lice, flies, mites, and keds	For ticks: dilution rate 2–3 ml/l water For mites: 4–6 ml/l water For lice: 1–2 ml/l water For flies: 2–3 ml/l water
Amitraz 12.5% w/v	Ticks, lice, flies, and mites	Dilute 2–4 ml/l water and spray or wash all over body Repeat application 3 times at 15-day intervals
Ivermectin 1% w/v	Mange	1 ml/50 kg body weight by subcutaneous route

skins; transmission of tick-borne diseases of various types; and predisposing animals to secondary attacks from other parasites such as screwworm flies and infection by pathogens such as *Dermatophilus congolensis*, the causative agent of streptothricosis. Other losses directly attributable to ticks include skin damage that greatly lowers value of the skin. Some of the tick-borne parasitic infections in sheep and goats include the following:

- *Babesia ovis*, transmitted by *Rhipicephalus bursa* and *Rhipicephalus evertsi*.
- *Babesia motasi*, transmitted by *Haemaphysalis* spp., *Dermacentor* spp., and *Rhipicephalus bursa*.
- *Theileria ovis*, transmitted by *Rhipicephalus bursa* and *Rhipicephalus evertsi*.
- *Anaplasma ovis*, transmitted by *Rhipicephalus bursa* and *Rhipicephalus evertsi*.
- Heartwater, transmitted by *Amblyomma herbarium* and *Amblyomma variegatum*.
- Tick paralysis, transmitted by *Ixodes rubicundus*, *Rhipicephalus evertsi*, *Amblyomma* spp., and *Dermacentor* spp.

21.3.1.1 Treatment, Prevention, and Control of Ticks

- The most effective and most widely used method of tick control is acaricide application.
- Chances of reinfection of the host are very high in areas where many ticks exist and therefore treatment must be repeated regularly.
- In sub-humid areas the period of highest tick activity is the wet season and only a few ticks are found on animals during the dry season. In lowland areas most ticks are active throughout the year and must be controlled continuously.
- Treat all newly arrived animals before adding them to the flock.
- Treat with acaricides only where ticks are present in large numbers. If tick numbers are not large, then use a needle or thorn to kill them.
- Knapsack spraying is the most practical method if more intensive control measures are needed for a small number of animals. The most efficient method of hand spraying is to spray along the entire length of the back, then spray the sides and flanks in a zigzag pattern. After that spray the brisket, each leg, belly, udder or scrotum, tail, and anal area. Finally spray the head, face, neck, and ears.
- External parasites can be removed by dipping. It is best to avoid dipping pregnant and sick animals (Ethiopia Sheep and Goat Productivity Improvement Program 2010, pp. 2–10).

21.3.2 Lice

Lice are small, wingless insects and are host specific. They can only survive for a very short period of time away from the host. Basically there are two types of lice: biting lice and sucking lice. Biting lice graze on epidermal tissue, hair, and other organic waste. They cause intense itching by their action. Sucking lice have mouthparts adapted for penetrating the skin of the host and sucking blood. Both immature and adult stages suck the blood or feed on the skin. Lice are generally transmitted from one animal to another by direct contact. There population increases greatly during the rainy season.

Lice have a tendency to multiply very fast and are responsible for causing anemia, unthriftiness, emaciation, reduced weight gain, and loss of production. The saliva and feces of lice contain substances capable of causing allergies and giving rise to severe irritation to the skin. This is usually shown by the animal rubbing itself against objects. Lice do not transmit a serious disease in goats.

21.3.2.1 Treatment and Control of Lice Infestation

Spraying or dipping with insecticides is effective, but it should always be carried out twice, the first time to kill the lice currently on the body, the second 14 days later to kill lice hatching from eggs present at the first treatment. Eggs are not affected by insecticides. If there is more than one goat, then all must be treated or the problem will keep reoccurring (Ethiopia Sheep and Goat Productivity Improvement Program 2010, pp. 2–10).

21.3.3 Mites

Mites are microscopic ectoparasites that remain in direct contact with the skin. All the stages of the mite stay on the animal, feeding on the epidermis, serum, and hair, and in some cases burrowing beneath the epidermis or into hair follicles. Mites spread from one animal to another mainly through direct contact. They do not survive very long when removed from the animal. They lead to skin inflammation, often accompanied by hair loss. High temperature, humidity, and sunlight favor mange mite infestation. Major mange mites may be psoroptic, sarcoptic, or demodectic, according to the species of infesting mite.

21.3.3.1 Psoroptic Mange

Psoroptic mange is a highly contagious disease of goats. *Psoroptes* are highly host specific, live on the surface of the skin, and are non-burrowing. They pierce the skin and suck the host's tissue fluids, causing irritation and inflammation, and discharging lymph fluid that dries to form yellowish crusts and scabs that often protect them. Psoroptic mites may be found even in the ear canal (ear mange). Affected skin is located in most areas of the body, such as shoulders, sides, and back, and is covered with exudate. This dries to form scabs. Massive loss of hair usually occurs. Mites are usually more active in winter and the oviposition rate is higher at lower temperatures.

21.3.3.2 Sarcoptic Mange

Sarcoptic mange is a very serious problem in goats and is even responsible for causing death of the animal. It is caused by infestation with *Sarcoptes scabiei* var. *capri* in goats and is more acute than the other forms of mange, in that it may involve the entire body surface in a short time. Sarcoptic mange is highly contagious. Its spread is mainly by close physical contact between infected and healthy animals. It usually starts on a relatively hairless part of the skin and may later generalize. The mites burrow into the skin and form tunnels, where they remain for the rest of their lives. They cause small red papules on the skin. The affected area is itchy and frequently damaged by scratching and biting. Loss of hair, thick brown scabs, and thickening and wrinkling of the surrounding skin are observed.

21.3.3.3 Demodectic Mange

Demodectic mange invades the hair follicles and sebaceous glands of all species of domestic animals. It is a very serious problem in goats and is even responsible for causing death of the animal. The lesions consist of thick scabs overlaying the skin, which is reddened and thickened, usually round the eyelids, nose, brisket, lower neck, forearm, shoulder, and the tips of the ears. In severe cases there may be general hair loss and thickening of the skin. Animals become immunocompromised with severe demodectic mange. The disease spreads slowly and transfer of mites takes place by contact. Demodectic mange causes small nodules and pustules that may develop into large abscesses. The contents of the pustules are usually white in color and cheesy in consistency. In large abscesses the pus is more fluid.

21.3.3.4 Control and Treatment Strategy for Mange Mites

- Treatment and control should focus on all animals in a flock to achieve control.
- If spraying, start at the head, finish at the tail, and spray all areas of the body thoroughly.
- There is no acaricide yet that readily destroys the eggs of mange mites; thus a second treatment is necessary after 7 days for psoroptic mange and 14 days for sarcoptic mange to deal with the newly hatching parasites.

- Thick scabs and crusts should be loosened or removed mechanically with a comb before spraying. The animal can be washed with soap and water to soften and remove the epidermal scales.
- Spray animal houses and pasture fences with acaricides.
- Animals newly introduced to a flock are the main source of infection.
- Quarantine newly bought animals and treat them twice before they join the herd.
- Dipping is more effective than spraying. Acaricides such as diazinon 60% and ivermectin injection (0.2 mg/kg) are effective (Ethiopia Sheep and Goat Productivity Improvement Program 2010, pp. 2–10).

21.4 Control of Protozoal Infections

21.4.1 Coccidiosis

Coccidia is a protozoan that infects various species of animals, including goats. *Coccidia* are host specific; some species are more pathogenic than others (*Eimeria ninakohlyakimovae* is the most pathogenic) (Figure 21.10 and Table 21.4). Resistance to infection increases with age, but is specific to the infecting species of *Coccidia* and depends on continuous exposure to the parasite. Adult goats normally shed low numbers of oocysts, but are usually resistant to clinical disease unless they are exposed to a new species, an overwhelming dose, and/or stressors such as shipping, weather or feed changes, lactation, or concurrent diseases.

Sporulated oocysts are ingested and immature stages go through a complex series of replications and changes in the wall of the intestine, which amplifies the infection and causes damage to the intestine. Clinical disease, which is usually seen in 3–5-month-old kids, starts two weeks after ingestion and is caused by destruction of the intestinal cell wall by the organisms. Kids are most susceptible at weaning, but coccidiosis can be seen as early as 2 weeks of age. Clinical signs in kids include abdominal pain, diarrhea +/− fresh blood (not as common in goats as in calves), anemia, weakness, weight loss, and dehydration. If kids survive clinical disease, compensatory weight gain occurs, but survivors can be unthrifty and require additional time to match weights of uninfected animals of the same age.

21.4.1.1 Treatment and Control of Coccidiosis

- Symptomatic and supportive treatment can be given to the animal, including oral or parenteral balanced electrolytes to prevent dehydration.
- In severe cases, antibiotics are advised to prevent bacterial invasion of the disrupted intestinal wall with subsequent septicemia.

Figure 21.10 Control measures for
protozoal infection.

Symptomatic and supportive
treatment

Maintenance of dehydration
Proper hygiene and
sanitation

Stress-free environment

Dry bedding

Fecal contamination –
prevention

Sunlight and drying of
premises

Nutrition and health
management

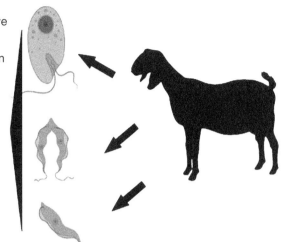

Table 21.4 *Eimeria* species identified in goats.

Species	Affinity site	Hosts
E. alijevi	Small and large intestines	Domestic goat
E. caprina	Small and large intestines	Domestic goat
E. ninakohlyakimovae	Small and large intestines	Domestic goat, Ibex, Persian gazelle
E. arloingi	Small intestine	Domestic goat, Ibex, angora
E. christenseni	Small intestine	Domestic goat
E. aspheronica	Unknown	Domestic goat
E. caprovina	Unknown	Domestic goat
E. hirci	Unknown	Domestic goat
E. jolchijevi	Unknown	Domestic goat

- Coccidiostats only control the early stages of development and may not be effective in animals showing clinical signs unless a mixed-species infection is present with some organisms still in the early stages of infection. Sulfonamides (avoid use in dehydrated animals) and amprolium given for 4–5 days can be used for treatment of clinical coccidiosis.
- Maintain good sanitation.
- A stress-free environment should be ensured, particularly avoiding overcrowding and handling stress.
- Certain management practices like dry bedding, prevention of fecal contamination of feed and water, and reduction or removal of feces will decrease the build-up of *Coccidia* in the environment.
- Sunlight and drying will decrease numbers; most disinfectants do not work.

- Provide adequate nutrition.
- Do not mix younger kids with older kids or raise them in an area where older kids have been. Try to limit the age spread in a group to two weeks.

Coccidiostats should be used for 30 days before anticipated outbreaks to control the severity of disease. Decoquinate (0.5–1 mg/kg body weight, or 2 lb 6% Deccox® [Zoetis, Parsippany, NJ, USA] to 50 lb salt) and monensin (20 g/ton of feed) are approved for use in goats. They can be incorporated into creep feed or salt, but uptake must be monitored to ensure the appropriate dose. Treatment failures occur if the dose is inadequate. Treatment of late-pregnant does will decrease oocyst shedding from dams and thus decrease contamination of the environment prior to kidding. Amprolium can be used by prescription in goats and sheep for prevention (25–50 mg/kg/day for 21 days) and treatment (5 days) (Stehman and Smith 2004, pp. 1–9).

21.4.2 Cryptosporidiosis

Cryptosporidiosis is a self-limiting clinical disease of goat that occurs at less than 4–6 weeks of age. Mostly kids are affected and show non-fatal diarrhea at 5–10 days old. Death mainly occurs due to dehydration and electrolyte imbalance. Treatment consists of supportive care against dehydration. Kids with diarrhea should be isolated and strict sanitation of feeding utensils, waterers, and pens should be implemented to prevent build-up of the organism in the environment and spread of the infection. People handling sick kids should not handle healthy kids without using sanitary precautions between groups and to prevent their own exposure (Stehman and Smith 2004, pp. 1–9).

21.4.3 Toxoplasmosis

Toxoplasmosis is mainly responsible for causing late-term abortion. There is no specific treatment, but transmission can be controlled by preventing contamination of feed and hay with feces from cats (especially young kittens).

21.5 Diseases of Nutrition and Metabolism

21.5.1 Mineral Deficiencies

Mineral deficiencies are rare in most goats grazing in the tropics, if they are able to select a wide range of feed. Localized mineral deficiencies do occur, such as the well-known deficiencies in copper, zinc, manganese, and cobalt in plants grown on the soils of the Rift Valley in East Africa. If they are known to occur, the appropriate supplements should, ideally, be fed. However, in practice it is often hard to do so. Common salt should be offered regularly, particularly in very hot climates (Peacock 1996, pp. 215–217) (Table 21.5).

21.5.2 Vitamin Deficiencies

Young, growing animals have a much higher demand for vitamins and minerals and are therefore more likely to exhibit signs of their lack. Provided that it is supplied with

Table 21.6   Vitamin deficiencies.

Vitamin	Deficiency symptoms	Source of vitamin
Vitamin A	Poor appetite, weight loss, night blindness, poor hair coat	Browse, leafy hay, sweet potato vines
Vitamin B1	Blindness, nervous signs	Synthesized in rumen, supplied from brewer's yeast
Vitamin B12	Weight loss, weakness	Synthesized in rumen, supplies cobalt to rumen
Vitamin D	Weak, deformed bones	Synthesized by skin, obtained from hay, fish meal
Vitamin E	Weak muscles, difficulties walking, poor fertility	Grains, leaves of green forage

the necessary ingredients, the goat itself can successfully synthesize many vitamins (Peacock 1996, pp. 215–217) (Table 21.6).

21.5.3 Milk Fever

Milk fever is caused by an acute shortage of calcium in a doe just before, or just after, kidding. It is quite rare. The doe will become very weak, perhaps unable to walk, and

Table 21.5   Mineral deficiencies.

Mineral	Deficiency symptoms	Source of mineral
Major minerals		
Calcium	Deformed bones (rickets) Retarded growth Milk fever	Milk, green feed, fish/bone meal, limestone
Phosphorus	Rickets, stunted growth, soil eating, deformed bones, low milk yield, poor fertility	Milk, cereals, fish/bone meal
Magnesium	Weight loss, excitability	Bran, cottonseed/linseed cake
Sodium	Loss of appetite, slow growth	Common salt, fish/bone meal
Sulfur	Salivation, baldness	Protein in feeds
Minor minerals		
Copper	Weight loss, weakness	Vitamin B12
Cobalt	Anemia, weight loss, poor appetite, nervous signs	Seeds
Iodine	Goiter, poor hair, birth of dead kids, poor growth and fertility	Fish meal, seaweed, iodized salts
Iron	Anemia, poor appetite	Green forages
Manganese	Difficulties in walking, deformed fore limbs, poor fertility	Rice/wheat bran
Selenium	Weak muscles, difficulties in walking	Vitamin E
Zinc	Stiff joints, salivation, swelling of feet, low libido	Cereal grains

may have difficulty delivering her kid. She may have an abnormally low temperature. This disease should be considered an emergency. In a severe case, if left untreated, the doe may enter a coma and die. Treatment involves the slow intravenous injection of calcium borogluconate (25%). An injection of 50–100 ml should be given cautiously, as the heart may be affected. Milk fever is rare in goats in the tropics, but may occur in high-yielding dairy goats.

21.5.4 Grass Tetany

Grass tetany, or grass staggers, occurs when the forage consumed has low levels of magnesium. It may occasionally occur if goats are grazing very fast-growing pastures. Goats with grass tetany show nervous signs at first that can look like milk fever. They may tremble and be unable to stand. Treatment involves the use of drugs containing magnesium.

21.5.5 Ruminal Acidosis

Ruminal acidosis is a common metabolic disorder in goats that occurs due to abrupt feeding of a large amount of a highly fermentable diet leading to change in the rumen pH (<6). The damage of the pH reduction to the ruminal mucosa allows fluid from the bloodstream to enter the rumen, causing severe dehydration and worsening metabolic acidosis. It is considered one of the most important clinical emergencies in small ruminants and results in high mortality (Constable et al. 2017).

Treatment of ruminal acidosis depends on its severity. It is primarily focused on addressing the plasma volume deficit, correcting acid–base disturbances, and restoring a normal rumen microenvironment. Intravenous administration of sodium bicarbonate has been the mainstay of the treatment of lactic acidosis. However, aggressive use of this therapeutic modality can lead to serious complications.

21.6 Poisonous Plants

There are several plants that are reported to poison goats if eaten. In most cases goats appear to know which plants are poisonous and avoid them, unless they are very hungry. The most common plants reported to poison goats are as follows:

- **Lantana (*Lantana camara*)**: Lantana is a common ornamental species in the tropics that often escapes from gardens and colonizes large areas if left unchecked. It is not liked by goats, except during severe dry periods, when it may be consumed. Large quantities have to be consumed before any symptoms are shown. The plant is reported to make the skin sensitive to light

(photosensitization) and may cause severe diarrhea, even resulting in death.
- **Castor bean plant (*Ricinus communis*)**: The castor bean plant contains the poison ricin in the leaves and stems as well as the bean.
- **Solanaceae family**: This includes the thorn apple and Sodom's apple. All are poisonous but are rarely eaten by goats.
- **Mimosine**: This is found in many legumes including *Leucaena*, and is toxic to most goats if consumed in large quantities (>50% of the diet). There are goats in some countries, such as Indonesia and Hawaii, that are very tolerant of high levels of mimosine in the diet. A procedure has been developed to inoculate mimosine-intolerant goats with rumen microorganisms from tolerant goats, enabling them to consume high levels of mimosine-rich legumes.
- **Cassava**: This has a high level of hydrogen cyanide in the skin that can poison goats. Cassava should never constitute >50% of the diet.

The sudden death of a goat from an unknown cause is often attributed to poisonous plants, for want of any other cause. In reality poisonous plants only rarely kill goats. Evidence of the suspected plant should be looked for in the rumen contents while carrying out a postmortem examination. It should be a large part of the rumen contents if a convincing case for poisoning is to be made.

21.7 Pregnancy Toxemia

Pregnancy toxemia mainly occurs in goats that are carrying twins or triplets and are very poorly fed during pregnancy. There are many reasons for the development of pregnancy toxemia. The uterus expands as the fetuses grow, reducing the capacity of the doe to consume a large quantity of forage. The multiple fetuses themselves also make high nutritional demands on the doe. If the forage is of very low quantity, the doe is in double trouble: she has a critical shortage of energy and will have to mobilize whatever body reserves she has. This rapid mobilization of body reserves at the end of the pregnancy results in the production of ketones as a byproduct; these are toxic in large numbers.

The main symptoms of pregnancy toxemia include depression, weakness, poor balance, and eventually inability to stand. If the condition is caught in the early stages, good feeding with a grain concentrate will help. If it is caught late, the doe is most likely to die in a few days. Intravenous glucose, together with good feeding, may save her, but the chances are slim (Peacock 1996, pp. 215–217).

Multiple-Choice Questions

1 What do you call a female goat of any age?
   A Doe
   B Sow
   C Ewe
   D Wether

2 What do you call a male goat castrated when young?
   A Buck
   B Steer
   C Wether
   D Doe

3 Which of the following species is resistant to botulism?
   A Goat
   B Horse
   C Sheep
   D Pig

4 What is the flea in relation to the tapeworm?
   A Intermediate host
   B Host
   C Dead-end host
   D Precursor

5 What is inflammation caused by?
   A Heat
   B Swelling
   C Redness
   D All of the above

6 What causes the defense system to decrease?
   A Sanitation
   B Vaccination
   C Exposure to infectious agent
   D All of the above

7 What is another name for tetanus?
   A Lockjaw
   B Strangles
   C Influenza
   D Poll evil

8 Which of the following is not an external parasite?
   A Lice
   B Bot
   C Mite
   D Pin worm

References

Constable, P.D., Hinchcliff, K.W., Done, S.H., and Grunberg, W. (2017). *Veterinary Medicine: A Textbook of the Diseases of Cattle, Horses, Sheep, Pigs and Goats*, 11e, 461–472. St. Louis, MO: Elsevier.

Ethiopia Sheep and Goat Productivity Improvement Program (2010). Control of External Parasites of Sheep and Goats. Technical Bulletin 41. Langston, OK: ESGPIP.

Peacock, C. (1996). *Improving Goat Production in the Tropics: A Manual for Development Workers*. Oxford: FARM-Africa and Oxfam. https://policy-practice.oxfam.org/resources/improving-goat-production-in-the-tropics-a-manual-for-development-workers-122995.

Stehman, S. and Smith, M.C. (eds.) (2004). Goat parasites: management and control. Taken from presentations during the ECA Symposium on Goat Health, June 3, 1995. http://goatdocs.ansci.cornell.edu/Resources/GoatArticles/GoatHealth/GoatParasites/Parasites-SM.pdf.

Answers

Chapter 1

Answers to Multiple-Choice Questions

1 Which among the following are ancestors of goats?
   A Bezoars
   B Aurochs
   C Hyracotherium
   D Wild boar

2 Currently, goats are spread globally, with more than 300 breeds living on every continent except which one?
   A Antarctica
   B Asia
   C Africa
   D Americas

3 Which among these species are highest in number worldwide?
   A Sheep
   B Goat
   C Cow
   D Pig

4 What is goat meat known as?
   A Mutton
   B Chevon
   C Venison
   D Beef

5 Where is the highest population of goat seen?
   A China
   B India
   C Pakistan
   D Bhutan

6 What is known as the poor man's cow?
   A Goat
   B Cow

C Buffalo
D Sheep

7 Which country contributes the highest production of goat milk?
   A India
   B China
   C Afghanistan
   D Estonia

8 Which country is the largest producer of chevon?
   A India
   B China
   C Nepal
   D Pakistan

9 What breed of goat produces mohair?
   A Angora
   B Cashmere
   C Gadi
   D Malabari

10 How much cashmere can each goat contribute annually?
   A 100–250 g
   B 500 g–1 kg
   C 1–2 kg
   D 2.5–5 kg

Chapter 2

Answers to Multiple-Choice Questions

1 What is dry matter intake in dairy goats?
   A 3% of their body weight
   B 4–6% of their body weight
   C 2–2.5% of their body weight
   D None of the above

2 What may flushing in goats result in?
A Increased kidding rate
B Increase chances of twins and triplets
C Decreased early embryonic mortality
D <u>All of the above</u>

3 What is the length of time required to bring a doe with BCS 2.0 up to the ideal body condition for breeding?
A Nine weeks
B Three weeks
C Two weeks
D <u>Six weeks</u>

4 Breeding should be delayed in female goats until they attain which body weight?
A 50% of their adult body weight
B <u>60–70% of their adult body weight</u>
C 40% of their adult body weight
D None of the above

5 What is the digestible crude protein (DCP) level of the concentrate mixture for feeding adult goats?
A <u>12%</u>
B 20%
C 10%
D 16%

6 At what age should kids be weaned?
A 60 days
B <u>90 days</u>
C 30 days
D 180 days

7 Which vitamin is not required to be supplemented in a goat's ration?
A Vitamin C
B Fat-soluble vitamins (A, D, E, K)
C <u>Vitamin B</u>
D Both a and b are correct

8 What might be a reason for castrating a kid?
A Higher body weight gain
B Selection of breeding males
C <u>Both a and b are correct</u>
D None of the above

9 What may regular grooming of goats be associated with?
A Better circulation
B Removal of ectoparasites
C Sleek and glossy hair coat
D <u>All of the above</u>

10 When should colostrum be fed to kids?
A <u>30 minutes after birth</u>
B 10 hours after birth
C 24 hours after birth
D 28 hours after birth

Chapter 3

Answers to Multiple-Choice Questions

1 Wh.at are the advantages of adaptation to handling before artificial insemination?
A Enhanced conception rates
B Decreased temperament
C Lowered cortisol levels
D <u>All of the above</u>

2 Shouting, slapping, and dragging result in lower milk yield compared to which of the following?
A Soft talking
B <u>Stroking in goats</u>
C Both of the above
D None of the above

3 During oral administration of medicines by drenching, using a balling gun, stomach tubing, or via an electuary, which of the following is it necessary to avoid?
A <u>Drenching pneumonia and choking</u>
B Stomatitis
C Facial paralysis
D Swallowing

4 What is the preferred intravenous route for a goat?
A Cephalic vein
B Saphenous vein
C Ear vein
D <u>Jugular vein</u>

5 Where can horned animals be restrained?
A Anywhere on the horn
B <u>Near the base of the horn</u>
C Tip of the horn
D Middle of the horn

6 What is the drug of choice for restraining goats?
A Magnesium sulfate
B Chloral hydrate
C Ketamine
D <u>Chlorpromazine hydrochloride</u>

7 What is rumping generally used for?
A Controlling the animal by holding the flank
B Controlling the animal by sitting it on its rump
C Controlling the animal by holding its legs
D Controlling the animal by holding its jaw

8 What material is generally used for halters for goats?
A Metal
B Leather
C Rope
D Chain

9 What is stockmanship?
A The stocking of products
B The art and science of proper handling of farm animals
C Using field knowledge in selling
D A profit policy

10 Where is the muzzle?
A Head
B Tail
C Neck
D Flank

11 What does a goat prefer during handling?
A Feed
B Scratching
C Both a and b
D Being held by its legs

12 What is holding the goat's chest closely with one hand and wrapping the animal with the other arm normal procedure for?
A Buck
B Doe
C Pregnant goat
D Kid

13 Which of the following is very easy to handle or manage?
A A herd of four goats
B A single goat
C Both of the above
D Goats with sheep

14 What are the purposes of handling and restraining?
A Physical examination
B Medication
C Increasing production
D All of the above

15 When approaching, a goat handler must not catch, lift, or pull which part of the goat?
A Leg
B Hair
C Head, ear, or tail
D All of the above

16 Why may kicking, dragging, yelling, etc. cause a frustrating experience for the goat during handling?
A They have strong reactions
B They have a good memory
C They have a vicious nature
D They have a tendency to run

17 What is the space requirement during transport for a 35 kg goat?
A $0.24\,m^2$
B $0.40\,m^2$
C $0.28\,m^2$
D $1\,m^2$

18 How does the goat experience segregation from its herd mates?
A As stressful
B As normal
C As encouraging
D As likely to increase playfulness

19 What does the adoption of good handling procedures do?
A Makes the situation easy for the handler
B Makes the situation easy for the animal
C Both a and b
D Makes no difference in handling

20 Which of the following behavioral tests evaluate animal behavior during routine handling and restraint?
A Chute scoring
B Pen scoring
C Aversion test
D All of the above

21 Before administration of a restraining drug, how long should a goat be starved for?
A 18–24 hours
B 48 hours
C 32 hours
D 4–8 hours

22 What is common practice when approaching an animal?
   A Calling the animal
   B Speaking before touching
   C <u>Both a and b</u>
   D Shouting

23 Who is a goat herd generally led by?
   A A dominant female
   B A dominant male goat
   C <u>Both a and b</u>
   D A kid

24 What does repeated improper handling of goats during transportation and related disturbances cause?
   A Increased production
   B <u>Serious weight loss</u>
   C Higher conception rate
   D Increased production of milk

25 Why should a goat's first experience of handling and restraint be positive?
   A Their nature is to be calm
   B Their nature is to be annoying
   C <u>Their memories of a negative handling situation can last a long time</u>
   D None of the above

Chapter 4

Answers to Multiple-Choice Questions

1 What cause of disease is suggested by papules with folliculitis?
   A Fungal
   B Bacterial
   C Parasitic
   D <u>All of the above</u>

2 What is pruritus caused by prion?
   A Lice
   B Sarcoptic
   C <u>Scrapie</u>
   D Photosensitization

3 What is lumpy wool disease caused by?
   A <u>*Dermatophilus congolensis*</u>
   B Photosensitization
   C Parasite
   D Fungus

4 Decoloration of hair is due to deficiency of which mineral?
   A Iron
   B Zinc
   C Cobalt
   D <u>Copper</u>

5 What is bilateral ventral distension in goats due to?
   A Fetus
   B <u>Acute duodenal obstruction</u>
   C Food
   D Gas

6 What is the cause of ascites?
   A <u>Hypoproteinemia</u>
   B Urinary bladder rupture
   C Peritonitis
   D Hydrometra

7 Which is an obstructive cause of abdominal pain?
   A Cecal torsion
   B <u>Urolithiasis</u>
   C *Escherichia coli*
   D Ileus

8 Deficiency of which mineral can lead to diarrhea in goats?
   A Zinc
   B <u>Copper</u>
   C Manganese
   D Calcium

9 When are pharyngeal-origin sounds loudest?
   A Inspiration
   B <u>Expiration</u>
   C Both of the above
   D None of the above

10 Hemoglobinuria is seen in a case of what?
   A Urolithiasis
   B Cystitis
   C Carcinoma
   D <u>Intravascular hemolysis</u>

11 Glucosuria is caused by which bacterial disease?
   A <u>*Clostridium perfringens* type D</u>
   B Anthrax
   C *Escherichia coli*
   D Salmonellosis

12 Of what is ketonuria diagnostic?
    A Amyloidosis
    B <u>Pregnancy toxemia</u>
    C Enterotoxemia
    D Muscular dystrophy

13 What is stranguria?
    A Difficulty in urination
    B Frequent urination
    C <u>Slow painful urination</u>
    D Absence of urination

14 What is uremia of renal origin due to?
    A Poor renal effusion
    B Dehydration
    C <u>Renal failure</u>
    D Urolithiasis

15 White muscle disease is due to deficiency of what?
    A <u>Selenium and vitamin E</u>
    B Calcium
    C Phosphorus
    D Iron

16 What does arthrogryposis refer to?
    A <u>Congenital fixation of multiple joints</u>
    B Severely flexed fore limbs
    C Overextended hind limbs
    D Contracted tendon

17 Polioencephalomalacia occurs due to deficiency of what?
    A Glucose
    B Magnesium
    C <u>Thiamine</u>
    D Copper

18 In a case of coenurosis, what clinical sign is seen?
    A <u>Convulsions</u>
    B Diarrhea
    C Dyspnea
    D Pruritus

19 In pregnancy toxemia, clinical signs observed are related to which system?
    A Lymphatic
    B <u>Nervous</u>
    C Musculoskeletal
    D Gastrointestinal

20 When are convulsions seen?
    A Hypoglycemia
    B Hypomagnesemia
    C Hepatoencephalopathy
    D <u>All of the above</u>

21 Nutritional anemia is caused by deficiency of what?
    A Iron
    B Copper
    C Cobalt
    D <u>All of the above</u>

22 What is gangrenous mastitis caused by?
    A *Streptococcus* spp.
    B <u>*Staphylococcus* spp.</u>
    C *Escherichia coli*
    D *Mycoplasma*

23 What is the cause of nonregenerative anemia in goats?
    A External parasites
    B Hypophosphotemia
    C <u>Chronic flurosis</u>
    D Haemoprotozoa

24 What does braken fern poisoning lead to?
    A Anemia
    B Thrombocytopenia
    C Pancytopenia
    D <u>All of the above</u>

25 When is the condition of hypermetria seen?
    A Scrapie
    B Gid
    C Enzootic ataxia
    D <u>All of the above</u>

Chapter 5

Answers to Multiple-Choice Questions

1 Which of the following is used as a preservative for tissues collected for histopathological examination?
    A <u>10% neutral buffered formalin</u>
    B Acetone
    C Ether
    D None of the above

2 If PPR virus is to be isolated, which preservative will be used for storage of pneumonic lungs?
    A Chloroform
    B Formalin
    C <u>50% buffered glycerine</u>
    D All of the above

3   If a goat is suffering from fungal infection of skin, which of the following examinations is needed?
    A   Histopathological examination
    B   Virological examination
    C   Skin scraping examination
    D   Toxicological examination

4   If a goat is suspected to have died due to ochratoxicosis, which of the following tissue samples must be collected for isolation of ochratoxin?
    A   Brain
    B   Skin
    C   Kidney
    D   Spleen

5   Why are clinical samples collected?
    A   To investigate an outbreak
    B   To estimate the prevalence of disease in an endemic situation
    C   To demonstrate freedom from infection or transmission
    D   All of the above

6   Which of the following is the sample of choice to diagnose FMD in goats?
    A   Vesicular lesions
    B   Liver tissue
    C   Urine
    D   None of the above

7   What should samples collected for bacteriological examination be transported on/in?
    A   Formalin
    B   Chloroform
    C   Ether
    D   Ice

8   In a case of abortion, particularly in brucellosis, which of the following is the sample of choice for diagnosis?
    A   Stomach contents of fetus
    B   Kidney contents of fetus
    C   Skin of fetus
    D   None of the above

9   What must ticks collected from the body of a goat with dermatitis be preserved in?
    A   70% ethanol
    B   10% formalin
    C   5% ether
    D   Both a and b

10 If a goat is suspected to have died due to arsenic poisoning, which of the following samples should be collected for diagnosis?
    A   Eye
    B   Hair
    C   Brain
    D   None of the above

11 For coccidial oocysts, which solution is the preferred transport medium?
    A   2.5% potassium dichromate
    B   2% ether
    C   1% sodium hypochlorite
    D   All of the above

12 For mycological studies, which solution are skin scrapings collected in?
    A   20% potassium hydroxide
    B   5% potassium hydroxide
    C   2% potassium hydroxide
    D   Saturated potassium hydroxide

13 For toxicological analysis, which preservative should be added to the sample collected?
    A   No preservative
    B   10% formalin
    C   5% ether
    D   Saturated sodium hydroxide

14 To diagnose Johne's disease antemortem, which of the following samples will be preferred?
    A   Rectal pinch
    B   Voided feces
    C   Urine
    D   Nasal swab

15 To diagnose mastitis in goats, which sample should be collected?
    A   Milk
    B   Tissue
    C   Feces
    D   Urine

Chapter 6

Answers to Multiple-Choice Questions

1   In goats heavily infected with ostertagiasis, what does the abomasum resemble?
    A   Morocco leather
    B   Dry paper
    C   Nodular
    D   Cotton candy

2 Is the life cycle of all *Oesophagostomum* species direct or indirect?
  A Indirect
  B <u>Direct</u>
  C Both direct and indirect
  D None of the above

3 How many eggs per day can mature adult flukes lay?
  A <u>20 000</u>
  B 40 000
  C 60 000
  D 80 000

4 What is the cause of dicrocoeliosis in goats?
  A *F. hepatica*
  B <u>*D. dendriticum*</u>
  C *F. gigantica*
  D *P. cervi*

5 How susceptible are goats to dicrocoeliosis compared to sheep?
  A Equally
  B <u>Less</u>
  C More
  D Highly

6 What are *Moniezia expansa* eggs present in feces ingested by?
  A <u>Oribatid mites</u>
  B Lizards
  C Ants
  D Snails

7 At what stage are *Stilesia globipunctata* worms highly pathogenic and form nodules in the intestine of the host?
  A Mature
  B <u>Immature</u>
  C Both
  D Adult

8 What is *Haemonchus contortus* also known as?
  A Barber worm
  B Pole worm
  C Lancet fluke
  D <u>Barber pole worm</u>

9 Which species of worms is commonly known as the thin-necked worm?
  A *Avitellina* sp.
  B <u>*Nematodirus* sp.</u>
  C *Haemonchus* sp.
  D *Fasciola* sp.

10 What does *Chabertia ovina* form at the site of attachment that alter the gut lining and lead to malabsorption?
  A Nodules
  B Tumors
  C <u>Ulcers</u>
  D Cysts

Chapter 7

Answers to Multiple-Choice Questions

1 Which is the current taxonomic name of *Mycoplasma* strain F38?
  A *Mycoplasma agalactiae*
  B *Mycoplasma ovipneumoniae*
  C <u>*Mycoplasma capricolum* subsp. *capripneumoniae* (Mccp)</u>
  D *Mycoplasma ovis*

2 Milk smells rotten in which causative agent of contagious agalactia?
  A *Mycoplasma agalactiae*
  B *M. mycoides* subsp. *capri*
  C *Mycoplasma capricolum* subsp. *capricolum*
  D <u>*Mycoplasma putrefaciens*</u>

3 For the growth of *Mycoplasma agalactiae*, which of the following is/are required?
  A Isopropanol
  B Sterol
  C *Pyruvate*
  D <u>All the above</u>

4 Pulmonary involvement is absent in which cause of contagious agalactia?
  A *Mycoplasma agalactiae*
  B *M. mycoides subsp. capri*
  C *Mycoplasma capricolum* subsp. *capricolum*
  D <u>*Mycoplasma putrefaciens*</u>

5 No invasins or toxins are produced by which *Mycoplasma* sp. for adhesion?
  A *Mycoplasma agalactiae*
  B *M. mycoides subsp. capri*
  C <u>*Mycoplasma capricolum* subsp. *capripneumoniae*</u>
  D *Mycoplasma putrefaciens*

6 Which of the following statements is/are correct?
  1 Hemotropic *Mycoplasmas* are also called hemoplasmas

2 Hemotropic *Mycoplasmas* affecting goats include *M. ovis* only

3 Hemotropic *Mycoplasmas* affecting goats are not transmitted by vectors
   - **A** 1 is wrong, 2 and 3 are correct
   - **B** 1, 2, and 3 are correct
   - **C** <u>1 is correct, 2 and 3 are wrong</u>
   - **D** All statements are wrong

7 Which of the following statements is/are false about *Mccp*?
   1 *Mccp* is a fragile bacterium
   2 *Mccp* is resistant and does not get inactivated at higher temperatures
   3 Aerosol spread of *Mccp* is possible at shorter distances
   4 *Mccp* is spread through fomites and arthropod vectors
   - **A** 1 only
   - **B** <u>2 and 4</u>
   - **C** 1, 2, and 3
   - **D** 1, 3, and 4

8 What is coughing syndrome?
   - **A** <u>A mild respiratory form of *M. ovipneumoniae* infection in kids</u>
   - **B** An infection caused by *M. putrefaciens* in adult goats
   - **C** A pneumonia caused by *M. agalactiae*
   - **D** A hemotropic mycoplasma causing pneumonia in goats

9 For diagnosis of contagious agalactia in goats, which of the following clinical samples is/are not recommended?
   - **A** Milk
   - **B** <u>Swab from ear canal</u>
   - **C** Joint fluid
   - **D** Blood

10 According to the OIE, contagious caprine pleuropneumonia can be documented in which of the following circumstances?
   1 Laboratory isolation of *Mccp* from suspected samples is successful
   2 Serological tests confirm the isolation of *Mccp*
   3 Lesions are confined to lung and pleura causing pleuropneumonia
   4 No enlargement of interlobular septa of lungs
   - **A** Statements 1 and 2 are true
   - **B** Statements 1, 2, and 3 are true
   - **C** Statement 2 is true
   - **D** <u>All statements are true</u>

11 How is *Ehrlichia ruminatium* transmitted?
   1 Vertical transmission
   2 Vector-borne transmission
   3 Transstadial transmission in ticks
   4 Transovarial transmission in ticks
   - **A** <u>1, 2, and 3</u>
   - **B** 4 only
   - **C** 2 only
   - **D** 3 and 4 only

12 Which developmental stage of *Ehrlichia ruminatium* is infectious?
   - **A** <u>Elementary bodies</u>
   - **B** Intermediate bodies
   - **C** Reticulate bodies
   - **D** Both elementary and reticulate bodies

13 What is microscopic examination of a horseshoe- or ring-shaped appearance of an organism close to the nucleus suggestive of?
   - **A** *Anaplasma ovis*
   - **B** *Mycoplasmsa agalactiae*
   - **C** <u>*Ehrlichia ruminatium*</u>
   - **D** *Chlamydia pecorum*

14 What is the gold-standard test for confirmation of anaplasmosis in goats?
   - **A** cELISA
   - **B** PCR and cELISA
   - **C** Indirect ELISA along with microscopic examination
   - **D** <u>cELISA along with microscopic examination</u>

15 During *Chlamydia abortus* infection, when can pregnant goats abort?
   - **A** Third stage of pregnancy
   - **B** <u>Any stage of pregnancy</u>
   - **C** First third of pregnancy
   - **D** Abortion does not occur

16 Which of the following features of *Anaplasma ovis* infection in goats is/are true?
   1 Presence of *Ixodes* sp. ticks in the environment
   2 Yellowish-brown distended gall bladder
   3 Purple-colored intraerythrocytic inclusion body in Giemsa-stained peripheral blood smear
   4 Hydropericardium
   - **A** 1 and 2
   - **B** 2 and 4
   - **C** 3 and 4
   - **D** <u>1, 2, and 3</u>

17 Which of the following is the primary postmortem lesion of heartwater disease?
  A <u>Hydropericardium along with hydrothorax</u>
  B Congested liver with fatty degeneration
  C Unilateral pleuropneumonia
  D Distended gall bladder

18 Elementary bodies of what against a blue background are confirmatory of *Chlamydia abortus* and what should they be differentiated from?
  A Red clumps, *Anaplasma ovis*
  B Purple clumps, *Ehrlichia ruminatium*
  C <u>Red clumps, *Coxiella burnetii*</u>
  D Green clumps, *Mycoplasma agalactiae*

19 What is the route of inoculation for isolation of *Chlamydia abortus* in embryonated chicken eggs?
  A Chorio allantoic membrane
  B <u>Yolk sac</u>
  C Amnio allantoic fluid
  D Intravenous route

20 What is swelling of joints in weaned kids and young goats suggestive of?
  A <u>*Chlamydia pecorum* infection</u>
  B *Chlamydia abortus* infection
  C *Ehrlichia ruminatium*
  D *Mycoplasma ovis*

Chapter 8

Answers to Multiple-Choice Questions

1 The milk ring test in milk/colostrum aids in detecting which disease?
  A Anthrax
  B <u>Brucellosis</u>
  C Salmonellosis
  D Caseous lymphadenitis

2 Crepitating swelling is a characteristic feature of which bacterial disease?
  A Anthrax
  B Foot rot
  C <u>Blackquarter</u>
  D Caseous lymphadenitis

3 Which disease can be prevented by the ATS vaccine?
  A Anthrax
  B <u>Tetanus</u>
  C Enterotoxemia
  D Foot rot

4 What does *Dichelobacter nodosus* cause?
  A Mastitis
  B Tetanus
  C Blackquarter
  D <u>Foot rot</u>

5 A carcass should never be opened at postmortem if it is suspected of what disease?
  A Pneumonia
  B <u>Anthrax</u>
  C Botulism
  D Johne's disease

6 Which etiological agent causes Johne's disease?
  A *Pasteurella* spp.
  B <u>*Mycobacterium avium*</u>
  C *Clostridium perfringens*
  D *Clostridium chauvoei*

7 Caseous abscesses in peripheral lymph nodes are a characteristic feature of which disease?
  A Anthrax
  B Foot rot
  C Blackquarter
  D <u>Caseous lymphadenitis</u>

8 What is pulpy kidney disease caused by?
  A <u>*Clostridium perfringens*</u>
  B *Escherichia coli*
  C *Salmonella dublin*
  D *Pasteurella* spp.

9 Which form of anthrax is known a wool sorters' disease?
  A <u>Pulmonary form</u>
  B Intestinal form
  C Cutaneous form
  D Cardiac form

10 What is bacterial pneumonia in caprines caused by?
  A *Clostridium chauvoei*
  B <u>*Pasteurella* spp.</u>
  C *Mycobacterium avium*
  D *Salmonella typhimurium*

Chapter 9

Answers to Multiple-Choice Questions

1 What is the most common fungal pathogen recovered from a respiratory tract infection?
    A *Histoplasma capsulatum*
    B <u>*Aspergillus niger*</u>
    C *Trichophyton rubrum*
    D *Malassezia furfur*

2 What are the most common laboratory culture media for fungi?
    A Sabouraud dextrose agar
    B Brain heart infusion agar
    C Thayer Martin medium
    D <u>a and b</u>

3 Which antifungal medicine is most effective for the treatment of rashes in athlete's foot or ringworm fungal infection?
    A Optochin
    B Bacitracin and zinc
    C <u>Clotrimazole</u>
    D Tobramycin

4 What is histoplasmosis caused by?
    A Protozoa
    B <u>Fungus</u>
    C Bacteria
    D Virus

5 Which of the following is used in routine microscopic laboratory methods of identifying fungal specimens?
    A 70% KOH mount
    B 50% H2O2
    C <u>10% KOH</u>
    D Formalin

6 In the 1920s Sir Alexander Fleming was able to discover an antibiotic from which mold?
    A *Aspergillus* spp.
    B *Mucor* spp.
    C *Fusarium* spp.
    D <u>*Penicillium* spp.</u>

7 What is a fungal disease that affects the internal organs and spreads through the body called?
    A Mycoses
    B <u>Systemic mycoses</u>
    C Mycotoxicosis
    D Superficial mycoses

8 Which of the following is the sun ray fungus?
    A <u>*Actinomyces irraeli*</u>
    B Chromoblastomycosis
    C *Streptomyces griseus*
    D Cryptococcosis

9 Who was mycorrhiza first observed by?
    A Funk
    B <u>Frank</u>
    C Crick
    D Fisher

Chapter 10

Answers to Multiple-Choice Questions

1 A natural form of PPR infection is present in which animals?
    A Wild sheep
    B Wild deer
    C Sahelian goat
    D <u>a and b</u>

2 PPR involves which system(s)?
    A Cardiac system
    B Alimentary system
    C Respiratory system
    D <u>b and c</u>

3 PPR-affected goats display which common clinical sign(s)?
    A Mucopurulent discharge
    B Matting of eyelids and nostrils
    C Necrotic lesions on oral mucosa and lips forming diphtheritic plaques
    D <u>All of the above</u>

4 Which live attenuated vaccine is available in India for PPR?
    A <u>Sungri 96</u>
    B Raksha-triovac
    C Raksha-ovac
    D None of the above

5 What is the morbidity and mortality rate of pox virus infection in young goats?
    A <u>6%</u>
    B <5%

6 The malignant form of goat pox virus infection is seen in which animals?
    A <u>Lambs</u>
    B Adult ewes
    C Adult rams
    D All of the above

7 What test is available for the detection of antibodies against CaPV?
A ELISA
B RT-PCR
C Virus neutralization tests
D <u>All of the above</u>

8 Which goat pox virus vaccination is considered safe for goats only?
A GPV Utterkashi
B GPV Mysore
C <u>Both a and b</u>
D GPV Gorgan

9 What are the most common signs of FMD in goats?
A Lameness, S. agalactiae
B Pyrexia, nasal discharge, and salivation
C <u>Both a and b</u>
D Myocarditis

10 How long do persistent FMDV infections in goats last?
A 3.5 years
B 9 months
C <u>4 months</u>
D 30 days

11 Dairy goats are challenged 28 days after which vaccination?
A <u>Emulsigen-D and aluminum hydroxide gel</u>
B Inactivated FMD vaccine
C Raksha-triovac
D None of the above

12 What are the manifestations of CAEV infection in adult goats and kids, respectively?
A Encephalitis and polyarthritis
B <u>Polyarthritis and encephalitis</u>
C Polyarthritis and diarrhea
D Encephalitis and dysentery

13 Multiple regions of which kind within the renal cortex and medulla of both kidneys are interpreted as infarcts in CAE infection?
A Whitish, oval-shaped regions
B Pale, oval-shaped regions
C <u>Pale, wedge-shaped regions</u>
D Whitish, wedge-shaped regions

14 In CAE, interspecies transmission occurs between which animals?
A Cattle and goats
B Goats and pigs
C Sheep and cattle
D <u>Sheep and goats</u>

Chapter 11

Answers to Multiple-Choice Questions

1 African swine fever first occurred in which country?
A Japan
B <u>China</u>
C USA
D Norway

2 African swine fever is a devastating transboundary disease of which species?
A Cattle
B Goat
C Horse
D <u>Pig</u>

3 Lumpy skin disease is an emerging transboundary infectious disease of animals with what degree of morbidity and mortality?
A <u>High morbidity and low mortality</u>
B Low morbidity and high mortality
C Low morbidity and low mortality
D None of the above

4 Capripoxviruses are an emerging worldwide threat to which species?
A Horse
B Pig
C Mule
D <u>Sheep</u>

5 The Black Death was speculated to be which disease?
A Leprosy
B Rabies
C <u>Plague</u>
D None of the above

6 Which of the following *cannot* be transmitted via infectious droplets?
A Influenza
B Common cold
C Rubella
D <u>None of the above</u>

7 *Nipah henipavirus* is carried by what means?
A <u>Bat</u>
B Air
C Water
D None of the above

8 Creutzfeldt-Jakob disease (vCJD) can be contracted only in which way?
  A Consuming water tainted with *E. coli*
  B <u>Consuming nerve tissues (brain and spine) of cattle infected with mad cow disease</u>
  C Consuming shrimp infected with *E. coli*
  D None of the above

9 What does the bacterium *Yersinia pestis* cause?
  A Measles
  B <u>Bubonic plague</u>
  C Roseola
  D Rubella

10 What was the 1918 flu pandemic, also called Spanish flu, caused by?
  A Simian virus 5
  B Influenza C virus
  C <u>H1N1 influenza A virus</u>
  D SARS coronavirus 2

Chapter 12

Answers to Multiple-Choice Questions

1 The body condition score of goats in a flock should be maintained around what level to prevent metabolic diseases?
  A 2
  B <u>3</u>
  C 4
  D 5

2 What biochemical alteration(s) are observed in pregnancy toxemia?
  A Hypoglycemia
  B Ketonemia
  C <u>Both hypoglycemia and ketonemia</u>
  D Both hyperglycemia and ketonemia

3 When is milk fever in goats mostly seen?
  A <u>Preparturient</u>
  B Postparturient
  C Equally pre- and postparturient
  D No correlation with parturition

4 Which of the following is false with regard to pregnancy toxemia?
  A Seen in late gestation
  B Occurs more in goats with multiple fetuses
  C Results in nervous signs, dystocia, and fetal mortality
  D <u>Hyperglycemia is seen as the main biochemical change</u>

5 Which of the following is false for hypomagnesemic tetany?
  A Goat milk contains magnesium at 14 mg/100 g of milk
  B High potassium decreases magnesium absorption
  C Magnesium plays a role in muscular conduction
  D <u>Deficiency of magnesium results in discharge of acetylcholine</u>

6 Which of the following is not a factor associated with milk fever?
  A Feeding a high-calcium diet during pregnancy
  B <u>High milk yield</u>
  C Oxalate in feed
  D High estrogen level after kidding

7 What is the range of total serum levels of calcium in cattle in mg/dl?
  A 2.2–6.6
  B <u>8.8–12.2</u>
  C 10.4–14.2
  D 6.4–10.6

8 By what route should the first injection of calcium in milk fever be given?
  A <u>Intravenous</u>
  B Subcutaneous
  C Intradermal
  D Intraperitoneal

9 How can milk fever be prevented?
  A Maintaining a negative dietary cation–anion balance
  B Avoiding excess phosphorous in the diet
  C Careful feeding of feeds with oxalates
  D <u>All of the above</u>

10 How is pregnancy toxemia associated with parasitism classified?
  A Primary
  B <u>Secondary</u>
  C Starvation
  D Stress induced

11 Where is magnesium absorbed in ruminants?
  A <u>Rumen</u>
  B Small intestine
  C Abomasum
  D Large intestine

12 How is hyperesthesia in hypocalcemia initially seen?
  A Increased muscular tone
  B <u>Muscle membrane instability</u>
  C Decreased muscular tone
  D Increased vascularity

13 Which of the following is milk fever in goats not associated with?
  A Decreased gastrointestinal tract motility
  B Decreased stroke volume
  C Tetany and flaccid paralysis depending on magnesium concentration
  D <u>Elevated body temperature</u>

14 Which of the following is false with respect to the body condition score?
  A Indicates fat cover/fat reserve of body
  B Reflects nutritional status
  C Reflects animal welfare management
  D <u>All of the above</u>

15 Which of the following is false with respect to milk fever?
  A Ionized calcium level is more important than non-ionized calcium level
  B Fever is not evident in milk fever
  C Increased fetal calcium demand leads to preparturient hypocalcemia
  D <u>Flaccid paralysis is evident in goats</u>

Chapter 13

Answers to Multiple-Choice Questions

1 Which is the toxic principle present in the *Lantana camara* plant?
  A <u>Lantadenes</u>
  B Dhurrin
  C Gossypol
  D Mimosine

2 *Lantana camara* can cause secondary photosensitization due to the accumulation of phylloerythrin in the system following compromise of which organ function?
  A Lung
  B Heart
  C <u>Liver</u>
  D Intestine

3 Which antidote is commonly used for cyanide poisoning in goats?
  A Sodium thiosulphate
  B Sodium nitrite
  C <u>Both a and b</u>
  D None of the above

4 A bitter almond-like smell is observed from the breath of the animal and during necropsy after opening the rumen due to poisoning by what?
  A Nitrate
  B Carbon monoxide
  C <u>Cyanide</u>
  D Phosphorous

5 What is the toxic principle present in subabul (*Leucaena leucocephala*)?
  A <u>Mimosine</u>
  B Dhurrin
  C Gossypol
  D Abrin

6 What can prolonged grazing by ruminants on some oxalate-rich tropical grasses result in?
  A <u>Hypocalcemia</u>
  B Hypercalcemia
  C Hyperphosphatemia
  D Anemia

7 In oxalate poisoning, oxalate is combined with which ion(s) to form insoluble oxalate crystals that may block urine flow and cause kidney failure in animals?
  A <u>Calcium and magnesium</u>
  B Iron
  C Sodium
  D Potassium

8 What is the toxic principle that is present in oleander (*Nerium oleander*)?
  A Mimosine
  B Dhurrin
  C <u>Cardenolides</u>
  D Abrin

9 What is the mechanism of action of toxicity due to the oleander plant?
  A <u>Inhibits cellular membrane Na^+/K^+ ATPase</u>
  B Inhibits Ca++ channel
  C Inhibits angiotensin-converting enzyme
  D All of the above

10 Which plant contains the toxic constituent gossypol?
  A Subabul
  B <u>Cotton-seed cake</u>
  C Oleander
  D Groundnut cake

11 Which insecticide is commonly used against ectoparasites (ticks, lice, and mites) in goats?
   A Type I pyrethroid
   B <u>Type II pyrethroid-flumethrin</u>
   C Benzene hexachloride
   D Lindane

12 Pyrethrin insecticide is obtained from the flowers of which plant?
   A *Nerium oleander*
   B *Leucaena leucocephala*
   C <u>*Chrysanthemum cinerariaefolium*</u>
   D *Heteromeles arbutifolia*

13 A chocolate brown-colored appearance of blood is seen in poisoning due to which compound?
   A Oxalate
   B Cyanide
   C <u>Nitrite</u>
   D Fluoride

14 Which antidote is used for nitrite and nitrate poisoning in animals?
   A <u>Methylene blue</u>
   B Acetic acid
   C Sodium sulfate
   D Sodium nitrite

15 Which drug is used for the treatment of urea poisoning in animals?
   A <u>Acetic acid</u>
   B Sodium sulfate
   C Sodium nitrite
   D Methylene blue

16 What causes mottling of teeth and osteosclerosis of the skeleton in poisoning?
   A Nitrite
   B Urea
   C <u>Fluoride</u>
   D Cyanide

Chapter 14

Answers to Multiple-Choice Questions

1 In which species are chromosomal defects of a structural nature (translocations) seen?
   A Cattle
   B Pig
   C Dog
   D <u>Goat</u>

2 In which species do transmissible spongiform encephalopathies (TSEs) occur?
   A Cattle
   B <u>Goat</u>
   C Pig
   D dog

3 How can genetic abnormalities for the carrier state be detected?
   A Enzymes
   B Surface protein markers
   C <u>Both a and b</u>
   D None of the above

4 What is it essential to do regarding congenital defects in order to determine their frequency and overall incidence?
   A Report
   B Document
   C <u>Both a and b</u>
   D None of the above

5 On what information are genetic tests becoming more and more reliant?
   A Quantity
   B Quality
   C <u>Both a and b</u>
   D None of the above

Chapter 15

Answers to Multiple-Choice Questions

1 What is gall sickness associated with?
   A <u>Anaplasmosis</u>
   B Babesiosis
   C Trypanosomiosis
   D Theileriosis

2 Rakshavac-T is a cell culture vaccine against what?
   A Coccidiosis
   B Babesiosis
   C Trypanisomiosis
   D <u>Theileriosis</u>

3 A shuttle programme is associated with the treatment of what?
   A <u>Coccidiosis</u>
   B Babesiosis
   C Trypanisomiosis
   D Theileriosis

4 Which of the following anticoccidials is a thiamine analog?
   A Sulphonamide
   B <u>Amprolium</u>
   C Salinomycin
   D Monensin

5 What is coffee-coloured urine associated with?
   A <u>Babesiosis</u>
   B Theileriosis
   C Toxoplasmosis
   D Trypanosomiosis

6 What are intermittent fever, nervous signs, and petechial haemorrhages associated with?
   A Babesiosis
   B Theileriosis
   C Toxoplasmosis
   D <u>Trypanosomiosis</u>

7 Which of the following is a rapidly dividing stage?
   A Bradyzoites
   B <u>Tachyzoites</u>
   C Oocysts
   D All of the above

8 Which is the infective stage of *Toxoplasma gondii*?
   A Bradyzoites
   B Tachyzoites
   C Oocysts
   D <u>All of the above</u>

9 How many sporocysts and sporozoites, respectively, are there in *Cryptosporidium parvum*?
   A 2, 4
   B 4, 2
   C <u>0, 4</u>
   D 0, 8

10 What is swelling of lymph nodes characteristic of?
   A Trypanosomosis
   B <u>Theileriosis</u>
   C Amoebiasis
   D Sarcocystosis

11 What are punched-out necrotic ulcers characteristic of?
   A Trypanosomosis
   B <u>Theileriosis</u>
   C Amoebiasis
   D Sarcocystosis

12 What is red-coloured urine characteristic of?
   A Trypanosomosis
   B <u>Babesiosis</u>
   C Amoebiasis
   D Sarcocystosis

13 What is neonatal diarrhoea in kids characteristic of?
   A Trypanosomosis
   B <u>Cryptosporidiosis</u>
   C Amoebiasis
   D Sarcocystosis

14 Buparvaquone is used in the treatment of what?
   A Trypanosomosis
   B <u>Theileriosis</u>
   C Amoebiasis
   D Sarcocystosis

15 Imidocarb is used in the treatment of what?
   A Trypanosomosis
   B <u>Babesiosis</u>
   C Amoebiasis
   D Sarcocystosis

16 Amprolium is used in the treatment of what?
   A Trypanosomosis
   B <u>Coccidiosis</u>
   C Amoebiasis
   D Sarcocystosis

17 Trypan blue is used in the treatment of what?
   A Trypanosomosis
   B Theileriosis
   C Amoebiasis
   D <u>Babesiosis</u>

18 Buparvaquone is used in the treatment of what?
   A Trypanosomosis
   B <u>Theileriosis</u>
   C Amoebiasis
   D Sarcocystosis

19 Parasitic infections are characterized by an increase in levels of what?
   A IgG
   B IgM
   C IgA
   D <u>IgE</u>

20 Rakshavac-T is prepared using what?
 A <u>Attenuated schizonts</u>
 B Attenuated sporozoites
 C Recombinant SPAG-1
 D Recombinant p67

21 What is the most important zoonotic species of *Cryptosporidium*?
 A *Cryptosporidium canis*
 B *Cryptosporidium felis*
 C <u>*Cryptosporidium parvum*</u>
 D *Cryptosporidium suis*

22 *Theileria annulata* infection in the salivary glands of tick can be visualized after what kind of staining?
 A Ponceau staining
 B Commassie brilliant blue staining
 C Acridine orange staining
 D <u>Pyronin methyl green staining</u>

23 Which of the following chemicals is used for cryo-preservation of parasites?
 A <u>Polyethylene glycol</u>
 B Glycerol
 C Calcium chloride
 D Magnesium hydroxide

24 The MASP culture technique is used for the culture of what?
 A <u>*Babesia* spp.</u>
 B *Theileria* spp.
 C *Anaplasma* spp.
 D *Cowdria* spp.

25 What species does the smallest coccidian oocyst come from?
 A <u>*Cryptosporidium* spp.</u>
 B *Sarcocystis* spp.
 C *Toxoplasma gondii*
 D *Eimeria tenella*

Chapter 16

Answers to Multiple-Choice Questions

1 What are the main causes of polioencephalomalacia in goats?
 A <u>Thiamine deficiency and excessive sulfur intake</u>
 B Copper poisoning and selenium deficiency
 C Fumonisin poisoning and biotin deficiency
 D Reduction in the movement of confined animals and excess body fat in late gestation

2 What is the specific therapy for polioencephalomalacia?
 A Amoxicillin (250 mg orally)
 B Ketamine (22 mg/kg intramuscularly)
 C <u>Thiamine (10 mg/kg intravenously)</u>
 D Fenbendazole (50 mg/kg orally)

3 Several factors are known to predispose goats to pregnancy toxemia. Which of these is *not* a predisposing factor?
 A Foods with low nutritional quality or unbalanced diets
 B <u>Young goats (less than 5 years old)</u>
 C Low body condition score
 D High body condition score

4 What does the best laboratory test to evaluate pregnancy toxemia seek to determine?
 A <u>Plasma β-hydroxybutyrate (BHB) levels</u>
 B Complete blood count
 C Plasma niacin levels
 D Presence of enterotoxins in urine

5 What is the typical clinical sign of periparturient hypocalcemia in goats?
 A Flaccid paralysis
 B Bilateral blindness
 C Teeth grinding, swollen limbs
 D <u>Hyperesthesia and tetany</u>

6 The specific therapy for periparturient hypocalcemia in goats consists of administering a solution of what substance?
 A Calcium hydroxyapatite
 B <u>Calcium borogluconate</u>
 C Magnesium chloride
 D Phosphorus pentasulfide

7 What are the clinical signs of hypomagnesemia?
 A Nystagmus, strabismus, lateral recumbency with opisthotonos, odontoprisis, muscle rigidity, and convulsions
 B Progressive impairment of consciousness, anorexia, apathy, difficulty in standing, and ataxia
 C <u>Ataxia, stiffness, hyperexcitability, tetanic spasms, recumbency, and paddling</u>
 D Excitability, staggering gait, head pressing, ataxia, apparent blindness, and muscle trembling

8 The prevention of hypomagnesemia includes avoiding heavy fertilization of pastures with what?
 A Sulfide and phosphorus
 B Phosphorus and potassium
 C Sulfide and nitrogen
 D <u>Potassium and nitrogen</u>

9 Diets with which dietary factors can contribute to urolith formation in goats?
   A <u>Altered calcium : phosphorus ratio</u>
   B Deficient in selenium
   C Deficient in magnesium
   D Rich in salt and carbohydrates

10 To prevent urolithiasis, confined male goats must be fed a balanced diet with what ratio?
   A Magnesium : phosphorus ratio of at least 2 : 1
   B <u>Calcium : phosphorus ratio of at least 1.5 : 1</u>
   C Phosphorus : magnesium ratio of at least 1.5 : 1
   D Phosphorus : calcium ratio of at least 2 : 1

Chapter 17

Answers to Multiple-Choice Questions

1 Excessive dietary intake of calcium and copper causes deficiency of what?
   A Magnesium
   B Cobalt
   C <u>Zinc</u>
   D Iron

2 What is the most common parenteral form of iron?
   A Iron fumarate
   B Iron glutamate
   C <u>Iron dextran</u>
   D Iron dextrose

3 What deficiency is congenital chondrodystrophy in kids associated with?
   A <u>Manganese deficiency</u>
   B Magnesium deficiency
   C Calcium deficiency
   D Zinc deficiency

4 Hopping gait occurs in kids due to deficiency of what?
   A Vitamin E
   B Selenium
   C Vitamin E and selenium
   D <u>Manganese</u>

5 Spectacle disease most often occurs due to deficiency of what?
   A Zinc
   B Iron
   C <u>Copper</u>
   D Cobalt

6 What is the most common source of iron in case of iron deficiency in a grazing goat?
   A Ferrous sulfate solution
   B Ferric ammonium citrate
   C Molasses
   D <u>Grass grown on fertile soil</u>

7 What are peat scour, falling disease, and pine examples of?
   A Primary copper deficiency
   B Chronic copper deficiency
   C Tertiary copper deficiency
   D <u>Secondary copper deficiency</u>

8 Parakeratosis-like skin lesions are produced in deficiency of what?
   A Zinc
   B Cobalt
   C Manganese
   D <u>Nickel</u>

9 Granulocytic hyperplasia of the endometrium in goat occurs due to deficiency of what?
   A <u>Vanadium</u>
   B Calcium
   C Cadmium
   D Magnesium

10 What does the presence of a high amount of fructans in pasture lead to?
   A Copper deficiency
   B Chromium deficiency
   C <u>Cobalt deficiency</u>
   D Choline deficiency

11 Why does hepatic lipidosis in goats mainly occur?
   A Deficiency of cobalt and vitamin A
   B Deficiency of copper
   C <u>Deficiency of cobalt and vitamin B12</u>
   D Deficiency of selenium and vitamin E

12 Spermatogenesis in bucks is directly linked to which mineral?
   A Selenium
   B <u>Zinc</u>
   C Cobalt
   D Iron

13 Grass tetany in kids occurs due to deficiency of what?
   A Manganese
   B <u>Magnesium</u>
   C Molybdenum
   D Calcium

14 What should the ratio of calcium and phosphorus in goat rations be?
- **A** 2:1
- **B** 2.2:1.1
- **C** 3:1
- **D** <u>1.5:2.1</u>

15 In nutritional muscular dystrophy, which muscles are commonly affected?
- **A** Smooth muscle
- **B** Cardiac muscle
- **C** <u>Skeletal muscle</u>
- **D** Abdominal muscle

16 What is absorption of copper directly related to?
- **A** Presence of zinc and iron in the rumen
- **B** <u>Presence of molybdenum and sulfur in the rumen</u>
- **C** Presence of calcium and zinc in the rumen
- **D** Presence of molybdenum and iron in the rumen

Chapter 18

Answers to Multiple-Choice Questions

1 What are Medusa-head colonies characteristic of?
- **A** <u>*Bascillus antracis*</u>
- **B** *E. coli*
- **C** *Brucella*
- **D** None of the above

2 What are fried-egg colonies characteristic of?
- **A** *Mycobacterium*
- **B** *Rickettsia*
- **C** <u>*Mycoplasma*</u>
- **D** None of the above

3 Lipopolysaccharide is present in the cell wall of what type of bacteria?
- **A** Gram +ve
- **B** <u>Gram −ve</u>
- **C** Both
- **D** None

4 On Gram staining how do Gram +ve bacteria appear?
- **A** <u>Purple</u>
- **B** Red
- **C** Blue
- **D** Gray

5 What is Ziehl-Neelson staining used for?
- **A** Anthrax
- **B** *Mycoplasma*
- **C** <u>*Mycobacterium*</u>
- **D** None of the above

6 Which of the following stains does not require fixing?
- **A** Gram stain
- **B** Giemsa stain
- **C** <u>Leishman's stain</u>
- **D** None of the above

7 What condition are gunmetal gray kidneys seen in?
- **A** Arsenic poisoning
- **B** Lead poisoning
- **C** <u>Copper toxicity</u>
- **D** None of the above

8 What concentration of dextrose is recommended for pregnancy toxemia treatment?
- **A** <u>50%</u>
- **B** 30%
- **C** 20%
- **D** None of the above

9 What plasma cortisol level indicates pregnancy toxemia?
- **A** 5 ng/ml
- **B** <u>10 ng/ml</u>
- **C** 20 ng/ml
- **D** All of the above

10 What does the Sulkowitch test detect in urine?
- **A** Magnesium
- **B** Protein
- **C** <u>Calcium</u>
- **D** Glucose

11 What is the serum magnesium level below which hypomagnesemia is indicated?
- **A** 4 mg/dl
- **B** 3 mg/dl
- **C** 2.5 mg/dl
- **D** <u>1.5 mg/dl</u>

12 What is the normal pH of rumen?
- **A** 4
- **B** 5
- **C** 6
- **D** <u>7</u>

13 Feeding what with the diet can stabilize propionate : acetate levels?
- **A** <u>Monensin</u>
- **B** Tylosin
- **C** Amprolium
- **D** None of the above

14 Calcium below what level can result in hypocalcemia?
   A 8 mg/dl
   B 10 mg/dl
   C 12 mg/dl
   D None of the above

15 What can be used to treat postparturient hemoglobinuria?
   A Sodium acid phosphate
   B Dicalcium phosphate
   C Both of the above
   D None of the above

16 What are two forms of pregnancy toxemia?
   A Nervous form and gastric form
   B Wasting form and taxemic form
   C Nervous form and wasting form
   D None of the above

17 What is Rothera's test used for?
   A Pregnancy toxemia
   B Milk fever
   C Acidosis
   D Alkalosis

Chapter 19

Answers to Multiple-Choice Questions

1 Which of the following steps of pain transmission is not affected by local anesthetics?
   A Transduction
   B Transmission
   C Modulation
   D Perception

2 Which of the following is/are concerns regarding the use of a transdermal fentanyl patch in a goat?
   A An external heat source altering absorption
   B The animal potentially consuming the patch
   C Human abuse of the patch
   D All of the above

3 Which of the following is not an identified benefit of acupuncture or electroacupuncture therapy?
   A Prostaglandin inhibition
   B Increases in regional microcirculation
   C Accelerated nerve injury healing
   D Increases in endogenous opioid production

4 What is the phenomenon of increased pain sensitivity that is observed after a painful stimulus?
   A Wash-out
   B Nociceptive wind-up
   C Drug withdrawal
   D Wind-down

5 What is the approximate absolute bioavailability of transdermal flunixin in meat goats (i.e. compared to intravenous administration)?
   A 100%
   B 75%
   C 50%
   D 25%

6 Which of the following analgesic drugs would not be expected to cause sedation in a patient?
   A Xylazine
   B Flunixin meglumine
   C Butorphanol
   D Ketamine

7 Which of the following is considered a toxic dose of lidocaine for goats?
   A 3 mg/kg
   B 2 mg/kg
   C 8 mg/kg
   D 1 mg/kg

8 How many mg of lidocaine are in 1 ml of 2% lidocaine solution?
   A 0.2 mg
   B 2 mg
   C 20 mg
   D 200 mg

9 Which of the following could be employed for management of a goat with chronic osteoarthritis?
   A Body weight reduction
   B NSAID administration
   C Padded floor surfaces
   D All of the above

10 Which of the following is considered a potential adverse effect from the NSAID drug class in goats?
   A Seizures
   B Decreased renal perfusion (decreased glomerular filtration rate)
   C Respiratory depression
   D Tachycardia

11 Which of the following could be used to treat suspected abomasal ulceration from NSAID administration in an adult goat?
   A <u>A proton pump inhibitor (e.g. pantoprazole)</u>
   B Lidocaine
   C Grapriprant
   D Morphine

12 Which of the following drugs do not influence the perception component of the physiology of pain?
   A Sedatives
   B <u>Local anesthetics</u>
   C Opioids
   D NSAIDs

13 Which of the following is not a component of pain from osteoarthritis?
   A <u>Nerve endings in the hyaline cartilage</u>
   B Thermal afferent receptors
   C Chemical afferent receptors
   D Mechanical afferent receptor

14 Which of the following routes would not be an effective way to deliver flunixin meglumine in a goat?
   A Intravenous
   B Subcutaneous
   C <u>Transdermal</u>
   D Oral

15 Which of the following NSAIDs is associated with residues that are harmful to scavenging wildlife?
   A <u>Diclofenac</u>
   B Meloxicam
   C Flunixin meglumine
   D Aspirin

16 Which of the following is/are receptor(s) that interact with opioids?
   A Mu (μ)
   B Delta(δ)
   C Kappa (κ)
   D <u>All of the above</u>

17 Which of the following receptors does morphine interact with?
   A <u>Mu</u>
   B Delta
   C Kappa
   D Omega

18 Which of the following opioids has the greatest potency?
   A Morphine
   B Butorphanol
   C <u>Fentanyl</u>
   D All have equal potency

19 Which of the following could be used to reverse an α_2 adrenergic agonist?
   A <u>Yohimbine</u>
   B Xylazine
   C Detomidine
   D Romifidine

20 Which of the following drugs has been demonstrated in livestock to have synergism for pain management when administered with gabapentin?
   A Butorphanol
   B Fentanyl
   C <u>Meloxicam</u>
   D Xylazine

21 Which of the following adverse effects could potentially occur with the use of opioids in goats?
   A Respiratory depression
   B Decreased gastrointestinal mobility
   C Hyperexcitation
   D <u>All of the above</u>

22 Which of the following drugs functions by direct action on the prostaglandin receptor?
   A Meloxicam
   B <u>Grapriprant</u>
   C Flunixin meglumine
   D Ketamine

23 Which of the following could be utilized to reverse an opioid?
   A Yohimbine
   B Tolazoline
   C <u>Naloxone</u>
   D Ketamine

24 Which of the following is not a mediator associated with pain from osteoarthritis?
   A Substance P
   B Bradykinin
   C Interleukin-1
   D <u>Gastrin</u>

25 Which stage of the pain pathway are opioids not thought to be effective in?
   A Transduction
   B <u>Transmission</u>
   C Modulation
   D Perception

Chapter 20

Answers to Multiple-Choice Questions

1 What is the most common cause of acceleration of antimicrobial resistance in small ruminants?
   A <u>Indiscriminate use of drugs</u>
   B Unchecked antimicrobial dosage
   C Inadequate diagnostics
   D Poor hygiene and sanitation practices

2 What must antibiotic dosing be aimed at?
   A Only the bacteria isolated
   B The most resistant subpopulation in the colony
   C Preventing the advent of further resistant infections
   D <u>All of the above</u>

3 What are the characteristics of natural antimicrobial resistance?
   A There can be intrinsic resistance
   B There can be induced resistance
   C It does not possess the target site for drugs
   D <u>All of the above</u>

4 Which of the following feature in acquired antimicrobial resistance?
   A <u>Microbes obtain the ability to resist the activity of an antimicrobial agent</u>
   B It does not possess the target site for drugs
   C Both a and b
   D None of the above

5 What is an example of acquired resistance?
   A Methicillin-resistant *Staphylococcus aureus* (MRSA)
   B Vancomycin-resistant *Staphylococcus aureus* (VRSA)
   C Polymyxin-resistant *Staphylococcus aureus*
   D <u>Both a and b</u>

6 If a microbe population becomes resistant to an active ingredient, what is it called?
   A <u>Side resistance</u>
   B Acquired resistance
   C Innate resistance
   D Cross-resistance

7 What are the features of antimicrobial cross-resistance?
   A <u>Microbes have the ability to survive therapeutic doses of chemically unrelated drugs with different modes of action</u>
   B Microbes obtain the ability to resist the activity of an antimicrobial agent
   C Microbes do not possess the target site for drugs
   D All of the above

8 When does multiple resistance or multiple drug resistance occur?
   A <u>Any drug is taken for longer than necessary or when it is not needed</u>
   B Microbes obtain the ability to resist the activity of an antimicrobial agent
   C Microbes do not possess the target site for drugs
   D None of the above

9 What are the mechanisms required for natural resistance?
   A Permeability barrier
   B Biofilm formation
   C <u>Both of the above</u>
   D None of the above

10 What are the characteristics of Gram-positive bacteria?
   A No extra layers outside their peptidoglycan layer
   B Increased susceptibility of bacteria to antimicrobial attack
   C Presence of lipid bilayer and lipopolysaccharide layer
   D <u>Both a and b</u>

11 What are the characteristics of Gram-negative bacteria?
   A Presence of lipid bilayer and lipopolysaccharide layer outside the outer membrane
   B Reduced susceptibility of bacteria to antimicrobial attack
   C Increased susceptibility of bacteria to antimicrobial attack
   D <u>Both a and b</u>

12 What are the characteristics of biofilm formation?
   A Important form of natural resistance in bacteria
   B Highly organized communities of bacteria cohabiting in extracellular polymeric substance (EPS) slime
   C EPS protects the biofilm community against threats from outside, such as biocides and topical antibiotics
   D <u>All of the above</u>

13 What is acquired resistance mediated through?
  A Vertical gene transfer
  B Horizontal gene transfer
  C <u>Both of the above</u>
  D Neither of the above

14 What is the common mechanism of acquired resistance?
  A <u>Modification of antimicrobial target</u>
  B Decrease in drug uptake
  C Modification of metabolic enzymes
  D None of the above

15 How is enzymatic modification of an antimicrobial agent achieved?
  A Addition of acetyl, adenyl, or phosphate groups
  B Inactivation of the antimicrobial agent
  C Inability to bind to the target site
  D <u>All of the above</u>

16 Which of the following are described correctly?
  A *tra* Genes enable the bacterium to form a mating pair with another organism
  B *ori*T (origin of transfer) sequences of the mobilizable plasmid enable the DNA to move through the conjugative bridge
  C Transposons or jumping genes are small pieces of DNA that encode enzymes that enable the transposon to move from one DNA location to another, either on the same molecule of DNA or on a different molecule.
  D <u>All of the above</u>

Chapter 21

Answers to Multiple-Choice Questions

1 What do you call a female goat of any age?
  A <u>Doe</u>
  B Sow
  C Ewe
  D Wether

2 What do you call a male goat castrated when young?
  A Buck
  B Steer
  C <u>Wether</u>
  D Doe

3 Which of the following species is resistant to botulism?
  A Goat
  B Horse
  C Sheep
  D <u>Pig</u>

4 What is the flea in relation to the tapeworm?
  A <u>Intermediate host</u>
  B Host
  C Dead-end host
  D Precursor

5 What is inflammation caused by?
  A Heat
  B Swelling
  C Redness
  D <u>All of the above</u>

6 What causes the defense system to decrease?
  A Sanitation
  B Vaccination
  C Exposure to infectious agent
  D <u>All of the above</u>

7 What is another name for tetanus?
  A <u>Lockjaw</u>
  B Strangles
  C Influenza
  D Poll evil

8 Which of the following is not an external parasite?
  A Lice
  B Bot
  C Mite
  D <u>Pin worm</u>

Index

Note: Page numbers followed by *f* and *t* indicate figures and tables.

Principles of Goat Disease and Prevention, First Edition. Edited by Tanmoy Rana.
© 2024 John Wiley & Sons, Inc. Published 2024 by John Wiley & Sons, Inc.